Cancer Drug Discovery and Development

Beverly A. Teicher, Series Editor

Tumor Models in Cancer Research

Edited by

Beverly A. Teicher

Lilly Research Laboratories
Indianapolis, IN

Humana Press ✳ Totowa, New Jersey

Dedication

For Joseph,
the Black Warrior

© 2002 Humana Press Inc.
999 Riverview Drive, Suite 208
Totowa, New Jersey 07512
humanapress.com

For additional copies, pricing for bulk purchases, and/or information about other Humana titles, contact Humana at the above address or at any of the following numbers: Tel.: 973-256-1699; Fax: 973-256-8341; E-mail: humana@humanapr.com or visit our Website: http://humanapress.com

Cover illustration: Background: A Comparison between the expression of 8-OhdG in Vitamin E and DMBA and DMBA-Induced oral carcinomas. (*See* Fig. 6, p. 153). Inset: External and internal images of liver lesions of AC3488-GFP. (*See* Fig. 9, p. 108)

Cover design by Patricia F. Cleary.

Production Editor: Mark J. Breaugh.

This publication is printed on acid-free paper. ∞
ANSI Z39.48-1984 (American National Standards Institute) Permanence of Paper for Printed Library Materials.

Printed in the United States of America. 10 9 8 7 6 5 4 3 2 1

Library of Congress Cataloging-in-Publication Data

Tumor Models in Cancer Research / edited by Beverly A. Teicher.
    p. ; cm. -- (Cancer drug discovery and development)
  Includes bibliographical references and index.
  ISBN 0-89603-887-4 (alk. paper)
  1. Tumors--Animal models. 2. Cancer cells. 3. Oncology, Experimental. I. Teicher, Beverly A., 1952- II. Series.
  [DNLM: 1. Neoplasms, Experimental. 2. Disease Models, Animal. QZ 206 T925 2001]
  RC267 .T855 2001
  616.99'4027--dc21
                                  2001024082

In Memoriam

In memory of Dr. Greg MacEwen, who passed away suddenly May 12, 2001. Greg was an internationally recognized leader in the field of comparative oncology for more than 25 years. Greg trained many young oncologists, some of whom have gone on to become leaders in the field. He also conducted numerous innovative clinical trials, particularly in the fields of immunotherapy, gene therapy, and experimental therapeutics. His leadership was central to the formation of the Veterinary Cancer Society, which provides a central forum for exchange of ideas and information regarding new frontiers in companion animal cancer therapy. Greg always had great concern for his patients, while at the same time not losing sight of the value his patients gave to the greater good of treating human patients with cancer. His leadership and friendship will be missed.

Preface

"My Nemesis rises to his full height, fixes me with a stern but pitying stare, and asks if I really believe all this work done in animals has anything whatsoever to do with the clinical problem? I would suggest that if past experience is any criterion, I would expect some, but certainly not all, of what has been observed in leukemic animals to carry over (in principle) to man. We are abundantly aware that many of the experiments we have carried out were under conditions far removed from the usual clinical situation; i.e., in most instances we have studied the effects of early treatment of animals bearing relatively small numbers of leukemic cells. In this particular research program we have been seeking fundamental scientific knowledge; I shall be surprised if some of it is not applicable." — **Howard E. Skipper**, 1965

Progress in a given field is often dependent upon the development of appropriate, accurate models. In modern times, cancer research has been engaged in a focused search for such models for more than 50 years. The foremost problem in developing such models is that cancer is many, many diseases arising from nearly every tissue and metastasizing to many. A major breakthrough for models in cancer research was the development of transplantable rodent tumors. Many of the early tumor lines were carcinogen-induced, but others arose naturally in elderly animals from inbred strains of mice. These syngeneic tumors grown in the inbred host of origin allowed reproducible tumor growth and reproducible response to anticancer agents to be achieved. These tumor lines also frequently allowed analysis of tumor metastasis in the host.

The mutual needs for as large an array as possible of tumor types and the expansion of true inbred strains of mice to carry these tumors led to the identification of mutant mice with characteristics of deficient immunity suitable for the growth of human tumors as xenografts. The most frequently used of these mutant mouse strains are nude mice and SCID mice. Human tumor xenograft models were established from the many human tumor cell lines developed in the 1970s and 1980s and from fresh tumor explants. Since techniques for genetic manipulation have become more routine, animals expressing "oncogenes" or missing "tumor suppressor" genes have been developed, allowing a new level of understanding of the process of malignancy and new models for testing anticancer agent efficacy. Through the use of these techniques for some diseases and targets, it has been possible to establish specific animal models.

Therapeutic index continues to be a critical variable for anticancer agents directed toward any cellular target related to proliferation. Animal models developed to determine potential normal tissue toxicities of new agents as well as the potential of normal tissue protectors have focused on proliferating normal tissues such as mucosa, gut, skin, and bone marrow although cardiac, renal, and lung toxicity can also be modeled. Still, it is the determination of meaningful experimental endpoints that defines the usefulness of models to a field. Increase-in-lifespan (survival) was an endpoint used by Dr. Howard E. Skipper and colleagues in their groundbreaking murine leukemia studies. Many current models, especially solid tumor models, are not amenable to a survival endpoint; therefore, other measures of tumor response, usually involving tumor volume measurements, are applied. Endpoints such as tumor growth delay and tumor growth inhibition closely mimic clinical endpoints such as response time and time to recurrence. Other endpoints, such as ratio of treated group to control group, log kill, percent apoptosis, and tumor cell survival, depend upon the availability of an untreated or vehicle-treated control group in the experiment.

An ideal tumor model would imitate in scale and mirror in response the human disease. Though no such ideal models exist for the diseases that are cancer, the models described herein represent the efforts of many investigators for many years and approach with closer and closer precision examples that can serve as guides for the selection of agents and combinations for the treatment of human malignancy.

Beverly A. Teicher

Contents

Contributors

RAJESH AGARWAL • *Department of Pharmaceutical Sciences, School of Pharmacy, University of Colorado Health Sciences Center, Denver, CO*

ENRIQUE ALVAREZ • *Division of Cancer Research, Lilly Research Laboratories, Indianapolis, IN*

CATHERINE BOOTH • *EpiStem Ltd., Manchester, UK*

ROD D. BRAUN • *Department of Anatomy/Cell Biology, Karmanos Cancer Institute, Wayne State University School of Medicine, Detroit, MI*

ANGELIKA M. BURGER • *Institute for Experimental Oncology, University of Freiburg, Freiburg, Germany*

MICHELE CARBONE • *Cardinal Bernardin Cancer Center, Loyola University, Maywood, IL*

WILLIAM E. CARSON III • *Division of Surgical Oncology, Arthur G. James Comprehensive Cancer Center, The Ohio State University, Columbus, OH*

ROBERT CLARKE • *Department of Oncology, Georgetown University School of Medicine, Washington, DC*

THOMAS H. CORBETT • *Prentice Cancer Research Center, Barbara Ann Karmanos Cancer Institute, Detroit, MI*

MARK W. DEWHIRST • *Department of Radiation Oncology, Duke University Medical Center, Durham, NC*

LAWRENCE A. DONEHOWER • *Department of Molecular Virology and Microbiology, Baylor College of Medicine, Houston, TX*

JULIAN D. DOWN • *BioTransplant Inc., Charlestown, MA*

DONALD J. DYKES • *Southern Research Institute, Birmingham, AL*

SUZANNE A. ECCLES • *McElwain Labs, Institute of Cancer Research, CRC Center for Cancer Therapeutics, Surrey, UK*

HEINZ-HERBERT FIEBIG • *Institute for Experimental Oncology, Tumor Biology Center, University of Freiburg, Freiburg, Germany*

DAI FUKUMURA • *Edwin L. Steele Laboratory, Department of Radiation Oncology, Massachusetts General Hospital and Harvard Medical School, Boston, MA*

BEPPINO GIOVANELLA • *Stehlin Foundation for Cancer Research, Houston, TX*

JOHN W. GREINER • *Laboratory of Tumor Immunology and Biology, National Cancer Institute, National Institutes of Health, Bethesda, MD*

XINBIN GU • *Department of Oral Maxillofacial Pathology, Howard University College of Dentistry, Washington, DC*

ORLIN HADJIEV • *Wayne State University, School of Medicine, Detroit, MI*

STEADMAN HARRISON • *EMD Pharmaceuticals Inc., Research Triangle Park, NC*

STUART HAZELDINE • *Karmanos Cancer Institute, Wayne State University School of Medicine, Detroit, MI*

GILDA G. HILLMAN • *Department of Radiation Oncology, Barbara Ann Karmanos Cancer Institute, Detroit, MI*

ROBERT M. HOFFMAN • *AntiCancer Inc., and Department of Surgery, University of California, San Diego, CA*

JEROME P. HORWITZ • *Karmanos Cancer Institute, Wayne State University School of Medicine, Detroit, MI*

PETER J. HOUGHTON • *Department of Molecular Pharmacology, St. Jude Children's Research Hospital, Memphis, TN*

STEPHEN D. HURSTING • *Division of Cancer Prevention and Center for Cancer Research, National Cancer Institute, National Institutes of Health, Bethesda, MD*

RAKESH K. JAIN • *Edwin L. Steele Laboratory, Department of Radiation Oncology, Massachusetts General Hospital and Harvard Medical School, Boston, MA*

PAUL E.G. KRISTJANSEN • *Institute for Molecular Pathology, University of Copenhagen, Copenhagen, Denmark*

JUIWANNA KUSHNER • *Karmanos Cancer Institute, Wayne State University School of Medicine, Detroit, MI*

ALFRED J. LAWSON • *Varian Medical Equipment, Bartlett, TN*

WILBUR R. LEOPOLD III • *Warner-Lambert/Parke-Davis Pharmaceutical Research, Ann Arbor, MI*

JOHN J. LETTERIO • *Laboratory of Cell Regulation and Carcinogenesis, National Cancer Institute, National Institutes of Health, Bethesda, MD*

RONALD A. LUBET • *Division of Cancer Prevention, National Cancer Institute, National Institutes of Health, Bethesda, MD*

E. GREGORY MACEWEN • *Department of Medicine, School of Veterinary Medicine, University of Wisconsin, Madison, WI*

KRISHNA MENON • *Lilly Research Laboratories, Indianapolis, IN*

ROBERT E. MEYER • *Department of Anatomy, Physiological Sciences, and Radiology, College of Veterinary Medicine, North Carolina State University, Raleigh, NC*

RAYMOND E. MEYN • *Department of Experimental Radiation Oncology, The University of Texas MD Anderson Cancer Center, Houston, TX*

RICHARD MOORE • *Department of Chemistry, University of Hawaii, Honolulu, HI*

LANCE L. MUNN • *Edwin L. Steele Laboratory, Department of Radiation Oncology, Massachusetts General Hospital and Harvard Medical School, Boston, MA*

HIROSHI NAKAGAWA • *Division of Gastroenterology, University of Pennsylvania School of Medicine, Philadelphia, PA*

OLIVER G. OPITZ • *Division of Gastroenterology, University of Pennsylvania School of Medicine, Philadelphia, PA*

JENNIFER PALUCH • *Karmanos Cancer Institute, Wayne State University School of Medicine, Detroit, MI*

HARVEY I. PASS • *Barbara Ann Karmanos Cancer Institute, Harper Hospital, Detroit, MI*

LISA POLIN • *Karmanos Cancer Institute, Wayne State University School of Medicine, Detroit, MI*

CHRISTOPHER S. POTTEN • *EpiStem Ltd., Manchester, UK*

JAMES RAKE • *Sanofi-Synthelabo Research, Malvern, PA*

BANDARU S. REDDY • *Division of Nutritional Carcinogenesis, American Health Foundation, Valhalla, NY*

Bill J. Roberts • *Warner-Lambert/Parke-Davis Pharmaceutical Research, Ann Arbor, MI*

Sara Rockwell • *Department of Therapeutic Radiology, Yale University School of Medicine, New Haven, CT*

Anil K. Rustgi • *Division of Gastroenterology, Department of Genetics, Cancer Center, University of Pennsylvania, Philadelphia, PA*

Joel Schwartz • *Department of Oral Maxillofacial Pathology, Howard University College of Dentistry, Washington, DC*

Martha G. Sensel • *Children's Cancer Group ALL Biology Reference Laboratory, Parker Hughes Institute, St. Paul, MN*

Rana P. Singh • *Department of Pharmaceutical Sciences, School of Pharmacy, University of Colorado Health Sciences Center, Denver, CO*

Stephen T. Sonis • *Division of Oral Medicine, Oral and Maxillofacial Surgery, and Dentistry, Brigham and Women's Hospital and the Dana-Farber Cancer Institute, Boston, MA*

Michael B. Sporn • *Department of Pharmacology, Dartmouth Medical School, Hanover, NH*

L. Clifton Stephens • *Department of Veterinary Medicine, The University of Texas MD Anderson Cancer Center, Houston, TX*

Clinton F. Stewart • *Department of Pharmaceutical Science, St. Jude Children's Research Hospital, Memphis, TN*

Beverly A. Teicher • *Lilly Research Laboratories, Indianapolis, IN*

Henry J. Thompson • *AMC Cancer Research Center, Denver, CO*

Joyce Thompson • *Department of Hematology-Oncology, St. Jude Children's Research Hospital, Memphis, TN*

Donald Thrall • *Department of Anatomy, Physiology, and Radiology, College of Veterinary Medicine, North Carolina State University, Raleigh, NC*

Stuart Tyner • *Department of Molecular Virology and Microbiology, Baylor College of Medicine, Houston, TX*

Fatih M. Uckun • *Parker Hughes Cancer Center, Parker Hughes Institute, St. Paul, MN*

Ronald van Os • *Department of Hematology, Leiden University Medical Center, Leiden, The Netherlands*

Sundaresan Venkatachalam • *Department of Molecular Virology and Microbiology, Baylor College of Medicine, Houston, TX*

Michael J. Walker • *Division of Surgical Oncology, Arthur G. James Comprehensive Cancer Center, The Ohio State University, Columbus, OH*

William R. Waud • *Southern Research Institute, Birmingham, AL*

Kathryn White • *Karmanos Cancer Institute, Wayne State University School of Medicine, Detroit, MI*

I INTRODUCTION

1

Perspective on the History of Tumor Models

Steadman Harrison, *PhD*

CONTENTS

"In spite of the fact that no animal tumor system has been demonstrated to reliably predict for response of any specific human tumor to drug treatment, we believe that laboratory studies indicating improved therapeutic responses in animals have been useful to clinical oncologists in improving cancer treatment in man, and the future promise of laboratory successes for indicating improved treatment of tumors of man is great" (1).[a]

1. INTRODUCTION

When I was a younger researcher working with Frank Schabel in the few years prior to his retirement and death, I would frequently join him in his office to talk science. Often he would be seated at a table with a manuscript he was reviewing spread before him. He would tap some tabulated data or a figure with his finger and then, to be certain of my attention, he would reach over with the same finger and tap me on the arm or knee and say, "We've *got* to teach 'em." Invariably, these data would be offered to support a claim of antitumor activity for a drug in a murine tumor model. Another

---

[a] After Frank Schabel's death in 1983, many whom he was pleased to consider his colleagues shared their perspectives on his career and contributions, but there are now fewer of us for whom Schabel's memory really lives. Although he possessed a towering ego, Schabel was a man who once humbly described himself to the author as "running along behind Howard [Skipper] with a teacup to catch the sloppings from Howard's bucket." He was in fact the genius for execution of Skipper's strategies for the cure of experimental leukemia. Dr. Vincent DeVita once introduced him as "the William Osler of mouse doctors." It is with overdue satisfaction that I dedicate this "perspective" to Frank M. Schabel, Jr., Ph.D. (1918–1983).

From: *Tumor Models in Cancer Research*
Edited by: B. A. Teicher © Humana Press Inc., Totowa, NJ

researcher would be reporting tumor-growth inhibition, but when the numbers were considered critically and analyzed by the standards that Frank insisted on, it would be obvious, even to me, that the tumor burden in the group of treated mice had actually increased during the course of treatment. The nadir of tumor mass suggested a therapeutic response, but the experiment had not been adequately designed to assess it. And so it went. And so it continues.

As I consider the history of antitumor drug discovery and development and the use of tumor models to support this endeavor, I view time as divided into three eras. First, there was the cure of childhood leukemia. Next, there has been the ongoing effort to do the same for the major solid tumors. I believe that the second era is likely to be viewed in retrospect more as an era of failure than as an era of success. But it is leading us to the third era, into which I believe we are already in transition. Seeing this new era clearly from the perspective of cancer treatment is like seeing the kids' soccer game as they mature from their elementary school years to college. The younger kids focus on one thing—smashing the ball. The older kids, tutored by experience and coaching, learn to set up the shots so that when the killer blow is delivered, it scores. In much the same way, I believe that the treatment of solid tumors is moving from an approach that has focused on smashing the tumor cell with a drug or drug combination—in the best tradition of leukemia treatment—to an approach that will allow us to set up the tumor cell so that when the killer dose is delivered, regression and cure occur with satisfying frequency.

The new approach is not meant to abandon the principles that have led to the cure of some cancers. Rather, I am referring to new targets and treatment approaches that are being added to the established, well-worked strategies. But how must we approach these targets and treatments experimentally with our tumor models? Here, at the end of just over 50 yr of experimental cancer chemotherapy research, we should be able to determine with some confidence what tumor models will and will not do for us, and what they predict and don't predict. The heterogeneity of cancer continues to impose pressures on our models that are not duplicated in any other disease setting. The goal of this chapter is to call attention to some of the important lessons of the first and present eras, because it's still important to "teach 'em," while I depend on the remainder of this book to describe the advent of a new era of triumph in cancer treatment.

1.1. The Scope of Modeling Tumor Behavior

When "model" is used in the cancer literature of the past five decades, it may refer to an experimental tumor growing in a nonhuman host, often a mouse. Alternatively, and often without the distinction of a clear context, it may refer to a mathematical description of tumor growth and regression. Because the mathematics have usually been applied to observations of experimental tumors, the mathematical "model" is really a subtype of the more broadly applicable sense of "model," where the experimental tumor may yield to a mathematical description as readily as to a biologic, biochemical, or genetic description. This distinction is important to avoid confusion, and is emphasized here as needed. In regard to the modeling of tumor growth *and regression,* the insights gained by early investigators have become much clearer in the last decade—namely, the importance of the processes underlying tumor regression. Before our present-day, more widely shared vision for cytostatic therapy, tumor regression following effective and potentially curative therapy was assumed as a given. Because an increas-

Table 1
Context for Tumor Models in Biology and Therapy of Cancer

- Discovery: Screening for new drugs
- Biology: Tumor proliferation, progression, programmed cell death
- Mechanisms: Drug interaction with target
- Development: Prediction of drug efficacy and safety

ing number of new treatment approaches aim to extend the time to disease progression and to produce stable disease, tumor regression in our models and in the clinic may be less frequently the end point of choice in the future to guide drug development and to describe positive clinical outcomes. But we must remain cautious here. There is recent evidence (Von Hoff DD, personal communication) that as we have insisted on complete regressions (CRs) and cures in preclinical models, we have seen that a concomitantly higher percentage of drugs entering the clinic ultimately exhibit clinical activity. The percentage of new drugs confirmed to be active in the clinic is higher than ever before. So while I emphasize—and even insist on—the general and historical importance of tumor regression in our models, I must acknowledge the challenge of modeling and predicting cytostatic responses.

1.2. "Our Major Tool is the Tumor-Bearing Animal" (2)

The contributions of tumor models to present-day therapy have been the usual point of departure for most previous efforts to place tumor models into a historical perspective. Simply stated, the argument has been made that tumor models of the past have led us to the drugs of the present (3,4). This is essentially Schabel's position in the quotation that begins this chapter (1). And in the broadest sense, there is no basis to dispute this. However, under critical examination, this argument becomes less satisfying, and leads to the controversy that has surrounded the various strategies for discovering new cancer drugs (i.e., screening) since 1985. Although aspects of this controversy are important and will be examined later, the preponderance of heat over light has been distracting, and has changed the focus of the discussion. It has been easy to forget that models have provided a means to study not only the therapy of cancer, but the biology of cancer as well (Table 1). And when one has examined the predictive fidelity of tumor models, it has been easy to emphasize their apparent failure to correlate with positive clinical outcomes—i.e. cancer therapy—and to overlook the success with which they have endowed our understanding of cancer biology.

2. CURE OF CHILDHOOD LEUKEMIA

So to pick a year, what did the cancer therapy landscape look like in 1970? From the perspective of tumor models, where was the focus? Answers may be discerned in a review by Scott (5), who mentioned little other than leukemias and lymphomas. Even the anthracyclines were characterized as antileukemic agents in 1970. Asparaginase was of theoretical importance. Less than three dozen active drugs were known (*see* Table 2, refs. 6,7). Cisplatin was not known yet. And only (or predominantly) patients with leukemia or lymphoma benefited from chemotherapy.

Table 2
History of Cancer Drug Availability

Decade	Number of currently used drugs that entered clinic[a]	Example
1940	6	Methotrexate
1950	14	Fluorouracil
1960	14	Doxorubicin
1970	4	Tamoxifen
1980	16	Taxol
1990	(55)[b]	Gemcitabine

[a] Ref. 6

[b] Ref. 7

The title of this section is also the title of an important and helpful work by Laszlo *(8)*. As a historical milestone, the cure of childhood leukemia marked an era identified in the Introduction. However, as the reader will have anticipated, the subject of this section is more properly the cure of *experimental* leukemia. Laszlo captures well the entrepreneurial spirit of the day among those at the heart of the cancer chemotherapy revolution. This was a clinical revolution led by outstanding clinical investigators. But at the periphery of this revolution was a vigorous program of applied research aimed at addressing critical clinical issues with work in tumor models. And within the context reflected by Scott *(5)*, the models of the day, like the clinical targets of the day, were *leukemias,*—most notably, the L1210 developed by Lloyd Law prior to 1949 *(9)*.

When the clinical groups confronted and described any one of a series of obstacles on the path to success, the mouse doctors, who were kept in close communication with the clinicians through Zubrod's network *(8)*, would launch L1210 experiments to explore the obstacle. One example was the challenge of central nervous system (CNS) relapse among the children who achieved initial remission of their leukemia. Goldin's group at the National Cancer Institute (NCI) modeled this aspect of the natural history of acute lymphocytic leukemia *(10)*. They wanted to know which route leukemia cells take to enter the brain, and the extent to which systemic chemotherapy affected leukemia cells in the CNS. The tumor model (L1210) provided insights into biological (anatomic) as well as therapeutic (pharmacokinetic) aspects of the clinical problem.

DeVita *(11)* refers to a cardinal rule of chemotherapy that has its roots in this era. "The cardinal rule of chemotherapy—the invariable inverse relation between cell number and curability—was established in this model [L1210] and applies to all others." One important lesson of this early era is *not* that tumor models have given us this or that drug, but that tumor models, including L1210, have given us cardinal rules that have guided the advancement of clinical experimentation in cancer treatment. And without question, more of these cardinal rules are based on the work of Lasker Award winner Howard Skipper *(8)* than any other experimental chemotherapist. I have not found a finer, more succinct and critical summary and appraisal of Skipper's work than that of Jackson *(12)*. As he recounts,

"In 1964, Skipper and colleagues published a long paper dealing with the curability of a mouse leukemia at different stages of advancement, with a variety of single drugs. Three major conclusions were stated: (1) There is an invariable inverse rela-

tionship between the total leukemia cell burden and curability with chemotherapy; (2) dose-response relationships are apparent for all classes of anticancer drugs and are reflected in both the survival time of treatment failures and cure rates; and (3) a given dose of a given drug will kill approximately the same percentage, not the same number, of widely different-sized leukemia cell populations—as long as their growth fraction and degree of phenotypic heterogeneity are similar."

The import of the third major conclusion warrants a subsection of its own (*see* Subhead: 2.1.).

Skipper went on to focus on the problem of drug resistance, and how the existence of or the emergence of drug-resistant clones within a tumor-cell population may account for clinical treatment failure. As stated by Jackson *(12)*, "The modeling studies of Goldie and Coldman and of Skipper provided a powerful tool for the study of why chemotherapy fails and how to prevent failure." The point is that in the era culminating in the cure of childhood leukemia, leukemia models permitted serious study of *big* questions of importance to the improvement of leukemia treatment. It is important to recognize that to this point, tumor models were more *generally* predictive for clinical outcomes vis-à-vis treatment *strategies* than they were specifically predictive for clinical activity of a particular drug in a particular setting. These accomplishments cannot be trivialized by familiarity or the passage of time. The 20 years from 1945 to 1965, when childhood leukemia was cured, saw the reduction to practice of a remarkable (at that time) concept—the drug-induced cure of a cancer. Leukemia models were important, and their contributions are hardly overshadowed by advances of the recent past two decades, impressive though they are.

2.1. Log-Kill or Log-Cell-Kill

"The Skipper-Schabel-Wilcox model or 'log-kill model' was the original, and is still the preeminent, model of tumor growth and therapeutic regression." So declared Dr. Larry Norton *(13)* in a thoughtful evaluation of clinical outcomes in breast cancer. This log-kill or log-cell-kill model was based on work in Skipper's group by Wilcox *(14)*. It is related to the third major conclusion in Skipper's work cited earlier *(12)*— that "a given dose of a given drug will kill approximately the same percentage, not the same number, of widely different-sized leukemia cell populations." Restated by their clinical counterparts (e.g., Blum and Frei, *15*), who referred to "this log cell kill concept,"

"In general, for homogeneous populations of tumor cells there is a log/linear relationship between tumor-cell destruction and dose."

Lloyd *(16)* provided a formal definition:

"The term 'log kill' is defined formally as $y = -log(F)$ where F is the fraction of tumor surviving treatment. It provides the means of accommodating a wide dynamic range of the variable (in this instance, F) in a dimensionless quantity of convenient magnitude. For example, if the fraction surviving is 0.1, then log kill = 1.0, or if the fraction surviving is 0.0000000001, then log kill = 10.0. Not only is a log kill easily converted to the fraction surviving, but it also represents the number of log units by which the tumor is reduced. If, for instance, a tumor size of 10^{10} cells is subjected to a treatment which results in a 4.5 log kill, then the number of cells remaining is $10^{5.5}$."

The tumor model that provided the basis of the log-cell-kill concept was L1210, the same tumor model whose value was emphasized in the preceding section. But Lloyd *(16)* and others extended the applicability of log-cell-kill to solid tumors as well.

There is a misconception that the log-cell-kill concept applies *only* to leukemias. Norton may be cited *(13)* as having challenged aspects or applications of the Skipper-Schabel-Wilcox model. And indeed, when one considers the principal assumption of this model, one recognizes the limitation emphasized by Norton. The assumption is that a fixed doubling time accurately reflects the proliferative behavior of a given tumor. But Norton points out, for example, that chemotherapy may alter the cytokinetics of residual tumor cells *(13)*. The Norton-Simon hypothesis *(12,13)* states that in solid tumors growing with Gompertzian kinetics, the rate of regrowth increases as the tumor shrinks, so that cure requires greater dose intensity than induction of regression. Skipper had expected that exponential growth and a fixed doubling time would characterize all tumor-cell populations that were sufficiently small, especially micrometastases. However, Norton points out that "clinical experience, unfortunately, has not *entirely* [emphasis added] confirmed these optimistic predictions" *(13)*. The failure of adjuvant chemotherapy of breast cancer to achieve expected tumor-burden reductions required an explanation, and Skipper's was mutation of cells to a drug-resistant phenotype *(12)*. However, for our purposes, one need not conclude that the log-kill model is generally inconsistent with clinical experience—quite the contrary. The log-kill model provides a useful *estimate* of the effect of treatment on cell number in solid tumors as well as in leukemias. What the model does not account for is the failure of residual tumor cells to maintain an unchanging genetic profile. The result is that over time, the fraction of solid tumor cells killed by a given dose is *not* constant because the cells change—i.e., the cells themselves are *not* constant *(13)*.

> The Skipper-Schabel-Wilcox model is so meaningful because it conceptualizes both tumor growth (exponential) and tumor regression (log-kill) in response to chemotherapy *(13)*. In my experience, one is far more likely to go wrong in interpreting experimental chemotherapy data from any tumor model by *not* applying the log-cell-kill concept than by relying on it to estimate the effect of a treatment on tumor burden in a mouse.

3. CYTOREDUCTION IN SOLID TUMORS

Just as antibacterial chemotherapy in 1945 broadly exposed the public to the concept of chemotherapeutic *cure* and raised the expectation that similar success could be ours with all diseases, including cancers, the success of L1210 leukemia as a model of acute lymphocytic leukemia in children raised the expectation, still prevalent today, that a murine solid tumor of a given histologic type will behave in a predictive way for a human solid tumor of the same histologic type. Schabel wrote:

> *"We clearly lack highly reliable predictive experimental tumor systems for most of the solid tumors in man..." (2),*

and his words remain as accurate a characterization of our situation today as they were in 1972. It cannot be overemphasized how common is the logical but uninformed belief that response of a given histologic type of cancer—e.g. ovarian, especially of a transplanted human tumor xenograft—in a preclinical setting is predictive or more-than-hopeful for a positive clinical outcome in the same histologic type of cancer. Why is this not the case? Schabel's assessment offers answers *(1)*. Here are four:

1. Lack of common etiology or natural history, including the program of progressive genetic changes that accompanies progressive neoplastic disease, between tumor models and human disease;
2. Ability to characterize tumors beyond histologic type is greater now than when Schabel wrote (23 years ago), but selection of the tumor cell to match the human disease does not necessarily solve the preceding etiology problem;
3. There is a tendency ***not*** to study advanced disease in models; and,
4. Drug exposure often differs among hosts, as does biochemistry—e.g. folate status.

So tumor models, especially solid-tumor models, have continued to exhibit important limitations. But the opposite extreme is no more fair an assessment of tumor-model usefulness than the previous one. Often, I have witnessed presentations of work in a tumor model, followed by a clinical investigator who asserts that *we all know* those models are not likely to be predictive for patient responses! Well, we most emphatically *do not* know this. We *suspect* that response in a single or a few models predicts little, with confidence, for patients. However, *as the number of responding models (by rigorous definition) increases, the confidence of predicting "some" response in patients also increases.* To quantitate or generalize this continues to be elusive, and the emphasis is on "response." It is noteworthy that in tumor models, aspects of experimental design where the end point is *not* response—such as drug kinetics or effects on a molecular target—have been far less contentious. Historically, most of the controversy that seems to have surrounded the usefulness of tumor models has focused on the issue of response.

3.1. Perspective on Predictive

Earlier, I stated that attempts to extend to common solid tumors the success that had been achieved by 1965 with leukemias and a few other high-growth-fraction tumors marked the second era in the development of cancer therapy—one that continues to the present day. This era has lacked the signal success(es) of its predecessor—a point not likely to be disputed. But what have we learned about tumor models in the past 35 years? Schabel made a compelling case, often ignored, for using tumor models in a way that reflects as closely as possible the realities of the clinical situation *(1)*. Dedrick has pointed out that "…the mouse is not just a little person" *(17)*. And the model is more than just the mouse. Realities of the clinical situation include orthotopic disease, advanced disease, disseminated disease, host metabolism, host kinetics, and a host of other variables in addition to the heterogeneity of the tumor-cell population, with all its implications.

With this in mind, what do the authorities say about the predictive reliability of tumor models? I have already cited Schabel *(1,2)*. Martin et al. wrote, "Many clinical investigators believe that murine tumor models are not relevant to the human cancer problem…" *(18)*. Grindey stated: "While none of the in vivo models currently available directly predict for overall clinical utility, they do provide very important information required for assessing probable clinical potential" *(19)*. And Fidler *(20)* said "No" to both of the following questions:

1. Are experimental tumor models predictive for therapeutic response of human cancer?
2. Is one tumor model predictive for response of a second tumor model?

Venditti went even farther: "…patients bearing tumors of a given type do not necessarily provide a perfectly predictive model for others with the same tumor type" *(21)*. But as Martin et al. pointed out, "The predictive value of animal tumor models could be readily improved simply by imposing more rigorous criteria for the selection of clinical candidates" *(18)*. And I might add that this is true regardless of whether the context is screening or more advanced drug development. But what *criteria? Response* criteria. We must consider, as an important aspect of the model, how we define "response." What demands should we make of our tumor models? Schabel *(1)*, Martin *(18)* and others would have us look at *clinical* criteria for response. And we shall. But unfortunately, we must recognize that even here there is a lack of uniformity.

Tonkin, Tritchler, and Tannock *(22)* analyzed the standard of practice for defining tumor response in clinical trials in 1985. They found that the criteria for tumor response were poorly defined and variable, and that differences in response criteria contributed to variability in reported response rates. One of the reasons that one patient seems to be a poor model for the next *(21)* is suggested here—lack of uniform end points for tumor response to treatment. Tonkin et al. noted that there was disparity in reported responses of patients with the same cancer treated with the same regimens. They found "heterogeneity in the criteria that are used by different investigators to determine tumor response. … it is evident that 'standard' criteria [of response] do not exist" *(22)*. Although "…all investigators require >50% shrinkage in cross-sectional area for partial response," even this is not without some variability *(22)*. For our purposes, there are two important points here. First, the clinicians themselves do not adhere uniformly to standard definitions of end points, complicating but not excusing our own shortcomings in applying "rigorous criteria" to the design and interpretation of experimental trials aimed at predicting clinical activity. Second, by 1985, certain definitions were at least *accepted* on a fairly broad scale, including "partial response" (PR) and "complete response" (CR). The case has been made eloquently and emphatically that these end points are the measures of choice for tumor models as well as for human cancer *(1,18)*. Recall that the log-cell-kill concept was worked out for leukemia, but that Lloyd *(16)* and others extended its applicability to solid tumors. Later I will examine how log cell-kill might best be used in this context. However, anyone uncomfortable with log cell-kill can have no complaint about recording >50% regression of measurable tumors. It is noteworthy that if one measures individual tumors in mice twice per week for an adequate time, both end points are available from the same data. One end point (PR or CR) provides clinically relevant and understandable information. The other (log cell-kill) permits estimation of a quantitative effect of treatment on a tumor-cell population that responded, perhaps with delayed growth, but did not regress sufficiently to qualify as a PR or CR, a population for which one may wish nevertheless to compare effects of two or more treatment regimens.

3.2. The Take-Home Message

If we wish to improve the predictive reliability of our solid-tumor models for drug activity in human cancer, we must certainly demand more rigorous criteria for declaring a drug to be active in the preclinical setting *(1,18)*. And in order to make decisions about the development of a new drug, what criteria must be applied? "Mere inhibition of solid tumor growth is usually used as the criterion for activity in the preclinical setting, whereas 50% or greater tumor regression, *requiring the killing of 2 or more logs of the clonogenic tumor cells* (emphasis added), is the acceptable criterion for activity in clinical trials" *(18)*. *That's pretty clear.*

> *Laboratory workers have reported anticancer treatment of animal tumors as being positive, and therefore effective by inference, if drug treatment held the growth of solid tumors to 50% or less of that of untreated controls. Even complete inhibition of tumor growth under treatment would be negative to the clinician, since he requires reduction of the tumor mass by greater than 50% for objective [cytoreductive] activity by drug treatment (23).*

If I am developing an antitumor drug and I am at any stage along the value chain from discovery to investigational new drug (IND) application and I want to say something about the activity of my drug, here's what I need to be saying. Partial regression (PR) of a tumor model is good. Complete regression (CR) is better. Cure—the disappearance of an established tumor and its failure to regrow during an observation period equal to several volume doubling times after cessation of treatment—is best. And the more models in which I do this, the better. Finally, a two-log reduction in tumor burden at the end of treatment is the minimally acceptable definition of antitumor activity when the expectation is cytoreduction. When the expectation is that the drug will produce cytostasis, one must show, at a minimum, that the tumor burden did not *increase* during the treatment period. Both conclusions require the same tumor staging at the start of treatment and the same serial tumor measurements during the course of the experiment.

The origin of this "two-log" rule is a bit difficult to determine. Martin et al. *(18)* mentioned it. Corbett *(24)* has employed it. It probably goes back again to the leukemia work. Blum and Frei *(15)* defined PR and then commented on the quantitative cell-kill (in logs) required. Although their context was drug combinations and the drug effects (cell-kill) required for therapeutic synergism, their correlation of log-kill and response is clear. A one-log reduction in the tumor burden in a host, man or mouse, will appear as a PR in leukemia. Whether it will be measurable as a PR in a solid tumor will depend on the kinetics of regression in that tumor and its host *(25)*. To effect a CR (in leukemia), at least a two-log reduction in tumor-cell number is required. If one observes a CR in a tumor model, at least two logs of cells will have been killed. If the kinetics of regression of a solid-tumor model are such that one only measures a delay in tumor growth, this delay (in days) may still be used to estimate log cell-kill. And if the log-kill is two or more, one may conclude that a CR is probably attainable, perhaps with extended treatment. James et al. *(26)* have estimated that a 50% reduction of tumor *diameter* equates to a tumor-volume reduction of 87% or a *tumor burden reduction of about one log*. Parenthetically, the paper by James et al. *(26)* serves to update the conclusions of Tonkin et al. *(22)* mentioned earlier, and there is still no standard for clinical response criteria, although World Health Organization (WHO) criteria are described as "most frequently used" now. However, experimental oncologists, faced with the challenges of new drug mechanisms, cannot afford to ignore standards for defining drug activity. The effect of treatment on tumor burden must be estimated and interpreted in tumor models at the end of treatment, and the minimum acceptable response suggesting clinically relevant drug activity is a two-log reduction of tumor burden, with CRs and prolonged tumor-free survival (cure) as the goal. "The accurate conversion of appropriate tumor measurement end-points or animal survival data into $\log_{10}$ tumor cell kill is essential for any meaningful evaluation of therapeutic effectiveness. In chemotherapy experiments with syngeneic tumor models, changes induced in tumor volume doubling time are rare. Thus, with correctly staged and well-controlled chemotherapy experiments, there is little trouble in the conversion of appropriate observable endpoints into $\log_{10}$ tumor cell kill" (27). Elsewhere, Corbett (24) concluded that "…the more tumors [tumor models] that respond, respond at more than one dose level, and respond markedly [>2-log kill, CR, or cure], the more likely the agent will be clinically useful." And Johnson (28) observed that "…drugs with a high degree of efficacy and a broad spectrum of activity in animal tumor models have generally proven to be useful in the treatment of human cancer." Indeed, said Grindey, "…it seems reasonable that therapeutic approaches [drugs] with a broad spectrum of antitumor activity in the preclinical tumor model might have the best clinical potential" (19).

3.3. The Search for New Drugs Active Against Solid Tumors

In the so-called screening controversy surrounding the discovery of new cancer drugs, my primary purpose is to re-emphasize that the perspective I wanted to capture here has less to do with using tumor models to detect or discover or screen for new drug activity, and more to do with using tumor models to make decisions about advancing to the clinic with a drug believed to have antitumor activity. Nevertheless, it was March 1980 when a watershed conference was held at Airlie House in Virginia to assess the state of tumor models (19–21). Partly because of the influence of that conference, by 1985 important changes were in place in the NCI drug screening program (29). These changes were sufficiently profound to precipitate a number of the articles from which this present perspective has been drawn (4,18,28), and others that provide additional insight (30), not to mention seemingly endless discussion. Most readers know this story. The NCI screen had been an in vivo screen composed of murine leukemia, syngeneic murine solid tumors, and three human tumor xenografts. It was replaced by an in vitro screen of 60 tumor-cell lines representing major human cancers for which new therapies were (and are still) needed (29). A secondary screen was eventually elaborated, consisting of solid-tumor xenografts derived from the 60 cultured-cell lines (31). And the clock began to run. That was 15 years ago. No one has published a definitive or conclusive evaluation of the 15-yr screening experience with the 60 cell lines. I can think of no clinically active drug whose discovery was linked exclusively to the NCI program during this period, but it may be too early. This is only one opinion and one recollection—mine. But this is *not* the point of the present perspective. New drugs can be discovered in numerous ways. To succeed in human patients, a new drug must modify the course of the disease it is intended to treat. Modifying the course of cancer can be tested in available tumor models. And if appropriate end points are used in the preclinical setting, experience suggests that the likelihood of seeing clinical activity can be maximized. However, it must be borne in mind that no amount of confidence in our models

> …will save the experimental and clinical investigator the pain of having to learn to 'translate' (emphasis added) in both directions" (18). "In the present context, transla-

*tion means the changes in regimen required to achieve a similar response in a second
tumor system when a given response to some therapeutic procedure is observed in one
tumor system... (32).*

Translational research will be discussed further in a later section.

3.4. An Example—Quinocarmycin

It is noteworthy that most published descriptions of tumor models only *describe* the
models or their evolution. They generally *do not* document "track record" or answer
the questions: For what are they useful? What will they tell us? What do they predict?
How well do they predict it? If it turns out that drug candidates taken into clinical
development lack activity, why might this be? Did our tumor models predict inaccu-
rately? The search for new cancer drugs—particularly for disease-specific drugs—over
the past 15 years has yielded opportunities to explore this question. Drawing from the
published NCI experience, the clearest example may be the quinocarmycin analog DX-
52-1 *(33).*

*This agent represents one of the first to be selected for preclinical development based
on disease-panel specificity [melanoma] discovered in the National Cancer Institute
cancer drug screen (33).*

Examination of a more detailed presentation of the tumor model data two years later
(34) is instructive. In this later article, Plowman et al. indicate that DX-52-1
"...demonstrated statistically significant antitumor activity against five of seven
melanoma xenografts" *(34),* but this activity was measured as *tumor-growth inhibition.*
Only two of seven melanoma xenografts responded with clinically relevant PRs or
CRs. Of seven xenograft models derived from cell lines that were sensitive to DX-52-1
in vitro, one would want at least four models to respond with PRs or CRs in order for
the drug to be accepted as active. So what has the clinical experience revealed? Herein
lies an example of a great historic weakness in the way cancer drugs have been developed—coordination of clinical trial design with data from preclinical models. Public
databases indicate (and personal communications confirm) that DX-52-1 was studied
in the United States in two NCI-sponsored Phase I trials. Although the results are not
yet public, available information indicates that *only one melanoma patient was
enrolled.* It is presumed that specificity for melanoma will be tested in Phase II. Venditti et al. indicated in 1984 that our progress in understanding the prediction of activity
in a specific histologic type of cancer had been hampered by limitations in the *clinical*
data for new agents. Overcoming these limitations "...will require considerable clinical
feedback on new agents entering clinical trial since 1976" *(3)* and to the present day.
Activity in a tumor type in vitro and in vivo has not been shown to correlate with
tumor-type activity (much less, specificity) in humans. In the main, this is more a failure to obtain the clinical data than an overall failure of an adequate test of the hypothesis. Where the clinical comparison *has* been done, the correlation looks surprisingly
good *(35).*

So even "...the first [agent] to be selected for preclinical development based on disease-panel specificity" (DX-52-1) and forwarded to the clinic on the basis of xenograft
"responses," seems not to have received an early evaluation in a melanoma setting
where disease specificity might have achieved preliminary support along with safety
and pharmacokinetics. And no early indication of clinical activity has been published.

Perhaps DX-52-1 will eventually prove to be active. But in the same period (1995–2000), other agents such as ecteinascidin and cryptophycin have entered the clinic supported by much stronger tumor-model data *(36,37)* than that presented for DX-52-1 *(33,34)*. For example, in a study of cryptophycin-8, Corbett et al. reported that four of six xenograft models yielded PRs or CRs *(37)*. The other of these drugs, ET-743 (ecteinascidin), which produced PRs or CRs in two of three xenograft models in one report *(36)*, has already demonstrated meaningful clinical activity *(38)*. These examples are offered to illustrate my point, not to prove it. Greater persuasion would be beyond the scope of this perspective, and the data simply are not available. But there has been little written in the last decade to remind us of earlier thinking about how we might best use our tumor models. Disappointing as it may be, progress has not been as robust as the models might have allowed. We *must* demand the same responses from our tumor models that we want to see in the clinic. However, these are labor-intensive, expensive preclinical trials to conduct, and experience is clear that many investigators prefer to measure tumor growth inhibition as their primary end point in assessing drug activity in tumor models. Which brings me back to Von Hoff's observation (personal communication): to the extent that we have insisted on CRs and cures in tumor models, we are seeing correspondingly more positive clinical results with new drugs!

4. TARGET-DIRECTED CANCER THERAPY

"A new era of cancer research dawned in 1984 when mice reared from eggs injected with genes implicated in cancer (oncogenes) proved to develop specific types of tumors" (39).

This is the third era identified earlier, into which I believe we are now moving. It is marked by new and distinctive tumor models, and by new challenges for their prudent use. By 1985, cancer-drug discovery programs were increasing in number among the major pharmaceutical companies, and more emphasis was being placed on mechanistically driven screens. The NCI responded with the National Cooperative Drug Discovery Grant program, and most of these grants focused on a discrete target, such as topoisomerase I or II, or on a molecular mechanism, such as calcium signaling. The advent of genomics has brought even higher resolution to the characterization of molecular targets. Research has focused increasingly on target validation, as practiced in the pharmaceutical industry, or target "credentialing" as referred to by Wittes and Klausner *(40)*. Target validation requires the stepwise linkage of target with disease by three critical tests. First, is the target associated with the disease, and what is the frequency of that association? Second, is the target linked mechanistically to the disease so that—to cite an increasingly common approach—knocking in, knocking out, or knocking down the target has the expected result regarding presence or absence of the disease? And third, does pharmacologic modulation of the target, at an appropriate level of specificity, modify the disease? Target validation begins at the cellular level, moves through tumor models in animals, and culminates in translation to the clinic.

Translational research *(41)* is the clinical extension of target validation, as just described. The current emphasis on translational research has grown out of the imperative *(42)* to show, in patients, the target effects of target-based drugs. From the preclinical end, the problem is more straightforward. Relevant tissues for target assessment are more readily available than in the clinical situation. Pharmacodynamic/pharmacokinetic modeling in animals offers a rational reference to guide clinical trial design. From the clinical end, tissues for target assessment are more problematic, and surrogate tissues and even surrogate markers or assays are often the only resort. I suspect that these problems will ultimately yield to the forward progress of genomics. But the take-home message with regard to the tumor model is not the choice of target, not the assessment of the target, and not the extrapolation of pharmacokinetics across species. The take-home message from the preclinical end of translational research is that *translation will be flawed unless the pharmacodynamic piece* (therapeutic response) *is based on clinically relevant response criteria.*

After more than a quarter of a century of engagement with the cancer problem, the one lesson that seems to me to stand above all others is that each new layer of complexity foreshadows the next layer of greater complexity. We are now embracing the notion that if we can demonstrate target modulation in a tumor model, this will more reliably indicate a positive clinical outcome. But the "next layer" seems to challenge the notion that therapy directed to a single target will have a meaningful impact on cancer in patients. "Tumor cells represent a highly evolving population of cells with multiple potential targets. Any cancer treatment must start with this recognition. It is unlikely that drugs aimed solely at a single target, however important it may be, would be effective in cancer management" *(43)*. Zhang et al. *(44)* looked at differential expression of genes, a possible clue to altered function and the targets involved, and found about 500 differences when they compared normal colon epithelium and primary human colon cancers. Stoler et al. *(45)* analyzed the extent of genetic mutations in colon cancer, which suggests the scope of genomic events that underlie malignancy, and found approx 10^4 such events per colon-cancer cell—an unexpected (at least by me) magnitude of genomic heterogeneity. How can we take the next step to target-directed therapy while assuring that our tumor models, in the face of such complexity, do not lead us into a new era of clinical disappointment?

Retain has pointed out that "for target-based anticancer drugs, it is critical to establish that the observed preclinical activity can be attributed to modulation of the target" *(42)*. Although a measurable effect on a molecular target has become a more critical piece of any proof-of-principle, an effect on a target in a tumor model may predict no better for clinical activity than our historical experience *unless* target effects are accompanied by robust therapeutic responses (CRs and cures) in the model. If single-agent activity fails to meet this requirement, then single-agent cytostasis, where one can show, at a minimum, that the tumor burden did not *increase* during the treatment period, will be imperative. Evidence of CRs and cures must then be obtained from studies of drug combinations. The question has been raised whether growth delay in xenografts will translate to stable disease in the clinic. It may be stated emphatically that if the answer is to be "Yes," the number of days of growth delay *must* equate to a net zero increase in the tumor burden over the treatment or observation period. We now need to develop data that will test the hypothesis that the longer the period during which the tumor burden remains static in xenografts, the higher the probability of observing stable disease in the clinic.

Can I illustrate what I mean by a tumor burden that, at a minimum, does not *increase* during treatment, i.e. remains static? It seems simple enough, but here are three examples of what one might encounter. Consider first a report of the preclinical activity of the MAP/ERK Kinase-1 (MEK) inhibitor, PD184352 *(46)*. The desired effect on the target is well-supported. Then one comes to the question of therapeutic response in a tumor model (their Fig. 5). In one of three experiments, they implanted murine colon-tumor fragments subcutaneously in syngeneic mice on d 0. Mice were treated orally every 12 h on d 1–14. Tumors were measured from the day they became palpable until d 17, when the experiment was terminated. The diluent-treated controls evidenced a tumor volume doubling time of 4 d and reached an equivalent mass of 1000 mg by d 14. It is obvious from inspection that treatment inhibited tumor growth, but that tumors in treated mice had begun to grow during treatment. In this example, quantitation of tumor growth delay *(1)* and estimation of the effect of treatment on tumor burden are not possible, because the observation period was not of sufficient length. Treatment would be required to have delayed tumors from reaching 1000 mg until d 27 to reflect a net change in tumor burden of zero (cytostatis) over the 14-d course of treatment. For the sake of further illustration, a one-log *reduction* of tumor burden in this experiment (which is a little more theoretical because the implanted fragments were small on the day of first treatment) would have resulted in an additional delay until d 40 for treated tumors to reach 1000 mg. It is obvious from inspection of the published data *(46)* and from these considerations that tumor measurements beyond d 17 would have been instructive.

Consider now the activity of CGP41251, a staurosporine analog that inhibits several protein kinase C subtypes. This molecule has shown "…for the first time that a PKC inhibitor can block in vivo cell signaling pathways in cancer patients" *(47)*. If one takes a look at some tumor-model data *(48)* for CGP41251, one finds the claim of "stable disease." It is apparent from inspection of these data (their Fig. 2) that tumor volume neither increased *during* the 10-d treatment period with the higher dosage *nor* during the subsequent 9-d observation period in a bladder carcinoma xenograft model. The vehicle-treated controls evidenced a tumor volume doubling time of 7 d. Again, calculation of the effect of treatment on tumor burden is not possible, because the observation period was too short. The experiment was terminated before tumors treated with the higher dosage evidenced any growth at all, and tumor growth *delay* is the parameter that must be measured, the parameter linked to tumor-burden change *(1)*. This is seen perhaps more clearly in the final example. In this example, an inhibitor of the protein kinase C beta isoform was evaluated in an hepatocellular carcinoma xenograft model engineered to include the tetracycline-inducible promoter upstream from the vascular endothelial growth factor (VEGF) gene *(49)*. This model permitted the demonstration "…for the first time that PKC, especially the β-isoform, is a major regulator of VEGF-mediated tumor development and angiogenesis" *(49)*. If we look at the therapeutic response data, their Fig. 2 reports a statistically significant difference in growth between treated and control xenografts. Mice were treated daily beginning either on the day of tumor implantation (d 0) or on d 18 and continuing for the 46-d duration of the experiment. Did the tumor burden increase during treatment? From inspection of the data, it is obvious that the tumor volume increased throughout the course of the experiment regardless of treatment. Calculation of the log change in tumor burden reveals that the increase was about one log at d 39.

So here were three reports in which the target was convincingly affected, but where the therapeutic response data were either insufficient to interpret *(46,48)* or fell short *(49)* of the *minimum* criterion suggested here for a claim of cytostasis in a tumor model. And these models were all transplanted tumors, not "real cancer" as judged by Klausner *(40).* A xenograft in an immunodeficient mouse cannot be rationalized as reflecting, with more than rudimentary fidelity, a human cancer growing in its human host. But transgenic models are not ideal either. For example, "…the phenotypes of genetically engineered mice cannot be easily extrapolated to humans" *(50).* And yet, "although genetic mutations in mouse and humans do not always lead to the same tumour spectrum, the underlying molecular mechanisms are frequently relevant to both species" *(51).* As set forth in this perspective, experience indicates that xenograft models and newer, transgenic models *can* provide important and even predictive information for those who are making decisions about the development of cancer drugs. As Fidler has insisted, "the failure of animal tumor systems to serve as predictive models for human cancer *does not diminish* (emphasis added) their usefulness but indicates the absolute necessity to precisely define the question that the model will be used to answer" *(20).* And as I have tried to remind us, looking forward from the foundations laid by Skipper, Schabel, Goldin, Martin, Frei, Freireich, and others, there is above all the absolute necessity to demand therapeutic responses in our tumor models that are as similar as possible to the responses that we expect to obtain clinically with new cancer treatments in the era of hope and challenge that lies ahead.

REFERENCES

1. Schabel FM Jr, Griswold DP Jr, Laster WR Jr, Corbett TH, Lloyd HH. Quantitative evaluation of anti-cancer agent activity in experimental animals. *Pharmacol Ther* 1977; 1:411–435.
2. Schabel FM Jr. Screening, the cornerstone of chemotherapy. *Cancer Chemother Rep* 1972; 3:309–313.
3. Venditti JM, Wesley RA, Plowman J. Current NCI preclinical antitumor screening in vivo: results of tumor panel screening, 1976–1982, and future directions. *Adv Pharmacol Chemother* 1984; 20:1–20.
4. Corbett TH, Valeriote FA, Baker LH. Is the P388 murine tumor no longer adequate as a drug discovery model? *Invest New Drugs* 1987; 5:3–20.
5. Scott RB. Cancer chemotherapy—the first twenty-five years. *Brit Med J* 1970; 4:259–265.
6. Krakoff IH. Cancer chemotherapeutic and biologic agents. *CA* 1991; 41:264–278.
7. Holmer AF. New medicines in development for cancer. *Pharmaceut Res Manuf Amer* 1999; 1–43.
8. Laszlo J. *The Cure of Childhood Leukemia—Into the Age of Miracles.* Rutgers University Press, New Brunswick, NJ, 1995.
9. Law LW, Dunn TB, Boyle PJ, Miller JH. Observations on the effect of a folic-acid antagonist on transplantable lymphoid leukemias in mice. *J Natl Cancer Inst* 1949; 10:179–192.
10. Thomas LB, Chirigos MA, Humphreys SR, Goldin A. Pathology of the spread of L1210 leukemia in the central nervous system of mice and effect of treatment with cytoxan. *J Natl Cancer Inst* 1962; 28:1355–1389.
11. DeVita VT Jr. Principles of cancer management: chemotherapy. In: DeVita VT Jr, Hellman S, Rosenberg SA, eds. *Cancer: Principles & Practice of Oncology,* 5th ed, vol. 1. Lippincott-Raven, Philadelphia, PA, 1997, pp. 333–347.
12. Jackson RC. *The Theoretical Foundations of Cancer Chemotherapy Introduced by Computer Models.* Academic Press, San Diego, CA, 1992, pp. 227–261.
13. Norton L, Surbone A. Cytokinetics. In: Holland JF, Frei E III, Bast RC, Kufe DW, Morton DL, Weichselbaum RR, eds. *Cancer Medicine,* 3rd ed., Lea & Febiger, Philadelphia, PA, 1993, pp. 598–617.
14. Wilcox WS. The last surviving cancer cell: the chances of killing it. *Cancer Chemother Rep* 1966; 50:541–542.
15. Blum RH, Frei E III. Combination chemotherapy. *Methods in Cancer Res* 1979; 17:215–257.
16. Lloyd HH. Estimation of tumor cell kill from Gompertz growth curves. *Cancer Chemother Rep* 1975; 59:267–277.
17. Dedrick RL. Toxicology lessons from cancer chemotherapy. *CIIT Activities* 1992; 12(7):1–7.
18. Martin DS, Balis ME, Fisher B, Frei E, Freireich EJ, Heppner GH, et al. Role of murine tumor models in cancer treatment research. *Cancer Res* 1986; 46:2189–2192.

19. Grindey GB. Multiple models of utility for the rational development of new concepts involved in metabolic modulation. In: Fidler IJ, White RJ, eds. *Design of Models for Testing Cancer Therapeutic Agents.* Van Nostrand Reinhold, New York, NY, 1982, pp. 206–214.

20. Fidler IJ. The role of host factors and tumor heterogeneity in the testing of therapeutic agents. In: Fidler IJ, White RJ, eds. *Design of Models for Testing Cancer Therapeutic Agents.* Van Nostrand Reinhold, New York, NY, 1982, pp. 239–247.

21. Venditti JM. The model's dilemma. In: Fidler IJ, White RJ, eds. *Design of Models for Testing Cancer Therapeutic Agents.* Van Nostrand Reinhold, New York, NY, 1982, pp. 80–94.

22. Tonkin K, Tritchler D, Tannock I. Criteria of tumor response used in clinical trials of chemotherapy. *J Clin Oncol* 1985; 3:870–875.

23. Schabel FM Jr, Griswold DP Jr, Corbett TH, Laster WR Jr, Mayo JG, Lloyd HH. Testing therapeutic hypotheses in mice and man. *Methods in Cancer Res* 1979; 17:1–51.

24. Corbett T, Valeriote F, LoRusso P, Polin L, Panchapor C, Pugh S, et al. In vivo methods for screening and preclinical testing—use of rodent solid tumors for drug discovery. In: Teicher BA, ed. *Anticancer Drug Development Guide: Preclinical Screening, Clinical Trials, and Approval.* Humana Press, Totowa, NJ, 1997, pp. 75–99.

25. Simpson-Herren L. Kinetics and tumor models. *Cancer Chemother Rep* 1975; 5:83–88.

26. James K, Eisenhauer E, Christian M, Terenziani M, Vena D, Muldal A, et al. Measuring response in solid tumors: unidimensional versus bidimensional measurement. *J Natl Cancer Inst* 1999; 91:523–528.

27. Corbett TH, Valeriote FA. Rodent models in experimental chemotherapy. In: Kallman RF, ed. *Rodent Tumor Models in Experimental Cancer Therapy.* Pergamon, New York, NY, 1987, pp. 233–247.

28. Johnson RK. Screening methods in antineoplastic drug discovery. *J Natl Cancer Inst* 1990; 82:1082–1083.

29. Boyd MR. The NCI in vitro anticancer drug discovery screen—concept, implementation, and operation, 1985–1995. In: Teicher BA, ed. *Anticancer Drug Development Guide: Preclinical Screening, Clinical Trials, and Approval.* Humana Press, Totowa, NJ, 1997; pp. 23–42.

30. Sikic BI. Anticancer drug discovery. *J Natl Cancer Inst* 1991; 83:738–740.

31. Dykes DJ, Abbott BJ, Mayo JG, Harrison SD Jr, Laster WR Jr, Simpson-Herren L, et al. Development of human tumor xenograft models for in vivo evaluation of new antitumor drugs. In: Fiebig HH, Berger DP, eds. *Immunodeficient Mice in Oncology.* Karger, Basel, 1992, pp. 1–22.

32. Skipper HE, Schabel FM Jr. Quantitative and cytokinetic studies in experimental tumor systems. In: Holland JF, Frei E III, eds. *Cancer Medicine,* 2nd ed. Lea & Febiger, Philadelphia, *PA* 1982, pp. 663–685.

33. Plowman J, Dykes DJ, Narayanan VL, Abbott BJ, Saito H, Hirata T, et al. Efficacy of the quinocarmycins KW2152 and DX-52-1 against human melanoma lines growing in culture and in mice. *Cancer Res* 1995; 55:862–867.

34. Plowman J, Dykes DJ, Hollingshead M, Simpson-Herren L, Alley MC. Human tumor xenograft models in NCI drug development. In: Teicher BA, ed. *Anticancer Drug Development Guide: Preclinical Screening, Clinical Trials, and Approval.* Humana Press, Totowa, NJ, 1997, pp. 101–125.

35. Fiebig HH, Burger AM. Target-directed in vitro and in vivo testing procedures for the discovery of anticancer agents (abstr). *Proc 1999 AACR-NCI-EORTC Intl Conference* 1999; 142.

36. Valoti G, Nicoletti MI, Pellegrino A, Jimeno J, Hendriks H, D'Incalci M, et al. Ecteinascidin-743, a new marine natural product with potent antitumor activity on human ovarian carcinoma xenografts. *Clin Cancer Res* 1998; 4:1977–1983.

37. Corbett TH, Valeriote FA, Demchik L, Polin L, Panchapor C, Pugh S, et al. Preclinical anticancer activity of cryptophycin-8. *J Exp Ther Oncol* 1996; 1:95–108.

38. Taamma A, Misset JL, Delaloge S, Guzman C, Di Palma M, Yovine A, et al. Ecteinascidin-743 (ET-743) in heavily pretreated refractory sarcomas: early results of the French experience (abstr). *Proc 1999 AACR-NCI-EORTC Intl Conference* 1999; 63.

39. Adams JM, Cory S. Transgenic models of tumor development. *Science* 1991; 254:1161–1167.

40. Goldberg KB. New treatment for CML could be model for molecular target-based therapeutics. *Cancer Lett* 1999; 25(47):1–4.

41. Chabner BA, Boral AL, Multani P. Translational research: walking the bridge between idea and cure—seventeenth Bruce F. Cain Memorial Award lecture. *Cancer Res* 1998; 58:4211–4216.

42. Retain MJ. Development of target-based antineoplastic agents. In: Perry MC, ed. *Amer Soc Clin Oncol Educational Book—35th Annual Meeting.* Alexandria, VA: ASCO. 1999:71–75.

43. Rao RN. Targets for cancer therapy in the cell cycle pathway. *Curr Opin Oncol* 1996; 8:516–524.

44. Zhang L, Zhou W, Velculescu VE, Kern SE, Hruban RH, Hamilton SR, et al. Gene expression profiles in normal and cancer cells. *Science* 1997; 276:1268–1272.

45. Stoler DL, Chen N, Basik M, Kahlenberg MS, Rodriguez-Bigas MA, Petrelli NJ, et al. The onset and extent of genomic instability in sporadic colorectal tumor progression. *Proc Natl Acad Sci USA* 1999; 96:15,121–15,126.

46. Sebolt-Leopold JS, Dudley DT, Herrera R, Van Becelaere K, Wiland A, Gowan RC, et al. Blockade of the MAP kinase pathway suppresses growth of colon tumors in vivo. *Nat Med* 1999; 5:810–816.

47. Thavasu P, Propper D, McDonald A, Dobbs N, Ganesan T, Talbot D, et al. The protein kinase C inhibitor CGP41251 suppresses cytokine release and extracellular signal-regulated kinase 2 expression in cancer patients. *Cancer Res* 1999; 59:3980–3984.

48. Meyer T, Regenass U, Fabbro D, Alteri E, Rosel J, Muller M, et al. A derivative of staurosporine (CGP41251) shows selectivity for protein kinase C inhibition and in vitro anti-proliferative as well as in vivo anti-tumor activity. *Int J Cancer* 1989; 43:851–856.

49. Yoshiji H, Kuriyama S, Ways DK, Yoshii J, Miyamoto Y, Kawata M, et al. Protein kinase C lies on the signaling pathway for vascular endothelial growth factor-mediated tumor development and angiogenesis. *Cancer Res* 1999; 59:4413–4418.

50. Zhou S, Kinzler KW, Vogelstein B. Going mad with Smads. *N Engl J Med* 1999; 341:1144–1146.

51. Macleod KF, Jacks T. Insights into cancer from transgenic mouse models. *J Pathol* 1999; 187:43–60.

II TRANSPLANTABLE SYNGENEIC RODENT TUMORS

2

Murine L1210 and P388 Leukemias

Donald J. Dykes, BS and William R. Waud, PhD

CONTENTS

INTRODUCTION
ROLE IN DRUG SCREENING
CHARACTERISTICS
SENSITIVITY TO CLINICAL AGENTS
PREDICTIVE VALUE
DRUG-RESISTANT LEUKEMIAS
CONCLUSION
ACKNOWLEDGMENTS
REFERENCES

1. INTRODUCTION

Mouse leukemia models were a central component of the initial drug discovery programs employed by the Division of Cancer Treatment (DCT) of the National Cancer Institute (NCI) during the early 1960s and 1970s. The L1210 and P388 leukemias, developed in 1948 *(1)* and 1955 *(2)*, respectively, played a major role in both screening and detailed evaluations of candidate anticancer agents. Today, 40 yr later, these models are still used to evaluate anticancer activity, although at a greatly reduced level, and to study mechanisms of drug resistance. This chapter reviews their past contributions, updates their present role in the evaluation of anticancer drugs, and summarizes data for the drug sensitivity of these two leukemias and various drug-resistant P388 sublines to clinically useful drugs.

2. ROLE IN DRUG SCREENING

Spontaneous tumors in animals were first used as models for screening potential anticancer agents. In fact, these types of studies occurred even prior to the beginning of the twentieth century *(3)*, and provided the basis for modern drug-screening programs. However, large-scale screening and the ability to conduct detailed drug-evaluation studies with anticancer agents increased greatly in the 1920s through the development of inbred strains of mice that allowed investigators to propagate tumor lines by serial transplantation in vivo *(4)*.

From: *Tumor Models in Cancer Research*
Edited by: B. A. Teicher © Humana Press Inc., Totowa, NJ

The US Congress became interested in cancer research when it was recognized in the 1940s that systemic cancer could be influenced by drug treatment. This was demonstrated at Memorial Sloan-Kettering, one of the first of several institutions in the United States and Europe to begin drug-screening programs. In this program, the mouse sarcoma SA-180 was used as its screening model. However, as drugs exhibited anticancer activity and the supply of new candidate agents exceeded the screening capacity of that program, the need for additional drug development capabilities became apparent. With this impetus, Congress directed NCI to implement a national drug development program, which went into effect in 1955 as the Cancer Chemotherapy National Service Center (CCNSC).

Initially, the CCNSC primary screening program consisted of L1210 leukemia, SA-180, and mammary adenocarcinoma 755 *(5)*. Over the years, the composition of the primary screen changed several times—i.e., from the original three tumors to L1210 and two arbitrarily selected tumors; to L1210 and Walker 256 carcinosarcoma; to L1210 and P388 leukemia; and finally, to L1210, P388, and either B16 melanoma or Lewis lung carcinoma (LLC) *(6)*. Several other models were also used during this period for special, detailed drug evaluation.

The primary screening program underwent a major change in 1976, when DCT incorporated the use of three human tumor xenograft models. The new screen now consisted of a panel of colon, breast, and lung tumors, both murine and human. However, all drugs intended this screen were still initially evaluated for activity against the sensitive P388 leukemia model *(7)*. During this period, the small number of drugs discovered with marked antitumor activity against human solid tumors led to a radical change in the screening program that had used murine leukemia models as the primary screen. In the mid-1980s, NCI developed a new primary screen based on the use of established human tumor-cell lines in vitro *(8)*. The new and old screen programs were to be conducted in parallel to permit a comparison; however, in early 1987, budget cuts at NCI forced an end to large-scale P388 screening *(9)*.

3. CHARACTERISTICS

Both L1210 and P388 leukemias were chemically induced in a DBA/2 mouse by painting the skin with methylcholanthrene *(1,2)*. Propagation of the leukemia lines occurs in the host of origin by intraperitoneal (ip) implantation of diluted ascitic fluid containing either 10^5 (L1210) or 10^6 (P388) cells per animal. Testing is generally conducted in a hybrid of DBA/2 (e.g., $CD2F_1$ or $B6D2F_1$), because the hybrids are somewhat heartier. However, DBA/2 mice may be used for special studies, and should be used for serial in vivo propagation of the leukemias. Frequently used implant sites are ip, subcutaneous (sc), intravenous (iv), or intracerebral (ic). For L1210 leukemia with an implant of 10^5 cells, the median days of death and the tumor doubling times for these implant sites are 8.8, 9.9, 6.4, and 7.0 d and 0.34, 0.46, 0.45, and 0.37 d, respectively. For P388 leukemia with an implant of 10^6 cells, the median days of death and the tumor doubling times for these implant sites are 10.3, 13.0, 8.0, and 8.0 d and 0.44, 0.52, 0.68, and 0.63 d, respectively.

Skipper and colleagues at the Southern Research Institute determined the rate of distribution and proliferation of L1210 leukemia cells using bioassays of untreated mice after ip, iv, and ic inoculation *(10)*. Following ip inoculation, most of the L1210 cells were found in the ascites fluid of the peritoneal cavity. Using the median day of death as the evaluation time-point, the most commonly infiltrated tissues were the bone marrow, liver, and spleen. Following iv inoculation, the majority of L1210 cells appeared in the bone marrow. On the median day of death from the iv implant, the most infiltrated tissues were also the bone marrow, liver, and spleen. After ic inoculation, most of the L1210 cells remained in the brain (for 3–5 d). On the median day of death from the ic implant, the spleen was heavily infiltrated (the extent of the leukemia in other tissues was not reported).

Southern Research was one of the first institutions to become involved in the CCNSC screening program, and was heavily involved in designing protocols for the program. One aspect essential to the operation of a screening program is the development of appropriate parameters for measuring antitumor activity. At Southern Research, antitumor activity for leukemia studies is assessed on the basis of percent median increase in lifespan (% ILS), net $\log_{10}$ cell-kill, and long-term survivors. Calculations of net $\log_{10}$ cell-kill are made from the tumor-cell population doubling time that is determined from an internal tumor titration consisting of implants from serial 10-fold dilutions *(11)*. Long-term survivors are excluded from calculations of % ILS and tumor-cell-kill. To assess tumor-cell-kill at the end of treatment, the survival time difference between treated and control groups is adjusted to account for regrowth of tumor-cell populations that may occur between individual treatments *(12)*. The net $\log_{10}$ cell-kill is calculated as follows:

$$\text{Net } \log_{10} \text{ cell-kill} = \frac{(\text{T-C}) - (\text{duration of treatment in days})}{3.32 \times \text{T}_d}$$

where (T-C) is the difference in the median day of death between the treated (T) and the control (C) groups, 3.32 is the number of doublings required for a population to increase 1-$\log_{10}$ unit, and T_d is the mean tumor doubling time (days) calculated from a log-linear least-squares fit of the implant sizes and the median days of death of the titration groups.

4. SENSITIVITY TO CLINICAL AGENTS

The majority of clinically useful compounds in current use was first detected in the murine leukemia models. The sensitivities of L1210 and P388 leukemias (ip implantation) to most of these agents (ip administration) are shown in Figs. 1 and 2 and Figs. 3 and 4, respectively. Overall, P388 leukemia is somewhat more sensitive than L1210 leukemia. For alkylating agents, the sensitivities are similar. Notable exceptions are chlorambucil, mitomycin C, and carboplatin, for which P388 is markedly more sensitive. For antimetabolites, the sensitivities are also similar. Exceptions are floxuridine (P388 being markedly more sensitive) and hydroxyurea (L1210 being markedly more sensitive). For DNA-binding agents, P388 leukemia is clearly more sensitive (e.g., actinomycin D, mithramycin, daunorubicin, teniposide, doxorubicin, and amsacrine). For tubulin-binding agents, P388 leukemia is again clearly more sensitive. The vinca alkaloids are active against P388 leukemia, but ineffective against L1210 leukemia.

Although most of the sensitivity data are for ip-implanted leukemia and ip-administered drugs, valuable information can be obtained from separating the implant site and the route of administration. Table 1 shows the activity of melphalan (ip administration) against both L1210 and P388 leukemias implanted through ip, iv, and ic meth-

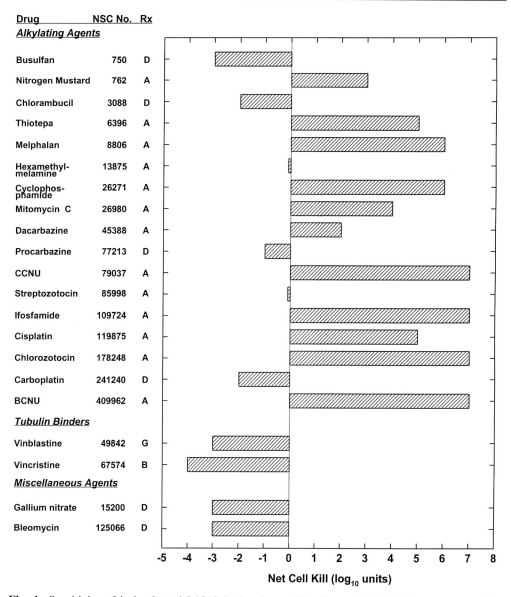

Fig. 1. Sensitivity of ip-implanted L1210 leukemia to clinically useful alkylating agents, tubulin binders, and other miscellaneous agents. L1210 leukemia (10^5 cells except for hexamethylmelamine, which used 10^6 cells) was ip-implanted on d 0. Beginning on d 1, the agents were ip-administered using the indicated schedules. Treatment schedule (R_x): A = d 1; B = d 1, 5, 9; C = d 1–5; D = d 1–9; E = d 1, 4, 7, 10; F = q3h × 8, d 1, 5, 9; G = d 1–15.

ods. The use of ip melphalan is very effective against both ip-implanted leukemias. The activity is reduced to less than one-half when changed to an iv implant site. The activity is further reduced with change to an ic implant site; however, melphalan can cross the blood-brain barrier to some extent. This principle is illustrated more fully with the data in Figs. 5 (L1210) and 6 (P388) for the leukemias with ic implantation, and various clinically useful agents with ip administration. Thiotepa, CCNU, BCNU, and ara-

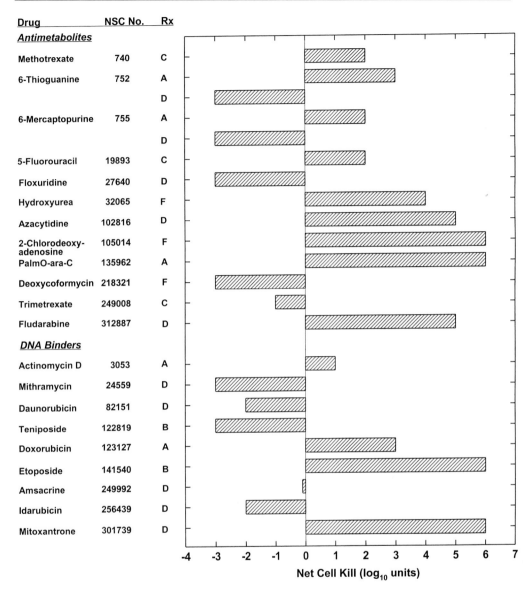

Fig. 2. Sensitivity of ip-implanted L1210 leukemia to clinically useful antimetabolites and DNA binders. L1210 leukemia (10^5 cells, except for hydroxyurea, which used 10^4 cells and 6-thioguanine (d 1-only treatment) and daunorubicin, which used 10^6 cells) was ip-implanted on d 0. Beginning on d 1 (d 2 for daunorubicin), the agents were ip-administered using the indicated schedules. Treatment schedule (R_x): see legend for Fig. 1.

C/palmO-ara-C, with ip administration, exhibit comparable activity against either ip- or ic-implanted leukemias. Cisplatin, cyclophosphamide, ifosfamide, and 6-mercaptopurine (L1210), in addition to melphalan, have reduced activity with an ic implant site. Several agents become inactive with an ic implant site—methotrexate (P388), 5-fluorouracil (5-Fu), floxuridine, actinomycin D, vincristine, doxorubicin, and etoposide. Comparisons among different treatment schedules can be misleading. Although all values have been expressed as net cell-kill (i.e., corrected for the treatment schedule),

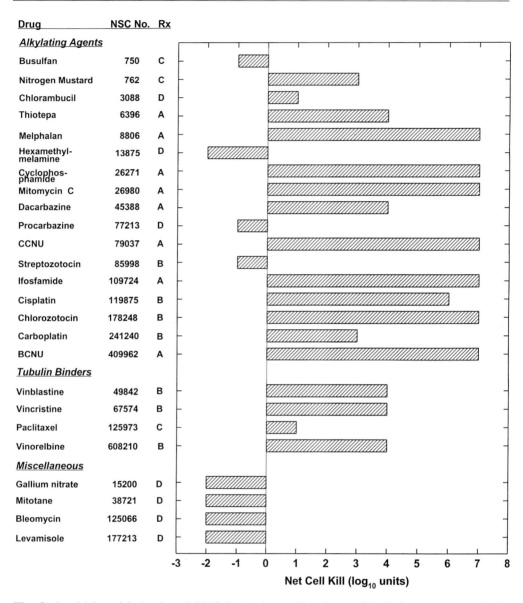

Drug	NSC No.	Rx
Alkylating Agents		
Busulfan	750	C
Nitrogen Mustard	762	C
Chlorambucil	3088	D
Thiotepa	6396	A
Melphalan	8806	A
Hexamethyl-melamine	13875	D
Cyclophos-phamide	26271	A
Mitomycin C	26980	A
Dacarbazine	45388	A
Procarbazine	77213	D
CCNU	79037	A
Streptozotocin	85998	B
Ifosfamide	109724	A
Cisplatin	119875	B
Chlorozotocin	178248	B
Carboplatin	241240	B
BCNU	409962	A
Tubulin Binders		
Vinblastine	49842	B
Vincristine	67574	B
Paclitaxel	125973	C
Vinorelbine	608210	B
Miscellaneous		
Gallium nitrate	15200	D
Mitotane	38721	D
Bleomycin	125066	D
Levamisole	177213	D

Net Cell Kill (log$_{10}$ units)

Fig. 3. Sensitivity of ip-implanted P388 leukemia to clinically useful alkylating agents, tubulin binders, and other miscellaneous agents. P388 leukemia (10^6 cells except for CCNU, which used 10^7 cells) was ip-implanted on d 0. Beginning on d 1 (d 2 for CCNU, streptozotocin, and chlorozotocin), the agents were ip-administered using the indicated schedules. Treatment schedule (R_x): see legend for Fig. 1.

one schedule can be optimal, whereas another schedule is suboptimal. For nitrogen mustard, no conclusion can be drawn from the data about its ability to cross the blood-brain barrier. The agent is active against the ip-implanted leukemia using a single ip injection (optimal), and is inactive against the ic-implanted leukemia using 15 daily ip injections (suboptimal). This is further illustrated by chlorambucil, which is active against ic-implanted L1210 (using a single ip injection), and inactive against ip-implanted L1210 (using nine daily ip injections).

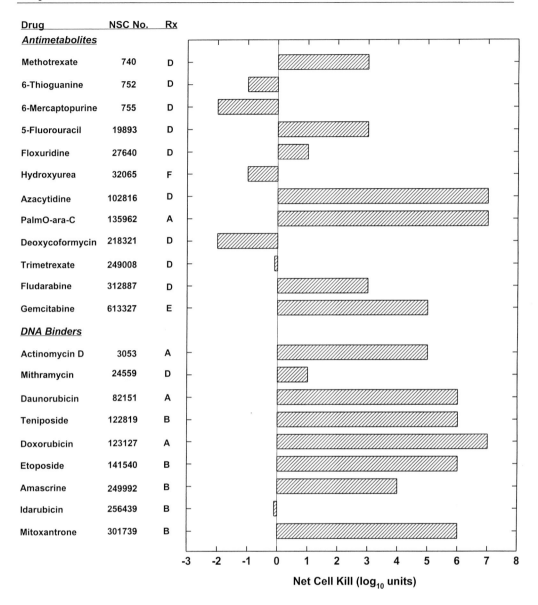

Fig. 4. Sensitivity of ip-implanted P388 leukemia to clinically useful antimetabolites and DNA binders. P388 leukemia (10^6 cells) was ip-implanted on d 0. Beginning on d 1, the agents were ip-administered using the indicated schedules. Treatment schedule (R_x): see legend for Fig. 1.

Studies with these screening models revealed that drug sensitivity was, in some cases, heavily dependent on drug concentration and exposure time, which in turn was impacted by the in vivo treatment schedule. As an example, studies conducted with 1-β-D-arabinofuranosylcytosine (ara-C) pointed out the need for concentration and time of exposure studies. Using L1210 leukemia in mice, it was shown that the optimal dosage and schedule for ara-C was 15–20 mg/kg/dose, given every 3 h for eight doses, then repeated three times at 4-d intervals (13). This regimen was "curative." The single-dose LD_{10} for mice was between 2500 and 3000 mg/kg, and using a single dose within

Table 1
Activity of Melphalan Administered as a Single IP
Injection Against L1210 and P388 Leukemias Implanted
ip, iv, and ic

Site	Inoculum size	Net cell-kill (log_{10} units)	
		L1210	P388
IP	10^6	4.7	>6.5
IV	10^6	2.0	2.9
IC	10^4	1.2	2.4

that range would effect a 3-log_{10}-unit reduction in L1210 cells but was not "curative." Although these in vivo results might give the appearance of a concentration-dependent effect, in vitro studies have clearly shown that cell-kill of L1210 in culture was time-dependent at the higher concentration levels employed. The apparent concentration dependence observed in vivo over a range of single doses resulted from the extended time of exposure of those extremely high dosage levels.

5. PREDICTIVE VALUE

Many investigators have questioned the use of experimental leukemias as primary screening models over the years. Some have argued that since L1210 or P388 leukemia was used for many years as the initial screening model, continued evaluation of compounds emerging from this screening configuration—even using solid-tumor models for secondary evaluation—would only produce antileukemic drugs *(14)*. If compounds active against solid tumors were being missed by the primary screen composed of leukemias, it would appear reasonable that in order to obtain agents that are active against specific tumor types or solid tumors in general, then the primary screen should consist of specific tumor types or solid tumors. Although this would appear to be a reasonable approach, it will depend on whether or not there are existing agents or whether agents can be developed that will selectively kill specific cancer histotypes.

The correlation between drugs active against L1210 or P388 leukemia and solid experimental tumor models has not been good. For example, only 1.7% of 1493 agents that were active against P388 leukemia were also active against murine LLC. Further, only 2% of 1507 agents active against P388 leukemia were also active against murine colon 38 adenocarcinoma. Finally, only 2% of 1133 agents that were active against P388 leukemia were also active against human CX-1 (HT29) colon tumor. However, when comparing leukemias, a correlation less than expected was obtained—only 15% of 1564 active agents against P388 leukemia were also active against L1210 leukemia *(15)*.

One common observation is that some drugs that are active against experimental solid tumors are inactive against P388 leukemia. For example, 15% of 84 agents that were inactive against P388 leukemia were active against at least one of eight solid tumors tested *(15)*. Flavone acetic acid has been cited as an example *(14)*. This compound was inactive in the initial P388 screen, although it was later shown to exhibit

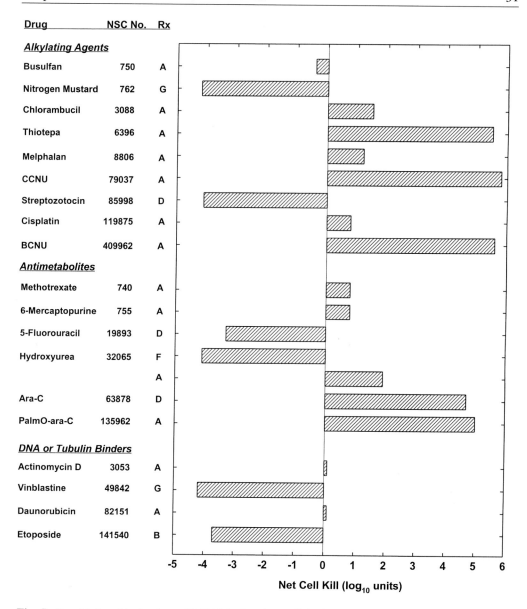

Fig. 5. Sensitivity of ic-implanted L1210 leukemia to clinically useful agents. L1210 leukemia (10^4 cells except for CCNU, which used 10^5 cells) was ic-implanted on d 0. Beginning on d 1 (d 2 for busulfan, chlorambucil, thiotepa, melphalan, hydroxyurea (single injection), cisplatin, BCNU, and daunorubicin), the agents were ip-administered using the indicated schedules. Treatment schedule (R$_x$): see legend for Fig. 1.

activity against the leukemia when the appropriate treatment schedule was used *(16)*. This example reveals a problem with large-scale screening programs—it is not logistically feasible to conduct preliminary schedule-dependency trials.

Another observation is that there are experimental solid tumors (e.g., murine pancreatic 02 ductal adenocarcinoma) that are not responsive in vivo to any clinically used agents, including many P388-active agents *(14)*. It may be noted, however, that this

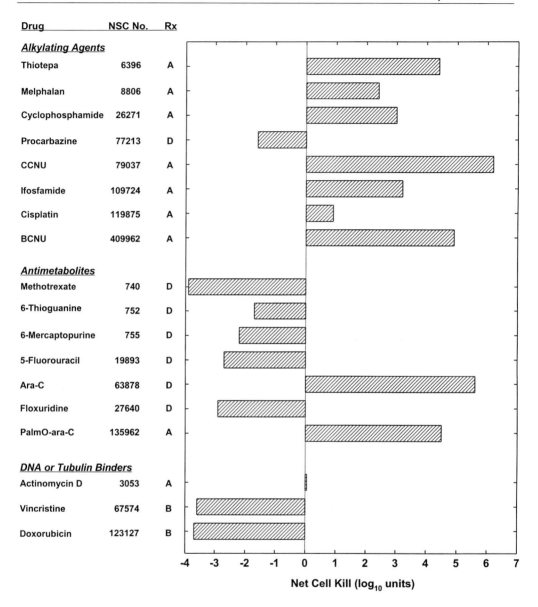

Fig. 6. Sensitivity of ic-implanted P388 leukemia to clinically useful agents. P388 leukemia (10^4 cells except for ifosfamide, methotrexate, 6-thioguanine, 6-mercaptopurine, 5-FU, and floxuridine, which used 10^3 cells and CCNU and ara-C, which used 10^5 cells) was ic-implanted on d 0. Beginning on d 1 (d 2 for ifosfamide), the agents were ip-administered using the indicated schedules. Treatment schedule (R_x): see legend for Fig. 1.

tumor is sensitive to numerous clinical agents in vitro after a 24-h exposure *(17),* suggesting that the in vivo insensitivity of this tumor may not be caused by cellular characteristics, but may be a result of physiological or architectural constraints of the animal.

Southern Research has evaluated a spectrum of compounds in the ip-implanted P388 model in order to evaluate this model as a predictor for the response of human tumor xenografts to new candidate antitumor agents (unpublished data). The P388 data collected were compared to the data for various sc-implanted human tumor xenografts, which were selected on the basis of the results of the NCI in vitro screen. In general, compounds that were active against P388 leukemia were active to a lesser degree in one or more of the xenografts in the in vivo tumor panel. However, there were isolated examples of a P388-active agent being inactive in the human tumor xenograft models tested, and vice versa. There was no indication that the P388 model could predict compound efficacy for specific tumor xenografts.

Whether or not the murine leukemias are poor predictors of activity in solid tumors is still somewhat questionable, and will only be determined with the availability of drugs without antileukemic model activity but with proven value in the treatment of human solid tumors.

6. DRUG-RESISTANT LEUKEMIAS

Panels of in vivo drug-resistant murine L1210 and P388 leukemia models have been developed at Southern Research for use in the evaluation of crossresistance and collateral sensitivity. These models have been used for the evaluation of new drugs of potential clinical interest. An extensive summary of in vivo drug resistance and crossresistance data has been published by Schabel and colleagues *(18)*. Their initial manuscript included results of in vivo crossresistance studies on 79 antitumor drugs in seven drug-resistant L1210 leukemias and 74 antitumor drugs in 12 drug-resistant P388 leukemias. Previously, we expanded this crossresistance data base for the drug-resistant P388 leukemias to include two new drug-resistant lines and more clinically useful drugs. Also, we updated the database to include new candidate antitumor agents entering clinical trials *(19)*. Recently, another drug-resistant P388 leukemia (P388/VP-16) was added to this database *(20)*. This section examines the crossresistance database for 16 drug-resistant P388 leukemias and many of the clinically useful agents.

6.1. Resistance to Alkylating Agents

The crossresistance profile of cyclophosphamide-resistant P388 leukemia (P388/CPA) to 14 different clinical agents is shown in Table 2. The P388/CPA line was crossresistant[1] to one of the five alkylating agents, no antimetabolites, no DNA-binding agents, and no tubulin-binding agents. Crossresistance of P388/CPA has also been observed for two other alkylating agents (chlorambucil and ifosfamide) *(20)*. Interestingly, there are differences among these three agents. Chlorambucil and ifosfamide, like cyclophosphamide, each have two chloroethylating moieties, whereas mitomycin C is from a different chemical class. Whereas ifosfamide, cyclophosphamide, and mitomycin C require metabolic activation, chlorambucil does not. Although P388/CPA is crossresistant to two chloroethylating agents, the line is not crossresistant to other chloroethylating agents (melphalan and BCNU). Therefore, P388/CPA appears to be crossresistant only to a select group of alkylating agents with differing characteristics. P388/CPA appeared to be collaterally sensitive to fludarabine.

---

[1] Crossresistance is defined as decreased sensitivity (by >2-$\log_{10}$ units of cell-kill) of a drug-resistant P388 leukemia to a drug compared to that observed concurrently in P388/0 leukemia. Similarly, marginal crossresistance is defined as a decrease in sensitivity of approx 2-$\log_{10}$ units. Collateral sensitivity is defined as increased sensitivity (by >2-$\log_{10}$ units of cell kill) of a drug-resistant P388 leukemia to a drug over that observed concurrently in P388/0 leukemia.

Table 2

Crossresistance of P388 Sublines Resistant to Various Alkylating Agents and Antimetabolites to Clinically Useful Agents

Drug	NSC No.	R_x^a	CPA	L-PAM	DPt	BCNU	MMC^b	MTX	5-FU	ARA-C
Alkylating Agents										
Melphalan	8806	A	−	+	−	−				±
Cyclophosphamide	26271	A	+	−	−	−				+
Mitomycin C	26980	A	±	+	−	−	+	−		+
Procarbazine	77213	D	−		−	−				
Cisplatin	119875	B	−	+	+	−	±[c]	−		+
BCNU	409962	A	−	−	−	+	−			−
Antimetabolites										
Methotrexate	740	D			−		−[d]	+	+	+
6-Thioguanine	752	A					−[d]	−		−
6-Mercaptopurine	755	D						−		
5-Fluorouracil	19893	D	−		−		−[d]		+	=
PalmO-ara-C	135962	A	−	−	−		−[d]	−	−	+
Trimetrexate	249008	D	−	±	−			−		−
Fludarabine	312887	D	=	=	=			−	=	+
Gemcitabine	613327	E	−	−	−			−		+
DNA Binders										
Actinomycin D	3053	A	−	±	−	−	±			−
Doxorubicin	123127	A	−	−	−	−	+			−
Etoposide	141540	B	−	−	−		+[c]			−
Amsacrine	249992	B	−	+	=		−[c]			−
Mitoxantrone	301739	B		+	=			−		−
Tubulin Binders										
Vinblastine	49842	A					+			
Vincristine	67574	B	−	+	−		+[c]	−		+
Paclitaxel	125973	C		−	−			−		−

CD2F₁ mice were ip-implanted with 10^6 P388/0 or drug-resistant P388 cells on d 0. Data presented are for ip drug treatment at an optimal ($\leq LD_{10}$) dosage. Symbols: resistance/crossresistance, +; marginal crossresistance, ±; no crossresistance, −; and collateral sensitivity, =.

a Treatment schedule (R_x): A = d 1; B = d 1, 5, 9; C = d 1–5; D = d 1–9; E = d 1, 4, 7, 10.

b Data from *In Vivo* 1987; 1:47–52.

c Treatment schedule was d 1.

d Treatment schedule was d 1 and 5.

The effect of 15 different clinical agents on melphalan-resistant P388 leukemia (P388/L-PAM) is shown in Table 2. The P388/L-PAM line was crossresistant to approximately one-half of the agents—2 of 4 alkylating agents, 1 of 4 antimetabolites, 3 of 5 DNA-binding agents, and 1 of 2 tubulin-binding agents. The alkylating agents involved in crossresistance represent different chemical classes. Similarly, the DNA-interacting agents involved in crossresistance include agents with different mechanisms of action—inhibitors of DNA topoisomerase II (amsacrine and mitoxantrone) and a DNA-binding agent (actinomycin D). However, the melphalan-resistant line did not exhibit crossresistance to other inhibitors of DNA topoisomerase II (e.g., doxorubicin and etoposide) or another DNA-binding agent (e.g., doxorubicin).

The sensitivity of cisplatin-resistant P388 leukemia (P388/DDPt) to 17 different clinical agents is shown in Table 2. The P388/DDPt line was not crossresistant to any of these agents. Interestingly, the cisplatin-resistant line was collaterally sensitive to three agents (fludarabine, amsacrine, and mitoxantrone). Of these three agents, the latter two have been reported to interact with DNA topoisomerase II *(21,22)*.

The crossresistance data for N,N′-*bis*(2-chloroethyl)-N-nitrosourea-resistant P388 leukemia (P388/BCNU) have been limited to the evaluation of alkylating agents. The crossresistance profile of P388/BCNU to four different clinical agents is shown in Table 2. The BCNU-resistant line was not crossresistant to melphalan, cyclophosphamide, mitomycin C, or cisplatin.

The crossresistance profile of mitomycin C-resistant P388 leukemia (P388/MMC) to 13 different clinical agents is shown in Table 2 *(23)*. The P388/MMC line was crossresistant to approximately one-half of the agents—1 of 3 alkylating agents, 0 of 4 antimetabolites, 3 of 4 DNA-binding agents, and two of two tubulin-binding agents. The pattern was similar to that observed for P388/L-PAM.

6.2. Resistance to Antimetabolites

The effect of 14 different clinical agents on methotrexate-resistant P388 leukemia (P388/MTX) is shown in Table 2. The P388/MTX line was not crossresistant to any of these agents.

The crossresistance data for 5-fluorouracil-resistant P388 leukemia (P388/5-FU) have been limited to antimetabolites. The sensitivity of the P388/5-FU to three different agents is shown in Table 2. The P388/5-FU line was not crossresistant to palmO-ara-C (a slow-releasing form of ara-C) or fludarabine (possible collateral sensitivity). Crossresistance was observed for methotrexate.

The crossresistance profile of 1-β-D-arabinofuranosylcytosine-resistant P388 leukemia (P388/ARA-C) to 16 different clinical agents is shown in Table 2. The P388/ARA-C line was crossresistant to members of several functionally different classes of antitumor agents—four of five alkylating agents, three of five antimetabolites, none of four DNA-binding agents, and one of two tubulin-binding agents. Interestingly, the line was collaterally sensitive to 5-FU.

6.3. Resistance to DNA- and Tubulin-Binding Agents

The effect of 17 different clinical agents on actinomycin D-resistant P388 leukemia (P388/ACT-D) is shown in Table 3. P388/ACT-D was not crossresistant to any alkylating agents or antimetabolites. However, it was crossresistant to all of the drugs tested that are involved in multidrug resistance, except for amsacrine.

Table 3
Crossresistance of P388 Sublines Resistant to Various DNA and Tubulin Binders to Clinically Useful Agents

Drug	NSC No.	R_x^a	ACT-D	ADR	AMSA	DIOHA	VP-16	CPT^b	VCR	PTX
Alkylating Agents										
Melphalan	8806	A	–	–	–		–		–	
Cyclophosphamide	26271	A	–	–	–		–		–	
Mitomycin C	26980	A	–	±	–			$–^e$	+	
Procarbazine	77213	D	–	–	–				–	
Cisplatin	119875	C	–	–	$–^c$		$–^c$	$–^e$	±	
BCNU	409962	A	–	–	–		–		–	
Antimetabolites										
Methotrexate	740	D	–	–	±	–	–		–	
6-Thioguanine	752	D	–	–					–	
6-Mercaptopurine	755	D	–	–					–	
5-Fluorouracil	19893	D	–	$–^d$	$–^d$		–			
PalmO-ara-C	135962	A	–	–	–					
Trimetrexate	249008	D		–						
Fludarabine	312887	D		=						
Gemcitabine	613327	E		–			–		–	
DNA Binders										
Actinomycin D	3053	A	+	+	+	–	+	$–^e$	–	
Doxorubicin	123127	A	±	+	+	–	+	$–^e$	–	+
Etoposide	141540	B	+	+	+	–	+		–	+
Amsacrine	249992	B	–	+	+	+	+	$–^e$	–	
Mitoxantrone	301739	B	+	+	+	+	+	$–^e$	–	
Tubulin Binders										
Vinblastine	49842	B	+	+	+		+		+	
Vincristine	67574	B	+	+	+	+	+		+	+
Paclitaxel	125973	C	±	±	+	–		$–^e$	–	+

CD2F$_1$ mice were ip-implanted with 10^6 P388 cells on d 0. Data presented are for ip drug treatment at an optimal ($\leq$LD$_{10}$) dosage. Symbols: resistance/crossresistance, +; marginal crossresistance, ±; no crossresistance, –; and collateral sensitivity, =.

[a] Treatment schedule (R_x): A = d 1; B = d 1, 5, 9; C = d 1–5; D = d 1–9; E = d 1, 4, 7, 10.

[b] Data from *Mol Pharmacol* 1990; 38:471–480.

[c] Treatment schedule was d 1, 5, 9.

[d] Treatment schedule was d 1–5.

[e] Treatment schedule was d 1 and 5.

The crossresistance profile of doxorubicin-resistant P388 leukemia (P388/ADR) to 21 different clinical agents is shown in Table 3. The P388/ADR line was not crossresistant to any of the antimetabolites, and was marginally crossresistant to only one alkylating agent (mitomycin C). Resistance was observed for all the drugs tested that are reported to be involved in multidrug resistance (actinomycin D, doxorubicin, etoposide, amsacrine, mitoxantrone, vinblastine, vincristine, and paclitaxel). P388/ADR was collaterally sensitive to fludarabine.

The sensitivity of amsacrine-resistant P388 leukemia (P388/AMSA) to 14 different clinical agents is shown in Table 3. P388/AMSA was not crossresistant to any of the alkylating agents, and was marginally crossresistant to only one antimetabolite. Crossresistance was observed for all the drugs tested that are involved in multidrug resistance.

The crossresistance data for mitoxantrone-resistant P388 leukemia (P388/DIOHA) have been limited mainly to agents involved in multidrug resistance. The sensitivity of P388/DIOHA to seven different clinical agents is shown in Table 3. The P388/DIOHA line exhibited mixed multidrug resistance—crossresistance to amsacrine and vincristine, but no crossresistance to actinomycin D, doxorubicin, etoposide, or paclitaxel.

The crossresistance profile of etoposide-resistant P388 leukemia (P388/VP-16) to 13 different clinical agents is shown in Table 3. The P388/VP-16 line was not crossresistant to any of the alkylating agents or antimetabolites. However, it was crossresistant to all of the drugs tested that are reported to be involved in multidrug resistance.

The sensitivity of camptothecin-resistant P388 leukemia (P388/CPT) to seven different clinical agents is shown in Table 3 (24). P388/CPT was not crossresistant to any of these agents.

The effect of 21 different clinical agents on vincristine-resistant P388 leukemia (P388/VCR) is shown in Table 3. The P388/VCR line was crossresistant to three of the agents—mitomycin C, cisplatin (marginal), and vinblastine. Unexpectedly, P388/VCR was not crossresistant to many of the drugs tested that are involved in multidrug resistance (e.g., actinomycin D, doxorubicin, etoposide, amsacrine, mitoxantrone, and paclitaxel).

The crossresistance data for paclitaxel-resistant P388 leukemia (P388/PTX) have been limited to agents involved in multidrug resistance. The sensitivity of P388/PTX to three different clinical agents is shown in Table 3. The P388/PTX line was crossresistant to drugs that are involved in multidrug resistance (doxorubicin, etoposide, and vincristine).

CONCLUSION

Currently, biotechnology appears to be advancing in an almost exponential fashion. Today, advanced techniques and tools allow us to conduct research that could not even be imagined 40 yr ago, when the L1210 and P388 leukemia models were first used extensively (e.g., sequencing the human genome). Utilizing molecular biology techniques, the emphasis is now on the development of compounds designed for a specific target. Current NCI strategy suggests that models for evaluating these compounds contain the specific target, either naturally or by gene transfection. Successful treatment of such models will theoretically provide the necessary proof-of-concept required for continued development. This is a radical departure from the empirical approach to mass screening of compounds against murine leukemias.

The L1210 and P388 leukemia models do have some advantages—they are rapid, reproducible, and relatively inexpensive (in comparison to human tumor xenograft models). However, as with any experimental animal tumor model, there are limitations. Neither leukemia is a satisfactory drug discovery model for either human cancer in general or human leukemia in particular. Of course, this could be said of any animal tumor model. Of the two leukemias, P388 is the more sensitive, but overpredicts drug activity for both preclinical human tumor xenograft models and the clinic. However, the question of whether P388 leukemia (or L1210) is a poor predictor for solid tumor-active drugs has not yet been sufficiently answered.

Although the murine leukemia models have serious limitations, these models have been very useful in anticancer drug development, in the development of a number of therapeutic principles, and in understanding the biologic behavior of tumor and host. These models are still useful today in conducting detailed evaluations of new candidate anticancer drugs (e.g., schedule dependency, route-of-administration dependency, formulation comparison, analog comparison, and combination chemotherapy).

Perhaps the greatest utility of the murine leukemias today is derived from the evaluations of the drug-resistant sublines for crossresistance and collateral sensitivity. Analysis of the crossresistance data generated at Southern Research for clinical agents has revealed possible noncrossresistant drug combinations. The P388 leukemia lines selected for resistance to alkylating agents (e.g., P388/CPA, P388/L-PAM, P388/DDPt, P388/BCNU, and P388/MMC) differed in crossresistance profiles, both with respect to alkylating agents and other functional classes. Similarly, P388 leukemia lines selected for resistance to antimetabolites (e.g., P388/MTX, P388/5-FU, and P388/ARA-C) differed in crossresistance profiles, both with respect to antimetabolites and other functional classes. Clearly, the spectrum of crossresistance of an alkylating agent or an antimetabolite will depend on the individual agent. P388 leukemia lines selected for resistance to large polycyclic anticancer drugs (e.g., P388/ACT-D, P388/ADR, P388/AMSA, P388/DIOHA, P388/VP-16, P388/CPT, P388/VCR, and P388/PTX) were not generally crossresistant to alkylating agents or antimetabolites. However, the crossresistance profiles to DNA- and tubulin-binding agents were variable.

Five of the 16 drug-resistant leukemias exhibited collateral sensitivity to one or more drugs. These observations of collateral sensitivity suggest that a combination of one of the five drugs plus one of the corresponding agents for which collateral sensitivity was observed may exhibit therapeutic synergism.

Crossresistance data, coupled with knowledge of the mechanisms of resistance operative in the drug-resistant leukemias, may yield insights into the mechanisms of action of the agents being tested. Similarly, crossresistance data, coupled with the mechanisms of action of various agents, may yield insights into the mechanisms of resistance operative in the drug-resistant leukemias (19). Furthermore, crossresistance data may identify potentially useful guides for patient selection for clinical trials of new antitumor drugs (19).

In conclusion, the role of L1210 and P388 leukemias in the evaluation of anticancer agents has diminished considerably. Nevertheless, the majority of clinical agents now in use was first detected by the murine leukemias. These models are clearly still appropriate for answering certain questions, and the drug-resistant sublines can provide valuable information concerning crossresistance and collateral sensitivity.

ACKNOWLEDGMENTS

The majority of this work was supported by Contracts NO1-CM-07315 and NO1-CM-47000 and predecessor contracts with the Developmental Therapeutics Program, DCT, NCI. The studies of gemcitabine and P388/VP-16 leukemia were supported by Eli Lilly and Company and by Burroughs Wellcome Company, respectively. The authors gratefully acknowledge the technical assistance of the staff of the Cancer Therapeutics and Immunology Department. J. Tubbs assisted with data management, and K. Cornelius prepared the manuscript.

REFERENCES

1. Law LW, Dunn DB, Boyle PJ, Miller JH. Observations on the effect of a folic-acid antagonist on transplantable lymphoid leukemias in mice. *J Natl Cancer Inst* 1949; 10:179–192.
2. Dawe CJ, Potter M. Morphologic and biologic progression of a lymphoid neoplasm of the mouse in vivo and in vitro. *Am J Pathology* 1957; 33(3):603.
3. Griswold DP Jr, Harrison SD Jr. Tumor models in drug development. *Cancer Metastasis Rev* 1991; 10:255–261.
4. Zubrod CG. Historic milestone in curative chemotherapy. *Semin Oncol* 1979; 6(4):490–505.
5. Goldin A, Serpick AA, Mantel N. A commentary, experimental screening procedures and clinical predictability value. *Cancer Chemother Rep* 1966; 50(4):173–218.
6. Carter S. Anticancer drug development progress: a comparison of approaches in the United States, the Soviet Union, Japan, and Western Europe. *Natl Cancer Inst Monogr* 1974; 40:31–42.
7. Goldin A, Venditti JM, Muggia FM, Rozencweig M, DeVita VT. New animal models in cancer chemotherapy. In: Fox BW, ed. *Advances in Medical Oncology, Research and Education.* Vol 5. Basis for Cancer Therapy 1. Pergamon Press, New York, NY, 1979:113–122.
8. Alley MC, Scudiero DA, Monks A, Hursey ML, Czerwinski MJ, Fine DL, et al. Feasibility of drug screening with panels of human tumor cell lines using a microculture tetrazolium assay. *Cancer Res* 1988; 48:589–601.
9. Boyd D. Budget cuts to force early end of P388 screening, DTP's, Boyd says. *The Cancer Letter* 1987; 13(2):5–7.
10. Skipper HE, Schabel FM Jr, Wilcox WS, Laster WR Jr, Trader MW, Thompson SA. Experimental evaluation of potential anticancer agents. XVII. Effects of therapy on viability and rate of proliferation of leukemic cells in various anatomic sites. *Cancer Chemother Rep* 1965; 47:41–64.
11. Schabel FM Jr, Griswold DP Jr, Laster WR Jr, Corbett TH, Lloyd HH. Quantitative evaluation of anticancer agent activity in experimental animals. *Pharmacol Ther* 1977; 1:411–435.
12. Lloyd HH. Application of tumor models toward the design of treatment schedules for cancer chemotherapy. In: Drewinko B, Humphrey RM, eds. *Growth Kinetics and Biochemical Regulation of Normal and Malignant Cells.* Williams & Wilkins, Baltimore, MD, 1977, pp. 455–469.
13. Skipper HE, Schabel FM Jr, Wilcox WS. Experimental evaluation of potential anticancer agents. XXI. Scheduling of arabinosylcytosine to take advantage of its S-phase specificity against leukemia cells. *Cancer Chemother Rep* 1967; 51:1625–1655.
14. Corbett TH, Valeriote FA, Baker LH. Is the P388 murine tumor no longer adequate as a drug discovery model? *Investig New Drugs* 1987; 5:3–20.
15. Staquet MJ, Byar DP, Green SB, Rozencweig M. Clinical predictivity of transplantable tumor systems in the selection of new drugs for solid tumors: rationale for a three-stage strategy. *Cancer Treat Rep* 1983; 67:753–765.
16. Trader MW, Harrison SD Jr, Laster WR Jr, Griswold DP Jr. Cross-resistance and collateral sensitivity of drug-resistant P388 and L1210 leukemias to flavone acetic acid (FAA, NSC 347512) in vivo (Abstr). *Proc AACR* 1987; 28:312.
17. Wilkoff LJ, Dulmadge EA. Sensitivity of proliferating cultured murine pancreatic tumor cells to selected antitumor agents. *J Natl Cancer Inst* 1986; 77(5):1163–1169.
18. Schabel FM Jr, Skipper HE, Trader MW, Laster WR Jr, Griswold DP Jr, Corbett TH. Establishment of cross-resistance profiles for new agents. *Cancer Treat Rep* 1983; 67:905–922 (see correction, *Cancer Treat Rep* 1984; 68:453–459).

19. Waud WR, Griswold DP Jr. Therapeutic resistance in leukemia. In: Teicher BA, ed. *Drug Resistance in Oncology.* Marcel Dekker, Inc., New York, *NY,* 1993, pp. 227–250.
20. Waud WR. Murine L1210 and P388 leukemias. In: Teicher B, ed. *Anticancer Drug Development Guide: Preclinical Screening, Clinical Trials, and Approval.* Humana Press, Totowa, NJ, 1997, pp. 59–74.
21. Ho AD, Seither E, Ma DDF, Prentice G. Mitoxantrone-induced toxicity and DNA strand breaks in leukemic cells. *Br J Haematol* 1987; 65:51–55.
22. Nelson EM, Tewey KM, Liu LF. Mechanism of antitumor drug action: poisoning of mammalian DNA topoisomerase II on DNA by 4'-(9-acridinylamino)methanesulfon-*m*-anisidide. *Proc Natl Acad Sci USA* 1984; 81:1361–1365.
23. Rose WC, Huftalen JB, Bradner WT, Schurig JE. *In vivo* characterization of P388 leukemia resistant to mitomycin C. *In Vivo* 1987; 1:47–52.
24. Eng WK, McCabe FL, Tan KB, Mattern MR, Hofmann GA, Woessner RD, et al. Development of a stable camptothecin-resistant subline of P388 leukemia with reduced topoisomerase I content. *Mol Pharmacol* 1990; 38:471–480.

3

Transplantable Syngeneic Rodent Tumors

Solid Tumors in Mice

Thomas H. Corbett, PhD, Lisa Polin, PhD, Bill J. Roberts, BS, Alfred J. Lawson, PhD, Wilbur R. Leopold III, PhD, Kathryn White, BS, Juiwanna Kushner, BA, Jennifer Paluch, BS, Stuart Hazeldine, PhD, Richard Moore, PhD, James Rake, PhD, and Jerome P. Horwitz, PhD

CONTENTS

1. INTRODUCTION

For many decades, the results from transplantable tumor models have been viewed with considerable skepticism. The perception has long been that these models are

From: *Tumor Models in Cancer Research*
Edited by: B. A. Teicher © Humana Press Inc., Totowa, NJ

excessively sensitive, and not predictive of the human disease. Although we do not intend to debate the many issues involved, it is our view that a better understanding of the transplant properties (e.g., take-rate) of the models—as well as a better understanding of the potential shortcomings in data presentation—will greatly aid the reader in the interpretation of these data. This chapter is an effort to summarize some of the basic operating characteristics of a wide range of solid-tumor models. Since this is a chemotherapy group, we can best explain some of the behavioral characteristics of these models within therapeutic experiments. Most of the data is drawn from the use of transplantable, syngeneic mouse tumors, but a few human tumors have been used for contrast.

2. COMPATIBILITY! COMPATIBILITY! COMPATIBILITY!

Why consider using mouse tumor models when there are so many human tumor models available? The reason is obvious: compatibility with the host animal. This one feature, above all else, allows the researcher a measure of dependability that can never be attained with the human tumor models in immune-deficient animals. Even if the researcher wishes to use the human tumor-xenograft models for a major portion of their studies, the ability to confirm a result in one or two syngeneic mouse tumor models and healthy immune-competent mice will usually eliminate the many pitfalls awaiting the unwary *(1–3)*.

3. COMPATIBLE BUT NOT PERFECT: INBRED MICE AND GENETIC DRIFT

An inbred mouse has >99% homozygosity, and is defined as a product of 20 or more generations of brother-sister mating (each generation reducing heterozygosity by 19%). However, many of the inbred strains were developed between 1905 and 1915, and have undergone genetic drift in various breeding facilities. As an example, the first and third authors well recall the variations in C3H/He mice from various breeders that came into the laboratory in the early 1970s. These mice had different shades of coat-color and snouts of different shape from various suppliers. Since obvious physical attributes were so varied, it was clear that the quality control in breeding was lacking. During that period, the National Cancer Institute (NCI) undertook a program to standardize the common inbred strains (e.g., C3H/He, C57B1/6, DBA/2, Balb/c), and all are now a product of over 150 brother-sister matings. This standardization was accomplished, but some of our long-used C3H mammary tumors failed to grow and metastasize adequately in the newly standardized C3H/He strain. Consequently, new tumor models were isolated and characterized—e.g., mammary adenocarcinoma-16/C and 13/C *(4)*. During the mid 1970s to early 1980s, we also developed various colon adenocarcinomas and pancreatic ductal adenocarcinomas for use in chemotherapy studies *(5–7)*. These tumor models have remained trouble-free in our laboratories and many other laboratories for over 20 y (using only the standardized mice purchased though NCI). This is not necessarily true for some of these same tumors used in other countries. In the late 1970s, we supplied Colon Adenocarcinoma-51 to a highly competent investigator in Europe, who found the tumor to be exceptionally drug-sensitive to a large number of different agents, and quite curable. In our hands, it was (and continues to be) among the least drug-sensitive tumor available (Table 1) *(6)*, and only curable with two agents (e.g., PCNU, Piposulfan). Likewise, Colon Carcinoma-26 has remained a drug-insensitive tumor in our laboratories (Table 1)*(6)*, but appears to be easily curable with a large number of agents in studies carried out

Table 1
In Vivo Activity of Standard and Investigational Agents Against Transplanted Tumors of Mice

In-vivo AGENT	Mam 44	Colon 38	Mam 16/C	Mam 16/C /adr	Mam 16/C/ taxol	Colon 51	Panc 02	Panc 03	Mam 17	Mam 17/ adr	Colon 26	Mel B16	Squam lung LC12	IV AML Leuk	IV Leuk L1210
Adriamycin	—	++	++++	±	+++	±	—	+++	++++	—	±	+	++++	++++	+
Taxol	—	++++	++++	—	—	+	—	++++	++++	—	±	±	—	—	—
Camp/CPT	—	+	++	NA	NA	+	—	++++	NA	NA	NA	+	++++	NA	NA
VP-16	++	++	++++	—	+	±	—	++	++	—	—	—	++++	NA	+++++
Vinbl/vinc	—	+++	++	—	—	—	—	—	+	—	—	—	—	—*	+
5-FU	—	+++	+++	+++	NA	—	—	+	++	+++	++	++	—	+*	+++
Ara-C	—	+++	++	NA	NA	—	—	—	++	NA	—	—	—	++++	++++
Gemzar	+	+++	++++	NA	NA	++	NA	NA	NA	NA	+++	NA	—	NA	+++++
Cytoxan	+	±	+++	+	NA	++	—	++	+++	+++	++	++	+++++	++++	+++++
cisDDPt	+	±	+	+	NA	++	—	++	+++	++++	++	++	++++	NA	++
BCNU	+++	—	—	±	NA	+++	+++	—	—	—	++++	++++	+	NA	+++++
Cryptophycin8	++++	++++	+++	+++	NA	+++	++++	++++	NA	++++	+++	++	+	+*	++**
SR271425	++	++++	++++	+	+++	++	++++	++++	++++	+	++++	++++	++++	++++	+++++
XK469	+++	++++	+++	+++	+++	+++	++++	++++	++++	+++	+++	+++	+++	+++	+++++

* SRI/NCI data for vinc and 5-FU against AML1498. **++ for Crypto52, no data for crypto8 against L1210 Mam44 data with close analog being considered for second generation clinical trials: The L1210 activity rating was expanded because of this tumor's higher sensitivity to a variety of agents (see methods for conversion of log kill to activity ratings). NA = not available

in Japan. One is never sure if the problem is tumor-host incompatibility or the development of deviant lines of tumors.

The implications are obvious: syngeneic tumor-model systems can be produced and maintained, but only with adequate quality controls and access to the mice of origin (discussed *vide infra*).

4. EVIDENCE OF TUMOR-HOST INCOMPATIBILITY AND CONSEQUENCES

This topic has been previously reviewed *(8,9),* but must be expanded, because so many manipulations are used to overcome the many problems encountered with incompatible models (especially in human tumor-xenograft studies). One suspects that incompatible systems are most frequently used because the treatment results are much more impressive, since the host immune system contributes substantially to the tumor-cell-kill *(8).* However, if such a tumor had a unique property required for study (and an appropriate syngeneic system could not be found), the investigator could use the mouse tumor in a (SCID) mouse host and probably eliminate much of the compatibility issue.

4.1. No-Takes

Failure to have 100% takes of 30–60-mg trocar tumor fragments may be ascribed to several factors:

1. infection;
2. one is using an extremely slow-growing, low malignancy, early-passage tumor
3. technical incompetence
4. substantial tumor-host incompatibility.

The investigator can certainly identify and eliminate the problem of infection *(9),* as well as technical incompetence. Furthermore, it is unlikely that an investigator would be using an extremely slow-growing, low-malignancy, early-passage tumor for most studies. Thus, a substantial no-take frequency (5% or more) is usually a signal of tumor-host incompatibility. Interestingly, to get around the problem, one often sees that the animals have been implanted and the tumors allowed to reach palpable size before they are entered onto the trial (e.g., 6–15 d postimplant, depending on the growth rate of the tumor). In this way, the no-takes are simply culled from the pool of trocared animals, and never entered onto the experiment (or mentioned).

4.2. Spontaneous Regressions or Tumors That Fail to Progress to Over 1000-mg Size

In a mouse-tumor model, the occurrence of either spontaneous regressions or a failure of the tumors to progress to over 1000 mg in size (even at a low frequency of 1/100 mice) would suggest marked tumor-host incompatibility, and thus an invalid model. In human tumor-xenograft systems, a spontaneous regression and no growth thereafter may be the result of a mouse that has regained immune capacity (leaky). This can be verified by reimplantation of the tumor in the presumed leaky mouse. If it fails to grow, the leaky nature of the mouse can be verified, and the regression explained. Human tumors that fail to progress in immune-deficient mice are more common in athymic nude mice than in severe combined immunodeficiency (SCID) mice (i.e., tumors that reach 250–500 mg and stay that size for many wk, or even regress to zero) (Table 2). These tumors are usually

Table 2
Comparison of the Behavior of Transplanted Human Tumors in Athymic Nude Mice and SCID Mice

Human tumor	Diffuse necrosis (determined by histology; H&E stained sides)		Exponential tumor volume doubling time in days SC tumors		Progressive tumor growth SC and spontaneous regression			
	Athymic nude mice	SCID mice	Athymic nude mice	SCID mice	Athymic nude mice		SCID mice	
	% Median necrosis (range)	% Median necrosis (range)	Median Td (range)	Median Td (range)	# of tumors reaching 250 to 500 mg but not getting any larger	# of these tumors regressing to zero	# of tumors reaching 250 to 500 mg but not getting any larger	# of these tumors regressing to zero
Colon H116	80 (60–90)	35 (10–50)	5.0 (3.0–5.0) 5 trials	4.0 (3.5–4.0) 5 trials	3/23	0/23	0/18	0/18
Colon H8	75 (70–80)	20 (15–20)	5.5 (4.0–6.0) 4 trials	3.0 (3.0–4.0) 5 trials	1/21	4/21	0/13	0/13
Lung H125	35 (30–40)	5 (0–5)	5.0 (3.0–8.8) 10 trials	3.0 (2.3–5.0) 14 trials	4/50	1/50	0/59	0/59
Prostate PC-3	20 (20)	0 (0)	6.0 (5.0–7.0) 2 trials	3.5 (3.0–5.0) 4 trials	2/7	4/7	0/11	0/11
Breast MX-1	50 (40–60)	0 (0–20)	4.0 (2.2–6.0) 16 trials	2.7 (1.8–4.5) 13 trials	4/91	3/91	0/62	0/62

AACR 36:303, 1995.

caused by extensive diffuse necrosis within the tumor mass, which can be easily verified with histology (Table 2). Based on one of the definitions of malignancy (a malignant tumor must be able to grow and kill the host), such a nonprogressing tumor model would be judged unusable. Failure to see plots of all tumors in all treatment cages to >1000 mg in size (or failure to provide data that include time to 1000 mg, with range) may suggest that such an invalid human tumor model was used for data collection.

4.3. Excessive Curability

Many tumor models of past decades were derived in random-bred mice or the original inbred strain subline is no longer available (e.g., Sarcoma 180, Ehrlich Ascites Carcinoma, Gardner lymphosarcoma). Clearly, these models are excessively curable, with a variety of antitumor agents, because the immune system of the host provides additional cell-kill. The immune system kills by zero-order kinetics (meaning that it can kill a finite number of cells; e.g., 3×10^8 tumor cells). If the drug treatment can reduce the population only slightly, the immune system can often handle the rest. One of the indicators of such an immunogenic system is that it is more curable by chemotherapy if the tumor is allowed to grow for about 7 d before treatment than if treatment is started 1–3 after implant (the total opposite of a syngeneic model). These 7 d of growth allow the mouse to see and process the cell-surface antigens and begin to develop an immune response.

Some tumor models have given rise to deviant sublines that are highly immunogenic. The most famous case was the deviant line of Lewis Lung Carcinoma (LLC) that was unfortunately widely distributed by NCI. This subline was highly curable by agents that historically had no activity against the tumor (8). At least one agent N-phosphoacylase L-aspartate disodium (PALA) was advanced to clinical trials on the strength that it was able to cure *LLC* at four dose levels, which should have provided skepticism by itself. Other lines of *LLC* behave as expected (8), and we still use this highly metastatic, drug-insensitive tumor for selected studies. However, the widespread use of the deviant line of *LLC* has given it such a bad reputation that few researchers believe any of the chemotherapy data derived from this famous old tumor model. This is unfortunate, since *LLC* is one of the most metastatic mouse tumors ever isolated.

Other tumor systems may or may not be immunogenic, and cures could simply be the result of treatment with a very effective agent. This is easily sorted out. The cures are simply rechallenged with 30–60 mg* subcutaneous (SC) trocar fragments of the original tumor. If they take and grow to 1000 mg* with the expected exponential volume doubling time, it is clear that immune factors were not involved in the original cure. No-takes of tumors implanted in the challenged mice are proof that immune factors were involved in the original cure. It is interesting to note how often tumor-free mice are declared cures without rechallenge. The time to rechallenge is sometimes an issue. The time for one tumor cell to populate to 1 g* = [3.32 Td × 9] can be added to the last day of treatment. If

---

*There is a relationship between tumor size and cell number. With syngeneic, transplanted mouse tumors, the tumor mass is usually >85% tumor cells while in exponential growth. A 1-g mass (1000 mg) = 1×10^9 cells; a 0.1-g mass (100 mg) = 1×10^8 cells; a 0.01-g mass (10 mg) = 1×10^7 cells; a 1-mg mass = 1×10^6 cells, and so on. Thus, a 30-mg mass = 3×10^7 cells (30 million cells). Human tumor cells and mouse tumor cells are approximately the same size, but only a few xenografted human tumors contain >80% tumor cells. Td = exponential tumor-volume doubling time. 3.32 = number of doublings per log. and cure is usually obtained when the population is reduced to approx 10 or 100 cells for most solid tumors.

the mouse is still tumor-free, a cure can be reasonably certain. This allows at least three doublings beyond detection (easy detection is 100 mg = 0.1 g = 10^8). However, some investigators (e.g., H. Skipper) point to the possibility of the survival of a slow Td cell or greater cell loss that can occur with low cell numbers, and the fact that some tumors can repopulate from one cell. For these reasons, they suggest that the time for one cell to grow to 1 g of cells be increased by 50% = 1.5 (3.32 × Td × 9) (which is then added to the last day of Rx) before cure is declared and the mouse can be rechallenged. Regardless, rechallenge of tumor-free survivors should be a prerequisite before an animal can be declared cured. This would clarify the nature of the model being used.

4.4. Lack of Invasion and Metastasis

The failure to invade and metastasize is often a sign of strong host-tumor incompatibility. In addition, these tumors will often grow to an unusually large size (>6000 mg) without affecting the health of the mouse. Most metastatic tumors will kill the mouse before they reach 6000 mg, and some tumors will kill before the tumors reach 2500 mg (e.g., Colon-26, Panc-02). A simple check for the metastatic capability of a tumor is as follows. The tumor (unilateral or bilateral) is allowed to reach approx 1500 mg in size (total burden). The mouse is sacrificed, and the lungs are removed though the back (with care to avoid the primary tumor). The lungs from each mouse are then implanted into a naive mouse of the same inbred strain. Growth of the lung tissue to a 1000-mg mass confirms that metastatic cells were present; a histologic check of the mass will verify the tumor of origin). Highly metastatic tumors can be propagated in this manner with only a 30–60-mg-size trocar fragment of the lung tissue. The invasive nature of the tumor is also verified by the metastasis check, since noninvasive (often immunogenic tumor models) have little or no capacity to metastasize. Finally, the number of tumor cells required to establish tumor growth closely correlates with the metastatic and invasive nature of the tumor. In virtually all cases, 3×10^5 tumor cells are sufficient to establish SC growth with a highly metastatic and highly invasive mouse tumor, and often 10^4 is sufficient (10,11). Poorly metastatic tumors often require more than 10^6 tumor cells to establish sc growth in 100% of the mice (11). All the mouse tumors we use are invasive and metastatic, although some are obviously more invasive and more highly metastatic (e.g., Pancreatic Ductal Adenocarcinoma 02, Mammary Adenocarcinoma-16/C, Colon Carcinoma-26, B16 melanoma, LLC, and Mammary Carcinoma 44). These six tumors can be used for surgery-chemotherapy adjuvant studies because lung metastasises are present in nearly 100% of the mice by the time the tumor reaches 1500 mg (4,6,7,10–14). The highly metastatic behavior can be encouraged and maintained by passaging lung fragments subcutaneously every passage or every few passages (instead of the primary sc tumor).

5. COMPATIBILITY PROBLEMS UNIQUE TO HUMAN TUMORS IN IMMUNE-DEFICIENT MICE

Without a doubt, the most evident problem with human tumors in athymic mice is a diffuse necrosis that can often make up 20–80% of the tumor mass, as determined by histology (Table 2). This diffuse necrosis (commonly referred to as shotgun necrosis) is evident even to the edges of the tumor mass, and even in tumors of small sizes (100- to 150-mg sizes). This type of diffuse necrosis is never seen in syngeneic mouse tumor models, or in human tumors in humans. The diffuse necrosis is less evident in SCID mice than in athymic nude mice, but still occurs (Table 2). Obviously, the extent of necrosis will explain the growth behavior of many human tumors in immune-deficient mice. If the cell loss from the diffuse necrosis matches or exceeds the cell gain from replication, one can have a nonprogressing or even a regressing mass. Examples of the marked differences in tumor volume doubling time of tumors implanted in SCID mice and athymic nude mice have been published (3), with other examples shown in Table 2. This lack of compatibility exerts considerable selective pressure on the tumor, and probably accounts for the marked biologic and drug-response variations in sublines of the same human tumor. For example, we have investigated four different sublines of human-prostate LNCaP from different sources, all totally dissimilar in terms of growth behavior and take-rate.

6. PASSAGE OF TUMORS IN CELL CULTURE: MAINTAINING GENOTYPE, HISTOLOGY, BIOLOGIC BEHAVIOR, AND DRUG-RESPONSE CHARACTERISTICS

The passage of tumors in cell culture may or may not alter the behavior of the tumors when reimplanted in mice. For example, one of the authors (Roberts) reimplanted Colon-26 in mice after 291 population doublings in culture (culture passage carried out by E. Dulmadge and L. Wilkoff of Southern Research Institute). This culture-passaged subline behaved similarly to the preculture tumor with respect to histology, growth behavior, and drug response to three agents (sensitive to MeCCNU and CisDDPt, and insensitive to PalmoAraC). On the other hand, Roberts found that Colon Adenocarcinoma-38 changed markedly after culture passage (culture passage carried out by E. Dulmadge and L. Wilkoff at the same time). On reimplantation in mice, the culture-passaged subline of Colon-38 was markedly less differentiated histologically, grew faster, and was unresponsive to 5-fluorouracil (5-FU) and Anguidine (both drugs were highly active against the preculture tumor). In other studies, we have seen substantial changes in modal chromosome number, as well as a marked increase in the distribution of chromosome numbers within the cells of culture passage of tumors, unlike the mouse-passaged tumors that had no genotypic changes. Finally, malignancy properties can change with longer-term culture passage. We have found that culture passage reduced the take-rate more than 10,000-fold for L1210 and P388 leukemias, as well as slowing the growth rate and markedly decreasing invasive and metastatic behavior on reimplantation into the host of origin (DBA/2 mice). Obviously, there is little reason for tumors to maintain high-malignancy properties in a culture setting; they only need to be able to survive and replicate in the artificial cell-culture environment. The substantial increase in genetic instability in culture has obvious implications for the fidelity of the tumor model after reimplantation in mice. With some effort, one can clone sublines of tumors from culture with widely differing properties. Some investigators (including the NCI) have been using long-term-culture-passaged human tumor lines for new drug discovery since the early 1980s (15).

7. CANCER: A CELLULAR DISEASE; TAKE-RATE; FEEDER EFFECT; IMPLICATIONS FOR CURE

Many of the behavioral characteristics of transplantable tumor models are controlled by the take-rate behavior of the tumor. To illustrate this fact, it is necessary to discuss the establishment and behavior of tumors from counted cell implants. Counted cell-implant experiments (by the routes of administration planned for using the model) are one of the first steps that an investigator can use to characterize a tumor.

Table 3
Comparison of Take-Rates of Mammary Adenocarcinoma-16/C by Various Implant Routes

Number of cells implanted	Number of tumor takes/number of mice implanted			
	Subcutaneous	Intravenous	Intracranial	Intraperitoneal
10^7	19/19			
10^6	19/20*	10/10	10/10	20/20
10^5	17/20	10/10	10/10	10/10
10^4	5/20	1/10	9/10	8/10
10^3	0/19	0/10	3/10	2/10
10^2				0/10
Take-Rate level	4×10^4	4×10^4	3×10^3	5×10^3

Note: One take-rate unit (by dilution) will establish a tumor in 63% of the mice $[100 \times (1-1/e)]$. This mammary adenocarcinoma is a highly invasive, highly metastatic, rapidly growing tumor.

* Leakage of the titered cell implant brei from the implant site probably accounts for the one no-take. Three logs of incomplete takes should not occur with technically perfect implants. Data of B.J. Roberts.

Table 4
Comparison of Take-Rates of Colon Adenocarcinoma-10
(A Low-Viability, Poor-Take-Rate Tumor) by Various Implant Routes

Number of cells implanted	Number of tumor takes/number of mice implanted			
	Subcutaneous	Intravenous	Intracranial	Intraperitoneal
10^8	8/9			10/10
10^7	2/10	6/9		6/10
10^6	1/10	1/10	10/10	0/10
10^5	0/10	1/10	9/10	0/10
10^4			6/9	0/10
10^3			3/10	0/9
10^2				
Take-Rate level	4×10^7	1×10^7	1×10^4	1×10^7

Note: One take-rate unit (by dilution) will establish a tumor in 63% of the mice $[100 \times (1-1/e)]$.

This colon adenocarcinoma was a slow-growing, low-viability tumor. It was in the 11th passage for this implant trial. Note that the tumor takes were 3 logs better by the ic route than by any other route of implant.

An example of the take-rate of a highly metastatic mammary tumor implanted by various routes is shown in Table 3. It should be noted that the take-rate varies, depending on the location. Historically, intracerebral implants have the best take-rates because the brain tissue acts as a feeder-layer. However, for this particular tumor, the intraperitoneal implants were almost as good (Table 3). An example of the take-rates of a low-viability, early-passage tumor is shown in Table 4. In this case, the (IC) take-rates were 3 logs better than the other three routes.

Take-rates vary enormously depending on the tumor used. Examples are shown in Table 5. In general, the take-rate correlates closely with the invasive and metastatic capability of the tumor. In these examples, Mammary Carcinoma 44 is the most metastatic and the most invasive (>90% metastasis to the lungs from 1000-mg-size sc

Table 5
Comparison of SC Take-Rates of Different Transplantable Tumors

Number of cells implanted	Number of tumor takes/number of mice implanted						
	Mam-44	Colon-26	Mam-16/C	Colon-51	Colon-09	Colon-10	Colon 36**
10^8					3/3	8/9	
10^7			19/19	10/10	9/9	2/10	2/10
10^6	10/10	10/10	19/20*	10/10	2/10	1/10	0/10
10^5	10/10	10/10	17/20	3/10	0/10	0/10	0/10
10^4	10/10	9/10*	5/20	1/10	0/10		
10^3	9/10	10/10	0/19	0/10			
10^2	not done	2/10					
63% take-rate level	$<10^3$	3×10^2	3×10^4	3×10^5	3×10^6	4×10^7	5×10^7

Note: One take-rate unit (by dilution) will establish a tumor in 63% of the mice [$100 \times (1-1/e)$]

* Leakage of the titered cell implant brei from the implant site probably accounts for the one no-take in each of these groups. Three logs of incomplete take should not occur with technically perfect implants (as occurred in Mam-16/C).

** In separate experiments, 2×10^7 cells SC produced 6/20 takes with ip implantation, confirming that this was a poor take-rate tumor.

tumors *(11)*. Colon 26 is virtually the same *(6,11)*. Mammary 16/C is reasonably close, with >80% metastasis to the lungs from 800–1000-mg-size sc tumors, and usually near 100% for tumors >1200 mg *(4,10,11)*. Colon-51 is metastatic to both the lungs and regional lymph nodes from a 1500-mg sc tumor in 80% of the mice, but has been used only occasionally for surgical studies *(11)*. Colon Adenocarcinomas-9, 10, and 36 were only marginally metastatic in the early passages studied (<10% from 1000-mg tumors).

It may be inferred from a casual reading of the literature that one tumor cell (1-cell) can be implanted, and will take and grow into a tumor mass that will kill the host. Although this is true for some tumors such as L1210 or P388 leukemias, these are exceptions. The lack of better tumor takes at a particular location (other than the brain) is caused by 1–3 log-cell loss of tumor cells at the implant site, which occurs within 24 h of implant *(16)*. This cell loss can be prevented by admixing X-ray killed tumor cells with the implants, or by admixing a brain-tissue brei with the tumor cells. An example is shown in Table 6. This phenomenon is known as the feeder-effect or the Revesz-effect, after the original investigator *(17–18)*. The feeder cells (radiation-killed cells) can be different from the titered tumor cells being assayed, but work best if they are from the same inbred strain and are derived from a highly metastatic/fast-growing/high-take-rate tumor (Table 7). The only normal tissue that provides the feeder effect to all tumors is brain tissue. The feeder effect provided by brain tissue probably accounts for some of the difficulty in curing intracranial malignancies, since an additional 1–3 logs of tumor-cell kill would be necessary to reduce the population below the take-rate level at that site. The feeder effect can only be provided by intact, metabolizing cells, and must be admixed with the titered cells and not at a distant location. Furthermore, greater than 10^6 X-ray killed cells are needed to produce the effect; with 5×10^7 to 1×10^8 used by most investigators. In selected cases, tumor cells killed

Table 6
Comparison of B16 Melanoma Tumor Takes With and Without Added Feeder Layers

Number of cells implanted	No feeder layer titered tumor cells only		Co^{60} killed B16 cells added to titered tumor cells		Brain brei from C57Bl/6 mice added to titered tumor cells	
	B16 tumor takes/number implanted*	Median time to 1.0 g	B16 tumor takes/number implanted*	Median time to 1.0 g	B16 tumor takes/number implanted*	Median time to 1.0 g
10^6	5/5	24				
10^5	4/5	30	4/4	18	4/4	17
10^4	1/10	34	10/10	21	10/10	22
10^3	0/10		9/10	27	10/10	26
10^2	0/10		5/10	(27–35 range)	6/10	(28–38 range)
10^1			0/10		1/10	
feeder-layer only			0/10			

* B16 tumors took and grew to 1.0 g in size. Feeder layers (approx 5×10^7 killed cells/implant) made with irradiated tumor cells or brain tissue and admixed with the titered tumor cells improved the take-rate by over 2 logs each.

Note: One take-rate unit (by dilution) will establish a tumor in 63% of the mice $[100 \times (1–1/e)]$. This is the take-rate level.

Table 7
Comparison of Adenocarcinoma 755 Tumor Takes in C57Bl/6 Mice
With and Without Added Feeder Layers

of cells implanted	No Feeder Layer Titered Tumor Cells only		10,000R Co^{60} Killed B16 cells added to Titered Tumor Cells		Brain Brei from C57Bl/6 mice added to Titered Tumor Cells	
	CA755 tumor takes/number implanted*	Median time to 1.0 g	CA755 tumor takes/number implanted*	Median time to 1.0 g	CA755 tumor takes/number implanted*	Median time to 1.0 g
10^6	5/5	18	5/5	11	5/5	16
10^5	5/5	24	5/5	14	5/5	17
10^4	0/10		10/10	16	5/5	22
10^3	0/10		10/10	20	5/5	33
10^2			7/8	26	3/5	38
10^1			0/10		0/5	
feeder-layer only			0/10			

*Adenocarcinoma 755 tumors took and grew to 1.0 g in size. Feeder layers made with irradiated tumor cells (of a different tumor) or brain tissue and admixed with the titered tumor cells improve the take-rate by more than 2 logs each.

Note: One feeder layer was made with Co^{60} Killed B16 cells; the other was made from a brain-tissue brei.

by an antitumor agent can provide feeder activity *(19)*. It is likely that some feeder-effect is taking place post-treatment with either chemotherapy or radiation treatment of any intact tumor mass. Immune-suppression does not change the take-rate of a syngeneic tumor model (Table 8). Thus the feeder effect is unrelated to subverting immune function. Other examples of the lack of influence of immune suppression on take-rates are available *(20)*.

As one approaches within 1 log of the take-rate level (or cure level), an accelerated tumor-cell loss is clearly taking place (compared to implants that are 3–4 logs above the take rate). This is evident in virtually any end point or tumor location *(10)*. There is also a consequent shift in the shapes of the curves (survival or time to a specific tumor size). At 3–4 logs above the take rate, curves are normal (i.e., Gaussian) *(10)*(Fig. 1). With a Gaussian curve, the top half of the curve can be inverted and can then be superimposed on the bottom half of the curve. At approx 0.5–1.5 logs above the take-rate, the curves become log-normal, in which case the data can be replotted using the log of time, and the curve will become normal or Gaussian-shaped *(10)*. Near the take-rate level, which yields 20–50% no-takes or survivors after therapy, the curve is first-order-kinetic *(10)* (Figure-1). This knowledge can be used to predict the outcome of a mouse experiment, or even a partially completed human trial. If the survival curve plunges in a Gaussian fashion, it is clear that one is far above the take-rate level, and no cures will be obtained. On the other hand, if the curve begins to bend-out in a first-order kinetic fashion, one can project that some cures will be obtained. Detailed examples of normal, log-normal, and first-order-kinetic plots, with explanations and mortality curve analyses have been published *(10)*. Other examples of first-order-kinetic behavior are common in physics and biology: e.g., light-bulbs burn out by first-order-kinetics (a constant fraction of the bulbs burn out per *u* time); most antitumor agents kill by first-order-kinetics (a constant fraction of the cells are killed per given dose of a drug) *(21)*; and disinfectants kill by first-order-kinetics (a constant concentration of the disinfectant in a test tube kills a constant fraction of the bacterial cells per *u* of time) *(21)*.

Once an investgator understands the take-rate behavior of a particular tumor, understands the relationship between tumor size and cell number, and understands the feeder effect, the meaning of cure for that particular tumor will become clear, regardless of the stage of the disease and the nature of the therapy. This knowledge can also be used in experimental planning and projecting the outcome of various treatment regimens.

With this perspective, we can now examine the results from treatment of high take-rate tumors and poor take-rate tumors. The first example is shown in Table 9. A total of 21 cures were produced in 77 mice with poor take-rate tumors by therapies that produced only one cure of 159 mice with high take-rate tumors; the log 10 tumor-cell kills were similar. A comparison of the curability, as a function of a three-fold increase in tumor size of a poor take-rate tumor, is instructive (Table 10). Clearly, the tumor (Colon-36) was slightly less sensitive at a larger size (note growth delay and net cell-kill), but not markedly less. Curability, however, decreased dramatically, with only a threefold increase in tumor-cell number. The calculations can be used to approximate the cure level (take-rate level and the feeder effect). Starting with the 200-mg masses, the median is 2×10^8 cells to start (8.3 logs). Treatment killed 2.9 logs, and thus the median population is reduced to 5.4 logs = 2.5×10^5 (producing 10/15 cures). At the 600-mg size masses, the median is 6×10^8 cells to start (8.78 logs). Treatment killed 2.1 logs. Thus, the median population is reduced to 6.68 logs = 4.8×10^6, and only 1/8

Table 8
Lack of Influence of Immune Suppression on the Take-Rate of B16 Melanoma Cells Implanted Intravenously in A Syngeneic Mouse

Host strain	# of B16 cells implanted iv on d 0	Nature of transplant	Immune-suppressive agent	Dosage; vol in ml/mouse/d	Schedule of treatment	Median day of tumor death (dying only)	Range of tumor deaths	Tumor-free survivors on d 205	Tumor takes/total
Controls									
BDF1	10^6	Syngeneic	none (saline)	0.075 mL	d –3 to d +7	34	26–41	0/17	17/17
BDF1	10^5	Syngeneic	none (saline)	0.075 mL	d –3 to d +7	52.5	45–60	17/19	2/19
BDF1	10^4	Syngeneic	none (saline)	0.075 mL	d –3 to d +7	56	56	19/20	1/20
BDF1	10^3	Syngeneic	none (saline)	0.075 mL	d –3 to d +7	none	none	19/19	0/19

One take-rate unit by dilution will establish a tumor in 63% of the mice: For the controls shown above, the take-rate level was calculated to be 6×10^5 B16 tumor cells

Immune-suppressed; Antilymphocyte serum (ALS) started 3 d before tumor implant and continued for 7 d after tumor implant

Host strain	# of B16 cells implanted iv on d 0	Nature of transplant	Immune-suppressive agent	Dosage; vol in ml/mouse/d	Schedule of treatment	Median day of tumor death (dying only)	Range of tumor deaths	Tumor-free survivors on d 205	Tumor takes/total
BDF1	10^6	Syngeneic	ALS	0.075 mL	d –3 to d +7	36	29–42	0/20	20/20
BDF1	10^5	Syngeneic	ALS	0.075 mL	d –3 to d +7	55.5	45–66	18/20	2/20
BDF1	10^4	Syngeneic	ALS	0.075 mL	d –3 to d +7	46	46	18/19	1/19
BDF1	10^3	Syngeneic	ALS	0.075 mL	d –3 to d +7	none	none	20/20	0/20

One take-rate unit by dilution will establish a tumor in 63% of the mice: For the immune-suppressed mice (ALS-treated) shown above, the take-rate level was calculated to be 6×10^5 B16 tumor cells; identical with that of the saline-treated controls.

Controls to determine the degree of immune suppression

Host strain	# of B16 cells implanted iv on d 0	Nature of transplant	Immune-suppressive agent	Dosage; vol in ml/mouse/d	Schedule of treatment	Median day of tumor death (dying only)	Range of tumor deaths	Tumor-free survivors on d 205	Tumor takes/total
C3H	B16, 60-mg fragments SC	Allogeneic	ALS	0.075 mL	d –3 to d +7			1/10	9/10
C3H	B16, 60-mg fragments SC	Allogeneic	No Rx	No Rx	No Rx			10/10	0/10
BDF1	B16, 60-mg fragments SC	Syngeneic	No Rx	No Rx	No Rx			0/8	8/8

Immune-suppression was sufficient to allow B16 melanoma to take and grow in a foreign (allogeneic) host mouse (C3H) in 9/10 mice (8/10 of these grew to over 1000 mg).

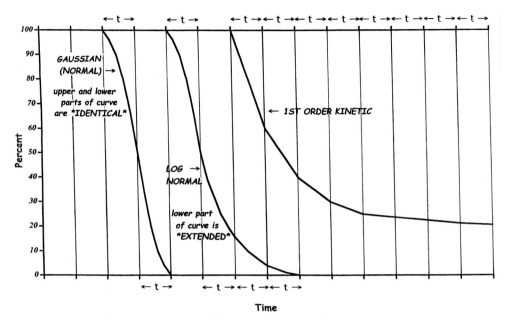

Fig. 1. Normal, log-normal, and first-order kinetic curves.

cures. The data can be plotted on semilog paper, and various results can be estimated. If the population is reduced to below 4×10^4, it should yield all cures. Above 1×10^7, there should be no cures. The 63% cure level is 3×10^5 cells. The feeder contribution for this dose-schedule of treatment and established tumors at the start of therapy was 2.22 logs (7.7 logs – 5.48 logs).

The cure of a poor take-rate tumor by chemotherapy is shown in Table 11. Again, the tumor-cell-kills were rather modest, considering the cures. Based on the last tumor to regrow in the treatment groups, it is possible to calculate that the cures produced by Procarbazine and Maytansine represent only slightly more than a 1.8 and 1.6 net log-kill, respectively.

The cure of a high take-rate tumor by chemotherapy is clearly a challenge. We have never obtained cures of 30 mg sc trocar-implanted tumors such as Mam-44 or Panc-02 with chemotherapy, even when treatment begins the day after implant. A more responsive tumor, such as Mam-16/C, has had only an occasional chemotherapeutic cure in hundreds of trials. Examples of treatment of Mam-16/C with highly active agents are shown in Table 12. The log-kill values were substantial, but cures were not forthcoming, except in one case. This cure was rechallenged on d 182, and grew to over 2 g in 11 d, indicating that immune factors were not involved in the cure. The log-kill values—gross and net—were also consistent with a cure. It should be noted that other dose-schedules of this agent failed to produce cures or this impressive log-kill (thus, even this one cure is an outlier).

In general, in order to obtain cures of such high take-rate tumors, surgery followed by chemotherapy has been successful, especially with highly active drug combinations *(6,7,10,11)*. However, in order to produce cures of such models as Mam-16/C without surgery, we would need to resort to some tricks. For example, we could ip-implant the

Table 9
Treatment of Transplantable Tumors of Mice with X-Irradiation

Tumor (SC) Size at 1st Rx	RADS per fraction (Q2dx3)	Total dosage in RADS	Treat- ment- related deaths	Median tumor growth delay in days	PR's, exclud- ing toxic deaths	CR's, exclud- ing toxic deaths	Log 10-kill per fraction	Log 10-kill gross	Log 10-kill net	Cures
Noncurable, High Take-Rate Tumors										
Mammary	1000	3000	3/26	13	12/26	8/26	0.9	2.8	1.7	0/26
adenocar-	750	2250	1/42	12	20/42	16/42	0.86	2.6	1.5	0/42
cinoma-16/C	500	1500	0/49	7	14/49	6/49	0.5	1.5	0.4	1/49
@100–400	200	600	0/18	3	0/18	0/18	0.23	0.7	–0.4	0/18
mg										

Time for median control-tumor mam-16/C to reach 750 mg post-trocar implant = 11–15 d. Exponential Td = 1.4 days
63% take-rate level = 3×10^4

Colon adeno-	845	2535	0/8	17	3/8	1/8	0.77	2.3	1.8	0/8
carcinoma-51	650	1950	0/8	12	3/8	0/8	0.55	1.64	1.2	0/8
@100–400	500	1500	0/8	10	0/8	0/8	0.46	1.37	1.0	0/8
mg										

Time for median control-tumor colon-51 to reach 750 mg post-trocar implant = 15 d. Exponential Td = 2.2 d (20 mice)
63% take-rate level = 3×10^5

Curable, Poor Take-Rate Tumors										
Colon adeno-	845	2535	0/15	37	13/15	10/15	1.07	3.2	2.9	10/15
carcinoma-36	650	1950	0/15	20	11/15	6/15	0.59	1.77	1.4	0/15
@100–400 mg	500	1500	1/15	17	4/15	4/15	0.50	1.5	1.15	2/15

Time for Median control-tumor Colon-36 to reach 750 mg post-trocar implant = 22 d. Exponential Td = 3.4 d
63% take-rate level = 5×10^7

Colon adeno	1100	3300	1/8	cures*	7/8	7/8	cures*	cures*	cures*	5/8
carcinoma-10	845	2535	0/8	48	8/8	7/8	0.8	2.4	2.2	2/8
@100–400 mg	650	1950	0/8	33	8/8	7/8	0.55	1.6	1.45	2/8
	500	1500	0/8	18	6/8	0/8	0.3	0.9	0.65	0/8

Time for median control-tumor colon-10 to reach 750 mg post-trocar implant = 36 d. Exponential Td = 6.0 d 63% take-rate level = 4×10^7
* only two mice regrew tumors, growth delay not meaningful (5 cured, 1 Rx death)

Curability was, in part, a function of the viability (take-rate) of a tumor. All tumor models were synegeneic.

tumor as a counted cell brei, and start ip treatment the next day. This would improve the tumor-cell-kill by approx 3 logs, and effect cures if the agent was highly active. This regimen has been successful for multiple agents, but does not reflect the usual clinical problem or treatment requirement. Likewise, we could implant the tumor only slightly above the take-rate, and begin treatment the next day by another route. Again,

Table 10
Treatment of Transplantable Colon Adenocarcinoma-36 in Mice with X-Irradiation Curability as A Function of Take-Rate and Tumor Size at First Treatment

Tumor (SC) Size at 1st Rx	RADS per fraction (Q2dx3)	Total dosage in RADS	Treat-ment-related deaths	Median tumor growth delay in days	PR's, exclud-ing toxic deaths	CR's, exclud-ing toxic deaths	Log 10-kill per fraction	Log 10-kill gross	Log 10-kill net	Cures
Colon-36 @100–400 mg **(200 mg median = 2 × 10⁸ cells)**	845	2535	0/15	37	13/15	10/15	1.07	3.2	2.9	10/15
@300–1000 mg **(600 mg median = 6 × 10⁸ cells)**	845	2535	0/8	27.3	6/8	1/8	0.8	2.4	2.1	1/8

Time for Median Control Tumor Colon-36 to reach 750 mg post-trocar implant = 22 d. Exponential Td = 3.4 d.

Curability was, in part, a function of the viability (take-rate) of the tumor. Note that the net log tumor-cell-kill for Colon 36 did not change markedly with the change in tumor size at first Rx (and the log-kill was not impressively large). The curability was simply related to the log-kill necessary to reduce the population below the take-rate level with a feeder.

some cures could be expected if the agent could produce a 1 log net cell-kill, but to what aim?

A casual reading of the literature may prompt the opinion that L1210 leukemia is a highly chemosensitive and curable tumor. It is indeed chemosensitive, but the cures have mainly been obtained with ip-implanted tumor and ip-drug administration the day after 10^5 cell implants. One can easily remove the possibility of a cure: the tumor can be iv-implanted with 10^6 cells, with treatment starting the next day. With this titer and implant route, cures are out of the question (Table 13). (In many respects, cure is the worst and most misleading end point that an investigator can use. In most cases, the reader will have no concept of the actual log-kill required to produce the cure.)

8. RESULTS TABULATION OF CHEMOTHERAPY TRIALS: DESIRED INFORMATION FROM A TUMOR MODEL

It is often said that a picture is worth a thousand words. However, the presentation of chemotherapeutic results in plots can be among the most misleading methods of presentation if all the information is not provided to the reader. Several examples follow.

The first example would seem to indicate self-evident antitumor activity of Gemzar against a very slow-growing, early-passage pancreatic adenocarcinoma. However, the

Table 11
Chemotherapeutic Treatment of A Poor Take-Rate Tumor

Experiment #	Treatment	Schedule (route)	mg/kg/ injection	% Body-wt loss at nadir (day of nadir)	Drug deaths	Median tumor mass on (day)	% T/C mass	Median time in days for tumors to reach 1000 mg (range)	Tumor growth delay in days	median log 10-kill gross	median log 10-kill net	tumor-free "cures"
Colon-36 (1564G1)	No Rx	—	—	not tabulated	—	1000 mg on d 21	—	21 (17.5–27.5)	—	—	—	0/20
	Ara-C	q3hx8 (IP) d 16,20	11.8	not tabulated	0/10	9/10 CR's	0%	48 (45–65)	27	2.5	2.2	4/10 d 208
	Palmo-AraC	qd16–23 (IP)	13.5	not tabulated	0/10	10/10 CR's	0%	55 (52–58)	34	3.2	2.5	8/10 d 208

The day of 1st treatment, the tumors were 231 mg median on d 16 (range 144–320) = 2.3×10^8 Exponential Tumor Volume Doubling Time (Td) = 3.2 days. The 63% take-rate level = 5×10^7

Experiment #	Treatment	Schedule (route)	mg/kg/ injection	% Body-wt loss at nadir (day of nadir)	Drug deaths	Median tumor mass on (day)	% T/C mass	Median time in days for tumors to reach 1000 mg (range)	Tumor growth delay in days	median log 10-kill gross	median log 10-kill net	tumor-free "cures"
Colon-36 (1499J1)	No Rx	—	—	not tabulated	—	1000 mg on d 25	—	25 (21–32)	—	—	—	0/10
	Procarbazine	qd3–8 (PO)	46	not tabulated	0/10	100 mg on d 25	10%	36 (28–51)	11	0.83	0.45	2/10 on d 67

Td = 4.0 days. Trocar SC-implanted on d 0.

Experiment #	Treatment	Schedule (route)	mg/kg/ injection	% Body-wt loss at nadir (day of nadir)	Drug deaths	Median tumor mass on (day)	% T/C mass	Median time in days for tumors to reach 1000 mg (range)	Tumor growth delay in days	median log 10-kill gross	median log 10-kill net	tumor-free "cures"
Colon-36 (1499Q1)	No Rx	—	—	not tabulated	—	1000 mg on d 23	—	23 (20–35)	—	—	—	0/10
	Maytansine	d 3,10 (iv)	0.44	not tabulated	0/10	63 mg on d 23	6%	37 (27–52)	14	1.2	0.6	2/10 on d 93

Td = 3.6 days: Trocar SC-implanted on d 0.

This is an excellent example of the utility of converting tumor-growth delay data to log10 tumor-cell-kill. The cures do not represent a huge log-kill. Only Ara-C and its depot form Palmo-Ara-C had substantial activity. The other two agents were only modestly active against this poor take-rate tumor.

Table 12
Chemotherapeutic Treatment Mammary Adenocarcinoma-16/C (A High Take-Rate Tumor)

63% Take-Rate evel = 3×10^4; The Exponential Tumor Volume Doubling Time = 1.0 days; Tumors Implanted as 30–60 mg fragments on day 0:

Tumor (exp)	Treatment	Schedule (route)	mg/kg/ injection	% Body-wt loss at nadir (day of nadir)	Drug deaths	Median tumor mass on (day)	% T/C mass	Median time in days for tumors to reach 1000 mg (range)	Tumor growth delay in days	median log 10-kill gross	median log 10-kill net	tumor-free "cures"
#2064 Passage 116	No Rx	–	–	unchanged d 8	–	1710(723–2232) on d 11	–	10(8.5–13)	–	–	–	0/5
	Cryptophycin #55	d1–8 (iv)	144	loss 7.5% (d 8)	0/5	0 (all zero) on d 11	0%	23 (20.5–24)	13	3.9	2.6	0/5
#1286 Passage 98	No Rx	–	–	gain 6% d 8	–	1539 (446–2440) on d 11	–	8 (8–14.5)	–	–	–	0/5
	Adriamycin	day 2,5,8 (iv)	18	loss 4% d 9	0/5	0 (all zero) on d 11	0%	24 (20–63)	16	4.8	3.0	0/5
#1361 passage 62	No Rx	–	–	gain 5%	–	1790 (1296–2537) on d 9	–	7.5 (4.5–8.5)	–	–	–	0/6
	Taxol	bid6,8,11,13 (iv)	124	loss 8%	0/7	0 (all zeros) on d 9	0%	21 (20–22)	13.5	3.3	2.0	0/7
	VP-16	d6,8,11,13 (iv)	84	loss 7%	0/7	0 (0–63) on d 9	0%	21 (20.3–22.5)	13.5	3.3	2.0	0/7
#2278 passage 118	No Rx	–	–	gain 7% d 8	–	1263 (735–1450) on d 9	–	8.6 (8.5–9.5)	–	–	–	0/5
	SR271425	qd 2–8 (po)	420	unchanged d 9	0/5	0 (all zero) on d 9	0%	22 (19.3–39)	13.4	4.0	2.2	0/5
#1620 passage 134	No Rx	–	–	gain 4% d 7	–	2460 (309–3560) on d 11	–	8.5 (7.5–14)	–	–	–	0/5
	XK469	d1,3,5,8,10, 12,14 (iv)	350	unchanged d 14	0/5	0 (0–95)	0%	41.7 (25.5–66.5)	33.2	10	6	1/5

With many dozens of trials, almost no cures could be found of this high take-rate tumor (indicating the difficulty in producing enough log-kill).

Table 13
Non-Curability of IV-Implanted L1210/0 A High Take-Rate Tumor

AGENT	Exp #	MTD total dosage mg/kg	L1210/0 Leukemia gross log-kill	Activity rating against L1210	Cures/no of mice implanted
XK469	2473	300	6.4	+++++	0/5
SR271425	2304	350	6.4	+++++	0/5
VP-16	2473	70	8.0	+++++	0/5
Palmo ARA-C	2443	140	5.7	+++++	0/5
Gemzar	2483	84	6.0	+++++	0/5
BCNU	2483	28	6.7	+++++	0/5
5-FU	2473	180	4.0	++++	0/5
Cisddpt	2473	12	2.4	++	0/5
Adriamycin	2304	17	1.6	+	0/6
Vinblastine	2473	6.0	1.6	+	0/5
Taxol	2304	63	0.4	–	0/6

Mice were iv-implanted on d 0 with 10^6 leukemic cells in the treatment groups (5 mice/group) and the corresponding control group. Titered controls were also included (10^4 and 10^2) in order to verify the tumor-doubling time and $\log_{10}$ kill. Treatment started on d 1. One cell will establish tumors with L1210.

plot is truncated in time to pick the best appearance, and we have provided very little information (intentionally). The following data are obviously missing: 1) What was the body-wt loss from the treatment? 2) What happened to the treated mice later in time? If the reader is not told what happened to all of the treated tumors to a size of 1000 mg, the presenter is remiss. Sacrifice for some assay or histology is not a valid explanation. Historically, if other findings are needed, extra mice are added to the trial, and the mice used for efficacy determination are not summarily killed until all the vital information is obtained. 3) What was the log-kill from the treatment? An unwillingness to do the log-kill can indicate that the presenter is attempting to conceal how poor the activity really is. If the treatment affects the tumor growth after cessation of Rx (e.g., radiation treatment of the tumor and tumor bed can slow regrowth), the exponential Td is taken from the treated tumors—and not the control tumors—for the purpose of the log-kill calculation.

This is the same trial presented in Fig. 2, but supplemented with additional information (including the details to the end of trial). The first important piece of information is the weight loss (–8.9% body-wt loss, with the nadir on d 89). Many antitumor agents and toxic agents make a mouse sufficiently sick that it fails to eat adequately or drink fluids sufficiently. This causes a nonspecific weight loss. It is well known that weight loss alone will cause substantial growth inhibition of a solid tumor (22). A –11% body-wt loss produced by 9 ds of caloric restriction will produce a tumor-mass inhibition (T/C) = 47% for mammary adenocarcinoma-16/C (with no deaths). Caloric restriction will have even greater affects on other solid tumors (22). The NCI cutoff for a minimum indication of antitumor activity is a T/C of 42%. This cutoff was adopted because of the various caloric restriction studies (ref. 22 is the most cited). Importantly, a T/C = 20% was possible with caloric restriction with no deaths (22), although the weight loss was punishing. A weight loss of –20% or more is considered frankly toxic by NCI stan-

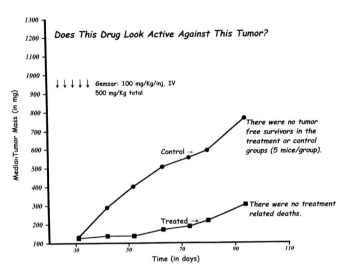

Fig. 2. Exp 2475: Treatment of a human pancreatic ductal adenocarcinoma.

dards, but weight losses of –15% are usually attended by some lethality. Historically, NCI requires a T/C (tumor mass) less than 10% to indicate high antitumor activity for a solid tumor. As an aside, weight loss does not add to survival improvement for a leukemia such as L1210 or P388, and is not an issue for survival testing. As Fig. 3 is examined, it is apparent that the treatment must have been near the lethal level, since the weight loss was –8.9% and the nadir occurred nearly 40 ds after treatment (indicating the treated mice were probably in relatively poor condition for an extended period). The T/C (mass) = 50% on d 129, which is inactive by NCI standards. Statistical significance values are often applied to solid-tumor treatment data. A T/C in the 42–50% range would usually meet statistical significance at the 5% level, but is hardly of biologic importance in light of weight-loss information.

In some cases, tumor-mass data can be presented as a mean value (average value). The mean provides greater proportional emphasis on the largest tumors in the group. In some cases it may be justified, but alternatively the presentation of a mean value may be done to place the best spin on the results, not the most conservative-spin. Historically, NCI prescribes that median values be used for tumor-mass information and mean values for weight-loss information.

The next item to note is the dispensation of all the treated mice up to a size of 1000 mg (Fig. 3). In this example, the median did not reach 1000 mg. One mouse died from tumor burden on d 136. Two mice had tumors over 1200 mg on d 143, and were sacrificed. The last measurement of all mice showed a median tumor mass of 580 mg (Fig. 3). The tumor-growth delay was 49 ds at this time-point. This is a substantial delay, until the weight loss and the slow Td of the tumor (Td = 22 d) are considered.

The last item is the conversion of the growth delay into gross log-kill (see Methods for additional details).

$$\text{Log-kill (gross)} = \frac{\text{tumor growth delay in days}}{3.32 \times (\text{exponential tumor-volume doubling time})}$$

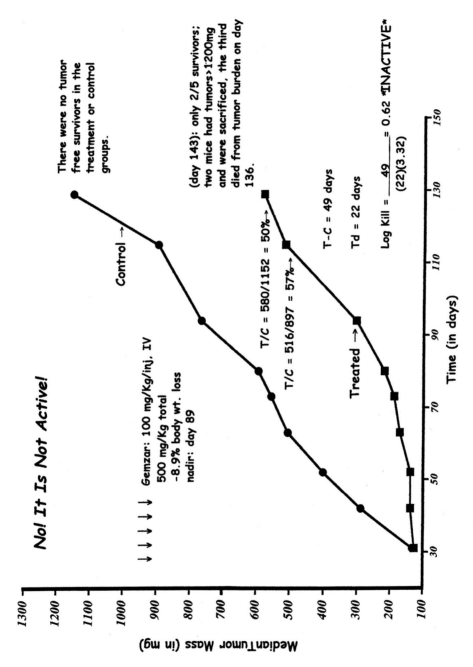

Fig. 3. Exp 2475: treatment of a human pancreatic ductal adenocarcinoma

$$\text{Log-kill (gross)} = \frac{49}{3.32(22)} = 0.62 \text{ (inactive)}$$

Now that the results are quantified and explained, the self-evident antitumor activity vanishes. This is a very good, highly active antitumor agent, but it does not work against this particular tumor.

Fig. 4: This is another example of an incomplete plot (treated tumors not plotted up to 1000 mg). On superficial examination, the agent may be considered active. If the mice are sacrificed on d 11, there would be no information to refute the purported activity. In actual fact, this is simply a truncated presentation of an agent that produced delayed lethality. The following actually occurred:

225 mg/kg total: all five mice were drug deaths, dying on d 11,12,13,13,14.

150 mg/kg total: all five mice were drug deaths, dying on d 13,14,16,16,16.

100 mg/kg total: there were two drug deaths (both d 16). The other three mice were sacrificed because of tumor burden. The optimum T/C mass = 700/1830 = 38% on d 9 (marginally active). The log-kill (gross) of this treatment group = 0.75 (marginally active).

Thus, in the final analysis of the agent used in Fig. 4, all treatment groups were toxic, and even the dose that produced 40% drug deaths was only marginally active. In many cases, mice are sacrificed if they are dying from toxicity (and this is not explained to the reader).

Delayed toxicity is an often overlooked topic in the use of tumor models (23). In some cases, the delayed lethality can occur 30–120 d after treatment, even with clinically available agents (23). It is for this reason that investigators will include nontumor toxicity control mice in some trials; i.e., nontumor normal mice injected with the maximum tolerated dosages (MTD based on short-term toxicity findings) of the drug and held for 150 ds posttreatment to verify that no long-delayed toxicity exists (23). Often, cured mice are held for the same purpose. One of the hallmarks of a delayed lethality drug is the failure of the mice to gain weight satisfactorily or to add skeletal mass. Normally, a mouse will continue to gain skeletal size throughout its life span, and at least reach 30 g within 3 mo posttreatment with most antitumor agents. If the mice stay in the 19–21-g size for an extended period of time, one can suspect serious nonreversible organ toxicities (e.g., lung, kidney). The use of nontumor toxicity-control mice to clearly separate tumor effects from treatment effects is standard practice (23).

It should be noted that the plot shown in Fig. 4, as well as the other plots, are done on Cartesian plots. This tends to give the appearance of more separation between the control and treated than there actually is (especially if the treatment groups are not plotted to 1000 mg). Historically, it is better to use semilog plots (with the median tumor masses plotted on the log axis). The exponential doubling-time portion of the growth curve will then be essentially linear, allowing the calculation of the exponential Td with more accuracy.

Fig. 5: This is NCI data. If it was not explained, it would appear that adriamycin was nicely active against the human breast adenocarcinoma MX-1 [T/C = 12%; 2/6 tumor-free mice cures; median of 1.7 log-kill among those not cured (++ activity rating)]. In fact, adriamycin is not active against this tumor in our testing (1,3), and furthermore, it is markedly more toxic in immune-deficient mice than in conventional mice (3). The dose used in the experiment shown in Fig. 5 is approx 3 times the MTD in immune-

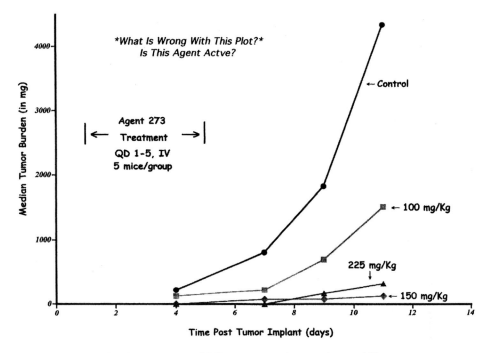

Fig. 4. Treatment of SC mammary adenocarcinoma 16/c.

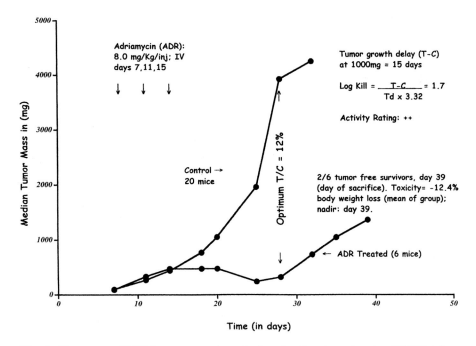

Fig. 5. Treatment of MX-1 mammary tissue in female athymic nude mice (NCI Data).

deficient mice *(3)*. This is a superb educational example because the weights of all the mice were provided up to and including the day of sacrifice (d 39). The first item to note is the large body-wt loss (–12.4% of body wt) occurred with the nadir on d 39 (the day of sacrifice). At face value, the tumors could be considered to cause some of the weight loss, except that the mice were continuously losing weight posttreatment, including two mice that were listed as tumor-free. Furthermore, the tumors in this cage were too small to cause the mice to lose weight (based on the controls). However, the actual weight losses of the tumor-free mice essentially tell the whole story. One lost 5.0 g (–26% of its body wt), and the other mouse lost –4.9 g (–22% of its body wt). The mice were obviously sacrificed because they were moribund and dying of drug toxicity. In addition, it is unacceptable to kill tumor-free mice so soon after treatment. These mice would need to be held for at least 2 more mo to be assured a cure. Lastly, the cures would have needed to be rechallenged with the tumor to prove that the cures were not the result of immune rejection in a leaky mouse.

The next lower dose of adriamycin was also a toxic dose, and had no antitumor activity (T/C = 103%; no log-kill).

9. CHARACTERIZATION OF A TUMOR MODEL AND QUALITY-CONTROL MONITORING

To a large extent, the types of characterization end points that the investigator needs depends on the usage of the model. Furthermore, the tumor model is not a static entity. The exponential tumor-volume doubling time usually shortens substantially during the first 10 transplant generations, and can shorten more with additional passage *(10)*. For example, Mam-16/C had a 4.5-d Td in the 4th passage and a 1.25-d Td in the 29th passage. The cause is a decrease in the cell-loss factor *(24)*, which is consistent with an observed improvement in the take-rate of a tumor with serial passage. Interestingly, the growth fraction and the intermitotic times do not change markedly with serial passage of new tumors *(24)*. Overall, it would appear that a transplantable tumor becomes fast-growing and less differentiated for two reasons: 1) the normal components that make up a portion of the original tumor and impart the highly differentiated character are lost in the first transplant (normal cells do not transplant well); and 2) the cell-loss factor decreases (either through an improvement in the fidelity of replication or by adapting to the implant environment). Either way, it is hard to envision that any of these changes could substantially alter the predictive worth of the model, other than making it more challenging. The Td has a bottom limit of 1.0 d for solid tumors of mice, and 0.35 ds for leukemias of mice.

We propose the following suggestions for using solid-tumor models for chemotherapy purposes. In most cases, this information will provide adequate characterization and quality-control monitoring.

1. Use tumors that have been in passage for over 10 serial passages (there is too much tumor to tumor-growth variability with fewer passages).
2. Use tumors from mouse passage and not culture passage. Tumors directly from culture tend to magnify responses, because they are less adapted to the mouse environment and thus more fragile.
3. Determine the take-rate of the tumor with titered tumor-cell implants at the various locations intended for use in the model. One should then use a titer for chemotherapy

that is at least 3 logs above the 63% take-rate level (more if high antitumor activity is expected).

4. Obtain histologic sections of the tumor at least every three or four passages (every passage if it is a human tumor because of the diffuse necrosis problem).

5. Determine the exponential tumor-volume doubling time, and monitor this every few passages (every passage if it is a human tumor, since human tumors can become contaminated with spontaneous lymphoma cells, resulting in a marked decrease in the Td; or undergo excessive diffuse necrosis and have a marked increase in the Td).

6. Determine the metastatic behavior of the tumor at various sizes.

7. Passage the tumors at a relatively small size (e.g., 600–1000 mg), while the animal is still healthy and the tumor is still in exponential growth. Passage at larger sizes increases the chance of passaging an infected tumor.

8. Passage mouse tumors in the inbred strain of origin only (F1 hybrids should not be used).

9. Passage mouse tumors in mice that have been in the laboratory for at least 2 mo (so that the mice are large and healthy and have well-developed immune systems). These older, larger mice have been exposed to, and have conquered, various extraneous bacteria and viruses. On the other hand, human tumors should be passaged in young immune-deficient mice (6–7 wk) to minimize development of leaky mice; and also to avoid the possibility of spontaneous lymphomas that will contaminate human tumors (athymic mice and balb/c SCIDs have less problems with spontaneous lymphomas than ICR SCIDs).

10. The texture and other appearance characteristics of the tumors should be noted. Photos are helpful if the tumor is being used for the first time (this is critical for human tumors which can, and do change easily over time).

11. Tumor fragments should be maintained in frozen storage vials in two different locations (10% dimethyl sulfoxide (DMSO) in media with 10% serum is standard).

12. Fragments of the tumor being passaged should be checked for bacterial contamination (incubate at 37°C for 72 h in a growth media).

13. The chemotherapeutic responses to standard agents should be determined.

14. Only syngeneic mouse tumors should be used. Verification can be done by treatment with IL-2, which is a simple and inexpensive technique *(25)*. More classic methods are also available *(26)*.

15. Simple vital statistics obtained: passage generation; histologic appearance and grade (degree of differentiation); host of origin; tissue and cell of origin; how induced; when induced; time required to reach 500 mg and 1000 mg from a trocar implant; unusual characteristics (e.g., mucin-producing; common metastatic sites that vary with implant location), appropriate references.

16. In the near future, molecular characterizations of the models will undoubtedly be critically important to a better understanding of the biologic and response behavior of the models.

Since each independently arising tumor is a separate and unique biologic entity, no one tumor model is a perfect predictor for any other model. For this reason, most investigators are forced to use multiple models for study *(1)*. Nonetheless, it is still better for the new investigator to understand a few models very well than many models superficially.

10. SUMMARY

Clearly, it is difficult to even introduce of the topic of solid-tumor models of mice. Many of the details can best be learned by an apprenticeship in a laboratory with an experienced staff, because only a small portion of the practical information and reasons for the various methodologies is published. Lastly, many of the issues are not covered at all, or only superficially, because of previous publications. As such, the following references are suggested for additional details in the use of tumor models *(1,3–11,21,23,27–38)*. Nonetheless, the information provided in this work concerning the transplant characteristics of the tumor models, as well as the few examples of data presentation pitfalls, should aid investigators in future readings. With these perspectives, the reader should not be misled into believing that transplantable mouse tumor models are exceptionally sensitive to everything. In fact, there are very few core molecules with substantial antitumor activity. One should consider the numbers: Worldwide, over 2,000,000 agents have been tested in tumor-bearing animals, and countless additional agents have been tested in culture or other assays to reduce the number to 2 million. Only about 60 agents are currently available for clinical use, of which less than 15 are used with regularity. Even fewer have substantial activity against common solid tumors of humans. Likewise, in our experience, fewer than 15 agents (clinically available and investigational) from separate chemical cores have a high antitumor ++++ rating against more than one of the highly metastatic, highly invasive, high-take-rate syngeneic solid tumor models of mice (Panc-02; Mam-16/C; Mam-44; Colon-51; Colon-26; B16 melanoma; LL Carcinoma; with the implant more than 3 logs above the take-rate and the drug and tumor injected by different routes, or both (Table 1) *(1,4,6,7,32,34,35)* and unpublished results. It should be noted that a ++++ rating only requires >2.8 log-kill (gross); *see* Methods Section for rating scale.

11. METHODS

The methods of protocol design, drug treatment, toxicity evaluation, data analysis, quantification of tumor-cell-kill, tumor-model systems, crossresistance behavior, and the biological significance of the drug treatment results with transplantable tumors have been presented previously *(1,3,9,26–29,31,33–37)*. A brief description of the methods as they apply to this work follows.

11.1. Tumor Maintenance

Tumors were maintained in the mouse strain of origin and were transplanted into the appropriate F_1 hybrid or inbred for the trials. Individual mouse body wts for each experiment were within 5 g, and all mice were more than 18 g at the start of therapy. The mice were supplied food and water *ad libitum*.

11.2. Origins of Mouse Tumors Used or Discussed

Colon Adenocarcinomas-26,38,51 *(5,6)*; Mammary Adenocarcinoma-16/C *(4)*; Mammary Adenocarcinoma-16/C/Adr *(37,39)*; Mammary Adenocarcinomas-17/0 and 17/Adr *(39,40)*; Mammary Adenocarcinoma-16/C/Taxol (induced in vivo with repeated Taxol treatments over 6 passage generations, first usage published in ref. *32*); Pancreatic Ductal Adenocarcinomas-02,03 *(7)*; Squamous-Cell Lung LC-12 *(41,42)*; B16 melanoma (1st chemotherapeutic treatment of) *(43)*; *LLC* (1st chemotherapeutic treatment of) *(43)*; L1210 Leukemia *(44)*; P388 Leukemia *(45)*; AML-C1498 leukemia (arose spontaneously in a 10 mo-old C57B1/6 female mouse at Jackson Memorial Labs in 1941 *(46)*.

11.3. Chemotherapy of Leukemias: L1210/0

The animals were pooled, iv-implanted with counted numbers of leukemic cells (10^6, 10^4, 10^2) prepared from a spleen brei containing approx 80% replacement of the spleen with leukemic cells (as judged by the eightfold enlarged size in the leukemic passage DBA/2 mice). Survival was the end point; with moribund mice sacrificed. Cause of death was verified by necropsy, and there were no drug deaths among the groups shown in Table 13. In all cases, treatment was started the day after implantation of the leukemic cells.

11.4. X-Irradiation of Solid Tumors

X-irradiation was delivered through a Picker Vangard X-ray unit operated at 280 kVp, 20 mA, 1.33 mm Cu HVL, and TSD of 47.5 cm. Anesthetized mice were irradiated (1.1 gy/min., 1 gy = 100 rads) through a treatment port of 1.2×4.1 cm that included the tumor site, axillary nodes, and 75% right-lung volume. Maximum scatter and leakage radiation to the shielded animal was less than 2.0%.

11.5. Chemotherapy of Solid Tumors

The animals were pooled, SC-implanted bilaterally with 30–60 mg tumor fragments by a 12-gauge trocar, and again pooled before unselective distribution to the various treatment and control groups. For early-stage treatment, chemotherapy was started within 1–3 d after tumor implantation, when the number of cells was relatively small (10^7 to 10^8 cells). For more advanced staged disease, the tumors were allowed to reach 100 to 800 mg (depending on the trial) before the start of treatment. Tumors were measured with a caliper twice weekly. Mice were sacrificed when their tumors reached 1500 mg. Tumor weights are estimated from two-dimensional measurements:

11.6. Tumor Weight = a (b²)/2

where a and b are the tumor length and width in (mm), respectively. In those cases in which bilateral sc tumors were used, both tumors on each mouse were added together, and the total mass per mouse was used for calculations of end points.

Note: Some investigators present data as measurements (partly because tumors masses are obtained by measurements). However, all NCI protocols of the past have mandated the use of tumor weights in mg. We have often found that readers do not relate to measurements, and in some cases the measurements obscure the fact that unusually small tumors are being shown and end points are obtained at sizes that are not acceptable in standard NCI protocols.

11.7. End Points Assessing Antitumor Activity Solid Tumors

The following quantitative end points are used to assess antitumor activity.

11.7.1. Tumor-Growth Delay (T-C value)

T is the median time (in days) required for the treatment group tumors to reach a predetermined size (e.g., 1000 mg), and C is the median time (in days) for the control group tumors to reach the same size. Tumor-free survivors are excluded from these calculations (cures are tabulated separately). In our judgment, this value is the single most important criterion of antitumor effectiveness because it allows the quantification of tumor-cell-kill.

11.7.2. PERCENT INCREASE LIFE SPAN (%ILS)

Leukemic mice only. The %ILS = [(T–C)/C] 100; in which C = The median day of death of the control group and T = The median day of death of the treated group. There were no cures in any of the trials shown herein.

11.8. Calculation Tumor-Cell-Kill

For subcutaneously growing tumors, and leukemic survival trials, the $\log_{10}$ cell-kill is calculated from the following formula:

$$\text{The } \log_{10} \text{ cell-kill total (gross)} = \frac{T - C \text{ value in days}}{(3.32)\,(Td)}$$

$$\text{The } \log_{10} \text{ cell-kill total (net)} = \frac{(T - C) - (\text{duration of treatment})}{(3.32)\,(Td)}$$

The $\log_{10}$ cell-kill/dose = log-kill gross/number of injections (if each injection has the same dose).

For solid tumors, the T-C is the tumor-growth delay described here, and Td is the tumor-volume doubling time (in days), estimated from the best-fit straight line from a log-linear growth plot of the control group tumors in exponential growth (100–800 mg range). The conversion of the T-C values to $\log_{10}$ cell-kill is possible because the Td of tumors regrowing posttreatment (Rx) approximates the Td values of the tumors in untreated control mice. If the regrowing tumors do not (e.g., irradiation of tumor and tumor bed), the Td value is determined from the regrowing tumors.

This equation for log-kill is also used for leukemia testing, where *T* is the median day of death for the treated group and *C* is the median day of death for the control group. The Td is determined from differences in the median days of death of the titered control groups. Four $\log_{10}$ dilution controls were included in all trials. There were five mice each in all treatment and control groups.

11.9. Activity Rating Solid Tumors

For comparison of activity with standard agents and comparisons of activity between tumors, the $\log_{10}$ kill values were converted to an arbitrary activity rating *(35)*. It should be noted that +++ or ++++ activity would be required to produce tumor regressions in most models. As such, ++ activity would not be scored by a clinician as more than stable disease.

Duration of Treatment
5–20 d

Antitumor Activity	Gross Log_{10} Tumor-Cell-Kill
Highly Active ++++	>2.8
+++	2.0–2.8
++	1.3–1.9
+	0.7 – 1.2
Inactive	<0.7

11.7.5. ACTIVITY RATING FOR LEUKEMIA L1210/0

Because the L1210 leukemia was markedly more sensitive to the antitumor agents than the solid tumors, an expanded activity rating was required (Tables 1,13).

Duration of Treatment
1–9 d

Antitumor Activity	*Gross Log$_{10}$ Tumor-Cell-Kill*
Highly Active +++++	≥5.0
++++	4.0–4.9
+++	3.0–3.9
++	2.0–2.9
+	1.0–1.9
Inactive	<1.0

11.10. Non-Quantitative Determination Antitumor Activity Tumor-Growth Inhibition (T/C Value)

The treatment and control groups are measured when the control-group tumors reach approx 700–1200 mg in size (median of group). The median tumor weight of each group is determined (including zeros). The T/C value in percent is an indication of antitumor effectiveness. A T/C equal to or less than 42% is considered significant antitumor activity by the Drug Evaluation Branch of the Division of Cancer Treatment (NCI). A T/C value <10% is considered to indicate highly significant antitumor activity, and is the level used by NCI to justify a clinical trial if toxicity, formulation, and certain other requirements are met (termed DN-2 level activity). A body-wt loss nadir (mean of group) of greater than 20% or greater than 20% drug deaths is considered to indicate an excessively toxic dosage.

ACKNOWLEDGMENTS

Supported by: CA12623, CA82341, CA53001, Sanofi Synthelabo Research, and Eli Lilly Corporation.

REFERENCES

1. Corbett, T., Valeriote, F., LoRusso, P., Polin, L., Panchapor, C., Pugh, S., et al. Tumor models and the discovery and secondary evaluation of solid tumor active agents. *Int J Pharmacogn* (Suppl.) 1995; 33:102–122.
2. LoRusso, P., Demchik, L., Dan, M., Polin, L., Gross, J.L., Corbett, T.H. Comparative efficacy of DMP-840 against mouse and human solid tumor models. *Investig New Drugs* 1995; 13:195–203.
3. Polin, L., Valeriote, F., White, K., Panchapor, C., Pugh, S., Knight, J., et al. Treatment of human prostate tumors PC-3 and TSU-PRI with standard and investigational Agents in SCID Mice. *Investig New Drugs* 1997; 15:99–108.
4. Corbett, T.H., Griswold, Jr., D.P., Roberts, B.J., Peckham, J.C., Schabel, Jr., F.M. Biology and therapeutic response of a mouse mammary adenocarcinoma (16/C) and its potential as a model for surgical adjuvant chemotherapy. *Cancer Treat Rep* 1978; 62(10):1471–1488.
5. Corbett, T.H., Griswold, Jr., D.P., Roberts, B.J., Peckham, J.C., Schabel, Jr., F.M. Tumor induction relationships in development of transplantable cancers of the colon in mice for chemotherapy assays, with a note on carcinogen structure. *Cancer Res* 1975; 35:2434–2439.
6. Corbett, T.H., Griswold, Jr., D.P., Roberts, B.J., Peckham, J.C., Schabel, Jr., F.M. Evaluation of single agents and combinations of chemotherapeutic agents in mouse colon carcinomas. *Cancer* 1977; 40(5):2660–2680.
7. Corbett, T.H., Roberts, B.J., Leopold, W.R., Peckham, J.C., Wilkoff, L.J., Griswold, Jr., D.P., et al. Induction and chemotherapeutic response of two transplantable ductal adenocarcinomas of the pancreas in C57BL/6 mice. *Cancer Res* 1984; 44:717–726.
8. Corbett, T.H., Valeriote, F.A. Rodent models in experimental chemotherapy In: *The Use of Rodent Tumors in Experimental Cancer Therapy: Conclusions and Recommendations.* Kallman RF, ed. Pergamon Press, New York, NY, 1987, pp. 233–247.

9. Corbett, T., Valeriote, F., LoRusso, P., Polin, L., Panchapor, C., Pugh, S., et al. In vivo methods for screening and preclinical testing; use of rodent solid tumors for drug discovery. In: Teicher B, ed. *Anticancer Drug Development Guide: Preclinical Screening, Clinical Trials, and Approval.* Humana Press Inc., Totowa, NJ, 1997, pp. 75–99.

10. Corbett, T.H., Griswold, Jr., D.P., Roberts, B.J., Schabel, Jr., F.M. Cytotoxic adjuvant therapy and the experimental model. In: Stoll BA, ed. *New Aspects of Breast Cancer.* Vol. 4, Systemic Therapy in Breast Cancer, William Heinemann Medical Books, Ltd., London, 1981, pp. 204–243.

11. Corbett, T.H., Roberts, B.J., Lawson, A.J., Leopold III, W.R. Curative chemotherapy of advanced and disseminated solid tumors of mice. In: Jacobs JR, Al-Sarraf M, Crissman J, Valeriote F, eds, *Scientific and Clinical Perspectives in Head and Neck Cancer Management: Strategies for Cure.* Elsevier Scientific Publishing Company, Inc., New York, NY, 1987, pp. 175–192.

12. Griswold, Jr., D.P., Corbett, T.H. Use of experimental models in the study of approaches to treatment of colorectal cancer. In: Lipkin M., Good RA, eds. *Gastrointestinal Tract Cancer,* Medical Book Company, New York, NY, 1978, pp. 399–418.

13. Karrer, K., Humphreys, S.R. Continuous and limited courses of cyclophosphamide (NSC26271) in mice with pulmonary metastasis after surgery. *Cancer Chemother Rep* 1967; 51:439–449.

14. Schabel, F.M. Jr. Concepts for treatment of micrometastases developed in murine systems. *Am J Roentgenol Radium Ther Nucl Med* 1976; 126:500–511.

15. Boyd, M.R. The NCI in vitro anticancer drug discover screen, concept, implementation, and operation, 1985 to 1995. In: Teicher B, ed. *Anticancer Drug Development Guide: Preclinical Screening, Clinical Trials, and Approval.* Humana Press Inc., Totowa, NJ, 1997, pp. 75–99.

16. Wallace, A.C. Effect of Delayed Addition of Irradiated Cells to Small Viable Tumor Inocula. *Cancer Res* 1965; 25:355–357.

17. Revesz, L. Effect of tumor cells killed by X-rays upon growth of admixed viable cells. *Nature* 1956; 178:1391–1392.

18. Revesz, L. Effect of lethally damaged tumor cells upon the development of admixed viable cells. *J Natl Cancer Inst* 1958; 20:1157–1186.

19. Dykes, D.J., Griswold, D.P. Jr., Schabel, F.M., Jr. Growth support of small B16 Melanoma implants with nitrosourea-sterilized fractions of the same tumor. *Cancer Res* 1978; 36:2031–2034.

20. Annual Progress Report to Division of Cancer Treatment, National Cancer Institute on Primary Screening and Development and Application of Secondary Evaluation Procedures for Study of New Materials with Potential Anticancer Activity. pgs 1–9. Lack of Influence of Immune Suppression on the Number of Cells Required to Establish Takes of Solid Tumors. Southern Research Institute, Contract NO1-CM-43756, March 15, 1982.

21. Skipper, H.E. The effects of chemotherapy on the kinetics of leukemic cell behavior. *Cancer Res* 1965; 25:1544–1550.

22. Laster, W.R., Jr., Schabel, F.M., Jr., Skipper, H.E., Wilcox, W.S., Thomson, J.R. Experimental evaluation of potential anticancer agents IV. Host weight loss as it related to false positives in drug evaluation. *Cancer Res* 1961; 21:895–906.

23. Annual Progress Report to Division of Cancer Treatment, National Cancer Institute on Primary Screening and Development and Application of Secondary Evaluation Procedures for Study of New Materials with Potential Anticancer Activity. Section 27, pgs 1–32. Unusual Toxicity Problems Encountered in the Evaluation of New Antitumor Agents: Implications for Data Analysis and Protocol Design. Southern Research Institute, Contract NO1-CM-43756, March 15, 1982.

24. Houghton, J.A., Taylor, D.M. Growth characteristics of human colorectal tumors during serial passage in immune-deprived mice. *Br J Cancer* 1978; 37:213–223.

25. LoRusso, P.M., Polin, L., Aukerman, S.L., Redman, B.G., Valdivieso, M., Biernat, L., et al. Antitumor efficacy of Interleukin-2 alone and in combination with Adriamycin and Dacarbazine in murine solid tumor systems. *Cancer Res* 1990; 50:5876–5882.

26. Motycka K, Bostik J, Danek PF, Chudomel V. Immunogenicity of the Gardner lymphosarcoma for the mice of the strain C3H (H-2k). I. The effect of the 60Co-irradiation of recipients and of the interval between the immunization and transplantation of the tumor on the antitumor resistance of immunized mice. *Neoplasma* 1986; 33(2):167–175.

27. Simpson-Herren, L., Corbett, T.H., Griswold, Jr., D.P. The cell population kinetics and response to an S-phase specific agent of three transplantable colon tumor lines. *Cell Tissue Kinet* 1980; 13:613–624.

28. Corbett, T.H., Leopold, W.R., Dykes, D.J., Roberts, B.J., Griswold, Jr., D.P., Schabel, Jr., F.M. Toxicity and anticancer activity of a new triazine antifolate (NSC-127755). *Cancer Res* 1982; 42:1707–1715.

29. Corbett, T.H., Roberts, B.J., Trader, M.W., Laster, Jr., W.R., Griswold, Jr., D.P., Schabel, Jr., F.M. Response of transplantable tumors of mice to anthracenedione derivatives alone and in combination with clinically useful agents. *Cancer Treat Rep* 1982; 66(5):1187–1200.
30. Corbett, T., Valeriote, F., Baker, L. Is the P388 murine tumor no longer adequate as a drug discovery model? *Investig New Drugs* 1987; 5:3–20.
31. Corbett, T.H., Bissery, M.-C., LoRusso, P.-M., Polin, L. 5-Fluorouracil containing combinations in murine tumor systems. *Investig New Drugs* 1989; 7:37–49.
32. Corbett, T.H., Valeriote, F.A., Demchik, L., Polin, L., Panchapor, C., Pugh, S., et al. Preclinical anticancer activity of cryptophycin-8. *J Exper Therapeutics and Oncology* 1996; 1:95–108.
33. Corbett, T.H., Valeriote, F.A., Demchik, L., Lowichik, N., Polin, L., Panchapor, C., et al. Discovery of Cryptophycin-1 and BCN-183577: Examples of strategies and problems in the detection of antitumor activity in mice. *Investig New Drugs* 1997; 15:207–218.
34. Corbett, T.H., LoRusso, P., Demchick, L., Simpson, C., Pugh, S., White, K., et al. Preclinical antitumor efficacy of analogs of XK-469: Sodium-(2-[4- (7-chloro-2-quinoxalinyloxy)phenoxy] propionate. *Investig New Drugs* 1998; 16:129–139.
35. Corbett, T.H., Panchapor, C., Polin, L., Lowichik, N., Pugh, S., White, K., et al. Preclinical Efficacy of thioxanthone SR-271425 against transplanted solid tumors of mouse and human origin. *Investig New Drugs* 1999; 17:17–27.
36. Schabel, Jr., F.M., Trader, M.W., Laster, Jr., W.R., Corbett, T.H., Griswold, Jr., D.P. Cis-dichlorodiammineplatinum (II): combination chemotherapy and cross-resistance studies with tumors of mice. *Cancer Treat Rep* 1979; 63:1459–1473.
37. Schabel, Jr., F.M. Skipper, H.E., Trader, M.W., Laster, W.R. Jr., Griswold, Jr., D.P., Corbett, T.H. Establishment of cross-resistance profiles for new agents. *Cancer Treat Rep* 1983; 67:905–922.
38. Skipper, H.E., Schabel, F.M., Jr., Wilcox, W.S. Experimental evaluation of potential anticancer agents XIII: on the criteria and kinetic associated with curability of experimental leukemias. *Cancer Chemother Rep* 1964; 35:3–111.
39. Kessel, D., Corbett, T.H. Correlations between anthracycline resistance, drug accumulation and membrane glycoprotein patterns in solid tumors of mice. *Cancer Let* 1985; 28:187–193.
40. Biernat, L., Polin, L., Corbett, T. Adaptation of mammary tumors of mice to a soft agar assay for use in drug discovery. Seventh NCI-EORTC Symposium on New Drugs in Cancer Therapy. Abstract #185, Amsterdam, March 1992; 17–20.
41. Smith, WE, Yazdi, E., Miller, L. Carcinogenesis in pulmonary epithelia in mice on different levels of Vitamin A. *Environ Res* 1972; 5:152–163.
42. Tapazoglou, E., Polin, L., Corbett, T.H., Al-Sarraf, M. Chemotherapy of the squamous cell lung cancer LC-12 with 5-fluorouracil, cisplatin, carboplatin or iproplatin combinations. *Investig New Drugs* 1988; 6(4):259–264.
43. Sugiura, K., Stock, C.C. Studies in a tumor spectrum. III. The effect of phosphoramides on the growth of a variety of mouse and rat tumors. *Cancer Res* 1955; 15:38–51.
44. Law, LW, Dunn, TB, Boyle, PJ, Miller, JH. Observations on the effect of folic-acid antagonists on transplantable lymphoid leukemias in mice *J Natl Cancer Inst* 1949; 10:179–192.
45. Dawe, C.J., Potter, M. Morphologic and biologic progression of a lymphoid neoplasm of the mouse in vivo and in vitro (abstr) *Am J Pathol* 1957; 33:603.
46. Bradner, W.T., and Pindell, M.H. Myeoid Leukemia C1498 as a screen for cancer chemotherapeutic agents *Cancer Res* 1966; April, (pt 2) 375–390.

4

B16 Murine Melanoma

Historical Perspective on the Development of a Solid Tumor Model

Enrique Alvarez, DVM, MA

CONTENTS

INTRODUCTION
HISTORICAL CONTEXT
B16 MELANOMA
CONCLUSIONS
REFERENCES

The determination of weight of a factor in producing metastases can not be judged from single experiences on man, as it is impossible to eliminate conflicting conditions. Only by the use of a homogeneous material which the size of the cells, their histological and biological qualities, and the vascularity of the surrounding tissue, etc., are practically constant can valid conclusions be drawn, and this elimination of variables is possible to obtain only by the use of animal tumors of a long transplanted strain, so that the morphological and biological characters are well known.

Dr. Leila C. Knox, 1922 (1)

1. INTRODUCTION

The development of reliable models of disease mechanisms largely depends on our understanding of the characteristic processes of the disease being modeled. Syngeneic tumors in mice offer an important model for oncology research. Although the use of murine models of neoplastic disease has been raised to the level of a fundamental paradigm in oncology research, it is to be considered with all the care and diligence afforded to us by any biological model. Syngeneic murine tumors offer potential advantages as well as limitations, which should always be present in the mind of the investigator. Every year, countless studies are published describing new models and/or new cell lines available to scientists. Many of these are highly specialized, and have a narrow application to the broad community. Through time, several models are developed, which present us with a newer tool to truly advance our understanding. In many instances, these models fill a specific unmet need. If fortunate enough, the model is

From: *Tumor Models in Cancer Research*
Edited by: B. A. Teicher © Humana Press Inc., Totowa, NJ

also relatively easy to reproduce, thus providing for rapid dissemination among the community. The overall relative importance of an experimental model depends largely on two important aspects. First, how does the model recapitulate the process it attempts to emulate? Second, how does the model itself offer the flexibility to expand our knowledge relating to the pathologic process being evaluated? This chapter pinpoints how the B16 murine melanoma line has proven itself a valuable model on both points. This tumor line provides researchers with the ability to model the process of solid-tumor formation and the following metastatic process seen in animals and man. Upon establishment of this model of metastasis, a more detailed understanding of the steps involved in tumor dissemination was gained. Astute manipulation of the cell line and a rational use of experimental animal models were essential for this process. Overall, this effort has helped the modern description of fundamental processes in metastasis, invasion, and anti-tumor drug development. The body of knowledge derived from the B16 murine melanoma line is ample, and even at present continues to grow. The emphasis of this overview is limited to its origin and to the seminal work attributable to the early work done with this tumor line and some of the tumor models that have arisen from it. In the span of biological research, this model is relatively new. But within one lifetime, it has helped shape our understanding of oncology. In science, many posed questions are old and numerous, but the tools we need to thoroughly explore them and ask new ones are in continuous evolution. These new tools encourage even more questions. The B16 melanoma is one of those tools.

2. HISTORICAL CONTEXT

The process of scientific discovery never occurs outside the context of contemporary knowledge. Contemporary knowledge is relative to the time of the work itself. In the early 1970s, at the time of the establishment of the B16 as a model for metastasis research, the state of metastasis research from a technical standpoint was immature when compared to today's standards. Although many recent developments in the area of metastasis have depended on the use of relatively recent technological advances (e.g., molecular biology, protein chemistry, and bioinformatics), many questions regarding the nature of metastasis are very old. Up to the early 1970s, there had been numerous qualitative (i.e., autopsies) and some quantitative studies (i.e., rodent models) relating to the natural history of the metastatic process, but a readily accessible murine model was lacking—specifically, a model that would offer a predictable metastatic pattern.

A periodic survey of the historical record serves to focus our attention to the correct context of the research. Within this context, the significance of the questions asked becomes clearer, as well as the importance of the techniques being used. The development and current use of the B16 melanoma line should be incorporated into a larger scope of oncology research by looking at a previous generation of researchers and their professional contributions to the field.

An often-quoted work by Dr. Stephen Paget was seminal in establishing our appreciation for the complexity of the processes involved in metastasis (2). The concept of Seed and Soil, as it applies to the tumor embolus and its potential site of invasion, is firmly entrenched in the minds of researchers in the field of metastasis. Simple, allegorical, yet effective at setting the concepts of a complicated pathological process, the idea of seed and soil has been fundamental for over 110 years. The careful evaluation of human autopsies derived from breast-cancer patients an obvious nonrandom pattern of metastasis, noted by Paget, demonstrated that breast-cancer patients had a notable predisposition for bony metastasis. This bony metastasis was nonrandom in its distribution, since, as Dr. Paget commented: "Who has ever seen the bones of the hands or the feet attacked by secondary cancer?" This observation is critical in two important aspects. First, the bony tissue clearly presents the tumor with a preferred invasion site (soil to the seed). Second, bones are not just bones; there appears to be further discrimination by the tumor embolus as to which bone offers an optimal site for colonization. Effective tools, such as animal models that could be used to experimentally understand the human condition, were not yet available to Paget. It would still be many years until such specific disease models were widely available for use. Our contemporary description of the specific relationship between the cell and its host tissue uses the term "tumor microenvironment" to essentially name the same phenomena described in 1889. Successful tumor metastasis is a complex, nonrandom, multifactorial event that requires contributing components from both the cancer cell and its host.

As with many areas in science, in oncology we also find a periodic re-evaluation of fundamental themes. The "Seed and Soil" concept has not been immune to this effect. In 1982, Hart specifically reflected on the mechanisms of metastasis as they apply to murine models *(3)*. This work reiterated the clear importance of circulation and physical-cell distribution on the outcome of a metastatic event. Hart concluded:

Patterns of metastasis primarily appear to be a direct consequence of the delivery of an optimal dose of tumor cells to the first organ encountered along the lymphatic or venous pathway. Nonetheless, the very same tumors that use this mechanism as a predominant mode of spread will, on other occasions, exhibit true organ tropism.

This conclusion did not exclude the already noted metastatic preference of tumors to certain organs, but gave a stronger importance to circulatory parameters in the final disposition of tumor metastasis. This attempt at revisionism occurred almost 100 years after the publication by Paget. What had transpired in that interval to call for the re-evaluation of the concept?

In the first half of the 1900s, there was a general effort to describe the nature of circulating tumor cells in man and rodent models. In 1913, while studying a carcinoma model of the Japanese waltzing mouse, Tyzzer found a correlation between the tumor size, duration of tumor presence, peculiar conditions furnished by the host, and the number of metastases *(4)*. These important clinically applicable correlations were being laid down by scientists using syngeneic models. In 1915, Iwasaki presented a paper, which when carefully read can serve to introduce today's researcher to many of the important areas of current interest *(5)*. By using microscopy to describe the tumor embolus-host interaction in necropsy cases, Iwasaki finely described the disposition of several tumor types in the vessels of patients. Most of the work presents the reader with a description of the relationship between the tumor embolus, thrombus formation/organization, and the formation of tumor metastasis. A particular description of tumor-vessel interaction by Iwasaki is of particular interest today:

The tumour cell mass is here covered by a thin layer of endothelium continuous with the intima. Though a small number of leucocytes may be found between the tumour cells, the latter appeared to be normal: no sign of degradation can be seen. Some con-

nective-tissues fibres from the wall, as well as cells from the covering endothelium, are thrust into the mass: these serve as stroma. I consider them as the first stage of metastases formation; at the same time, I consider that the penetration of the wall by the tumor cells from inside can sometimes occur without such an endothelial cover.

Eighty-five years ago we find an accurate description of the process of extravasation by a metastatic cell, while at the same time describing a relationship between tumor cells and endothelium. In the same paper Iwasaki also studied the fate of intravenous (iv)-injected tumor cells in rats and mice.

In the cases of mouse carcinoma I again observed the appearances of which I have described in cases of human sarcoma, that is, the tumour cell group on a vessel wall, having a single endothelial layer directly covering it. The carcinoma cells of such fixed emboli appear to be in healthy condition in every respect, and in the cases where connective tissue bundles thrust into and divide them up, they have the common appearance of alveolar carcinoma and are not to be considered as degenerating or organizing at all.

This statement serves to offer initial validation of the use of murine models from a comparative and histological perspective. When comparing his own tumor implantation results with that of fellow researchers (who obtained a lower tumor take-rate than himself) Iwasaki concluded:

From my results I hold that it is not difficult to cause tumours by inoculating foci directly into vessels. Nevertheless, all tumor cells introduced into blood vessels do not necessarily disintegrate, as several authors believe, but if the technique is suitable, the lung will be attacked in a very considerable number of cases.

Iwasaki's work was important in describing the lung as the preferred site of tumor takes after iv injection. Much work followed to determine the reasons for this apparent affinity.

Warren and Gates clearly demonstrated that the successful establishment of tumors in rodent lungs after iv injection is strongly correlated with the cell viability of the sample being used *(6)*. At that time, the authors were attempting to standardize the procedure of iv tumor-cell implantation. This was demonstrated using the Walker 256 carcinoma line in rats. Cloudman in 1947 studied the—as they were formerly called—organophilic tendencies of murine hepatic tumors *(7)*. At that time, the author specifically looked at the dissemination patterns of two tumor lines (C954 liver carcinoma and C198 reticuloendothelioma). The work employed the use of subcutaneous (SC) implantations using a trochar as well as the use of parabiosis in mice. Interestingly, Cloudman's method of tumor passage may have contributed to the organophilic tendencies noted. The mode of tumor maintenance for the C198 line required that tumor-affected pieces of liver from mice be SC-implanted in naive hosts. This SC tumor would lead to disseminated disease in the mice. When the initial line was being established, simple SC implantation led to poor tumor-take. But the hepatic metastatic spread of the tumor offered an optimal tissue for reproducibly metastatic tumor whenever this tissue was SC-implanted. In the case of the C954 tumor line, it was maintained via simple SC passage. The C954 had no metastatic properties. Retrospectively, it appears that Cloudman unintentionally selected for a tumor-line variant by only using the tumor stock from metastatic sites. The research compared the metastatic potential of the C198 line vs the nonmetastatic C954 line. In addition to a direct comparison between both tumor lines, by using various mouse strains, there was a demonstration of the different metastatic patterns (organophilic tendencies) attributable to the mouse strain being used. This led to the conclusion:

The appearance of tumor metastasis within a specific internal organ is probably dependent upon a host-tumor interrelationship rather than upon either the tumor type or the host type alone.

This is an important holistic approach to in vivo modeling. But strictly speaking, it was probably not a comparison of equal lines. The successful establishment of the tumor is attributed to both the tumor cell and the selected host.

In 1949, Coman et al. presented work, which in the context of Paget's hypothesis, discussed the apparent inability of the V2 rabbit carcinoma to metastasize to muscle *(8)*. By injecting tumor cells into the arterial circulation and demonstrating tumor growth in the muscle mass, the authors confirmed the ability of the tumor to recognize the tissue as favorable. In their conclusion, the reason for the apparent lack of tumors in certain organs was the result of a filtering effect by the lungs.

In 1950 and 1952, Zeidman studied important parameters for the use of a murine tumor line in vivo at the University of Pennsylvania *(9,10)*. Zeidman specifically studied the relationship between the number of viable tumor emboli iv-implanted and the total number of resulting metastatic nodules. In 1950, using the mouse Sarcoma 241 line, Zeidman concluded:

That the number of metastases is directly proportional to the number of viable tumor cell emboli released into the circulation. The longer a primary tumor existed the greater the number of emboli released, as judged by the number of metastases appearing in the lungs (9).

In his studies, the author also compared two rabbit tumor lines (V2 squamous-cell carcinoma (SCC), Brown-Pearce carcinoma) and one rat tumor line (Walker 256 carcinoma). One matter that still had to be resolved regarding iv injections of tumor cells related to the pulmonary disposition of tumor cells. Were the lungs acting as a mere sieve? To test this hypothesis, rabbits received an iv injection of tumor cells, while aortic outflow was captured. This collected blood was then iv-injected into a naive host; this second animal was then followed for tumor formation. Tumor formation in the second hosts demonstrated that tumor cells successfully passed through the pulmonary circulatory system. All three tumors were able to pass through the pulmonary vasculature and form tumors in the second host, thus negating the pulmonary sieve hypothesis.

In 1961, Zeidman used microcinematic techniques to further evaluate the flow patterns of tumor cells in circulation *(11)*. In this work, he demonstrated the higher degree of membrane flexibility/deformability of the Brown-Pearce tumor vs the V2 tumors. This work was done by studying the vascular patterns in the mesenteric vessels of rabbits. It illustrated how the Brown-Pearce cells, upon reaching an arteriolo-capillary junction, could deform and pass more freely than the V2 cells. This added to the body of evidence for the tumor's enhanced ability for transpulmonary passage, thus highlighting an intrinsic cellular difference between both lines.

Descriptive pathology and in vivo work, as many of the works presented here have been, continue to be essential for the development of our understanding of metastasis.

Even at the present time, in the era of genomics an attempt to elucidate the underlying biological forces involved in the dissemination of prostatic carcinoma required the careful evaluation of autopsies over 19,000 patients *(12)*. Approximately 1,500 cases of prostatic carcinoma were identified in this cohort. Of those cases, 35% showed evidence of metastatic spread. Interestingly, over 100 years after the seminal work of Dr. Paget, this paper offers an attempt to describe in detail the common metastatic patterns of dissemination found in prostatic carcinoma patients using autopsy records.

3. B16 MELANOMA

In the context of the Seed-Soil hypothesis, the use of the B16 murine melanoma line as a model for both solid-tumor formation and metastasis was an important development in oncology research. Although the introduction of this model for metastasis research can be traced to 1970, the cell line itself had been identified and characterized as a tumorigenic line years before. The B16 murine melanoma cell line originated in 1954. The tumor spontaneously arose in a C57BL/6J mouse at the Jackson Laboratories in Maine. There is no record of the sex of the originating mouse. The initial neoplastic lesion arose in the skin at the base of the ear. The following is a histological description of the tumor from the *Handbook on Genetically Standardized Jax Mice* by Dr. Earl Green:

> *Gross: soft gray tissue, frequently hemorrhagic. Microscopic: tumor cells polyhedral or spindle-shaped, arranged in perivascular mantles and diffuse masses; some cells contain fine pigmented granules, a few are obscured by large, very dark globules of pigment; stoma delicate and vascular. Pigment greatly decreased in comparison with early-transplant generation (13).*

This offers the first histological description of the tumor line in its host. The tumor line was maintained at the Jackson Laboratories by continuous passage in vivo. At the time of the report, the tumor is described as metastatic to lung, liver, and spleen. This metastatic pattern was present after sc implantation.

Using the B16 melanoma line from the Jackson Laboratories, Dr. Isaiah Fidler carefully documented the final disposition of the melanoma cells after iv injection in mice in 1970 *(14)*. A number of protocols used before this time to aid in the understanding of the metastatic process proved to be either cumbersome, unreliable, or both. There was an unmet need for a mouse line, and this line offered an important opportunity for the field. In the 1970 study, B16 murine melanoma cells were initially cultured in vitro. The cells used for iv injection were labeled with ^{125}I-5-iodo-2-deoxyuridine. This radioactive label provided a clear and specific way to monitor the organs in which tumor cells arrested. This ability to monitor cells was specifically caused by the affinity of the radioactive label for viable cells. Cell death would lead to the excretion of the label from the animal, thus precluding the possibility of labeling the host's tissues. The iv injection of killed labeled B16 cells served to demonstrate the inability of the host to reutilize the radioactive label, thus preventing a false-positive reading. In vitro, 200,000 labeled cells would produce an average of 40,000 counts per min. After inoculating the cells into naive hosts, the number of viable tumor cells in each organ was determined from radioactivity count, by the use of the ratio of cpms to cells in the original inoculum. Simple and efficient, the labeling of B16 murine melanoma cells could now open the door for the description of a complex tumor-host interaction. The B16 melanoma cells could now be iv-implanted and followed

Table 1
Fate of ^{125}IUDR-Labeled Tumor Emboli Organ Distribution of 200,000 ^{125}IUDR-Labeled
Melanoma Cells Injected Intravenously into C57BL/6J Mice

Time of death	Number of cells*					
	Lung	Liver	Spleen	Kidney	Blood+	Urine++
1 min	136,750	2,230	200	300	3,750	–
2 min	128,500	5,500	230	270	1,590	–
5 min	106,700	7,600	260	270	2,200	–
7 min	103,500	7,570	280	290	2,300	–
10 min	130,500	9,350	270	310	2,600	100
15 min	122,800	8,390	310	310	3,340	350
30 min	117,900	4,260	250	370	3,500	4,300
45 min	105,000	4,140	390	460	3,900	4,100
1 h	100,550	3,570	330	370	3,800	10,000
2 h	89,590	5,830	680	530	4,300	7,000
4 h	46,700	5,300	870	770	4,660	33,900
8 h	18,000	1,340	320	300	4,500	23,500
12 h	5,500	700	580	230	1,050	10,500
1 d	1,700	600	140	130	580	1,700
2 d	610	260	160	130	140	1,400
3 d	450	200	90	20	40	20
7 d	450	230	40	0	0	0
14 d	400	0	0	0	0	0

* Mean number of cells (20 mice per time interval)

+ 1.0 cc of blood

++ Urinary bladder and contained urine

in the host animal, providing a faster, less cumbersome method than the previously used histopathological approaches.

Tables 1 and 2 from the 1970 paper show the final organ of cellular arrest and temporal distribution of the viable/dead and labeled B16 murine melanoma cells after a single iv injection (14). From the table, it can be easily established that in the earliest postinjection time-points, the majority of the cells find themselves in the pulmonary tissue, but some are also localized in other organs. After 14 d, only the lungs contain labeled cells, now seen as tumor nodules. Liver, spleen, kidneys, and blood all showed the early presence of the labeled cells, but none of these tissues show the establishment of tumors at 14 d postinjection. Intravenously-injected B16 melanoma cells in mice could lead to rapid accumulation of cells in the pulmonary tissue, lead to early high levels of tumor cells in circulation caused by transpulmonary passage, or ultimately produce a very low rate of tumor formation in the animals. In the case of the B16 line, this tumor formation was limited to the pulmonary tissue. As a control, the author used killed B16 cells, which had had also been labeled with ^{125}I-5-iodo-2-deoxyuridine. Some of the obvious questions presented by this work include: Why are so few cells if the injected cells able to form tumors? Why such apparent inefficiency? How do the cells select the target organ for colonization? Again, in the case of the B16 tumor, the lungs were not acting as a passive sieve. This work demonstrated that the mere pres-

Table 2
Fate of [125]IUDR-Labeled Tumor Emboli Organ Distribution of 200,000 [125]IUDR-Labeled
Melanoma Cells Injected Intravenously into C57BL/6J Mice

Time of death	Number of cells*					
	Lung	Liver	Spleen	Kidney	Blood+	Urine++
1 min	96,700	4,860	40	120	2,314	–
2 min	97,250	5,420	100	570	845	–
5 min	99,600	4,810	90	120	1,190	–
10 min	91,700	5,700	300	270	2,070	345
15 min	64,400	4,000	220	200	2,600	380
30 min	41,500	9,300	420	590	5,600	3,530
45 min	19,500	12,430	900	930	6,790	20,060
1 h	2,100	8,800	940	740	9,340	25,000
2 h	550	1,700	450	435	13,200	24,500
4 h	200	2,310	640	360	4,010	22,290
8 h	0	750	330	0	1,950	7,260
24 h	0	40	120	0	100	190
2 d	0	30	40	0	0	120
7 d	0	0	0	0	0	60
14 d	0	0	0	0	0	0

* Mean number of cells (10 mice per time interval)

+ 1 cc of blood

++ Urinary bladder and contained urine

ence of neoplastic cells in the circulation of the mice is not a guarantee of successful tissue colonization by the tumor, confirming earlier work done with mouse Sarcoma 241 tumors in 1950 by Zeidman. *(9)*. The work with the B16 line is a good example of how research is done in the context of an already established scientific framework.

But strictly speaking, the process recapitulated in the B16 model is only representative of what happens to neoplastic cells, which have escaped a primary tumor into circulation. At this point in time, the iv model was not truly representative of the entire set of steps now established as requirements for a cell to leave the primary tumor and successfully colonize a distal site. In 1973, Dr. Fidler published another paper, which described a model for metastatic neoplasia using B16 melanoma cells iv-injected in syngeneic mice *(15)*. Until this time, metastatic tumor models usually relied on the desegregation of cells from solid tumors (a heterogeneous mixture of neoplastic and normal cells). This study focused on the relationship between the number of implanted cells, tumor emboli size, and the resulting pulmonary metastatic nodules. Cell selection was aided by the use of in vitro culturing of the cells in order to select the most optimal cell population for implantation. Building upon prior work by Zeidman, the author studied the effects of cell viability and cell clumping in the formation of pulmonary nodules (Tables 3 and 4). The value of this effort was as important as it was simple. Using the B16 line, the results demonstrate a proportional increase in lung metastasis formation in animals injected with higher numbers of cells. Although this is a rather intuitive point (and one previously tested) it served to solidify a base of knowledge around the B16 as a murine model. In the context of the contemporary studies, this

Table 3
Relationship of the Number of Viable B_{16} Melanoma Cells Injected I.V.
in C_{57} Mice to the Number of Resultant Pulmonary Metastases

Number of viable B_{16} cells iv-injected	Average number of pulmonary metastases* ± S.D.	
100	0.3	(0–1)
1,000	12.1 ± 3.4	(9–18)
10,000	71.6 ± 16.2	(52–96)
50,000	205.5 ± 34.3	(166–260)
100,000	394.8 ± 51.6	(338–502)

* Nine mice per each group. Pulmonary metastases were counted on d 14 post iv injection with the aid of a dissecting microscope

Table 4
The Effect of B_{16} Melanoma Embolic Sze
on Resultant Pulmonary Metastases in C_{57} Mice

Total number of embolic B_{16} cells iv-injected	Number of cells per embolic clump	Average number of resultant pulmonary metastases*± S.D.
50,000	1	11.5 ± 3.4 (5–14)
10,000–12,000	4–5	33.3 ± 8 (21–41)

* Eight mice per each group. Pulmonary metastases were counted on d 14 post iv injection with the aid of a dissecting microscope

effort established a standard to be followed by contemporary scientists. The careful selection of viable single cells in this model was again shown to be essential for the establishment of a reproducible model of in vivo metastasis. These 1970 and 1973 papers presented what should be considered, an introduction of the B16 tumor line to the scientific community (14,15). Importantly, the works themselves clarified an optimal protocol for the establishment of metastatic lesion in the lungs of C57-black mice, using a relatively simple technical procedure.

Also published in 1973, the process that gave rise to the B16 (F1, F10) sublines with different metastatic potentials. This was a short two-page paper with important ramifications (16). The work describes the in vivo-in vitro selection process used to identify cell variants with a high degree of preference for metastatic growth in the lungs. The experimental protocol started by sc implantation of the tumor cells into mice. The cells would grow into a tumor and spontaneously metastasize. The author then selected a resulting metastatic nodule from the lung. This tumor was dissociated and cultured as a monolayer in vitro. Upon expansion of the selected cells, these were then iv-implanted into a new host. Again, the resulting pulmonary nodules were harvested and cultured in vitro. After five cycles through the selection process, a line was derived. At this point the B16-F10 melanoma line had been specifically selected to metastasize to the lungs after iv injection. Table 5 shows the illustration used to explain the selection process. In 1973 Fidler concluded:

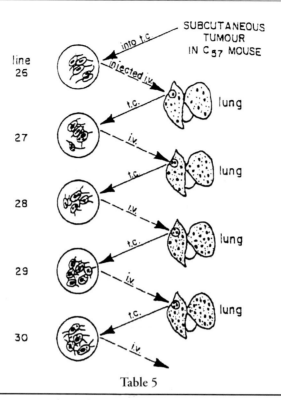

Table 5

Schematic representation of the tissue culture and animal transplantation system. The SC B_{16} melanoma tumor in the syngeneic mouse, C57Bl/6J, was adapted to grow in tissue culture as described previously *(2,3)*. Confluent monolayers of tumour cells were collected by 2-min treatment of 0.25% trypsin and vigorous shaking. Cell suspensions were diluted to give an inoculum dose of 50,000 viable cells (trypan blue excluding cells) in 0.25 ml. Hank's basic salt solution (HBSS). Mice were injected iv and were killed with ether 3 wk later, and submerged in consecutive washes of 7% iodine, 70% ethanol and sterile saline, and then placed in a laminar air flow hood. Their lungs, which contained melanoma nodules, were removed aseptically. Several pulmonary metastases were dissected free of the lungs, gently pressed through a number 70 stainless-steel mesh sieve and filtered through gauze. After centrifugation, the cells were resuspended in supplemented media[2], plated in several Petri dishes, and incubated at 37° C, 5% CO_2. Three to four days later, small colonies could be observed with the aid of an inverted microscope; one to five colonies with melanin granules were selected in each dish and their position marked. All other cells or colonies were removed by scraping and washed off with media. The selected attached colonies were incubated for an additional 3–5 d, then trypsinized, combined, and replated into $75C^2_m$ Falcon flasks (Falcon Plastics). When the cultures became confluent, cells were collected, diluted to 25,000 cells 0.25 ml.[-1], and injected iv into new C57 mice. Three weeks later, these mice were killed, and their pulmonary metastases adapted to grow in culture as described above. This procedure was repeated five times. The original line was designated as line No. 26 (our melanoma clone 26), and its daughter lines and their progenies designated as lines 27, 28, 29 and 30. T.c., Grown in tissue culture; injected intravenously.

As the tumour cell viability, size and homogeneity, and the syngeneic recipient did not change from one preparation to another, the differences in metastatic incidence could only be attributed to properties intrinsic to the various tumour cell lines. The clonal selection of tumours from successive metastases apparently results in cells better capable of survival and formation of secondary growths. This indicates that survival of circulating tumour emboli is not a random phenomenon (16).

Fifty years had passed since Dr. Leila Knox had proposed the criteria for an experimental murine model of metastasis.

The B16 model system was incorporated into the American Type Culture Collection in June 1978 (Mr. Andrew Redman personal communication). In the 1983 edition of the Catalog of Transplantable Animal and Human Tumors published by the Division of Cancer Treatment, National Cancer Institute (NCI) (Maryland, USA) a letter by Dr. Fidler is included *(17)*. This letter approves the distribution of the deposited B16 melanoma lines by the NCI. The catalog shows on the summary sheets for each tumor line that on October 11, 1979 the B16-F1, -F10, -F10[LR-6] and -BL-6 were incorporated into the tumor repository. At this point, this important model was available to the entire scientific community.

After the demonstration of the lung-colonizing ability of the B16-F10 lines, many in vivo lines were derived, using a similar selection approach. This approach of intravenous tumor cell administration would be followed for target organ seeding. Those tumors arising at the target organ would be selected and again reimplanted into fresh hosts, this would force a selection process. Examples of this methodology can be found in Brunson et al. 1978, Nicolson et al. 1978, and Nicolson 1978 *(18–20)*. These particular examples show how the selected lines would preferentially metastasize to the brains of C57 mice. The brain-colonizing lines were shown to invade the meninges or the forebrain (lines were designated B16-B10b or B10n). Line B16-B10n showed preference for cerebral vasculature. By this route, the cells would gain access to the cerebral cortex. In 1979, Brunson and Nicolson selected another variant of the B16 melanoma line. This time the selected lines would invade the ovarian tissue when implanted in mice *(21)*. An observation was made that the selection process produced a less melanotic cell line than the originating cells. This ovary-colonizing variant was designated the B17-010 line. In 1980, Raz and Hart used the cytochalasing B and colchicines as selection agents in the B16 melanoma to promote the cytoskeletal changes, which the authors suspected believed to be important in the development of differential patterns of metastases in this particular line *(22)*. The selected lines (designated B16-F10-B1, B2, and B3) the selected lines in addition to showing a higher capacity for brain colonization. The cells also showed an increased mean number of chromosomes when compared to the originating parental line. In addition to this selection process, which led to a line with higher propensity for brain colonization, the line also demonstrated a much higher rate of pulmonary growth when iv-injected. In 1988, another model of brain metastasis was presented using the B16 melanoma line *(23)*. This time, the B16 clones used produced metastatic spread to the brain parenchyma from the vessels found in the leptomeninges.

In 1988, Arguello et al., using the B16 melanoma line, were able to modify its injection into mice to produce a model of bone-marrow metastasis *(24)*. Injection of a relatively small number of cells into the left ventricle produced a metastatic pattern strongly directed to the axial skeleton and bone marrow. In the description of the metastatic pattern of the line, the authors commented: *Metastases were also commonly found in the proximal large bones of the extremities. No metastases were ever seen in the most distal small bones such as carpals and tarsals.*

This pattern of dissemination is reminiscent of the pattern described by Paget *(2)*. Now a model closely resembling the seminal work of Pagewas available with the B16 melanoma line.

In a recent publication by Dithmar et al., a novel selection of the B16 model was again demonstrated *(25)*. In this study, the B16-LS9 line selected by Rusciano et al. is used to establish a model of uveal melanoma in mice *(26)*. The transcorneal implantation method used produces extra-ocular metastasis to lung and liver tissue. This pattern is similar to the human uveal melanoma condition. Again, the use of the B16 line helped in the development of a model for human pathology.

Another area of cancer research that has directly benefited from the development of the B16 tumor line as a model for metastatic disease is cancer immunology. In some of the earliest work with the B16 melanoma line, Fidler and Ziedman studied the effect of host irradiation on the line's metastatic rate *(27)*. At that time, the increased metastatic rate of the cells in mice that had received whole-body irradiation was not attributed to immunodepression, but to endothelial-cell damage. This increased colonizing ability was referred to as "enhanced trapping effect." Interestingly, in their own discussion, the authors cite how previous work had demonstrated that the use of cortisone could also increase the metastatic ability of cells. It is likely that both the use of whole-body radiation and cortisone treatment of the animals also led to a degree of immunosuppression, which enhanced lung colonization by tumor cells. In some of the earliest studies of B16 melanoma cells and immune cells, the relationship between lymphocytes, macrophages, and B16 melanoma cells *(28–31)*. The direct repercussion of this work can be seen in the development of various methods used to activate the patient's own immune system against the circulating cancer cells. Specifically, it is seen in protocols that use muramyl dipeptide or muramyl tripeptide in a liposome-based vehicle for iv administration *(32–34)*. Through activation of tissue macrophages, an immune-mediated antitumor effect was elicited in vivo. This has led to a better understanding of the complex host-immune response to tumor cells.

The B16 melanoma line was also instrumental in expanding our knowledge of the ability of metastases to spread. With the use of parabiosis systems in mice, it was demonstrated that metastatic spread can originate from a metastatic nodule. In a clever experiment, a mouse was sc-implanted with B16 melanoma, and if this first animal underwent surgical removal of the primary tumor site (leg amputation) and was then surgically joined to a naive host, the naive host developed lung tumors. These lung tumors originated from metastatic nodules present in the first animal. This finding offers proof that once a solid tumor has successfully spread to other tissues, the metastatic cascade perpetuates itself in the host. This problem can serve to emphasize the basic problem with solid tumors: metastases present the biggest therapeutic challenge.

CONCLUSIONS

A recurring theme of this chapter is that the work that we now see as a final product is the summation of many people working at various points in time. This is evident from Paget's hypothesis in the late 1800s to the current development of newer models

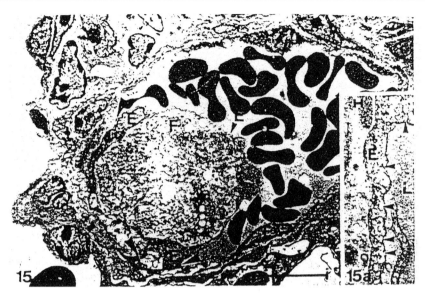

Fig. 1. An endothelialized thrombus attaching to the vessel wall (arrow heads), 24 h after inoculation of tumor cells. Part of a tumor cell (*) and E, endothelium.

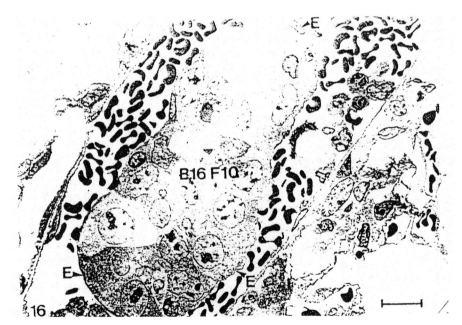

Fig. 2. A group of tumor cells completely surrounded by an endothelial covering (E) in the lumen of an arteriole, 2 wk after inoculation of tumor cells. Scale bar: 10μm, × 1060.

of metastasis *(2)*. As a final example, I would like to offer an image giving a visual description of the now commonly accepted tumor-cell endothelialization extravasation steps for the B16-F10 melanoma line (Figs. 1 and 2). Lapis et al. published this sophisticated microscopy work in 1988 *(35)*. This is a clear example of how a new technology

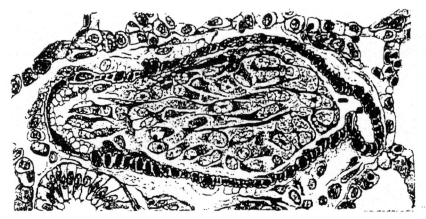

Fig. 3. Experiment 37/189 E: iv inocoulation, March 3, 1915; killed 3 d later. Commencing growth of a young sarcoma embolus. Vacuolation of endothelial cells is seen at one point, and early distension of the artery is indicated by flattening of the folds of the elastic laminoe. Cells resuming spindle shape. (×525.)

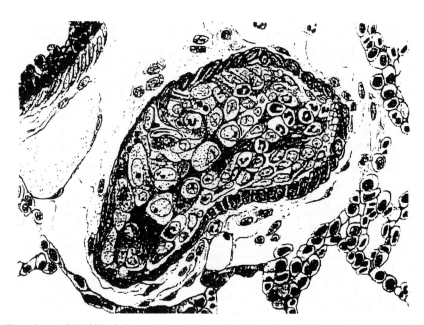

Fig. 4. Experiment 37/189B: iv inoculation, March 3, 1915; killed 5 d later. A later stage than Fig. 3. Increasing distension of vessel and entrance of capillaries into ombolus on left upper surface. (×525).

was able to shed light on ongoing scientific research. But microscopy work—specifically, studying the relationship between the endothelium and circulating tumor cells in a rodent model—can be traced to work presented in 1915 by Iwasaki (Fig. 3 and 4) *(5)*. While Iwasaki mostly studied human samples, a series of images were drawn of murine tumors cells interacting with the vasculature. Back in 1915, Iwasaki recognized that the importance of the tumor-endothelial interactions as essential for the establishment of the tumor embolus. In Lapi's paper, newer technologies are applied to answer old questions. Over 70 yrs had passed since the Iwasaki's description of extravasating tumor cells. At that time, two different reactions of the endothelium were noted, and contact of the tumor cell with the vessel wall would lead to either a separation of endothelial cell or an engulfment by the endothelial lining. The images here present us with a visual representation of works separated by many years, but of equal impact to our knowledge.

In conclusion, the success of the B16 melanoma tumor model is clearly evident today. As an in vivo model for solid tumor formation and metastasis, the B16 has fulfilled two important criteria presented earlier. The model has been instrumental in the dissection of the many steps now associated with tumor establishment and the metastatic cascade. A wide range of disciplines have originated from the use of this tumor line. The eventual relevance of the many sublines that have been selected so far still remains unclear. The development of the solid-tumor model is a dynamic process, and one that attempts to produce a very close representation of the disease process itself. Currently, orthotopic tumor implantation appears to be gaining favor in the scientific community. Knowledge regarding embolization, tumor-cell viability, cell number, organ of arrest, and host strain are all important basic concepts required for the refinement of solid-tumor models. Another important topic in the ultimate development of metastatic models is how the site of implantation of tumor cells in the host animal will influence the metastatic pattern in murine models. Whereas many of the murine tumors that are sc-implanted spread to limited organs (mostly lungs), tumors implanted orthotopically generally behave in a manner more consistent with the natural metastatic progression of the human counterpart for in-depth coverage on this topic. An argument has recently been made regarding the need to use the advanced orthotopic tumor models for the screening and development of chemotherapeutic agents (36,37). While the orthotopic models might provide the researcher with a model that more accurately depicts the natural history of the tumor, the model itself is more technically demanding and costly than syngeneic metastatic systems.

The knowledge gained from these efforts has directly led to the use of the B16 model to ask more questions regarding the nature of metastasis, with the added benefit of time to provide newer tools to answer such questions. It is also important to keep in mind that the overall selection and the acceptance of the model in the scientific community has been influenced by the already existing scientific framework of the time. The B16 melanoma tumor line has most definitely made a profound impact in the field of oncology research. It has served as a model for basic biological research, and has helped in the identification of distinct pathways now available as potential therapeutic targets.

DEDICATION

In memory of E. Gregory MacEwen, a dedicated teacher and friend. Your enthusiasm will live in us.

REFERENCES

1. Charlton Knox L. (1922). The relationship of massage to metastasis in malignant tumors. *Ann Surg* 1922; 75(2): 129–142.
2. Paget, S. Distribution of secondary growths in cancer of the breast. *Lancet* 1889; 571–573.

3. Hart I. 'Seed and soil' revisited: mechanisms of site-specific metastasis. *Cancer Metastasis Reviews* 1982; 1: 5–16.

4. Tyzzer E. Factors in the production and growth of tumor metastases. *Journal of Medical Research* 1913; 28: 309–333.

5. Iwasaki T. Histological and experimental observations on the destruction of tumor cells in the blood vessels. *J Pathol Bacteriol* 1915; 20: 85–105.

6. Warren S, Gates O. The fate of intravenously injected tumor cells. *American Journal of Cancer* 1936; 27: 485–492.

7. Cloudman A. Organophilic tendencies of two transplantable tumors of the mouse. *Cancer Res* 1947; 7: 585–591.

8. Coman D, Eisneberg RB, McCutcheon M. Factors affecting the distribution of tumor metastases experiments with V2 carcinoma of the rabbit. *Cancer Res* 1949; 9: 649–654.

9. Ziedman I, McCutcheon M, Coman DL. Factors affecting the number of tumor metastases. Experiments with a transplantable mouse tumor. *Cancer Res* 1950; 10: 357–359.

10. Ziedman I., Buss JM. Transpulmonary passage of tumor cell emboli. *Cancer Res* 1952; 12: 731–733.

11. Ziedman I. The fate of circulating tumor cells I. Passage of cells through capillaries. *Cancer Res* 1961; 21: 38–39.

12. Bubendorf L, Schopfer A, Wagner U, Sauter G, Moch M, Willi N, et al. Metastatic patterns of prostate cancer: an autopsy study of 1589 patients. *Hum Pathol* 2000; 31(5): 578–583.

13. Green E. *Handbook of genetically standardized JAX mice.* The Jackson Laboratory, Bar Harbor, ME, 1968, p. 57, 58.

14. Fidler I. Metastasis: quantitative analysis of distribution and fate of tumor emboli labeled with 125I-5-iodo-2′-deoxyuridine. *J Natl Cancer Inst* 1970; 45(4): 773–782.

15. Fidler I. The relationship of embolic homogeneity, number, size and viability to the incidence of experimental metastasis. *Eur J Cancer* 1973; 9: 223–227.

16. Fidler I. Selection of successive tumour lines for metastasis. *Natl New Biol* 1973; 242(148–149).

17. National Cancer Institute, Division of Cancer Treatment Tumor Repository: Catalogue of transplantable animal and human tumors. Frederick, National Cancer Institute, 1983.

18. Brunson K, Beattie G, Nicolson GL. Selection and altered properties of brain-colonising metastatic melanoma. *Nature* 1978; 272: 543–546.

19. Nicolson G, Bronson KW, Fidler IJ. (1978). Specificity of arrest, survival and growth of selected metastatic variant lines. *Cancer Res* 1978; 38: 4105–4111.

20. Nicolson G. Experimental tumor metastasis: characteristics and organ specificity. *BioScience* 1978; 28: 441–447.

21. Brunson K, Nicolson GL. Selection of malignant melanoma variant cell lines for ovary colonization. *J Supramo Struct* 1979; 11: 517–528.

22. Raz A, Hurt IR. Murine melanoma: a model for intracranial metastasis. *Br J Cancer* 1980; 42: 331–341.

23. Alterman A, Stackpole CH. B16 melanoma spontaneous brain metastasis: occurrence and development within leptomeninges blood vessels. *Clin Expl Metastasis* 1989; 7(1): 15–23.

24. Arguello F, Baggs RB, Frantz CN. A murine model of experimental metastasis to bone and bone marrow. *Cancer Res* 1988; 48: 6876–6881.

25. Dithmar S, Rusciano D, Grossniklaus HE. A new technique for implantation of tissue culture melanoma cells in a murine model of metastatic ocular melanoma. *Melanoma Res* 2000; 10: 2–8.

26. Rusciano D, Logenzoni P, Burger MM. Murine models of liver metastasis. *Invasion Metastasis* 1994; 14: 349–361.

27. Fidler I, Ziedman I. Enhancement of experimental metastasis by x-ray: a possible mechanism. *J Med* 1972; 3: 172–177.

28. Fidler I. Inhibition of pulmonary metastasis by intravenous injection of specifically activated macrophages. *Cancer Res* 1974; 34: 1074–1078.

29. Fidler I. Immune stimulation-inhibition of experimental cancer metastasis. *Cancer Res* 1974; 34: 491–498.

30. Fidler I, Darnell JH, Budmen MB. Tumoricidal properties of mouse macrophages activated with mediators from rat lymphocytes stimulated with concanavalin A. *Cancer Res* 1976; 36: 3608–3615.

31. Fidler IJ, Bucana C. Mechanism of tumor cell resistance to lysis by syngeneic lymphocytes. *Cancer Res* 1977; 37: 3945–3956.

32. Fidler IJ. Therapy of disseminated melanoma by liposome-activated macrophages. *World J. Surg* 1992; 16: 270–276.
33. Killion J, Fidler IJ. Systemic targeting of liposome-encapsulated immunomodulators to macrophages for treatment of cancer metastasis. *Imm Meth* 1994; 4: 273–279.
34. Killion J, Fidler IJ. Therapy of cancer metastasis by tumoricidal activation of tissue macrophages using liposome-encapsulated immunomodulators. *Pharmacol Ther* 1998; 78(3): 141–154.
35. Lapis K, Paku S, Liotta LA. Endothelialization of embolized tumor cells during metastasis formation. *Clin Expl Metastasis* 1988; 6(1): 73–89.
36. Kerbel R. What is the optimal rodent model for anti-tumor drug testing? *Cancer Metastasis Rev* 1999; 17: 301–304.
37. Killion J, Radinsky R, Fidler IJ. Orthotopic models are necessary to predict therapy of transplantable tumors in mice. *Cancer Metastasis Rev* 1999; 17: 279–284.

III HUMAN TUMOR XENOGRAFTS

5

Xenotransplantation of Human Cell Cultures in Nude Mice

Beppino Giovanella, PhD

The first successful xenotransplant of cultured human cells in nude mice was achieved by Giovanella et al. (1), who inoculated a suspension of melanoma cells subcutaneously in a nude mouse. This result was confirmed and extended by the same author (Giovanella et al. (2,3) and by others (4–9).

Further studies demonstrated that cultured tumor cells had a much higher rate of takes when inoculated into nude mice than human solid tumors of the same histological type that were transplanted directly from the patient. For example, human breast carcinoma has a 6% take-rate in Swiss nude mice (Giovanella et al.) *(10)*, but cell lines derived from human breast carcinomas took in 50% of the cases. The quantitation of such procedures has been limited. By inoculating serial dilutions of cell suspensions, Giovanella demonstrated that human tumors require at least 1×10^3 cells and frequently more for a significant percentage of takes, whereas 1×10^2 or less is sufficient with murine tumors.

Malignant cells grow in nude mice, but normal cells do not. This definition of cell malignancy was put forth by Giovanella in 1974 *(11),* based on a series of experiments that demonstrated lack of growth of actively proliferating cell cultures derived from normal tissues vs active growth of many tissue-cultured cell lines derived from human tumors after inoculation of both into nude mice. This observation was confirmed on many more cell cultures and cell lines by Giovanella and others *(2,5,12–15).*

A logical corollary of this finding was to use subcutaneous (sc) inoculation of human or animal cells into nude mice to test for their neoplastic transformation. If these cells grew into a tumor, they were considered neoplastic. If they did not grow, they were classified as nonneoplastic. This test greatly helped the oncological virologists and the molecular biologists to differentiate between viruses and plasmids that produced only morphological and/or biological transformation of a cell line or culture from the ones that were capable of full malignant transformation. These characteristics made the nude mouse into one of the most used tools for the study of in vitro carcinogenesis.

However, it is important to caution against too literal an interpretation of such results. Thus, if a cell line produces a tumor after sc inoculation of $\sim1\times10^6$ cells in nude mice, it is undoubtedly neoplastic. However, several cell lines derived from malignant tumors do not grow in this manner after inoculation in nude mice. Others do

From: *Tumor Models in Cancer Research*
Edited by: B. A. Teicher © Humana Press Inc., Totowa, NJ

not grow if early passages are inoculated, but later passages produce tumors. The most extensively studied of these cell lines is PA 1, a teratocarcinoma line derived from the ascitic fluid obtained from a terminal patient with an ovarian germline tumor *(2,16–17)*. Cultured in vitro, these ascites cells exhibited the characteristics of embryonal cell lines. Early passages grew slowly in culture, and sometimes formed slow-growing tumors when 1–3 million cells were inoculated into nude mice. These tumors histologically resemble more well-differentiating teratomas than teratocarcinomas. The growth rate of these cells in vitro increased with successive passages, until they grew very rapidly. However, from passage 30–90, they did not produce tumors in nude mice, even after inoculation of 10 million cells. After passage 90, PA 1 cells again became tumorigenic, forming malignant teratocarcinomas in 100% of the inoculated nude mice. All the cells of this line are near-diploid. The spontaneous transformation is a reproducible phenomenon.

Transfection experiments with DNA from passage 100 or higher reproducibly gave rise to highly transformed foci of (NIH-3T3) cells. Conversely, transfection experiments with DNA from nontumorigenic early passages never produced transformed foci. The transforming oncogene was identified as N-*ras,* with an activating point mutation at amino-acid position 12 *(18–20)*. Finally, a nontumorigenic clone of PA 1 isolated at passage 63 became highly tumorigenic when transfected with the activated *ras* gene obtained from the DNA of PA 1, passage 330 *(18–20)*. In this case, the inoculation in nude mice clearly differentiated fully neoplastic cells from cells that were only immortalized and preneoplastic before N-*ras* activation.

A similar yet lesser-known cell line is HBL 100 *(21–24)*. This cell line, unlike PA 1, was obtained from presumably normal human cells. It originated from a culture of human epithelial breast cells obtained by centrifuging the normal milk of a lactating woman with no history of cancer. Normal milk cells attach, but do not reproduce, when cultured under standard conditions. Afterwards, they survive and metabolize. However, this particular culture proliferated and expanded, was passaged, and proved to be aneuploid and immortal. Cancer was never detected in the donor. Early passages did not give rise to tumors after inoculation into nude mice, but later passages did. This cell line is now rapidly growing in vitro and tumor-producing in vivo.

It is probable that a similar mechanism applies to other cells obtained from malignant tumors that grow well in tissue culture, but do not take as tumors after inoculation into nude mice. For example, Cailleau grew human breast-carcinoma cells from pleural effusates in tissue culture *(25,26)*. These cells are derived from a malignant tumor, are metastatic, and are adapted to life in an effusate. In every sense, they should be considered highly malignant cells. However, when we inoculated 14 such cell lines into nude mice, only seven gave rise to progressively growing tumors. Seven did not grow at all *(10)*. Lack of growth in nude mice is a fairly common occurrence in breast-cancer-derived cell lines (apart from the Cailleau series, 5 of 15 of the breast-cancer-derived cell lines in our repository do not grow in nude mice), and even more in ovarian-cancer-cell lines. It is, however, a rare occurrence in cell lines derived from other cancers. Should these cells be considered homologous to preneoplastic aneuploid cells as Li-Fraumeni fibroblasts *(27)?* Probably, but we cannot be certain because of a further complicating factor. Cells, in order to form tumors, must be "neoplastic," but they also must not be immunologically rejected. It is not easy to differentiate between the two events.

For example, human lymphocytes are nondividing and nonneoplastic under normal conditions. However, if they are cultured in presence of transforming Epstein-Barr Virus (EBV) *(28),* they divide indefinitely, becoming immortalized lymphoblasts. These lymphoblasts do not grow when inoculated subcutaneously into nude mice *(29–30).* However, if they are inoculated intracerebrally, they give rise to rapidly lethal B-cell lymphomas in 100% of the inoculated animals *(31).* If the same cells are inoculated in the brain of nonnude mice, no growth is observed, suggesting immunological rejection as an explanation for their failure to grow subcutaneously in adult nude mice. This hypothesis is supported by the observation that newborn nude mice inoculated subcutaneously with LCL develop tumors which regress at age 7–10 d when Natural Killer (NK) cells become active.

Lymphoblastoid cell lines (LCL) are diploid. However, after some time in culture, they become aneuploid. At this point, some LCL become capable of producing tumors after sc inoculation in nude mice. Are they doing this because they have lost the antigen that caused their rejection or because they have become more "malignant?"

Tumor cells growing in culture frequently have a good plating efficiency, and are relatively easy to clone. Cloning ability is considered to be related to the ability to metastasize. Metastases originate from single cells or small groups of cells. Using suspensions of human cultured cancer cells, artificial metastases have indeed been produced.

Inoculation of human tumor-cell suspensions into the spleen produces liver metastases with a high frequency using tumors (colon carcinoma in the specific case) selected for liver implantation (intrasplenic inoculation, which produces a few liver metastases—one of them is cultured and these cells re-inoculated into the spleen). With proper selection, it is possible to obtain cell lines that will metastasize almost exclusively to the liver and cause numerous micrometastases. Such metastases grow rapidly and kill the animal in 2–3 wk by almost complete replacement of the hepatic parenchyma with neoplastic cells *(32).*

The iv inoculation of cultured cell suspensions has been widely used in the hope of obtaining pulmonary metastases. Curiously, this rarely happens. The majority of cell lines do not give rise to pulmonary metastases after iv inoculation of several millions of cells. Only a few cell lines produce metastases, most with very low frequency. No sustained effort to select for highly metastatic cells has ever been made.

Inoculation in to the left heart has proven to be a very useful route for determining the specific organotropism of the inoculated cells *(33).* After left-heart inoculation of radiolabeled cells, these were distributed through the body according to the volume of blood flowing through the peripheral capillary bed of the organ studied. However, the appearance of metastases and their location did not depend on the distribution of the cancer cells, but purely on their biological characteristics. Using a melanoma clone, not a single metastases was observed in muscle, liver and lung, the three sites where the largest number of tumor cells was detected. On the contrary, it was possible to isolate two subclones—one specific for the adrenals and another for the brain—both derived from the same tumor. By serial dilutions, it was possible to demonstrate that such metastases originated from only one—or at most, a few—cells. Because the same cells will grow almost everywhere in the body when more than 1×10^5 cells are inoculated, but only in the adrenals or the brain, if less than 10 are used, the only logical explanation is that in this location there is present a growth factor necessary for the growth of such cells. A corollary of this hypothesis is that such a factor is secreted also by the cells themselves, but at very low levels. Thus, only when more than 1×10^5 are present is an effective concentration reached.

REFERENCES

1. Giovanella BC, Yim SO, Stehlin JS, Williams LJ, Jr. Development of invasive tumors in the "nude" mouse after injection of cultured human melanoma cells. *J Natl Cancer Inst* 1972; 48: 1531–1533.
2. Giovanella BC, Stehlin JS, Williams LJ. Heterotransplantation of human malignant tumors in "nude" mice. II. Malignant tumors induced by injection of cell cultures derived from human solid tumors. *J Natl Cancer Inst* 1974; 52: 921–930.
3. Giovanella BC, Stehlin JS, Santamaria C, Yim SO, Morgan AC, Williams LJ Jr., et al. Human neoplastic and normal cells in tissue culture. I. Cell lines derived from malignant melanomas and normal melanocytes. *J Natl Cancer Inst* 1976; 55: 1131–1142.
4. Freedman V, Shin S. Cellular Tumorigenicity in nude mice: correlation with cell growth in semi-solid medium. *Cell* 1974; 3: 355–359.
5. Freedman V, Shin S. Isolation of human diploid cell variants with enhanced colony-forming efficiency in semi-solid medium after a single-stem chemical mutagenesis. *J Natl Cancer Inst* 1977; 58: 1873–1875.
6. Freedman VH, Shin S. In: Fogh J, Giovanella B, eds. *Use of Nude Mice for Studies on the Tumorigenicity of Animal Cells,* Vol. 1. Academic Press, New York, NY, 1978, pp. 353–384.
7. Stiles D, Desmond W, Sato G, Saier M Jr. Failure of human cells transformed by simian virus 40 to form tumors in athymic nude mice. *PNAS* 1975; 72: 4971–4975.
8. Shin S, Freedman VH. Neoplastic growth of animal cells in nude mice. In: Nomura, T, Ohsawa N, Tamaoki N, Fujiwara K, eds. *Proc. 2nd* Int. Workshop on Nude Mice. pp. 337–349; U Tokyo Press, Tokyo, 1977.
9. Stiles CD, Kawahara AA. The Growth Behavior of Virus-Transformed Cells in Nude Mice. In: Fogh J, Giovanella BC, eds. *The Nude Mouse in Experimental and Clinical Research.* Academic Press, NY, 1978, pp. 385–409.
10. Giovanella, BC, Vardeman DM, Williams LJ, Taylor DJ, PD, et al. Heterotransplantation of human breast carcinomas in nude mice: correlation between nude takes, poor prognosis and overexpression of the HER-2/neu Oncogene. *Int J Cancer* 1991; 47: 66–71.
11. Giovanella BC, Stehlin JS. Assessment of the Malignant Potential of Cultured Cells by Injection in "Nude" Mice. In: Rygaard J, Povlsen C, eds. Proceedings of the 1st International Workshop on "Nude" Mice. Fischer Verlag, Heidelburg, Germany 1974, pp. 279–284.
12. Giovanella BC, Fogh J. Present and future trends in investigations with the nude mouse as a recipient of human tumor transplants. In: Fogh J, Giovanella BC, eds. *The Nude Mouse in Experimental and Clinical Research.* Academic Press, New York, NY, 1978, pp. 282–312.
13. Stiles CD, Desmond W, Chuman LM, Sato G, Saier MH Jr. Growth control of heterologous tissue culture cells in the congenitally athymic nude mouse. *Cancer Res* 1976; 36: 1353–1360.
14. Belewo J, Freedman VH, Shin S. Growth of murine sarcoma-virus transformed rat kidney cells in nude mice. *J Natl Cancer Inst* 1977; 58: 1691–1694.
15. Chen LB, Galimore PH, McDougall JD. Correlation between tumor induction and the large external transformation sensitive protein on the cell surface. *PNAS* 1976; 73: 3570–3574.
16. Giovanella BC, Stehlin JS, Yim SO. Establishment and characterization of a permanent cell line from a human teratocarcinoma. *In Vitro* 1974; 10: 382.
17. Zeuthen J, Norgaard JOR, Aner P, Fellous M, Wartiovaara J, Vaneri A, et al. Characterization of a human ovarian teratocarcinoma cell line. *Int J Cancer* 1980; 25: 19–32.
18. Tainsky MA, Cooper CS, Giovanella BC, Vande Woude GF. An activated ras^N gene: detected in late but not early passage human PA 1 teratocarcinoma cells. *Science* 1984; 225: 643–645.
19. Tainsky F, Shamanski D, Blair D, Giovanella BC. Causal Role for an Activated N-ras Oncogene in the Induction of Tumorigenicity Acquired by a Human Cell Line. *Cancer Res* 1987; 47: 3235–3238.
20. Tainsky MA, Krizman DB, Chiao PJ, Yim SO, Giovanella BC. PA-1A human cell model for multistage carcinogenesis: oncogens and other factors. *Anticancer Res* 1988; 8: 899–914.
21. Gaffney E, Polanowski FP, Blackburn SE, Lambiase JP. Origin, concentration and structural features of human mammary cells cultured from breast secretions. *Cell Tissue Res* 1976; 172: 269–279.

22. Giovanella BC, Gaffney EV, Yim SO, Stehlin JS. Increase of malignant potential of human line HBL 100 with long-term Passage in vitro. *In Vitro* 1980; 16: 211.

23. Gaffney EV. A cell line (HBL 100) established from breast milk. *Cell tissue Res* 1982; 227: 563–568.

24. Dhaliwal MK, Giovanella BC, Pathak S. Cytogenetic characterization of two human milk-derived cell line (HBL-100) passages differing in tumorigenicity. *Anticancer Res* 1990; 10: 113–118.

25. Cailleau R, Olive MD, Cruciger QV. Long-term human breast carcinoma cell lines of metastatic origin: preliminary characterization. *In Vitro* 1978; 14: 911–915.

26. Cailleau R, Young R, Olive M, Reeves WJ, Jr. Breast tumor cell lines from pleural effusates. *J Natl Cancer Inst* 1974; 53: 661–674.

27. Bischoff FZ, Yim SO, Pathak S, Grant G, Siciliano MJ, Giovanella BC, et al. Spontaneous abnormalities in normal fibroblasts from patients with Li-Fraumeni Cancer Syndrome: aneuploidy and immortalization. *Cancer Res* 1990; 50: 7979–7984.

28. Nilsson K. Establishment of permanent human lymphoblastoid cell lines in vitro. In: David J, Bloom BR, eds. *In Vitro Methods in Cell Mediated Tumor Immunity.* Academic Press, New York, NY, 1976, pp. 713–721.

29. Nilsson K, Giovanella BC, Stehlin JS, Klein G. Tumorigenicity of human hematopoietic cell lines in athymic nude mice. *Int J Cancer* 1976; 19: 337–344.

30. McCormick KJ, Giovanella BC, Klein G, Nilsson K, Stehlin JS. Diploid human lymphoblastoid and Burkitt lymphoma cell lines: susceptibility to murine NK cells and heterotransplantation to nude mice. *Int J Cancer* 1981; 28: 455–458.

31. Giovanella BC, Nilsson K, Zech L, Yim SO, Klein G, Stehlin JS. Growth of diploid, Epstein-Barr Virus carrying human lymphoblastoid cell lines heterotransplanted into nude mice under immunologically privileged conditions. *Int J Cancer* 1979; 24: 103–113.

32. Potmesil M, Vardeman D, Kozielski AJ, Mendoza J, Stehlin JS, Giovanella BC. Growth inhibition of human cancer metastases by camptothecins in newly developed xenograft models. *Cancer Res* 1995; 55: 5637–5641.

33. Verschraegen C, Giovanella BC, Mendoza JT, Kozielski AJ, Stehlin JS, Jr. Specific organ metastases of human melanoma cells injected into the arterial circulation of nude mice. *Anticancer Res* 1991; 11: 529–536.

6

GFP-Expressing Metastatic-Cancer Mouse Models

Robert M. Hoffman, PhD

CONTENTS

INTRODUCTION
METHODS
REFERENCES

1. INTRODUCTION

The visualization of tumor invasion and micrometastasis formation in viable fresh tissue or the live animal is necessary for a critical understanding of tumor progression and its control. However, the visualization of individual tumor cells in vivo has not been possible because of the lack of a sufficient marker. Previous studies used transfection of tumor cells with the *Escherichia coli (E. coli)* beta-galactosidase (lacZ) gene to detect micrometastases *(1,2)*. Detection of lacZ, however, requires extensive histological preparation, and therefore it has not been possible to detect and visualize tumor cells in viable fresh tissue or the live animal at the microscopic level.

To allow visualization of micrometastases in fresh tissue, we have utilized the green fluorescent protein (GFP) gene, cloned from the bioluminescent jellyfish *Aequorea victoria (3)*. GFP has demonstrated its potential for use as a marker for gene expression in a variety of cell types *(4,5)*. The GFP cDNA encodes a 283-amino-acid polypeptide with a mol wt of 27 *K*d *(6,7)*. The monomeric GFP requires no other *Aequorea* proteins, substrates, or cofactors to fluoresce *(8)*. Recently, GFP gene gain-of-function mutants have been generated by various techniques *(9–12)*. For example, the GFP-S65T clone has the serine-65 codon substituted with a threonine codon, which results in a single excitation peak at 490 nm *(9)*. Moreover, to develop higher expression in human and other mammalian cells, a humanized hGFP-S65T clone was isolated *(13)*. The much brighter fluorescence in the mutant clones allows for easy detection of GFP expression in transfected cells.

We have isolated more than 50 GFP transfectants of human and animal cancer cells that are stable in vitro and in vivo *(14–19)*. The transfectants are highly fluorescent in vivo in tumors formed from the cells. Using these fluorescent transfectants, orthotopic-transplant animal models *(18–22)* were utilized for visualizing the metastatic processes in fresh tissue down to the single-cell level, as well as by whole-body imaging that was not previously possible.

From: *Tumor Models in Cancer Research*
Edited by: B. A. Teicher © Humana Press Inc., Totowa, NJ

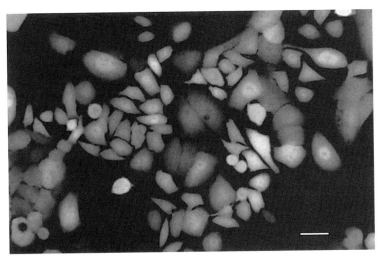

Fig. 1. Confocal micrograph of subclone of lung-cancer-cell line ANIP epxressing GFP in vitro. Cells were transfected with the dicistronic GFP expression vector pED-MTX^r. Cells were selected in methotrexate (MTX). GFP-expressing cells pictured above were able to growth in 50 nm MTX *(15)*.

1.1. Isolation of Stable High-Level Expression GFP Transductant Tumor-cell Lines

For isolation of very bright GFP-expressing tumor cells, the concentration of a selective agent, such as G418, is increased gradually up to 800–1200 µg/ml for selection of clones with increased expression of GFP. Bright GFP clones are then selected in the absence of antibiotic (Fig. 1) as a basis for stable high GFP expression in vivo *(18)*.

The stability of CHO-K1-GFP cells maintained in the presence vs absence of a selective agent over a 24-d period in vitro has been quantified. For cells grown in the presence of the selective agent, the median fluorescence intensity at d 3 was 105 (arbitrary units) compared to 81 *u* at d 24. In the absence of selective agents, cells showed a median fluorescence intensity of 95 *u,* similar to that of cells maintained under selective pressure at d 24. Thus, the GFP expression of the cells was sufficiently stable to permit visualization in vivo, even in the absence of selective pressure. Nonfluorescent cells were not detected among cells maintained with or without selective agents *(28)*.

1.2. GFP-Expressing Macro- and Micrometastases Using CHO Cells in Orthotopic Models

Nude mice were implanted into the ovary with 1-mm^3 cubes of stable-high-GFP-expression CHO-K1, that previously grew subcutaneously in nude mice *(14)*. All mice had tumors in the ovaries. The tumor subsequently spread throughout the peritoneal cavity, including the colon, cecum, small intestine, spleen, and peritoneal wall. The primary tumor and peritoneal metastases were strongly fluorescent. Numerous micrometastases were detected by fluorescence on the lungs of all mice. Multiple micrometastasis were also detected by fluorescence on the liver, kidney, contralateral ovary, adrenal gland, para-aortic lymph node, and pleural membrane down to the single-cell level. Single-cell micrometastases could not be detected by standard histological techniques. Even multiple-cell small colonies were difficult to detect by hematoxylin and eosin staining, but they could be detected and visualized clearly through GFP fluorescence.

Chinese homster ovary cells (CHO) proved to be highly metastatic from both the subcutaneous (sc) and orthotopic sites, as brightly visualized by GFP fluorescence. Metastases were visualized by GFP expression in the lung, pleural membrane, spleen, kidney, ovary, adrenal gland, and peritoneum after orthotopic implantation in nude mice. Metastases were visualized by GFP expression, mainly in the lung and pleural membrane after sc implantation in nude mice. Metastases were visualized in the lung and pleural membrane, liver, kidney, and ovary after sc implantation in (SCID) mice *(23)*.

1.3. Patterns of Contralateral and Regional Lung Tumor Metastases Visualized by GFP Expression in Orthotopic Models

The primary tumor grew in the implanted left lung in all mice after surgical orthotopic implantation (SOI) of GFP-transfected ANIP–973. GFP expression allowed visualization of the advancing margin of the tumor spreading throughout the ipsilateral lung. All animals explored had evidence of chest-wall invasion, and local and regional spread. Metastatic contralateral tumors involved the mediastinum, contralateral pleural cavity, and the contralateral visceral pleura. While the ipsilateral tumor had a continuous and advancing margin, the contralateral tumor seems to have been formed by multiple seeding events. These observations were made possible by the stable, high-GFP fluorescence of the tumor cells *(15,16)* (Fig. 1). Contralateral hilar lymph nodes were also involved, as well as cervical lymph nodes visualized by GFP expression *(15,16)*. When non-GFP-transfected ANIP was compared with GFP-transformed ANIP for metastatic capability similar results were seen *(15)*.

1.4. GFP-Expressing Bone Metastases of Lung Cancer in Orthotopic Models

Nude mice were implanted in the left lung by SOI with 1-mm^3 cubes of H460-GFP tumor tissue derived from an H460-GFP sc tumor *(18)*. The implanted mice were sacrificed at 3–4 wk at the time of significant decline in performance status. GFP fluorescence demonstrated metastases in the left lung, the contralateral lung, the chest wall, and the skeletal system. It was determined by GFP fluorescence that the vertebrae (Fig. 2) were the most involved skeletal site of metastasis. Metastasis could also be visualized in the tibia and femur marrow by GFP fluorescence *(18)*.

1.5. Prostate-Cancer Bone and Visceral Metastasis Visualized by GFP in Orthotopic Models

A stable high GFP expression clone of human prostate carcinoma PC-3 was orthotopically implanted surgically in nude mice. Subsequent skeletal metastasis included the skull (Fig. 3), rib, pelvis, femur, and tibia. All the tumors metastasized to the lung, pleural membrane, and kidney. Four of five tumors metastasized to the liver, and two of five tumors metastasized to the adrenal gland. In two mice, cancer cells or small colonies were seen in the brain, and in one mouse, a few cells could be seen in the spinal cord by GFP fluorescence *(19)*.

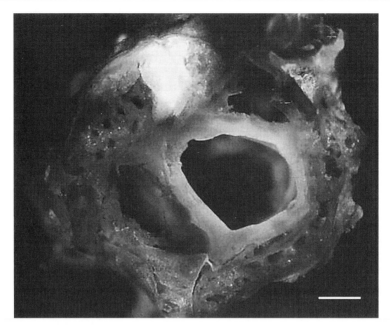

Fig. 2. Lumbar vertebral metastasis in nude mouse after orthotopic transplantation of GFP-express-ing human lung-cancer line H-460 transfected with GFP retrovirus pLEIN and selected in G418 *(18)*.

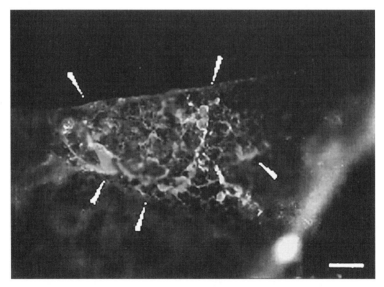

Fig. 3. Skull metastasis of GFP-expressing human prostate carcinoma PC-3 orthotopically trans-planted in nude mice. PC-3 was transduced with the GFP retrovirus pLEIN and selected in G418 *(19)*.

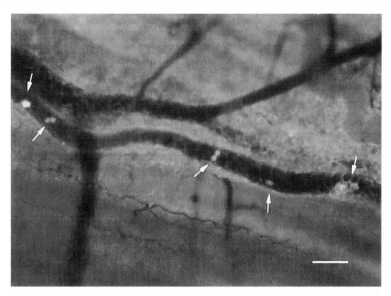

Fig. 4. GFP-expressing CHO-K1 cells in a peritoneal vessel 2 min after tail-vein injection in nude mice. CHO-K1 cells were transduced with the dicistronic GFP vector. pED-MTX^r and selected in MTX *(14).*

1.6. GFP-Expressing Experimental Metastases in Nude Mice

CHO-K1 GFP transfectants injected via the tail vein were visualized by GFP expression in the peritoneal wall vessels down to the single-cell level *(14)* (Fig. 4). These cells formed emboli in the capillaries of the lung, liver, kidney, spleen, ovary, adrenal gland, thyroid gland, and brain.

ANIP GFP cells were injected into the tail vein of nude mice, which were sacrificed at 4 and 8 wk. In both groups, numerous micrometastatic colonies were detected in the whole-lung tissue by GFP expression in fresh tissue *(16).* Even 8 wk after injection, in most of the mice colonies were not obviously further developed as compared to mice sacrificed at 4 wk *(16).* Numerous small colonies, which ranged in size down to less than 10 cells, were detected at the lung surface in both groups. After 8 wk, metastases in the brain (Fig. 5), the submandibular gland, the lung, the pancreas, the bilateral adrenal glands, the peritoneum, and the pulmonary hilum lymph nodes were visualized by GFP expression. Actively colonizing as well as dormant tumor cells were visualized in the lung *(16).* Dormant micrometastasis is one of the most important steps in tumor progression *(24).* In recent studies, the mechanism of this important phenomenon was studied with regard to angiogenesis and other chemical regulators of tumor colonization *(24).* However, these experimental models did not allow direct observation of the dormant colonies in fresh, live tissue as it occurs over time, as do the GFP studies.

1.7. Genetically Fluorescent Melanoma Bone and Organ Metastasis Models

We have characterized metastatic properties of bright, highly stable GFP-expression transductants of the B16 mouse malignant-melanoma cell line and LOX human melanoma line *(29).* The highly fluorescent malignant-melanoma cell lines allowed the

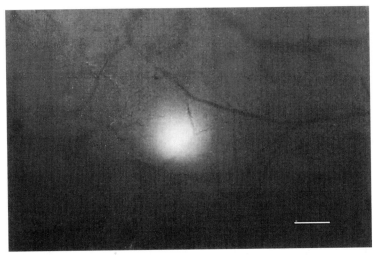

Fig. 5. Brain metastasis of GFP-expressing ANIP-973 human lung-cancer cells 8 wk after tail-vein injection in nude mice *(16)*.

visualization of skeletal and multi-organ metastases after intravenous (iv) injection of B16 cells in C57BL/6 mice and intradermal (id) injection of LOX in nude mice. The melanoma cell lines were transduced with the pLEIN-expression retroviral vector containing the GFP and neomycin resistance genes. Extensive bone (Fig. 6) and bone-marrow metastases of B16F0 were visualized by GFP expression when the animals were sacrificed after 3 wk after cell implantation. This is the first observation of experimental skeletal metastases of melanoma, which was made possible by GFP expression. For both cell lines, metastases were visualized in many other organs, including the brain, lung (Fig. 7), pleural membrane, liver, kidney, adrenal gland, lymph nodes (Fig. 8), muscle, and skin by GFP fluorescence.

1.8. Whole-Body Fluorescence Optical Tumor Imaging of Tumor Growth and Metastasis

Whole-body optical images visualized metastatic lesions of GFP-expressing tumors in the brain, liver (Fig. 9), pancreas, lymph nodes, and bone in transplanted mice. These images were used for real time, quantitative measurement of primary and metastatic tumor growth in each of these organs. Imaging was with either a transilluminated epi-fluorescence microscope or a fluorescence light box and thermoelectrically cooled color charged–coupled device (CCD) camera. The depth to which metastasis and micrometastasis could be imaged depended on their size. The simple, noninvasive, and highly selective imaging of growing tumors, made possible by the strong GFP fluorescence, enabled the detailed visualization of tumor growth and metastasis formation, even in freely moving animals. This new GFP imaging technology will facilitate in vivo high-throughput screening of antitumor and antimetastatic drugs *(25)*.

1.9. Selective In Vivo Tumor Delivery of the Green Fluorescent Protein Gene to Report Future Occurrence of Metastasis

The GFP gene was administered to intraperitoneally growing human stomach cancer in nude mice in order to visualize future regional and distant metastases. GFP retroviral

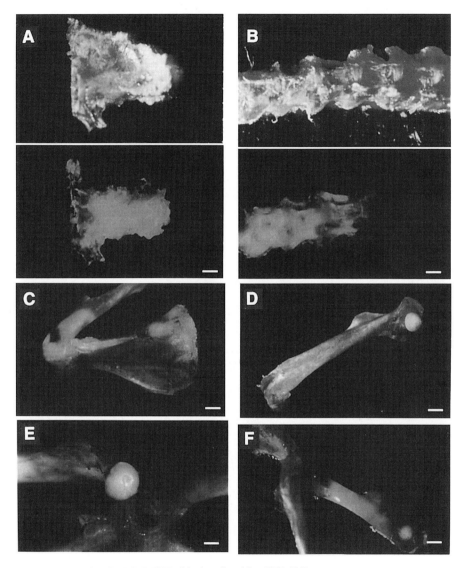

Fig. 6. Bone metastasis of B16F0 GFP C1 visualized by GFP *(29)*.
a: Skull, Top: no metastasis was detected under bright-field microscopy. Bar = 640 μm. Bottom: shows same area as top part, bone metastasis visualized in the skull under fluorescent microscopy.
b: Vertebral body, Top: no metastasis was detected under bright-field microscopy. Bar = 1280 μm. Bottom: shows same area as top part, bone metastasis visualized in the vertebral body under fluorescent microscopy.
c: Bone metastases visualized by GFP expression in humerus and scapula. Bar = 1280 μm.
d: Bone metastases visualized by GFP expression in the distal end of the femur. Bar = 1280 μm.
e: Bone metastases visualized by GFP expression in the head of the femur. Bar = 800 μm.
f: Bone metastases visualized by GFP expression in pelvis. Bar = 1280 μm.

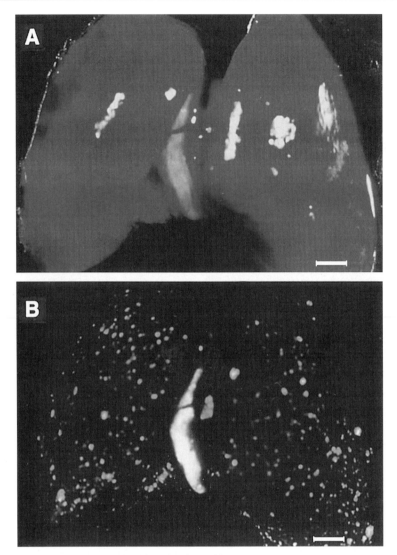

Fig. 7. Lung metastasis of LOX visualized by GFP *(29)*.
a: Shows the surface of the lung of nude mouse. No metastasis was detected under bright-field microscopy. Bar = 1280 μm.
b: Same field as **a.** Numerous micro-metastases and metastases are visualized by GFP expression in the lung under fluorescence microscopy. Bar = 1280 μm.

supernatants were ip-injected from d 4 to d 10 following ip implantation of the cancer cells. Tumor and metastasis fluorescence was visualized every other wk with the use of fluorescence optics via a laparotomy on the tumor-bearing animals. No normal tissues were found to be transduced by the GFP retrovirus. Within 2 wk after retroviral GFP delivery, GFP-expressing tumor cells were observed in gonadal fat, greater omentum, and intestine, indicating that these primary intraperitoneally growing tumors were efficiently transduced by the GFP gene and could be visualized by its expression. At the second and

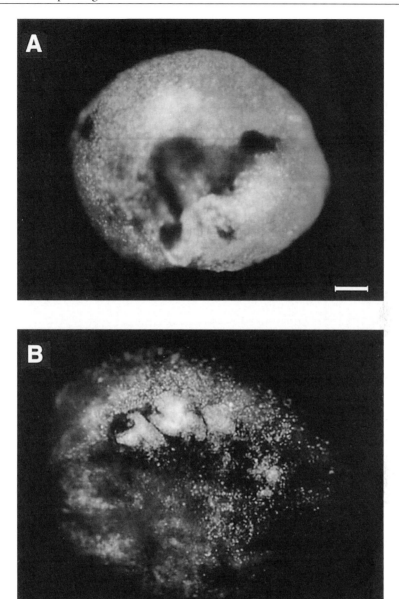

Fig. 8. Lymph-node metastasis of LOX visualized by GFP *(29)*
a and b: Tumor metastasized to the lymph nodes visualized by GFP expression. Bar = 200 μm.

third laparotomies at 4 and 6 wk, respectively, GFP-expressing tumor cells were found spreading to lymph nodes in the mesentery. At the fourth laparotomy at 8 wk, widespread tumor growth including liver metastasis was observed. Thus, reporter-gene transduction of the primary tumor enabled detection of its subsequent metastasis. This gene-therapy model could be applied to primary tumors before resection or other treatment in order to have a fluorescent early detection system for metastasis and recurrence *(26)*.

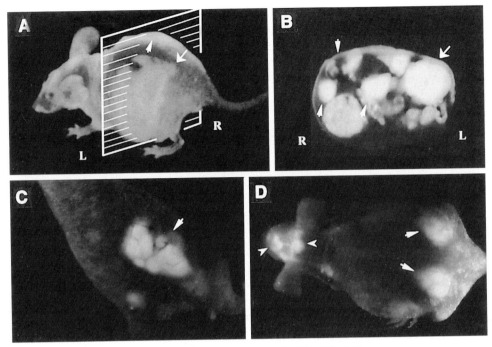

Fig. 9. External and internal images of liver lesions of AC3488-GFP *(25)*.

a: Lateral, whole-body image of metastatic liver lesions of a GFP-expressing human colon cancer in the left and right lobes of a live nude mouse at d 21 after surgical orthotopic transplantation (SOI).

b: Cross-section of mouse shown in Fig. 9A corresponding to the level of the external image of the tumor in the liver that was acquired (Fig. 9A). Arrows show metastatic lesions in the various lobes of the liver.

c: Fluorescent whole-body ventral image of primary colon tumor.

d: Dorsal external image of metastatic tumor in the caudal region of the left and right lobes of the liver (thick arrows), and skull metastasis (arrowheads).

2. METHODS

2.1. Imaging Apparatus

A Leica fluorescence stereo microscope, model LZ12, equipped with a 50W mercury lamp, was used for high-magnification imaging of GFP-expressing tumors and metastasis *in situ* or for whole-body imaging of animals with GFP-expressing tumors. Selective excitation of GFP was produced through a D425/60 band-pass filter and 470 DCXR dichroic mirror. Emitted fluorescence was collected through a long-pass filter GG475 (Chroma Technology, Brattleboro, VT) on a Hamamatsu C5810 3-chip cooled color CCD camera (Hamamatsu Photonics Systems, Bridgewater, NJ). Images were processed for contrast and brightness and analyzed with the use of Image Pro Plus 3.1 software (Media Cybernetics, Silver Springs, MD) Images of 1024×724 pixels were captured directly on an IBM PC or continuously through video output on a high-resolution Sony VCR model SLV-R1000 (Sony Corp., Tokyo, Japan). Whole-body imaging that visualized the entire animal at lower magnification was carried out in a light box illuminated by blue light fiberoptics (Lightools Research, Inc., Encinitas, CA) and imaged using the thermoelectrically cooled color CCD camera *(25)*.

2.2. Retroviral DNA Expression Vector

The RetroXpress vector pLEIN was purchased from CLONTECH Laboratories, Inc. (Palo Alto, CA). The pLEIN vector expresses enhanced green fluorescent protein (EGFP) and the neomycin resistance gene on the same bicistronic message that contains an internal ribosome entry site (IRES) *(18,19)*.

2.3. Retroviral Production

PT67, an NIH-3T3-derived packaging cell line, expressing the 10-Al viral envelope, was purchased from CLONTECH Laboratories, Inc. PT67 cells were cultured in Dulbecco's Modified Eagle's Medium (DME) (Irvine Scientific, Santa Ana, CA) supplemented with 10% heat-inactivated fetal bovine serum (FBS) (Gemini Bio-products, Calabasas, CA). For vector production, packaging cells (PT67), at 70% confluence, were incubated with a precipitated mixture of DOTAP™ reagent (Boehringer Mannheim), and saturating amounts of pLEIN plasmid for 18 h. Fresh medium was replenished at this time. The cells were examined by fluorescence microscopy after 48 h. For selection of GFP transductants, the cells were cultured in the presence of 500 µg/mL–2000 µg/mL of G418 (Life Technologies, Grand Island, NY) for 7 ds *(18,19)*.

2.4. Retroviral Transduction of Tumor Cells

For GFP gene transduction, 20%-confluent cancer cells were incubated with a 1:1 precipitated mixture of retroviral supernatants of PT67 cells and RPMI-1640 (GIBCO-BRL) containing 10% FBS (Gemini Bio-products, Calabasas, CA) for 72 h. Fresh medium was replenished at this time. Cells were harvested by trypsin/EDTA 72 hs postinfection, and subcultured at a ratio of 1:15 into selective medium containing 200 µg/mL of G418. The level of G418 was gradually increased to 800–1000 µg/mL. Stable GFP-expressing clones were then isolated in the absence of selective agent. Clones expressing GFP were isolated with cloning cylinders (Bel-Art Products, Pequannock, NJ) by trypsin EDTA and were amplified and transferred by conventional culture methods *(18,19)*.

2.5. Subcutaneous Tumor Growth

Three 6-wk-old Balb/c *nu/nu* female mice were injected subcutaneously with a single dose of 10^7 stable GFP transductants. Cells were first harvested by trypsinization, and washed three times with cold serum-containing medium, then kept on ice. Cells were injected in a total vol of 0.4 mL within 40 min of harvesting. The nude mice were sacrificed to harvest the tumor fragments 3 wk after tumor-cell injection *(14–19)*.

2.6. Experimental Metastasis

Nude mice were injected in the tail vein of mice with a single dose of 1×10^7 stable GFP-expressing cancer cells. Cells were first harvested by trypsinization, and washed three times with cold serum-containing medium, then kept on ice. Cells were injected in a total vol of 0.8 mL of serum-free medium within 40 min of harvesting. After various times, the mice were sacrificed, and fresh visceral organs and the skeleton were analyzed by fluorescence microscopy.

2.7. Surgical Orthotopic Implantation

2.7.1 OVARIAN CANCER

Tumor fragments (1 mm^3) derived from the nude mouse sc CHO-K1-GFP tumors were implanted by SOI on the ovarian serosa in six nude mice *(14,27)*. The mice were anesthetized by isofluran inhalation. An incision was made through the left lower abdominal pararectal line and peritoneum. The left ovary was exposed, and part of the serosal membrane was scraped with a forceps. Four 1-mm^3 tumor pieces were fixed on the scraped site of the serosal surface with an 8–0 nylon suture (Look, Norwell, MA). The ovary was then returned into the peritoneal cavity, and the abdominal wall and the skin were closed with 6–0 silk sutures. Four weeks later, the mice were sacrificed, and the lungs and the other organs were removed. All procedures of the operation described above were performed with a ×7 magnification microscope (Olympus) *(14)*.

2.7.2. LUNG CANCER

Tumor fragments (1 mm^3) derived from the ANIP-GFP or H460-GFP sc tumor growing in the nude mouse were implanted by SOI on the left lung in nude mice *(15,18)*. The mice were anesthetized by isofluran inhalation. The animals were put in a position of right lateral decubitus, with the four limbs restained. A 0.8-cm transverse incision of the skin was made in the left-chest wall. Chest muscles were separated by sharp dissection, and costal and intercostal muscles were exposed. A 0.4–0.5-cm intercostal incision between the third and fourth rib on the chest wall was made, and the chest wall was opened. The left lung was taken up by a forceps and tumor fragments were promptly sewn into the upper lung with one 8–0 suture. The lung was then returned into the chest cavity. The incision in the chest wall was closed by a 6–0 surgical suture. The closed condition of the chest wall was examined immediately, and if a leak existed, it was closed by additional sutures. After closing the chest wall, an intrathoracic puncture was made by using a 3-mL syringe and 25 and II gauge needle to withdraw the remaining air in the chest cavity. After the withdrawal of air, a completely inflated lung could be seen through the thin chest wall of the mouse. Then the skin and chest muscle were closed with a 6–0 surgical suture in one layer. All procedures of the operation described here were performed with a ×7 magnification microscope (Olympus).

2.7.3. PROSTATE CANCER

Two tumor fragments (1 mm^3) from a high-GFP-fluorescent sc tumor from a single animal were implanted by SOI in the dorsolateral lobe of the prostate in five nude mice *(19)*. After proper exposure of the bladder and prostate following a lower midline abdominal incision, the capsule of the prostate was opened, and the two tumor fragments were inserted into the capsule. The capsule was then closed with an 8–0 surgical suture. The incision in the abdominal wall was closed with a 6–0 surgical suture in one layer *(7,8)*. The animals were kept under isoflurane anesthesia during surgery. All procedures of the operation described here were performed with a × 7 magnification microscope (Olympus).

2.8. Analysis of the GFP-fluorescent Metastases at Autopsy

Mice were sacrificed when their performance status began to decline and the systemic organs were removed. The orthotopic primary tumor and all major organs, as well as the whole skeleton, were explored *in situ* by fluorescence microscopy. The fresh samples were then sliced at approx 1-mm thickness and further observed under fluorescence microscopy.

REFERENCES

1. Lin WC, Pretlow TP, Pretlow TG, Culp LA. Bacterial lacZ gene as a highly sensitive marker to detect micrometastasis formation during tumor progression. *Cancer Res* 1990; 50: 2808–2817.
2. Lin WC, Culp LA. Altered establishment/clearance mechanisms during experimental micrometastasis with live and/or disabled bacterial lacZ-tagged tumor cells. *Invasion Metastasis* 1992; 12: 197–209.
3. Morin J, Hastings J. Energy transfer in a bioluminescent system. *J Cell Physiol* 1971; 77: 313–318.
4. Chalfie M, Tu Y, Euskirchen G, Ward WW, Prasher DC. Green fluorescent protein as a marker for gene expression. *Science* 1994; 263: 802–805.
5. Cheng L, Fu J, Tsukamoto A, Hawley RG. Use of green fluorescent protein variants to monitor gene transfer and expression in mammalian cells. *Nat Biotechnol* 1996; 14: 606–609.
6. Prasher DC, Eckenrode VK, Ward WW, Prendergast FG, Cormier MJ. Primary structure of the *Aequorea victoria* green-fluorescent protein. *Gene* 1992; 111: 229–233.
7. Yang F, Moss LG, Phillips GN Jr. The molecular structure of green fluorescent protein. *Nat Biotechnol* 1996; 14: 1246–1251.
8. Cody CW, Prasher DC, Welstler VM, Prendergast FG, Ward WW. Chemical structure of the hexapeptide chromophore of the *Aequorea* green fluorescent protein. *Biochemistry* 1993; 32: 1212–1218.
9. Heim R, Cubitt AB, Tsien RY. Improved green fluorescence. *Nature* 1995; 373: 663–664.
10. Delagrave S, Hawtin RE, Silva CM, Yang MM, Youvan DC. Red-shifted excitation mutants of the green fluorescent protein. *Bio/Technology* 1995; 13: 151–154.
11. Cormack B, Valdivia R, Falkow S. FACS-optimized mutants of the green fluorescent proten (GFP). *Gene* 1996; 173: 33–38.
12. Crameri A, Whitehorn EA, Tate E, Stemmer WPC. Improved green fluorescent protein by molecular evolution using DNA shuffling. *Nat Biotechnol* 1996; 14: 315–319.
13. Zolotukhin S, Potter M, Hauswirth WW, Guy J, Muzycka N. 'Humanized' green fluorescent protein cDNA adapted for high-level expression in mammalian cells. *J Virology* 1996; 70: 4646–4654.
14. Chishima T, Miyagi Y, Wang X, Yamaoka H, Shimada H, Moossa AR, et al. Cancer invasion and micrometastasis visualized in live tissue by green fluorescent protein expression. *Cancer Res* 1997; 57: 2042–2047.
15. Chishima T, Miyagi Y, Wang X, Baranov, E, Tan Y, Shimada H, et al. Metastatic patterns of lung cancer visualized live and in process by green fluorescent protein expression. *Clinical & Experimental Metastasis* 1997; 15: 547–552.
16. Chishima T, Miyagi Y, Wang X, Tan Y, Shimada H, Moossa AR, et al. Visualization of the metastatic process by green fluorescent protein expression. *Anticancer Res* 1997; 17: 2377–2384.
17. Chishima T, Miyagi Y, Li L, Tan Y, Baranov E, Yang M, et al. The use of histoculture and green fluorescent protein to visualize tumor cell host interaction. *In Vitro Cell Dev Biol* 1997; 33: 745–747.
18. Yang M, Hasegawa S, Jiang P, Wang X, Tan Y, Chishima T, et al. Widespread skeletal metastatic potential of human lung cancer revealed by green fluorescent protein expression. *Cancer Res* 1998; 58: 4217–4221.
19. Yang M, Jiang P, Sun FX, Hasegawa S, Baranov E, Chishima T, et al. A fluorescent orthotopic bone metastasis model of human prostate cancer. *Cancer Res* 1999; 59: 781–786.
20. Kaufman RJ, Davies MV, Wasley LC, Michnick D. Improved vectors for stable expression of foreign genes in mammalian cells by use of the untranslated leader sequence from EMC virus. *Nucleic Acids Res* 1991; 19: 4485–4490.
21. Astoul P, Colt HG, Wang X, Hoffman RM. A "patient-like" nude mouse model of parietal pleural human lung adenocarcinoma. *Anticancer Res* 1994; 14: 85–92.
22. Wang X, Fu X, Hoffman RM. A new patient-like metastatic model of human lung cancer constructed orthotopically with intact tissue via thoracotomy in immunodeficient mice. *Int J Cancer* 1992; 51: 992–995.
23. Yang M, Chishima T, Wang X, Baranov E, Shimada H, Moossa AR, et al. Multi-organ metastatic capability of Chinese ovary cells revealed by green fluorescent protein (GFP) expression. *Clin and Exp Metastasis* 1999; 17: 417–422.
24. Holmgren L, O'Reilly MS, Folkman J. Dormancy of micrometastases: balanced proliferation and apoptosis in the presence of angiogenesis suppression. *Nat Med* 1995; 1: 149–153.

25. Yang M, Baranov E, Jiang P, Sun F-X, Li X-M, Li L, et al. Whole-body optical imaging of green fluorescent protein-expressing tumors and metastases. *Proc Natl Acad Sci USA* 2000; 97: 1206–1211.

26. Hasegawa S, Yang M, Chishima T, Shimada H, Moossa AR, Hoffman RM. *In vivo* tumor delivery of the green fluorescent protein gene to report future occurrence of metastasis. *Cancer Gene Ther* 2000; 7: 1336–1340.

27. Fu X, Hoffman RM. Human ovarian carcinoma metastatic models constructed in nude mice by orthotopic transplantation of histologically-intact patient specimens. *Anticancer Res* 1993; 13: 283–286.

28. Naumov GN, Wilson SM, MacDonald IC, Schmidt EE, Morris V, Groom AC, et al. Cellular expression of green fluorescent protein, coupled with high-resolution *in vivo* videomicroscopy, to monitor steps in tumor metastasis. *J Cell Sci* 1999; 112 (12): 1835–1842.

29. Yang M, Jiang P, An Z, Baranov E, Li L, Hasegawa S, et al. Genetically fluorescent melanoma bone and organ metastasis models. *Clin Can Res* 1999; 5: 3549–3559.

7

Human Tumor Xenografts and Explants

Heinz-Herbert Fiebig, MD, PhD,
and Angelika M. Burger, PhD

CONTENTS

1. INTRODUCTION

1.1. Historical Perspective

Since the first report of the successful xenografting of a human tumor into nude mice in 1969, there have been numerous studies conducted throughout the world using the nude mouse as a tool to answer a variety of questions regarding the cause, prevention, and therapy of cancer. Thus, the role of immunodeficient animals in oncology has continuously increased, and the athymic nude mouse has proven to be an outstanding host for many human solid-tumor xenografts *(1,2)*. These mice are now extensively used in the development of potential anticancer drugs, new antineoplastic treatment modalities, and studies of tumor biology *(3–7)*. Moreover, mice with severe combined immunodeficiency (SCID) have enlarged the spectrum of possible applications in cancer research and enabled engraftments of human tumors that were previously difficult to explant, such as those of the hematopoietic system *(8)*.

Prior to the discovery of immunodeficient mice, syngeneic transplantable mouse tumor systems or autochtonous rat tumors were employed as the main—or the only—tools in the development of antitumor agents *(5,7,9)*. Most of the chemotherapeutic agents currently used in the clinic have been developed in these rodent tumor models (reviewed in chapters 1–4). The most frequently used murine tumors were the leukemias L1210 and P388, the melanoma B16, and the Lewis Lung cancer *(LLC)* model. Yet the classes of agents found active in the mouse tumor models, however, were limited, and mainly comprise alkylating agents, and some other DNA interacting drugs *(5,10,11)*.

From: *Tumor Models in Cancer Research*
Edited by: B. A. Teicher © Humana Press Inc., Totowa, NJ

Table 1
Human Tumor Xenograft Models Established in Freiburg (XFs)

- more than 1600 tumors of cancer patients have been sc-implanted into nude mice
- more than 300 human tumors of the following tumor types have been established:

bladder	breast	colon	cervix uteri
CNS	gall bladder		head and neck
leukemias	liver	lung	lymphoma
melanomas	pleura mesothelioma		ovarian
pancreas	prostate	renal	sarcoma
stomach	testicle	thymoma	uterus

60 models have been well characterized (see following tables)

Nevertheless, today transplantable syngeneic murine-tumor models remain particularly valuable for studying biological response modifiers or certain agents that need to be evaluated in a syngeneic environment, such as those targeting distant organ metastasis (9).

In the late 1980s and early 1990s, new drug development moved from applying general cytotoxic principles to molecular target-directed treatment strategies (12). Consequently, there was a need to identify tumor types/individual patient tumors that express the target and could benefit from more selective therapies in phase II/III clinical trials. Thus, the in vivo models used in preclinical development today are "disease-oriented" and target-characterized, and are either human-tumor explants/xenografts or specifically bred transgenic mice (13). However, because of their high running costs and limited availability, transgenic mice are not suitable for large-scale drug testings. Thus, xenografts/human explants have become the gold standard in cancer-drug development. Their use is highly recommended by regulatory agencies such as the EMEA (European Agency for the Evaluation of Medicinal Products) in the "note for guidance on the pre-clinical evaluation of anticancer medicinal products" (14).

1.2. The Strength of Human Xenografts Derived from Patient Explants

Whilst the spectrum of transplantable and autochtonous murine tumor models is confined to certain entities such as melanoma, colon, breast, bladder, or lung carcinomas, and genetically engineered mouse models cannot cover all human cancers, patient explants and stably growing xenografts derived thereof can be generated from the vast majority of malignancies. Table 1 shows the broad panel of human tumor types included in the Freiburg xenograft collection.

Moreover, the use of fresh surgical patient material or human-tumor engraftments growing subcutaneously in nude mice enable chemosensitivity screening procedures in vitro and in vivo, and thus can be used to predict clinical response (10,15–17). Human-tumor xenografts established in serial passage have demonstrated a particularly high correlation of drug response compared to that in the clinic (Table 2). If evaluated in the nude mouse in vivo the correct prediction for response (positive predictive value) was 90% (16,17). If tested in vitro using the clonogenic assay, the correct prediction was 60%. The prediction for resistance was 97% in vivo

Table 2
Comparison of Drug Response in Human Tumors Growing
Subcutaneously in Nude Mice and in the Patient

Mouse/patient	Total
remission/remission	19
no remission/remission	2
no remission/no remission	57
remission/no remission	2

80 comparisons were obtained in 55 tumors. Xenografts predicted correctly for:
   → response in 90% (19/21)
   → resistance in 97% (57/59)

and 92% in vitro respectively. This allows for preselection of responsive tumor types in follow-up studies.

It will be crucial for a new drug to demonstrate a differential selectivity against human tumors compared to the most sensitive normal tissue. In this respect, human-tumor xenografts are being considered as the most relevant models, since the patient-derived tumors grow as a solid tumor and ii) they develop a stroma and iii) vasculature, as well as iv) central necrosis. They show v) more or less differentiation, and have clinically relevant response rates (17). The tumor-xenograft architecture, the cell morphology and molecular characteristics mirror in most of the cases the original patient cancers (Fig. 1). This is in marked contrast to xenografts derived from cell lines, which in general show a homogeneous undifferentiated histology and as a result, are very resistant to most of the standard agents (10,14) (Fig. 2). This is most likely a result of the high selection pressure in vitro during long-term culture resulting in aggressive subclones.

In this chapter, we report on our experience with the growth of more than 1.600 patient tumors, the correlation of drug response against clinically used agents, the molecular characterization of parameters/factors relevant for tumor development, growth and dissemination, and examples of target-directed compounds discovered by our group.

2. MATERIALS & METHODS

2.1. Establishment of Human-Tumor Xenografts from Patient Explants

All animal experiments were performed according to the project license number G-97/30 following German Animal License regulations (Tierschutzgesetz), which closely reflect the recently published United Kingdom Coordinating Committee on Cancer Research (UKCCCR) guidelines for the welfare of animals in experimental neoplasia (18).

2.1.1. ANIMALS

Outbred athymic nude mice of the NMRI genetic background developed by our own breeding facility were used for all studies described here. The mice were kept in Macrolon™ cages on laminar-flow shelves. In the first passage, tumors derived from

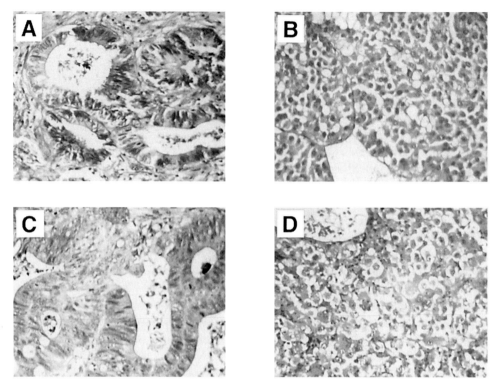

Fig. 1. Histological appearance of the colon carcinoma CXF 158 and the large-cell lung carcinoma LXFL 529 as original patient tumors depicted in **A** and **B** respectively, and xenografts established thereof as sc solid fragments in serial passage shown in **C-D. 1C** represents the CXF 158 human-tumor xenograft in passage 10 (P+10), **1D** the LXFL 529 explant in passage 5. Although stromal parts and blood supply are derived from the murine host, architecture and morphology of the tumors closely resemble the original patient specimens (H&E sections ×400).

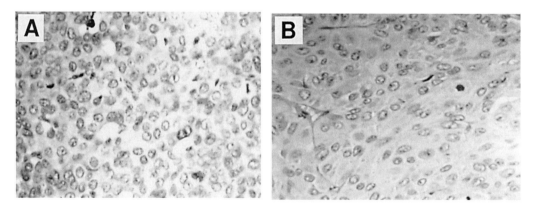

Fig. 2. Histological appearance of cell-line-derived human-tumor xenografts established by sc injection of **A** COLO 205 colon-cancer cells obtained from the NCI Central Repository or **B** DU145 prostate-cancer cells obtained from ATCC (American Type Culture Collection). Both human-tumor xenografts are undifferentiated and only sparsely vascularized. They lost morphological elements that would help to identify them as either colon- or prostate-cancer histologies (H&E sections ×400).

human male cancer patients were implanted into male nude mice, and tumors from women were inplanted into female mice. All therapeutic experiments, with the exception of testicular and prostate cancers, were carried out in female mice.

2.1.2. Tumors

Over the past 12 yr, more than 1.600 resected human solid malignancies were implanted subcutaneously into nude mice. Tumor slices of approx $5 \times 5 \times 0.5$ to 1.0 mm in diameter were implanted in the flanks of the animals. From patient material (first passage), 16 fragments were grafted into four mice. For therapeutic experiments, two tumor fragments of 1.5–2 mm in diameter were implanted subcutaneously between the fore- and hind flank of each mouse near the *arteria mammaria interna*.

2.1.3. Tumor-Growth Measurements

Tumor growth was followed weekly or bi-weekly (fast-growing tumors) by serial caliper measurements determining two perpendicular diameters. The product of the two diameters was taken as a measure for tumor size. Drug treatment efficacy was evaluated as tumor volume, and calculated according to the formula: $1 \times w^2/2$, where 1 is the longer and w is the perpendicular diameter. Relative tumor values were calculated for each individual tumor according to tumor size on day_x divided by tumor size on day_0 at the time of randomization multiplied by 100. The median tumor size was taken for evaluation.

2.2. Experimental Design of Drug Testing

2.2.1. Study Design

Drug testing was performed in serial passage when the tumor growth was regular. Drug response in the nude mouse vs that in the patient was compared using xenografts in passages between 2 and 10.

In vivo testing of novel agents was performed with human-tumor xenografts, which had not been propagated beyond 10 passages from the frozen master stock. Mice were selected randomly for vehicle control or test groups after 3–6 wk, when tumors were palpable and had reached mean diameters of greater than 4 mm. Tumors with a yellow color—indicating a high amount of fibrous tissue—were excluded. Using these criteria, we did not observe spontaneous regressions or stationary growth behavior in the controls. Each test group consisted of 5–6 animals comprising between 6–10 available tumors. Experiments were terminated when tumors reached a diameter of 1.5 cm.

2.2.2. Chemotherapy

Treatment regiments used in nude mice were adopted to clinically employed schedules with the exception that intermittent treatment was repeated in mice after 2 wk instead of 3–4 wk in patients. Drugs, dose, schedule, and route of administration are shown in Table 4. A dose around the LD_{10} after 14 d and around the LD_{20} 28 d after initiation of therapy was considered the maximum tolerated dose (MTD) in tumor-bearing nude mice. If available, agents were used as clinical formulation, experimental drugs were either dissolved in normal saline or prepared e.g. in 10% dimethyl sulfoxide/phosphate-buffered saline (DMSO/PBS) and 0.05% Tween-80™.

2.2.3. EVALUATION PARAMETERS FOR TUMOR RESPONSE

For comparing tumor responses in nude mice and in patients, the product of the two diameters was taken as a measure of tumor size. Tumors in nude mice were evaluated after maximum tumor regression or after 21–28 d in nonregressing tumors. The effect of treatment was classified in the xenograft system and in the patient as remission (the product of 2 diameters <50% of initial value), minimal regression (51–75%), no change (76–124%), and progression (>125%) of initial value. All patients enrolled in these studies had measurable lesions, and evaluation was usually performed after two treatment cycles or after maximal tumor regression. The evaluation of tumor response in nude mice and in the patients was performed by different physicians.

For testing new compounds, the in vivo evaluation was performed using tumor volume obtained by the formula 0.5 * length * (width)^2 according to Geran et al. *(19)*. Relative tumor volumes were calculated for individual tumors by dividing the tumor volume on day$_t$ by the tumor volume on day$_0$ multiplied with 100 for all timepoints. The *minimum* test/control in % is considered as the optimal value (optimal T/C%).

2.3. Molecular Target Characterization of the Freiburg Human-Tumor Xenograft Panel

A panel of approx 60 human-tumor xenografts has been extensively studied for the expression of novel, validated targets for cancer-drug development. The total of 29 molecular targets include several classes of tumor-associated proteins/physiologies. Target expression was determined either at the RNA (Northern blotting) or protein level (enzyme-linked immunosorbent assay [ELISA], Western blotting, immunohistochemistry).

Two examples for new targets for cancer-drug development are described in more detail in this chapter, namely matrix metalloproteinases (MMPs) and determinants of angiogenesis [vascular endothelial growth factor (VEGF) and vascular permeability/porosity (VP)], which are important for tumor neovascularization and dissemination.

Matrix metalloproteinases: MMP-2, MMP-9, and MMP-3, and the tissue inhibitor of matrix metalloproteinases TIMP-2 were measured as pro-MMPs or free tissue inhibitor of matrix metalloproteinase (TIMP) respectively in xenograft-tissue homogenates by an ELISA method (Amersham International, UK). MMP/TIMP-activity was measured in 20 µg total cellular protein of a tumor extract (lysis buffer: 10 mM Tris-HCI pH 7.5, 1 mM MgCI$_2$, 1 mM ethylene glycol-*bis* (β-aminoethylether-) -N,N,N′,N′-tetraacetic acid, 0.1 mM phenylmethylsulfonyl-fluoride, 5 mM β-mercaptoethanol, 0.5% v/v 3-[(3-cholamidopropyl)-dimethyl-ammonio]-1-propanesulfonate, 10% v/v glycerol) determined by Bradford assay (BioRad, Munich, FRG) and quantified in ng/mL relative to the individual MMP-standards provided by the manufacturer of the kit. The primary MMP-antibodies were human and mouse-specific. The MMP-activity was detected by using a immunoperoxidase methodology with TMB (trimethoxybenzoic acid) as substrate. The developing yellow color of the peroxidase reaction was read at 450 nm using a Dynatech MR 5000-plate reader (DPC Biermann GmbH, Germany).

Determinants of angiogenesis (VEGF/VPF and VP): VEGF was evaluated by using the human VEGF Quantikine Elisa kit (R&D Systems, Wiesbaden, FRG). VEGF was measured in 20 μg total cellular protein as previously described, and the kit was developed following the manufacturer's instructions. Peroxidase/TMB was used as detection system. VP was evaluated by Miles assay *(20)* with modifications to accommodate the tumor physiology described by Schüler et al. *(21)*. In brief, the Miles assay is based on the enhanced permeability and retention effect (EPR) of tumor-tissue vasculature, which is able to retain macromolecules. Thus, Evans blue dye is injected into the tail vein of a mouse (100 mg/kg) and forms albumin-conjugated macromolecules. The latter are retained in tumors because of EPR, and tumors are excised 30 min after Evans blue injection. Evans blue is then extracted from tissue in Aceton/NaCl 5% (7:3), quantified by spectroscopy (620 nm) and VP calculated as % dose of dye retained per g tumor *(21)*.

2.4. Clonogenic Assay

A modification of the double-layer soft-agar or clonogenic assay as described by Hamburger and Salmon was used *(10)*. The target-cell population of this assay is composed of tumor stem cells that are responsible for the unlimited growth of a tumor. An excellent correlation of drug response in the patient and in the clonogenic assay has been published by various groups *(15,22,23)*.

2.4.1. PREPARATION OF A SINGLE-CELL SUSPENSIONS

Solid human-tumor xenografts were mechanically disaggregated and subsequently incubated with an enzyme cocktail consisting of collagenase 0.05%, DNase 0.07%, and hyaluronidase 0.1% in RPMI-1640 at 37°C for 30 min. The cells were washed twice and passed through sieves of 200-μm and 50-μm mesh size. The percentage of viable cells was determined in a hemocytometer using trypan blue exclusion.

2.4.2. CULTURE METHODS

The tumor-cell suspension was plated into 24-multiwell plates over a bottom layer consisting of 0.2 mL Iscoves's Modified Dulbecco's Medium (IMDM) with 20% fetal calf serum (FCS) and 0.7% agar. 20,000–100,000 cells were added to 0.2 mL of the same culture medium, in 0.4% agar, and were plated onto the base layer. Drugs were added after 24 h (drug overlay) in 0.2 mL medium. In each assay, six control plates received the vehicle only, drug-treated groups were plated in triplicate in three or six concentrations.

Cultures were incubated at 37°C and 7% CO_2 in a humidified atmosphere for 6–18 d and monitored closely for colony growth using an inverted microscope. Within this period, in vitro tumor growth led to the formation of colonies with a diameter of >50 μm. At the time of maximum colony formation, vital colonies were stained with a tetrazoliumchloride dye 24 h before counting them with an automated image analysis system (Bausch & Lomb, OMNICON FAS IV).

Drug effects were expressed as percentage of survival, obtained by comparison of the mean number of colonies in the treated plates with the mean colony count of the untreated controls (colony count T/C × 100). A compound was considered active if it reduced colony formation to less than 30% of the control group value (T/C ≤ 30%).

Furthermore, inhibitory concentrations IC50, IC70 and IC90 were calculated corresponding to T/C values of 50, 30 and 10%. Using these evaluation parameters, the majority of clinically established anticancer agents was active at a concentration of <1 µg/mL. 5-FU was used as positive reference compound at ultra pharmacological doses of 100–1000 µg/mL. The coefficient of variation in the control group was <50%. The average cloning efficiency was 0.07%.

3. RESULTS AND DISCUSSION

3.1. Take Rates and Growth Behavior of Patient Tumor Explants in Nude Mice

Of 1.600 patient tumors, the growth behavior of 1.227 different human malignancies growing subcutaneously in nude mice has been characterized in detail, and is presented in Table 3. Histological examination of the tumors showed that 79% contained viable tumor tissue. However, only 41% of the tumors showed a rapid growth, with tumor diameters of more than 8 mm after 90 d (Table 3) equal to length × width of more than 60 mm². Thus, only these rapidly growing tumors were suitable for establishing stably growing models and for further investigations. Nonetheless, it must be noted that the growth of human tumors of the previously described category is still much slower than that seen in established murine models. Four hundred (33%) of the 499 "rapid" growing human tumor explants were successfully transferred in serial passage, and most of them were cryopreserved in liquid nitrogen with a recovery of 90% (Table 3).

Tumors in serial passage can be divided into three categories. The rate was highest (40–60%) in tumors of the esophagus, cervix, and corpus uteri, colon, small-cell lung, and melanomas. Intermediate growth rates between 20 and 40% were observed for carcinoma of the lung (non-small-cell) soft-tissue sarcoma, and carcinoma of the ovaries, head and neck, pancreas, testicle, pleuramesothelioma, stomach, and bladder. The lowest rates (5–19%) were observed in renal-cell cancers (RCC) and in the hormone-dependent mammary and prostate carcinomas. The growth of breast and prostate cancers was increased when intramuscular estrogen or dihydrotestosterone depots were given every 2 wk.

Among the 400 models, 246 have been selected for further characterization—e.g., a chemosensitivity profile. These models showed a regular growth behavior and typical characteristics in terms of histology and differentiation. Rapid- and slow-growing tumors were included, as well as sensitive and resistant models against standard agents. All the tumors can and have been frozen in liquid nitrogen, with a recovery rate of 90%.

At the University of California, in a similar effort to establish human-tumor models from surgical specimens, a total of 323 patient explants were collected (4). These yielded the development of only 27 (8%) of transplantable models. Although the California group had similar positive results with respect to retaining patient characteristics, their markedly lower success rate (8%) in obtaining stable, transplantable models vs that of our program (33%) however, might be a result of the processing of the specimens. The California group minced and then injected the tumor suspensions subcutaneously into nude mice without paying attention to the gender of the patient from which the tumors were derived or the age of the mice. We established our models from tumor fragments in very young mice (4 wk of age) of the same gender as the donor

Table 3
Growth Behavior of Human Tumors in Nude Mice

Tumor origin	Total	Rapid growth[a]		Serial passage[b]	
	N	N	[%]	N	[%]
Esophagus	10	7	70	6	60
Cervix uteri	10	7	70	6	60
Colorectal	152	88	58	78	51
Corpus uteri	8	4	50	4	50
Melanomas	63	39	62	27	43
Lung, small cell	39	14	36	16	41
Lung, NSC	227	118	52	87	38
Sarcomas, soft t.	79	36	46	29	37
Ovary	22	7	32	8	36
Head & neck	47	16	34	16	34
Pancreas	6	2	33	2	33
Brain	6	2	33	2	33
Hepatocell.	3	1	33	1	33
Neuroblastoma	3	1	33	1	33
Osteosarcoma	13	5	38	4	31
Testicle	48	14	29	12	25
Mesothelioma	36	14	39	9	25
Stomach	68	17	25	17	25
Bladder	44	17	39	10	23
Renal	124	37	30	24	19
Mammary	74	13	18	13	18
Prostate	41	7	17	2	5
Miscellaneous	129	42	33	34	26
Total	1.227	499	41 %	400	33%

[a] Tumor size $(a \times b) > 60$ mm^2 90 d after sc implant

[b] at least 3 passages

patient. Thus, we assured that the xeno-engrafted tumor specimens were provided with the most optimal environment such as their own extracellular matrix, appropriate hormonal conditions, high exposure to murine endogenous growth factors, and lowest probability of graft rejection.

3.2. Comparison of Drug Response of Tumors Growing in the Nude Mouse and in the Patient

In 55 tumors, 80 comparisons have been performed (Table 2). The patients and the xenotransplanted tumors were treated with similar schedules at their respective MTD. In the nude mouse, two treatment cycles were given.

In colorectal cancers, 24 comparisons were evaluated using single-agent chemotherapy with 5-fluorouracil (5-FU) or a nitrosourea and in three tumors a combination chemotherapy. The other tumor types were treated in 40 cases with combination chemotherapy, and in 13 cases with single-agent chemotherapy. Mammary cancers were initially treated with tamoxifen, and after progression with the combination of cyclophosphamide, methotrexate, and 5-FU, or adriamycin and cyclophosphamide. Stomach cancers were treated with 5-FU + adriamycin + mitomycin-C and small-cell lung cancers (SCLC) with the combination of adriamycin + vincristine + cyclophosphamide, and after progression with cisplatin and etoposide. The overall results are given in Table 2. A total of 21 patients reached a remission. The same result was observed in 19 tumors growing in the nude mouse. A total of 59 patients did not respond to treatment, and the same result was found in 57 cases in the nude mouse system. Overall, xenografts gave a correct prediction for resistance in 97% (57 of 59) and for tumor responsiveness in 90% (19 of 21).

Combination chemotherapy was more successful than single-agent therapy. Of the 43 combinations studied, 16 (37%) effected a remission in the patient, as compared to 5 of 35 (14%) of single-agent chemotherapies. Single-agent therapy was successful in four patients with colorectal cancer and in one with stomach cancer.

An example of a particular interesting case where mouse data translated into clinical response of an anaplastic thyroid cancer is shown in Fig. 3. The patient presenting with lung metastases responded well to the cyclophosphamide + vincristine + adriamycin + dacarbazine (CYVADIC) combination as did the explanted tumor XF 117 in serial passage 5 in the nude mouse (Fig. 3A and B). Furthermore, the nude mouse model enabled to identify the single-agent component responsible for the response of the thyroid cancer. By comparing drug efficacy of CYVADIC against that of cyclophosphamide, vincristine adriamycin, and dacarbazine (DTIC) monotherapy, it became obvious, that DTIC was the only active component of the combination (Fig. 3B).

3.3. Novel Clinically Used Agents Identified in the Freiburg Xenograft Panel

A second approach to validate the xenograft system as a model for drug development is retrospective chemosensitivity profiling. Thus, xenografts were analyzed in view of their ability to identify compounds active in the clinic. Here, we report on the response pattern of taxol, gemcitabine, taxotere, vindesine, and topotecan (Table 4) in clinically responsive and resistant tumor types. A more detailed analysis of 10 standard agents of the older generation of cytotoxic drugs studied in 508 different tumors are reported elsewhere (10,17).

Criteria for evaluation were the same as in the clinic. Each agent was evaluated in tumor types considered to be sensitive (CR + PR rate > 20%) or resistant (PR rate < 10%).

Overall, the 5 "novel" standard agents studied here (Table 4) induced remissions in 24% (45 of 187), and minor regressions or no change in 13% (25 of 187) of the cases examined. Yet 117 of 187 tumors (63%) progressed. Thus, the overall response rate is similar to what is observed with monotherapy regimens in the patient. In the subgroup of sensitive tumors, the five compounds effected remissions in 37%. In contrast, only 4% remissions were seen in the resistant tumor entities. A progression was observed in 49% of the sensitive tumor types compared to 84% of the resistant tumor types (Table 5). An outlined example of this analysis is shown for the tubulin-binding agent vindesine in Table 6.

In the responsive tumor entities of the lung (small- and non-small-cell), breast, leukemias, lymphomas, gastric cancers, and melanomas, vindesine effected a complete or

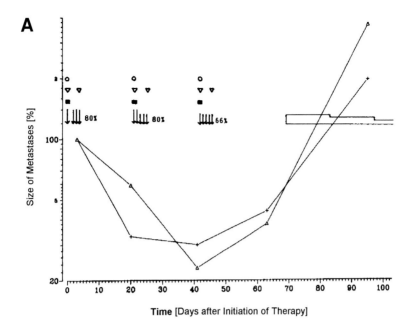

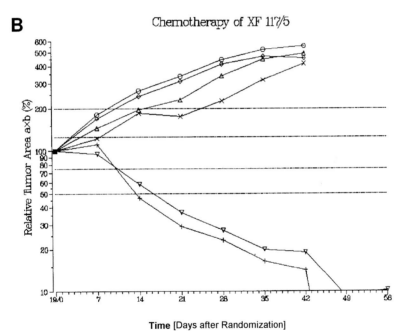

Fig. 3. A. Chemotherapy of a patient with thyroid carcinoma. Shown is the growth of two lung metastases under combination therapy with CYVADIC (○ cyclophosphamide 500 mg/m², Ⅴ vincristine 1 mg/m², ■ adriamycin 50 mg/m², and ↓ dacarbazine/DTIC 200 and 133 mg/m², respectively). The open box from d70–100 indicates prednisone treatment for oedema associated with brain metastases. **B.** Response of the xenograft XF 117 in passage 5 in the nude mouse, which was derived from the patient treated in A. The same chemotherapy protocol was employed using CYVADIC, as well as the single-agent components alone. CYVADIC caused tumor regression, as seen in **A.** The only active component of the CYVADIC combination in the XF 117 thyroid carcinoma was DTIC. ○ Control; Ⅴ vincristine (VCR) 0.5 mg/kg d 1,8,15 ip; + DTIC 70 mg/kg d1–4, 15–18; × cyclophosphamide (CY) 250 mg/kg 1,5 ip; ✧ adriamycin (ADR) 8 mg/kg d 1, 15 iv; Ⅴ CYVADIC: ADR 3 mg/kg, d1, 15 ip; CY 50 mg/kg d1, 15 ip; VCR 0.4 d1, 15 ip, DTIC 40 mg/kg d1–4, 15–^8 ip.

Table 4
Maximum Tolerated Doses* of Selected Anticancer Drugs
in Tumor-Bearing Nude Mice

Drug	Dose [mg/kg/d]	Schedule	Route
Gemcitabine	300	1,8,15	iv
Taxol, Paclitaxel	20	1,8,15	iv
Taxotere	20	1,8,15	iv
Topotecan	2.5	1–3	iv
Vindesine	1.5	1,8,15	iv

* until 7–10 days [d] after last therapy

Table 5
Anticancer Activity of 5 Drugs in Clinically Responsive* and Resistant Tumor Types

Drug	Responsive tumors				Resistant tumors			
	total	CR**+PR	MR+NC	P	total	CR**+PR	MR+NC	P
Gemcitabine	17	1	5	11	10	0	2	8
Taxol	13	7	1	5	6	0	0	6
Taxotere	3	2	1	0	6	1	5	0
Topotecan	8	3	1	4	11	0	0	11
Vindesine	72	29	8	35	41	2	2	37
Total	113 (100%)	42 (37%)	16 (14%)	55 (49%)	74 (100%)	3 (4%)	9 (12%)	62 (84%)

* for definition see text; **CR-complete remission; PR-partial regression; MR-minor regression; NC-no change; P-progression, for further details see methods

partial remission in 29 of 72 tumors (40%), a minor regression or no change was noted in 8 (11%), and a progression in 35 (49%) of the tumors studied. In marked contrast, in the resistant tumor types—including cancer of the bladder, colon, cervix uteri, ovary, prostate, and kidney only two remissions were observed. These occurred in kidney cancer and in soft-tissue sarcoma, and of 41 tumors, two with no change were found (5%). Thirty-seven (90%) of the tumors grew progressively. Overall, vindesine may have a slightly higher efficacy in the xenograft model, with a remission rate of 40% which is higher than observed in the clinic. This can be explained by the fact that the MTD in mice is 50% higher than in men based on body surface (Table 4). The MTD in mice is 1.5 mg/kg—equal to 4.5 mg/m^2—while in patients it is 3.0 mg/m^2. Nonetheless, this analysis clearly indicates that vindesine has a similar response pattern with sensitive tumors in the xenograft system, as in the clinic. Based on our data, gastric cancers appear to be a vindesine-responsive tumor entity, with 5 of 14 xenografts showing remissions (Table 6). Vindesine has thus far not been included in standard regimes for chemotherapy of stomach cancers, but further phase II studies of this tumor type are strongly recommended.

These in vivo chemosensitivity data demonstrate the strength of the human-tumor xenograft model as a predictor of clinical response. Thus, this patient explant-based model system provides a valuable tool to screen novel experimental agents for respon-

Table 6
Activity of Vindesine in 113 Human Tumor Xenografts*

	Tumor type	number	CR+PR**	MR+NC	P
Responsive					
	Lung – SCLC	6	5	1	
	NSCLC	22	4	3	15
	Breast	10	7		3
	Head & neck	2	1	1	
	Leukemia	1	1		
	Melanoma	11	2	2	7
	NHL	1	1		
	Gastric	14	5	1	8
	Testis	5	3		2
Total *n*		**72 (100%)**	**29 (40%)**	**8 (11%)**	**35 (49%)**
Resistant					
	Bladder	3			3
	Colon	6			6
	Cervix uteri	1			1
	CNS	1			1
	Hepatoma	1			1
	Mesothelioma	4			4
	Ovary	5			5
	Pancreas	2			2
	Prostate	3		2	1
	Renal	8	1		7
	STS	7	1		6
Total *n*		**41 (100%)**	**2 (5%)**	**2 (5%)**	**37 (90%)**

* Dose in nude mice: 4.5 mg/m^2 = 1.5 mg/kg, on ds 1,8,15 iv; **CR-complete remission; PR-partial regression; MR-minor regression; NC-no change; P-progression; n-number. NHL-non-Hodgkin's lymphoma; CNS-central nervous system, STS-soft-tissue sarcoma.

sive tumor types prior to entering phase II clinical trials. One example of a successful procedure is the development a human serum albumin metothrexate conjugate (MTX-HSA), which is described later.

The sensitivity and predictivity data of human-tumor explants growing subcutaneously in nude mice generated with the Freiburg xenograft panel, in recent years, have not always been mirrored in other programs using xenograft models such as that of the US National Cancer Institute (NCI) *(5,6,11)*. Status reports of latter institution about human tumor xenograft testings have not been favorable, and as a result, large scale in vivo screening have been recently dramatically reduced. The NCI xenograft systems established from patients in nude mice, which were initially used, were partly able to identify compounds active in the clinic *(11)*, the mammary tumor MX-1 10 of 21, the lung cancer LX-1 7 of 21, and the colon cancer CX-1 0 of 22. Xenografts established from cell lines of the NCI 60-cell-line panel were less successful. They only responded well to the alkylating type of agents and were otherwise very resistant. Tumor remission was an extremely rare event *(10,11)*. An explanation for this phenomenon could be found in the undifferentiated histology of the vast majority of cell-line-derived xenografts, as shown in Fig. 2. Compared to directly patient-derived

Table 7
Validated and Novel Molecular Targets Characterized in the 60 Human Tumor Xenograft Panel

Category	Target	Category	Target
Oncogenes		*Tumor-suppressor*	
	k-*ras*	*genes*	
	c-*myc*		*p53*
	cerb-B2		
	Di12		
Growth factors		*Enzymes*	
and receptors			DT-diaphorase
	Estrogen receptor (ER)		Telomerase
	Progesterone receptor (PR)		
	EGF-R		
	TFGα	*Metastasis-related*	
	TGFβ		nm23
	EGF		CD44v6
	bFGF		uPA
			cathepsin D
			MMP-2
			MMP-3/MMP-9
Drug resistance			TIMP-2
	Mdr1		
	Mdr3		
	GST (glutathione S-transferase)		
Angiogenesis		*Structural proteins*	
	Angiogenin		cytokeratin
	VEGF		
	Vascular porosity		
	Microvessel density		

explants, these tumors lost most differentiation and tissue architecture, vascularization was minimal, and it appeared that only one homogenous subclone persisted. The patient tissue-derived xenografts maintained donor characteristics at the morphological and molecular level (Fig. 1), and the clinical response characteristics. Whenever xenografts were established from fresh patient material—such as in our labs and at the Institute for Cancer Research in London, where six different tumor types (teratoma, small-cell lung, breast, melanoma, colon, and non-small-cell lung) were studied for chemotherapeutic response—xenografts were shown to be predictive and valuable for new drug development *(7,24)*.

3.4. Molecular Characterization of Human Tumor Xenografts for Target-Oriented Drug Discovery

The development of anticancer agents is now focusing on new molecular targets and the biological characteristics of human tumors. Thus, this approach requires disease-oriented models/molecularly defined systems, which could discriminate between specific and general cytotoxic antitumor activity. We have therefore characterized 60 xenografts from our collection for 29 validated or emerging new targets for cancer

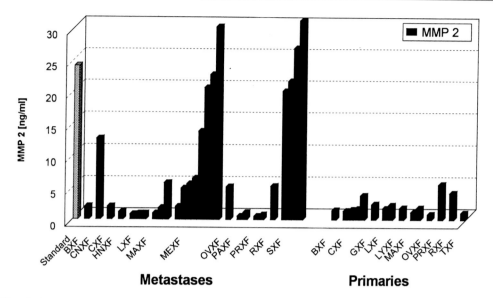

Fig. 4. Expression of the matrix metalloproteinase MMP-2 in a panel of xenografts comparing tumors established from metastases and primaries. BXF-bladder cancers; CNXF-CNS cancers; CXF-colon tumors; GXF-gastric cancers; HNXF-head & neck cancers; LXF-lung cancers; LYXF-lymphomas; MAXF-breast tumors; MEXF-melanomas; OVXF-ovarian carcinomas; PAXF-pancreatic cancers; PRXF-prostate tumors; RXF, renal-cell carcinomas; SXF-soft-tissue sarcomas; TXF-testicular germ-cell tumors. Standard = recombinant MMP-2. Melanomas and sarcomas show up to 10-fold and higher MMP-2 levels than other tumor types. Metastases-derived xenografts have in general higher MMP-2 expression than those established from primary tumors.

therapy listed in Table 7. Since it was not possible to extend this characterization to all of our 400 established human-tumor xenografts, we selected the 60 models most frequently used for routine drug-testing procedures and capable of growing in soft agar for an in vitro prescreen. These patient explants resemble a broad spectrum of histological types and sensitivity profiles. The tumor types presented are bladder (n=3), breast (n=7), cervical (n=2), colon (n=6), gastric (n=3) head and neck (n=3), lung (n=9), ovary (n=5), pancreas (n=2), prostate (n=4), renal-cell (n=6), testis (n=1), and uterus (n=1) cancers, as well as sarcomas (n=4), and melanomas (n=4).

Molecular analyses showed that target expression in human-tumor xenografts can be tumor-type-specific or random, and this also closely mimics data reported for patient specimens.

For example, the expression of the metastasis-associated protein CD44v6 showed inter- and intratumoral heterogeneity. Matrix metalloproteinase 2 (MMP 2) in contrast, was expressed at 10-fold higher levels in melanoma and sarcoma xenografts than in most other tumor types (Fig. 4) *(25)*. Similar results for both CD44v6 and MMP-2 are reported in studies performed with patient specimens *(26,27)*. Moreover, MMP-2 (also called gelatinase A) expression was in average up in tumors established from distant organ metastasis compared to those originating from primaries (Fig. 4). Because part of the extracellular matrix MMP-2 contributes significantly to normal tissue/stroma destruction, and thus to tumor-cell invasion and dissemination, it is possible to distinguish—on a molecular basis, by measurement of metastasis-associated proteins—

Table 8
VEGF and VP Expression in Human Tumor Xenografts

Tumor type	Designation	Vascular permeability* [% Dose/g Tumor]	VEGF-expression [pg/μg]**
Bladder	BXF 1299	2.4	3.5
	BXF 1301	3.1	5.0
Colon	CXF 158	4.0	1.1
	CXF 280	2.3	1.2
	CXF 1103	2.8	6.6
Stomach	GXF 97	4.8	0.7
	GXF 209	2.7	0.4
Lung	LXFA 629	1.9	0.3
	LXFA 983	2.9	ND
	LXFL 529	2.5	1.8
	LXFS 538	2.0	0.3
Breast	MAXF 401	3.8	7.3
	MAXF 449	**0.7**	**0.3**
	MAXF 857	2.0	0.3
	MAXF 1162	2.9	20.7
	MAXF 1322	4.0	0.7
Renal	RXF 393	8.2	36.9
	RXF 944LX	**8.6**	**41.8**
	RXF 1220	8.7	13.4
	RXF 486	2.5	1.1
	RXF 631	1.9	3.5

* Evans Blue dose retained per g tumor; **total protein

between xenografts derived from primaries and metastases (25). Although dissemination into organs of the host by subcutaneously growing human-tumor explants is a very rare event (4), they still appear to be good models for studying tumor biology of invasion and metastasis or for evaluation of inhibitory agents in this cascade. Our experience with MMPs and other metastasis-associated proteins suggests that the molecular information leading to the dissemination processes in patients is conserved in subcutaneously growing xenografts.

Another demonstration of the excellent correlation between molecular characteristics of grafted human tumors in our collection and fresh patient material are the determinants of angiogenesis and tumor neovascularization. The determination of VEGF and VP showed that renal carcinomas are a tumor type particularly high in these angiogenic factors (Table 8) (28). On the contrary, colon and lung carcinomas appeared much less angiogenesis-dependent. Although stroma and blood supply/vessels in a human-tumor xenograft are provided by the host (nude mouse), vessel density and tissue architecture as well as molecular-marker expression—here human VEGF—remained nearly identical with that of the human donor specimen.

All of our molecular data are available in a database and we are capable to correlate the expression of potential molecular targets with in vitro effective dose levels derived from the clonogenic assay using the xenograft material. This bioinformatic approach is based on the COMPARE algorithm developed by the NCI (29), and allows to determine if there is any statistical interaction (Spearman rank coefficient) with the potential molecular target, thus providing a hint of a possible mechanism of action of a drug.

3.5. Assessment of In Vivo Efficacy of Anticancer Agents—Drug Discovery Using the Freiburg Xenograft System

In recent years, we have developed a combined in vitro/in vivo testing procedure for anticancer drug development *(16,17)*. Broad in vitro testings using fresh human-tumor xenograft tissues in the clonogenic assay, or slow-growing permanent cell lines derived thereof have been employed in our laboratory as a prescreen preceding the in vivo testings in nude mice in order to identify the most sensitive tumor types, thus reducing the number of mouse experiments. The clonogenic assay offers the advantage of tumor cells growing in three dimensions, and only tumor stem cells are capable to proliferate. Furthermore, the tumor source—the in vivo growing xenograft or the initial patient explant—resembles the tumor as it would grow in a patient. In addition, the clonogenic assay has been well validated in the past in terms of response rates of fresh tumor explants vs that of patients in the clinic with a highly accurate prediction found for drug resistance and an intermediate predictivity for drug sensitivity *(15,17)*.

The first stage of the in vitro/in vivo xenograft model system is the evaluation of new compounds in 6, and the second stage in 20, human-tumor xenografts for their effect on colony growth in soft agar. The 2–3 most sensitive xenografts in vitro are used for subsequent in vivo testing against subcutaneously growing tumors in nude mice. One of the limitations of the clonogenic assay is its labor intensity. Nevertheless, it is very valuable as a secondary screen for testing several hundred compounds per year, and for significantly reducing the number of animal tests.

3.6. Selected Examples of Anticancer Agents in Clinical Trials Which Have Been Discovered in a Target-Oriented Approach

For the past 10 yr, our group has received compounds from academia, the European Organization for Research and Treatment of Cancer (EORTC), the NCI, and the pharmaceutical industry *(30,31)*. They belong to various structural classes and act by different mechanisms. An overview of compounds that showed activity in our models and where we contributed to the decision to develop the compounds clinically is shown in Table 9.

Compounds that have now entered clinical trials are methotrexate coupled to human serum albumin (MTX-HSA) as synthesized at the German Cancer Research Center, pH-sensitive salicylic-acid derivatives from the University of Freiburg; flavopiridol, spicamycin, and 17-allylamino-geldanamycin obtained from the NCI; ecteinascidin and rhizoxin from the EORTC, recombinant mistletoe lectin (rML), and various other compounds from the pharmaceutical industry.

Examples of novel compounds developed by a target-oriented approach using molecularly characterized tumor-model systems and by employing a combined in vitro/in vivo xenograft testing procedure are described in the next section.

3.6.1. 17-AAG

17-allylaminogeldanamycin (17-AAG, NSC 330507, Fig. 5) is a novel semisynthetic antitumor agent identified by the NCI in vitro screening program. The compound exhibits a differential cytotoxicity profile against several tumor types in the NCI 60

Table 9
Anticancer Drugs Discovered as Active in the Freiburg Human Tumor Xenograft Panel

		Mode of action	*Reference*
from Academia:	MTX - HSA,	antimetabolite, EPR effect	*36,38*
	lip. NOAC,	antimetabolite	*40*
	pH-sensitive SA	apoptosis	*41*
from the US-NCI:	Flavopiridol,	cyclin-dependent-kinase inhibition	*42*
	Quinocarmycin,	DNA binding	*43*
	Spicamycin,	glycoprotein synthesis	*44*
	17-AAG	heat-shock protein 90 modulation	*34,35*
from the EORTC:	ET743	DNA minor grove alkylation	*45*
	Rhizoxin,	tubulin binder	*46*
	EO9	bioreductive alkylating	*47*
from Companies:	Lobaplatin,	DNA cross-linking and adducts	*48*
	D21266,	PKC and PLC inhibition	*49*
	BAY 38-3441,	topoisomerase II inhibition	*50*
	RML,	RIP, ribosome inactivation/apoptosis	*51*
	several discrete compounds		

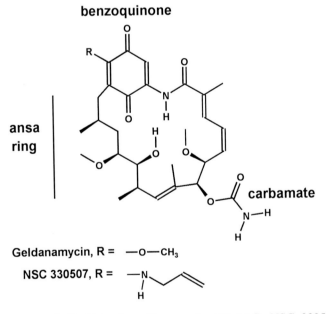

Fig. 5. Molecular structure of 17-allylaminogeldanamycin (17-AAG, NSC 330507) and gel-danamycin, respectively.

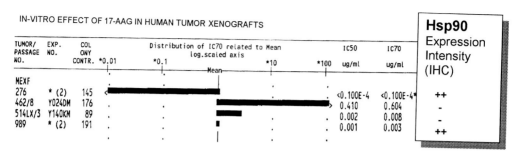

Fig. 6. Bar graph presentation of 17-AAG activity in the Freiburg melanoma xenograft panel in the clonogenic assay in vitro. Bars to the left indicate the more sensitive tumors compared to the mean IC70 value. Bars to the right are the more resistant tumors. MEXF 276 was more than two logs more sensitive towards 17-AAG than e.g. MEXF 514 or 462. Comparing 17-AAG activity against melanoma xenografts in vitro with the expression of its molecular target Hsp90, it is obvious that target expression as determined by immunohistochemistry (IHC) is highest in the more sensitive and low in the resistant melanomas. Colony contr. = mean number of colonies in the vehicle-treated wells. IC50, inhibitory concentration 50%; IC70, inhibitory concentration 70% in μg/mL. IHC expression ++ = high; + = moderate; – = low-to-negative.

human-cell-line panel, including melanomas (mean Gl_{50} = 84 nm). To evaluate whether these data would translate into preclinical activity in predictive xenograft systems, and whether in vivo efficacy could be related to target inhibition, 17-AAG was tested in four of our subcutaneously growing human melanoma xenografts (MEXF 276, MEXF 989, MEXF 462, and MEXF 514), in the clonogenic assay in vitro and in nude mice in vivo.

The heat-shock protein Hsp90 has been previously identified as molecular target for geldanamycins. Antitumor effects of this class of agents have been found to result from degradation of signaling proteins and nuclear-hormone receptors by binding their activator Hsp90 *(32,33)*. To allow the correlation between sensitivity to 17-AAG and expression of Hsp90 in our xenograft models, we determined Hsp90 expression in tissue specimens by immunoperoxidase staining and Western blot analysis. The pattern of Hsp90 expression and response of the four melanomas to 17-AAG treatment is depicted in Fig. 6.

In the clonogenic assay, 17-AAG was most active in MEXF 276 Gl_{50} < 0.02 nm, followed by MEXF 989 with Gl_{50} = 2 nm. MEXF 462 was least sensitive (μM range) in vitro (Fig. 5). In vitro activity in the soft agar assay was mirrored by in vivo efficacy of 17-AAG in the subcutaneously growing human tumor xenografts. The drug was administered intraperitoneally at 40, 30, and 20 mg/kg/d given twice daily (0 and 8 h) on ds 1–5 and 8–12. Partial tumor regression was seen in the MEXF 276 and 989 models, with optimal T/Cs at the MTD (80 mg/kg/d) of 6% or 13% respectively, whereas no significant effects were found in MEXF 462 (optimal T/C = 59%) and MEXF 514 (optimal T/C = 57%).

It is striking that high levels of Hsp90 expression in melanoma xenografts correlate with higher sensitivity toward 17-AAG treatment (Fig. 6), and that a marked decline of Hsp90 levels in MEXF 276 tumors under 17-AAG therapy and a subsequent response was observed. In marked contrast, these effects were not seen in the resistant MEXF 514 xenograft model *(34)*. Thus, the availability of a human melanoma xenograft panel with a differential in-target/Hsp90 expression enabled the preclinical development of 17-AAG and proof of its potential for clinical investigations in view of a specific antitumor activity in relation to target modulation *(35)*.

3.6.2. MTX-HSA

The rationale for combining MTX with the macromolecular carrier human serum albumin was a selective uptake of albumin in tumors that have a large energy demand and thus utilize proteins as a nitrogen source, and the enhanced permeability and retention effect (EPR) caused by tumor neovascularization *(36,37)*. Tumor vasculature has a higher porosity than normal tissue endothelium, and is responsible for the enhanced retention of macromolecules in tumors *(21,37)*. Previous kinetic studies in rats have demonstrated a selective uptake in tumors based on the energy supply hypothesis, yet we have studied MTX-HSA activity in relation to parameters of tumor vascularization in 21 solid human tumors of nine different histologies and two leukemias.

By comparing MTX-HSA efficacy in a xenograft of low (MAXF 449) and high (RXF 944) VP/EPR effect, the renal-tumor xenograft RXF 944LX responded to treatment (T/C 11%) and the mammary carcinoma MAXF 449 did not (T/C 82%). Fig. 7 shows that in vivo antitumor activity of the MTX-HSA macromolecule correlates well with VP and VEGF also named VPF, (vascular porosity factor) expression as a measure of neovascularization. The Evans blue retention/VP of 8.6% of the administered dose in RXF 944 tumors is 12 times higher than in MAXF 449 (0.7%), VEGF levels in RXF 944 (41 pg/µg) are more than 100-fold higher than in MAXF 449 (0.3 pg/µg) (Table 8), indicating that RCC are more angiogenesis-dependent than breast tumors.

Interestingly, the data of the very recent phase I clinical study appear to support the xenograft results *(38)*. Of 17 patients studied, three responses were seen. Of these, two occurred in patients with RCC *(38)*.

Other tumor types that responded to MTX-HSA at the MTD (12.5 mg/kg/d free MTX) in the nude mouse, and had a higher antitumor activity than MTX alone (given at 50 mg/kg/d), were cancers of the bladder and prostate and a sarcoma. These histologies should therefore be included in the upcoming phase II trials *(39)*.

In conclusion, MTX-HSA is a promising novel compound, and we have demonstrated its specific accumulation in human tumors. This finding supports the rationale on which it was developed, and an approach that targets tumors by employing their specific physiology—the phenomenon of tumor angiogenesis.

3.7. Possible Future Impact of Human Tumor Xenografts and Explants

Inasmuch as new drug development is already focused on target-oriented and tumor-cell-specific approaches based on currently available knowledge, there is still an ongoing demand for a better understanding of tumor biology. Thus, basic research is directed toward genetic tumor profiling and the finding of novel, more promising, tumor-type-specific therapeutic targets, or even individualizing cancer therapy. In accomplishing this, DNA array technology now provides a large amount of possible new gene candidates for therapeutic intervention, but the validation of these genes in a wide range of human tumor specimens seems to prove the bottleneck. In particular, the lack of sufficient tumor-tissue material to perform and thoroughly repeat a set of confirmatory analyses, such as Northern or Western blots, is often problematic. Here, our

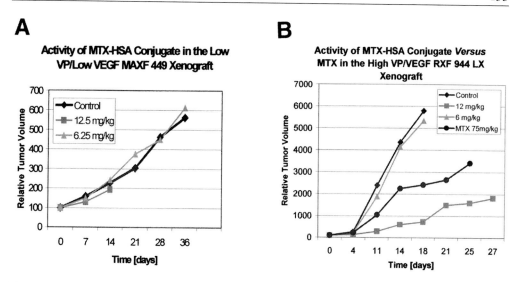

A

Activity of MTX-HSA Conjugate in the Low VP/Low VEGF MAXF 449 Xenograft

B

Activity of MTX-HSA Conjugate *Versus* MTX in the High VP/VEGF RXF 944 LX Xenograft

Fig. 7. Antitumor activity of MTX-HSA in the human mammary-tumor xenograft MAXF 449, **A**, and the RCC xenograft RXF 944, **B**. MAXF 449 is resistant against MTX-HSA conjugate therapy (T/C = 82%), and has low levels of VEGF (0.3 pg/µg protein), as well as a low rate of vascular permeability (0.7%/g dose). In contrast, RXF 944, shown in **B**, is responsive toward MTX-HSA at the MTD of 12 mg/kg (T/C = 11%), and this is accompanied by a high macromolecule retention capacity (*VP* = 8.6 %/g dose) and marked VEGF expression (41.8 pg/µg). Free MTX given at an equitoxic dose was much less effective.

xenograft collection not only provides a rich source of the human genome, but also provides material of persistent quality. Tissues can be collected freshly and immediately flash-frozen, which results in extremely high total RNA and mRNA quality. Moreover, the optimal tissue-processing procedure can be evaluated, and later on, novel treatments—either small molecules or gene therapy—can be tested in the same tissue from which a target was isolated and validated. In addition, pre- and posttreatment specimens for a pharmacogenomic approach can be easily collected. In view of these possibilities, the usefulness of human tumor xenografts and explants will steadily increase.

SUMMARY

In Freiburg, we have implanted more than 1.600 human tumors during the past 15 yr, and experimental models have been developed for all major solid human tumor types by engrafting patient tumors into immunodeficient mice. The percentage of tumors established in serial passage was highest (40–60%) for cancers of the esophagus, cervix, and corpus uteri, colon, SCLC, and melanomas. Take-rates from 20–39% were found for non-small-cell cancers of the lung (NSCLC), ovary, head and neck, pancreas, testicle, stomach, bladder, soft-tissue sarcomas, and pleuramesothelimas. Only 5–19% of cancers of the kidney, breast, and prostate could be transferred into serial passage. Sixty tumors were characterized in detail for sensitivity against standard agents, as well as expression of oncogenes, suppressor genes, growth factors and their receptors, parameters of angiogenesis, invasion, and metastasis, and resistance-associated proteins. The response of human-tumor xenografts to standard agents in the nude mouse in comparison to patient tumors was very similar—identical results were found in 90% (19 of 21) of sensitive and 97% (57 of 59) of resistant tumors. This highly accurate rate of predictivity validates the xenograft system for drug development. Moreover, since xenografts retain most of the molecular and pathophysiological patient-tumor characteristics, they are suitable tools to study target-oriented therapeutic approaches.

We have used these models for both biological and therapeutic investigations. Thus, initial testings are performed in vitro using the clonogenic assay and xenograft as donor material for fresh tissue specimens. Novel compounds are initially tested in six and then up to a total of 20 human-tumor xenografts. The dose that effects a 70% growth inhibition in vitro (IC70) is correlated against expression of potential molecular targets (e.g., k-*ras*, c-*myc*, *p53*, EGF-R, TGFα, TGFβ, VEGF, telomerase), as well as resistance-associated proteins (mdr1, mdr3, glutathione-S-transferase). The COMPARE algorithm allows the determination of any statistical interaction with a potential molecular target. The in vitro testings further allow the determination of the most sensitive tumors for subsequent in vivo studies, thus reducing the number of in vivo experiments. Compounds in clinical trial that have been discovered as active by our xenograft systems include a broad spectrum of agents with various modes of action and very specific targets, such as methotrexate coupled to human serum albumin (MTX-HSA), flavopiridol, 17-AAG, quinocarmycin, spicamycin, ecteinascidin, rhizoxin, rML, and EO9.

ACKNOWLEDGEMENTS

We are grateful to our colleagues Cornelia Steidle, Julia Schüler, and Anke Klostermeyer for their important contributions to this project. We thank Hildegard Willmann and Wolfgang Dengler for software development and data evaluation. The work was supported by grants from the German Ministry for Research and Technology (HHF); the US National Cancer Institute, Biological Testing Branch (HHF); and the Deutsche Froschungsgemeinschaft DFG (AMB).

REFERENCES

1. Rygaard J, Povlsen CO. Heterotransplantation of a human malignant tumour to the mouse mutant "nude." *Acta Pathol Microbiol Scand* 1969; 77: 758–760.
2. Povlsen CO, Sordat B, Tamaoki N. Human tumors serially transplanted in nude mice. Report. Copenhagen: The Nude Mouse Secretariat, 1977.
3. Houchens DP, Ovejera AA. Proceedings of the symposium on the use of athymic (nude) mice in cancer research, Gustav Fischer Verlag, New York, Stuttgart, 1978.
4. Reid LM, Holland J, Jones C, Wolf B, Niwayama G, Williams R, et al. Some of the variables affecting the success of transplantation of human tumors into the athymic nude mouse. In: Houchens DP, Ovejera AA, eds. Proceedings of the symposium on the use of athymic (nude) mice in cancer research, Gustav Fischer Verlag, New York, Stuttgart, 1978, pp. 107–122.
5. Ovejera AA. The use of human tumor xenografts in large scale drug screening. In: Kallman RF, ed. Rodent tumor models in experimental cancer therapy. Pergamon Press, New York, Oxford, 1987, pp. 218–220.
6. Venditti JM, Weseley RA, Plowman J. Current NCI preclinical antitumor screening in vivo: results of tumor panel screening, 1976–1982, and future directions. In: Garattini S, Goldin A, Hawking F, eds. *Advances in Pharmacology and Chemotherapy*, vol. 20, Academic Press, New York, NY 1984, pp. 2–20.

7. Staquet MJ, Byar DP, Green SB, Rozencweig M. Clinical predictivity of transplantable tumor systems in the selection of new drugs for solid tumors. Rationale of a three-stage strategy. *Cancer Treat Rep* 1983; 67: 753–765.

8. Fichtner I, Goan S, Becker M, Baldy C, Borgmann A, Stackelberg A, et al. Transplantation of human haematopoietic of leukaemic cells into SCID and NOD/SCID mice. In: Fiebig HH, Burger AM, eds. *Relevance of tumor models for anticancer drug development. Contrib Oncol,* vol 54, Basel, Karger, 1999, pp. 207–217.

9. Bibby MC. Transplantable tumours in mice—the way forward. In: Fiebig HH, Burger AM, eds. Relevance of tumor models for anticancer drug development. *Contrib Oncol* vol 54, Basel, Karger, 1999, pp. 1–13.

10. Fiebig HH, Dengler WA, Roth T. Human tumor xenografts: predictivity, characterization and discovery of new-anticancer agents. In: Fiebig HH, Burger AM, eds. Relevance of tumor models for anticancer drug development. *Contrib Oncol,* vol 54, Basel, Karger, 1999, pp. 29–50.

11. Goldin A, Venditti JM, MacDonald JS, Muggia FM, Henney JE, DeVita VT. Current results of the screening program at the division of cancer treatment, National Cancer Institute. *Eur J Cancer* 1981; 17: 129–142.

12. Sausville EA, Feigal E. Evolving approaches to cancer drug discovery and development at the National Cancer Institute. *Ann Oncol* 1999; 10: 1287–1292.

13. Malakoff D, Vogel G, Marshall E. The rise of the mouse, biomedicine's model mammal. *Science* 2000; 288: 248–257.

14. Note for guidance on the pre-clinical evaluation of anticancer medicinal products," *(http://www.eudra.org/emea.html).*

15. Scholz CC, Berger DP, Winterhalter BR, Henss H, Fiebig HH. Correlation of drug response in patients and in the clonogenic assay using solid human tumor xenografts. *Eur J Cancer* 1990; 26: 901–905.

16. Fiebig HH, Schmid JR, Bieser W, Henss H, Löhr GW. Colony assay with human tumor xenografts, murine tumors and human bone marrow. Potential for anticancer drug development. *Eur J Cancer Clin Oncol* 1987; 23: 937–948.

17. Fiebig HH, Berger DP, Dengler WA, Wallbrecher E, Winterhalter BR. Combined *in vitro/in vivo* test procedure with human tumor xenografts. In: Fiebig HH, Berger DP, eds. *Immunodeficient Mice in Oncology.* Contrib Oncol, vol 42, Karger, Basel 1992, pp. 321–351.

18. Workman P, Twentyman P, Balkwill F, Balmain A, Chaplin D, Double J, et al. United Kingdom Co-Ordinating Committee on Cancer Research (UKCCCR) guidelines for the welfare of animals in experimental neoplasy, 2nd ed. *Br J Cancer* 1998; 77: 1–10.

19. Geran RI, Greenberg NH, MacDonald MM, Schumacher AM, Abbott BJ. Protocols for screening chemical agents and natural products against tumor and other biological systems. *Cancer Chemother Rep* 1972; 3: 1–103.

20. Miles AA, Miles EM. Vascular reactions to histamine, histamine liberator and leukotaxine in the skin of guinea pigs. *J Physiol* 1952; 118: 228–257.

21. Schüler JB, Fiebig HH, Burger AM. Development of human tumor models for evaluation of compounds which target tumor vasculature. In: Fiebig HH, Burger AM, (eds). *Relevance of tumor models for anticancer drug development.* Contrib Oncol, vol 54, Karger Verlag, Basel 1999, pp. 181–190.

22. Von Hoff DD. In vitro predictive testing: the sulfonamide era. *Int J Cell Cloning* 1987; 5: 179–190.

23. Hamburger AW, Salmon SE. Primary bioassay of human tumor stem cells. *Science* 1977; 197: 461–463.

24. Steel G. How well do xenografts maintain the therapeutic response characteristics of the source tumor in the donor patient? In: Kallman RF, ed. Rodent tumor models in experimental cancer therapy. Pergam on Press, New York, Oxford, 1987, pp. 205–208.

25. Klostermeyer A, Schüler JB, Fiebig HH, Burger AM. Expression patterns of metastasis associated proteins (MMPs, CD44) in a panel of human tumor xenografts. *Ann Hematol* 1998; 77: 220.

26. Salmi M, Gron-Virta K, Sointu P, Grenman R, Kalimo H, Jalkanen S. Regulated expression of exon v6 containing isoforms of CD44 in man: downregulation during malignant transformation of tumors of squamocellular origin. *J Cell Biol* 1993; 122: 431–442.

27. Dome B, Somlai B, Tamasy A, Peter L, Tovari J, Horvath A, et al. Prognosis and invasion marker expression of cutaneous melanoma. Metastasis-associated genes (nm23, CD44v3, MMP2). *Orv Hetil* 1999; 140: 235–240.

28. Paradis V, Lagha NB, Zeimoura L, Blanchet P, Eschwege P, Ba N, et al. Expression of vascular endothelial growth factor in renal cell carcinomas. *Virchows Arch* 2000; 436: 351–356.

29. Paull KD, Shoemaker RH, Hodes L, Monks A, Scudiero DA, Rubinstein L, et al. Display and analysis of patterns of differential activity of drugs against human tumour cell lines: development of mean graph and COMPARE algorithm. *J Natl Cancer Inst* 1989; 81: 1088–1092.

30. Fiebig HH, Berger DP, Winterhalter BR, Plowman J. In-vitro and in-vivo evaluation of US-NCI compounds in human tumor xenografts. *Cancer Treat Rev* 1990; 17: 109–117.

31. Hendriks HR, Berger DP, Dengler WA, Drees M, Winterhalter BR, Lobbezoo MW, et al. New anticancer drug development: interim results of the cooperative program between the Freiburg preclinical anticancer drug development group and the EORTC new drug development office. *Contrib Oncol* 1996; 51: 108–114.

32. Stebbins CE, Russo AA, Schneider C, Rosen N, Hartl FU, Pavletich NP. Crystal structure of an Hsp90-geldanamycin complex: targeting of a protein chaperone by an antitumor agent. *Cell* 1997; 89: 239–250.

33. Schnur RC, Corman ML, Gallachun RJ, Cooper BA, Dee MF, Coty JL, et al. erbB-2 oncogene inhibition by geldanamycin derivatives: synthesis, mechanism of action, and structure-activity relationships. *J Med Chem* 1995; 38: 3813–3820.

34. Burger AM, Fiebig HH, Newman DJ, Camalier RF, Sausville EA. Antitumor activity of 17-allylaminogeldanamycin (NSC 330507) in melanoma xenografts is associated with decline in Hsp90 protein expression. *Ann Oncol* 1998; 9(Suppl 2): 132.

35. Burger AM, Sausville EA, Camalier RF, Newman DJ, Fiebig HH. Response of human melanomas to 17-AAG is associated with modulation of the molecular chaperone function of Hsp90. *Proc Am Assoc Cancer Res* 2000; 41: 447.

36. Stehle G, Sinn H, Wunder A, Schrenk HH, Stewart JCM, Hartung G, et al. Plasma protein (albumin) catabolism by the tumor itself—implications for tumor metabolism and the genesis of cachexia. *Crit Rev Oncol Hematol* 1997; 26: 77–100.

37. Matsumara Y, Maeda HA. A new concept for macromolecular therapeutics in cancer chemotherapy: mechanism of tumoritropic accumulation of proteins and the antitumor agent smancs. *Cancer Res* 1986; 46: 6387–6392.

38. Hartung G, Stehle G, Sinn H, Wunder A, Schrenk HH, Heeger S, et al. Phase I trial of methotrexate-albumin in a weekly intravenous bolus regimen in cancer patients. *Clin Cancer Res* 1999; 5: 753–759.

39. Fiebig HH, Roth T, Hartung G, Sinn H, Stehle G. In vivo activity of a methotrexat-albumin-conjugate (MTX-HSA) in human tumor xenografts. *Eur J Cancer* 1997; 9: 33(Suppl 8), 174.

40. Fiebig HH, Dengler WA, Drees M, Schwendener RA, Schott H. In vivo activity of N4-Octadecyl-Ara-C in human solid tumors and leukemias. *Proc Am Assoc Cancer Res* 1995; 36: A2434.

41. Burger AM, Steidle C, Fiebig HH, Frick E, Schlmerich J, Kreutz W. Activity of pH-sensitive salicylic acid derivatives against human tumors in vivo. *Clin Cancer Res* 1999; 5: 205.

42. Drees M, Dengler W, Roth T, Labonte H, Mayo J, Malspeis L, et al. Flavopiridol (L86-8275): selective antitumor activity *in vitro* and *in vivo* for prostate carcinoma cells. *Clin Cancer Res* 1997; 3: 273–279.

43. Fiebig HH, Berger DP, Dengler WA, Drees M, Mayo J, Malspeis L, et al. Cyanocyclin A and the Quinocarmycin analog NSC 607 097 demonstrate selectivity against melanoma xenografts in-vitro and in-vivo. *Proc Am Assoc Cancer Res* 1994; 2794.

44. Burger AM, Kaur G, Hollingshead M, Fischer RT, Nagashima K, Malspeis L, et al. Antiproliferative activity *in vitro* and *in vivo* of the spicamycin analog KRN5500 with altered glycoprotein expression *in vitro*. *Clin Cancer Res* 1997; 3: 455–463.

45. Hendriks HR, Fiebig HH, Giavazzi R, Langdon SP, Jimeno JM, Faircloth GT. High antitumor activity of ET743 against human tumour xenografts from melanoma, non-small-cell lung and ovarian cancer. *Ann Oncol* 1999; 10: 1233–1240.

46. Winterhalter BR, Berger DP, Dengler WA, Hendriks HR, Mertelsmann R, Fiebig HH. High antitumors activity of rhizoxin in a combines in-vitro and in-vivo test procedure with human tumor xenografts. *Proc Am Assoc Cancer Res* 1993; 34: 376.

47. Hendriks HR, Pizao PE, Berger DP, Kooistra KL, Bibby MC, Boven E, et al. E09, a novel bioreductive alkylating indoloquinone with preferential solid tumor activity and lack of bone marrow toxicity in preclinical models. *Eur J Cancer* 1993; 29: 897–906.

48. Klenner T, Voegeli R, Fiebig H, Hilgard P. Antitumor effect of the platinum complex D-19466 (Inn: Lobaplatin) against the transplantable osteosarcoma of the rat and other experiments. *J Cancer Res Clin Oncol* 1992; 118 (Suppl): 149.

49. Maly K, Uberall F, Schubert C, Kindler E, Stekar J, Brachwitz H, et al. Interference of new alkylphospholipid analogues with mitogenic signal transduction. *Anicancer Drug Des* 1995; 10: 411–425.

50. Fiebig HH, Steidle C, Burger AM, Lerchen HG. Anticancer activity of novel camptothecin glycoconjugates in human tumor xenograft models. *Clin Cancer Res* 1999; 5: 667.
51. Burger AM, Mengs U, Schüler JB, Zinke H, Lentzen H, Fiebig HH. Recombinant mistletoe lectin (rML) is a potent inhibitor of tumor cell growth *in vitro* and *in vivo*. *Proc Am Assoc Cancer Res* 1999; 40: 399.

IV CARCINOGEN-INDUCED TUMORS
Models of Carcinogenesis and Use for Therapy

8

Hamster Oral Cancer Model

Joel Schwartz, DMD, DMSc
and Xinbin Gu, MD, PhD

CONTENTS

1. INDUCTION OF ORAL CARCINOGENESIS

1.1. Historical Perspective

The primary focus of any experimental model for oral cancer is to gain an understanding of the mechanisms of neoplasia, and to gather data that will help the clinician to provide more effective treatment for cancer patients. The characteristics of the model must duplicate human disease as closely as possible (e.g., oral cancer). The hamster (Mesocricetus auratus) oral-cancer model system is widely used and extensively studied. The hamster oral-cancer model was originally developed through the studies of Salley. Morris produced later work in 1961, which was continued in many investigations by Shklar (1–4).

All animal models have advantages and disadvantages, and the hamster buccal mucosa oral-cancer model also has these characteristics. Various reviews have documented these aspects of the model (5). The advantages are:

1. The technique for carcinoma induction is simple to use.
2. The induction does not require any anesthesia.
3. Easy access to evaluate the development of oral cancer.

From: *Tumor Models in Cancer Research*
Edited by: B. A. Teicher © Humana Press Inc., Totowa, NJ

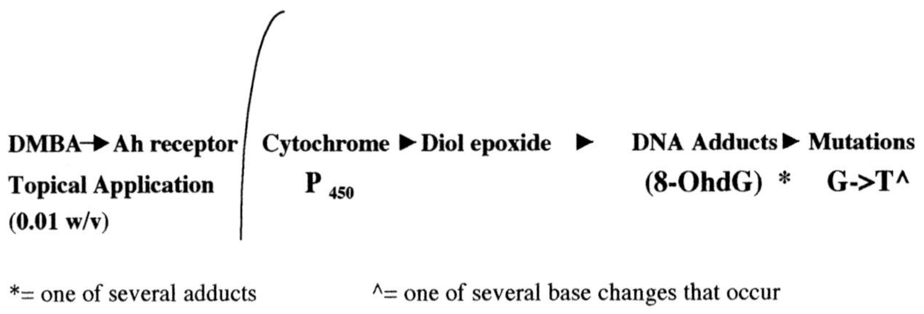

DMBA→Ah receptor	Cytochrome ▶ Diol epoxide ▶	DNA Adducts ▶ Mutations
Topical Application	P_{450}	(8-OhdG) * G->T^
(0.01 w/v)		

*= one of several adducts   ^= one of several base changes that occur

Fig. 1. DMBA Metabolism and Adduct Formation Pathway
The pathway for metabolic and mutation development after applying the carcinogen dimethylbenz(a)anthracene DMBA is shown. DMBA binds to the Ah membrane receptor, which is then processed through the membrane. The cytochrome P_{450} oxidative system acts upon this complex, forming diol-epoxide. The oxidized derivatives produce DNA adducts such as 8-hydroxy-2-deoxyguanine (8-OhdG), which is associated with the induction of mutations such as G->T transversions in tumor-suppressor genes exemplified by *p53*.

4. The surface areas of the pouch is relatively large, allowing easy visibility of changes in the mucosa.
5. Histopathologic changes consistent with those seen in human patients are found.
6. Biochemical and molecular similarities to human oral cancers (e.g., γ-glutanyl-transpeptidase (GGT), transforming growth factors (TGFs), tumor necrosis factors (TNFs), such as single-base mutations changes in *p53* and or the *ras* proto-oncogene.
7. Responses to chemopreventives and chemotherapeutic agents (e.g., tocopherols, retinoids, carotenoids, and alkylating and anti-metabolites).
8. A large body of information examining the staging of oral carcinogenesis in the buccal pouch is also available.

The disadvantages include:

1. Reduced antigenic recognition and cytotoxic T-cell response in the hamster *(6,7)*.
2. A delay in vascular drainage and a lack of lymphatics in the buccal pouch *(8)*.
3. The lack of anatomic facsimile in humans.

To reduce these liabilities, the use of both the tongue and buccal mucosa models in the hamster enhances the specificity of the relationship between chemical carcinogenesis, chemoprevention, and genetic and molecular expression. The details of these relationships are discussed in subsequent sections.

2. CHEMICAL INDUCTION OF ORAL CANCER

2.1. 7,12 Dimethylbenz(a)anthracene (DMBA)

DMBA is a polycyclic aromatic hydrocarbon (PAH) that is believed to induce oral carcinoma through an oxidation process that begins after the binding of DMBA to the Ah receptor located on the membrane of the oral keratinocyte (Fig. 1.) *(9)*. The direct contact of the carcinogen to the keratinocyte is required to produce the development of oral carcinoma. In one study, dimethyl sulfoxide (DMSO) was applied with DMBA. Shklar showed that carcinoma generation was retarded, and induced sarcomas in the underlying connective tissue *(10)*.

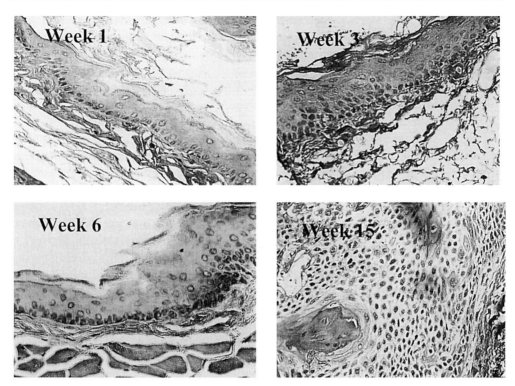

Fig. 2. Expression of 8-OhdG. During DMBA-Induced Oral Carcinogenesis During wk 1, DMBA (0.5%) is applied (three times) per wk. Hyperkeratosis and a slight hyperplasia in the number of oral keratinocytes are noted. Using the polyclonal antibody (1:25) for the antigen 8-OhdG and avidin-biotin peroxidase detection, a few darkly staining cells (6% ± 11.5) in the stratum basilis (proliferative zone) can be found. Wk 3: the hyperkeratosis is present, and an increase in the amount of hyperplasia is also observed. The number of darkly staining cells (53% ± 32.5) in the proliferative zone of the mucosa is found. Wk 6: more cells in the proliferative zone (76% ± 28.5) are positive, with a few supra basal cells also positive for the presence of this adduct. Week 15: in oral squamous-cell carcinoma (SCC) a high percentage of the cells (83% ± 33.5) in all layers of the mucosa are positive for the presence of 8-OhdG adduct formation (200X). The results indicate that with continual application of DMBA, more cells are exposed to the carcinogen and produce adduct formation that persists and accumulates in all layers of the mucosa.

The oxidation of the DMBA-Ah complexes occurs through the activation of the cytochrome P450 system. The further oxidation of DMBA produces a diol-epoxide that results in the formation of DNA adducts. One of these is 8-hydroxy-2-deoxyguanine (8-OhdG) *(11)*. (Fig. 2). The formation of the 8-OhdG adduct appears early in the process of oral carcinogenesis, before the appearance of dysplasia (wk 1). The amount of adduct accumulates as the histopathology changes from normal, mild, moderate, and severe dysplasia to invasive oral carcinoma (Fig. 2). The adducts that form are associated with mutation and genotoxicity of the hamster genome *(12)*.

2.2. Application, Induction and Development of Oral Carcinoma

The carcinogen is applied using a #4 sable brush with each application containing 0.25 mg in 0.25 mL (0.5% dissolved in mineral oil). DMBA is applied 3 d per wk for 16 wk to produce oral squamous-cell carcinoma (SCC) in the mucosa.

The hamster—which has been used in the majority of published studies—is outbred, but this is limited because the hamsters available are derived from a small number of breeding pairs. Passage viruses such as cytomegalovirus have been found among various rodent experimental models, but levels in the hamster population are very low. Another positive aspect to the use of the hamster is the lack of spontaneous carcinoma in the mucosa. Spontaneous tumor development can complicate the interpretation of the numbers of tumors induced by the chemical carcinogen. Reiskin and Berry (1968) studied the cell turnover of the oral keratinocyte population, and noted an increase following DMBA application *(13)*. More recent studies have shown that the cell proliferation markers were expressed as oral carcinogenesis, and progressed from normal and dysplastic to invasive carcinoma *(14)*. In a study by Safour et. al., the surgical manipulation of the primary site of oral carcinoma formation could also enhance the growth of the primary tumor and the metastatic spread of the cancers *(15)*.

2.3. Histopathology of Oral Carcinoma Induction in Buccal Mucosa

After one treatment of DMBA, oral mucosa change does not seem to occur. However, markers appear at this early stage. The DNA adduct 8-OhdG has been noted, and may be an early indicator of DMBA application. After 3 wk of DMBA applications the normal mucosa appears to express mild dysplasia. This state is characterized by hyperchromatism in the proliferative zone of the mucosa (stratum basilis). One or two bizarre mitoses per high-power field may also be seen. Hyperkeratosis and hyperplasia are also noted in the mucosa. After 6 wk of DMBA treatment, a moderate dysplasia with increases in the previously mentioned characteristics is noted. A period of 8–12 wk of treatment results in the appearance of carcinoma-*in-situ*. During this stage, increases in keratosis, the number of oral keratinocytes, hyperchromatism, and pleomorphism in cells of the stratum basilis extending into the stratum granulosa (spinosum) and 10–15 bizarre mitoses can be found in a high-power field. A period of 8–10 wk of treatment begins to produce papillary histology, with the other previously noted changes. A papillary surface to the developing leukoplakic (white) lesion is found. The clinical appearance of the surface lesions is predominantly white, with small areas of erthyroplakia (red). After 10 wk of treatment, the invasion into the underlying connective tissue and hyalinization (protein deposition) of the basement membrane is observed, with a dense lymphocytic infiltration. These morphologic changes are indicative of profound biochemical and molecular changes associated with extracellular matrix proteins. After 10–12 wk of treatment, histologic identification of extensive local invasion, with the appearance of surface necrosis, is commonly observed. These histological changes are also consistent with the lesions found in the biopsies of human patients. For example, Santis et al. showed that the sequence of lesions—from hyperkeratosis and dysplastic leukoplakia, to well-differentiated invasive oral carcinoma—was also found during DMBA-induced hamster oral carcinogenesis *(16)*.

The differences in oral cancers between buccal mucosa and the lateral border of the tongue have been identified *(17)*. The differences include the growth pattern of oral carcinomas induced by DMBA in the buccal mucosa and the lateral border of the tongue. The growth pattern of oral carcinomas of the tongue is not exophytic and papillary, as observed in the buccal mucosa—it is endophytic. The cancers on the lateral border of the tongue rapidly metastasize, and there are clear differences in the expression of markers such as the DNA adduct, 8-OhdG (Figs. 3 and 4) for programmed cell death and mutations in the tumor-suppressor gene *p53 (17)*.

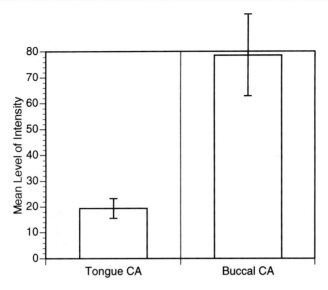

Fig. 3. A Comparison of 8-OhdG Expression in the Tongue and Buccal Mucosa. Indicated in Fig. 2, DMBA is applied to the hamster buccal pouch for 15 wk, and produces an oral SCC. In comparison, DMBA is also applied to the hamster tongue mucosa for 22 wk, and produces an oral SCC. The adduct is found to be present in all layers of the buccal mucosa oral carcinoma. In the tongue oral carcinoma, the positive stained cells are predominantly in the proliferative zone, and a few supra basal cells are also positive (20.5 ± 8.5) (X200). The lower number of DNA adduct cells in the tongue may indicate a lower level of cell death and a greater potential to produce the more aggressive endophytic carcinoma that is observed.

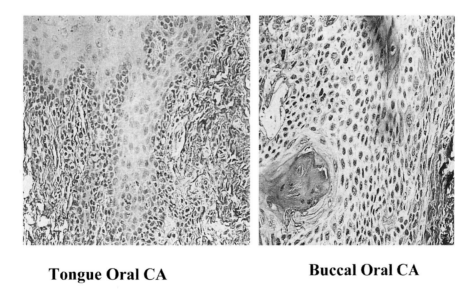

Tongue Oral CA   **Buccal Oral CA**

Fig. 4. Quantification of the Expression of 8-OhdG in Oral Carcinoma. The oral carcinomas depicted in Fig. 3 were quantified using a digital imaging system. The system is equipped with a CCD camera and imaging processing software (IMAGE PRO PLUS). Ten randomly selected sites were quantified per slide in at least two oral cancers per slide. Ten slides were analyzed for each anatomic site. The mean level of intensity for the antigen-antibody complex and a standard deviation were determined. The results indicate that a significant (Student's T Test) difference ($p < .01$) exists between the expression of 8-OhdG in the tongue and the buccal oral carcinomas.

The buccal-pouch mucosa is an excellent tissue surface to study in vivo the carcinogenic potential of various substances. Potential oral carcinogens can be applied to the hamster pouch for periods up to 6–12 mo. Unlike the lateral border of the tongue, the hamster buccal mucosa can provide a clear indication for the activity of a carcinogen because of the lack of appendages such as sebaceous glands or hair follicles. A recent development using in vitro cell growth to analyze the level of transformation in the oral keratinocytes following in vivo treatment has extended the possible use of the buccal mucosa, and could also be applied to tongue oral carcinogenesis studies *(18)*.

2.4. Staged Carcinogenesis-Initiation-Promotion Studies

Berenblum (1941) originally defined the concept of two phases in carcinogenesis *(19)*. The hamster buccal pouch has been used to test this idea. Odukoya and Shklar reported that DMBA could be used as the initiator and promotor of oral carcinogenesis *(20)*. The buccal mucosa was painted with a 0.1% soln of DMBA in mineral oil for 10 wk, but the mucosa did not develop tumors when left untreated for 6 wk. The treatment for an additional 4 wk with an 0.5% soln of DMBA acting as a promotor produces a oral carcinoma *(20)*. In another study, Suda et al. *(21)* and Odukoya and Shklar *(22)* treated hamster buccal mucosa for 10 wk, three times a wk with a 0.1% DMBA soln, followed by a period of rest of 6 wk of no application. A treatment period of 6 wk with the noncarcinogenic agent 40% benzoyl peroxide (40%) promoted the growth of oral carcinomas. Gimenez-Conti and Slaga later confirmed this relationship in their study by initiating oral keratinocyte transformation with DMBA (2 µmols), then promoted with benzoyl peroxide (40 mg) *(23)*.

3. OTHER CARCINOGENS AND ETIOLOGIES

3.1. Alcohol

One of the leading causes of oral cancer is the consumption of alcohol. The association between alcohol intake and oral cancer has been well established through a study by Rothman and Keller in 1992 *(24)*. More recent studies, which confirm these earlier findings, indicate that alcohol is not a carcinogen, but probably acts as a cofactor for carcinogenic activity by drying the oral mucosa and allowing carcinogens to contact the mucosa *(25)*. Friedman and Shklar studied, which the ingestion of alcohol during DMBA-induced oral carcinogenesis augmented the growth of oral carcinomas while hepatic damage was also observed *(26)*. Alcohol may also potentiate the effects of betel nut (pan masala), leading to the development of oral carcinoma in the hamster *(27)*.

3.2. Smoking

Smoking produces several potent carcinogens, which include polycyclic aromatic hydrocarbons (PAHs) such as benz(a)pyrene(3,4-benzpyrene) and nitroamines *(28)*. Condensates of tobacco smoke have been used to induce oral carcinomas in the buccal pouch, as identified by Kendrick and Moore and Miller *(29,30)*. The carcinogen BP has also been identified as a carcinogen in the buccal pouch, inducing oral carcinomas in a similar manner to methylcholanthrene *(31)*. The nitrosoamines, N'-nitrosonornicotine (NNN) and 4-(methylnitrosoamino-1-(3-pyridyl)-1-butanone (NNK) are not capable of inducing oral carcinomas when used as primary carcinogens in the hamster buccal mucosa *(32)*. After the application of an initiation dose of DMBA (0.1%) treatment for

6 wk with the additional applications for NNN for 16 wk produced oral carcinomas in a few hamsters *(33)*. In another study by Chen et al., hamster buccal mucosa were treated with either 0.01% NNN, 0.01% NNN and 6% nicotine, 0.01% NNK, 0.01% NNK and 6% nicotine, 6% nicotine, or sesame oil. The animals were treated three times per wk for 13 mo. The treatment of the buccal mucosa with nicotine combined with NNN showed more frequent histologic changes, including hyperplasia, hyperkeratosis. In one hamster, moderate dysplasia was noted, but no cancers were found *(28)*.

In several epidemiology studies, the use of smokeless snuff has been associated with an increased incidence of oral cancer *(34)*. No carcinogenic activity has been observed when snuff was inserted into the hamster pouch or spread over the oral mucosa. This result has been repeated in a number of experiments regardless of the application time—only once and left in place for several mo, or inserted repeatedly for up to 2 yr. In contrast, a few tumors were found in artificial lip canals following snuff application *(35)*. The extract enriched by the addition of 10 times the naturally occurring amounts of NNN and NNK produced only a few benign papillomas at the site of application, but the application of these agents directly enhanced the number of papillomas. Hamsters fed diets containing snuff at a concentration of 20% for 2 yr produced only fore-stomach papillomas, but this rate of benign tumor growth was also found when the hamsters were fed only cellulose *(36)*. In another study, the application of snuff produced no tumorigenic activity, and required the combination with DMBA to induce a 10–15% incidence of tumors in the buccal pouch *(37)*. The histologic effects of smokeless tobacco have been explored in a study by Summerlin et al. In addition to the previously mentioned benign papilloma formation, this study observed significant acanthosis with no indication of carcinoma formation *(38)*.

Using the hamster oral-carcinoma-cell line, HCPC-1 derived from a DMBA-induced oral carcinoma *(39)*, the growth potential of these cells was enhanced following treatment with smokeless tobacco extract. The growth of the oral carcinoma cells was associated with bradykinin expression *(40)*.

3.3. Viruses

The use of the hamster-tumor model to explore the role of virus infection was first explored during the 1960s. The relationship between adenovirus infection and oral pharyngeal carcinoma formation was studied by Rangan et al. *(41)*. Viral infection has also been shown to be occur through a transplacental infection and parenteral inoculations *(31)*.

3.3.1. HUMAN PAPILLOMA VIRUS

The human papilloma virus (HPV) serotypes 16 and 18 have been shown to be a cofactor in the formation of oral carcinoma *(42)*. The HPV expresses early proteins such as E6 and E7 that are linked to the suppression of the tumor-suppressors *p53* and retinoblastoma (Rb) activities *(43)*. The role of HPV in the induction of human oral carcinoma remains unclear, and the specific relationship to HPV infection and the induction of oral carcinoma through the activity of chemical carcinogenesis is also unresolved.

3.3.2. HERPES VIRUS

Rajacani et al. (1975) initially described the induction of a latent herpes virus type 1 infection in the trigeminal ganglia of the hamster *(44)*. The development of a herpes simplex Type 1 infection in the hamster buccal pouch was followed by an oral carcino-gensis study by Park et al. The study focused upon the relationship between the application of snuff and herpes infection, because snuff dipping had an association with an increased incidence of oral cancer and inactivation of herpes simplex virus (HSV), which appeared to induce malignant changes in oral keratinocytes (45). Mock and HSV inoculations were done once per mo for 6 consecutive mo. Snuff was placed in a consistent manner into the buccal pouch, using the diagonal cut off end of a straw. Simulated snuff dipping was continued for 6 mo after the initial treatment of viral inoculation, which continued for 4 wk. Simulated snuff dipping and HSV infection alone did not induce neoplastic changes in hamster buccal pouches, but HSV infection in *combination* with simulated snuff dipping resulted in epithelial dysplasia and invasive oral carcinoma in more than 50% of the animals in this group (46). In vitro studies have indicated that snuff may interfere with the DNA synthesis and the cytolytic activity of HSV (47). The expected result is the accumulation of mutation or an alteration in DNA repair, resulting in the increased growth of oral carcinomas. It is interesting to note that the HSV-2 induced cancers may be reduced in growth by reducing the immune response through cortisone treatment (48). Monoclonal antibodies (MAbs) to HSV have also been used to detect the presence of infection, and possibly to provide a means to lyze these infected keratinocytes (49).

Latent HSV-1 infection also appears to be enhanced during DMBA-induced carcinogenesis, increasing the tumor burden and the histopathologic changes associated with severity (50). The infection of HSV-1 was assumed to produce enhanced oncogene, proto-oncogene expressions and their products. HSV-1 immunization was attempted to reduce the formation of oral carcinomas induced by DMBA. In a study by Park et al., HSV-1 immunization did not alter the carcinogenic activity of DMBA, but it completely obstructed the co-oncogenic effect of HSV-1 in the oral cavity of the hamster (51).

To review, HSV alone is not carcinogenic in the hamster oral-cancer tumor model. HSV demonstrates a cocarcinogenicity. Viral inoculation enhances the oncogenic capacity of chemical carcinogens, most likely by altering tumor-suppressor, oncogene, and proto-oncogene expressions. These changes in gene expression result in enhanced programmed cell death, and in DNA repair activation.

4. GENETIC AND MOLECULAR DIFFERENCES IN ORAL CANCER FORMATION

4.1. Site-Specific Growth and Pathology

As previously noted, there are two oral carcinoma models that are induced by the application of DMBA. The oral carcinomas described here have different growth patterns, and exhibit fundamental differences in their genetic and molecular biology (17).

Fujino et al. produced lingual carcinomas in mice using 4-nitro-quinoline-N-oxide (52). Dachi later produced lingual carcinomas after 13 wk of application of DMBA in dimethyl sulfoxide (53). Fujita et al., using DMBA in acetone, produced carcinomas in four of 15 hamsters (54). These carcinomas were more readily formed in the middle one-third of the tongue, as compared to other areas of the tongue (54). Marefat and Shklar later demonstrated that the application of DMBA in acetone could be used to consistently produce oral carcinomas of the tongue in the hamster (55). The addition of trauma to the applications accelerated the growth of the oral carcinoma. Trauma, or trauma and acetone application to the tongue, did not produce carcinomas—only hyperkeratosis and some dysplasias *(55)*. The oral carcinomas induced in the tongue were endophytic, less differentiated, and spread earlier to the draining lymph nodes than the buccal oral carcinomas *(56)*.

4.2. Genetics and Molecular Biology Differences

4.2.1. DNA ADDUCT FORMATION

The identification of 8-OhdG in tongue and buccal oral carcinoma indicates a difference in the distribution of the oral keratinocytes that express this adduct. In the buccal oral carcinoma, the oral keratinocytes expressing this adduct were found throughout the mucosa, while in the tongue oral carcinoma the adduct-expressing cells were distributed primarily along the stratum basilis (Figs. 3 and 4). The differences in distribution could indicate a difference in the metabolism of the carcinogen in the two anatomic sites.

4.2.2. TUMOR SUPPRESSOR AND OTHER MARKERS FOR CARCINOGENESIS

Molecular and genetic markers can enhance our understanding of the process of oral carcinogenesis by providing valuable details concerning cell-biologic mechanisms. Biomarkers can also assist in determining the level of effectiveness for a particular agent or treatment during the development of carcinogenesis. The use of genetic and molecular markers also reduces the number of animals required to assess the function of a genetic pathway. Various types of markers have been analyzed during DMBA-induced oral carcinogenesis. The following section discusses some of these genetic indicators and their relationship to the formation of oral cancer.

4.2.3. TUMOR SUPPRESSOR (P53)

The expression of various tumor suppressors has been found to be expressed during oral carcinogenesis induced by DMBA. Specifically, the overexpression of *p53* was first noted through immunohistochemistry in 1993 in a study by Schwartz et al *(57)*. Oreffo et al. analyzed for mutations in *p53* in an NNK-induced hamster lung carcinoma, but none were found *(58)*. In a later study, Oreffo et al. again investigated hamster NNK-induced lung carcinomas, and found only one point mutation *(59)*. Chang et al. studied mutation expression in exons 5–8 of the *p53* gene in transplantable adenocarcinomas and N-methylnitrosourea (MNU)-induced hamster pancreatic ductal adenocarcinomas. Direct sequencing revealed an A→C transversion in codon 135, a frameshift in exon 7 *(60)*. These studies indicated that *p53* was involved in the process of hamster carcinogenesis.

In 1996, two groups observed and quantified mutation changes in the *p53* gene during DMBA or N-methyl-N-benzylnitrosamine (MBN) oral carcinogenesis. One group led by Chang et al. identified G→ A transitions at codon 248 *(61)*, and Gimenez-Conti et al. used single-stranded conformational polymorphisms (SSCP) to examine exons 5–8. They detected shifted bands in 17 oral carcinomas using SSCP. They sequenced eight bands to reveal four mutations. These were two G→T transversions in codons 216 and 252, one G→C transversion in codon 282, and a frameshift mutation in codon 251. These mutations are consistent with those revealed in human oral carcinomas *(62)*. In 1999 and 2000, Schwartz and Gu reported the detection of mutations of the

Table 1
Sequence Analysis of Mutations in the *p53* Gene[a]

exons DMBA	DMBA + VES[1]
5*$_{13095}$TGA→GGG	$_{13255}$TGA→TGG
7frame shift	
inserts $_{(1406)}$G→C, $_{(14063)}$C→A	$_{(14164)}$T→C
9inserts T→C, delete T	TT→GG
C→A, TTT→A, G→T (variable)	

(Sequencing of other exons 2,4,6,8, is in progress)

*( ) =nucleotide positions

[a] Gel separations from SSCP studies were analyzed using an automated ABI 370 sequencer. Smaller and fewer mutations were found for the VES+DMBA group compared to the DMBA group.

p53 gene after analyzing SSCP gels for exons 2–9. These mutations were sequenced from the oral carcinomas from five separate hamsters. The mutations were consistent with the previously known mutations, with the additional identifications for mutations in exons 6 and 8 (Table 1) *(17)*. The *p53* mutation and protein expression was compared in a recent study by Schwartz et al. in the formation of oral carcinoma in the hamster lateral border of the tongue and the buccal mucosa following DMBA application *(17)*. Using a SSCP method of mutation detection and sequence analysis, they observed that mutations in exon 4,6, and 8 appeared only in the buccal mucosa, but a mutation that appeared in the oral carcinomas of the tongue did not appear in the buccal oral carcinomas in exon 9. This mutation encoded a change in the amino acid alanine to valine (ala→ val) codon 307 *(17)*.

During DMBA-induced oral carcinogenesis, there appears to be hypermutability of the *p53* gene in the buccal mucosa *(63)*. This is not observed in the oral carcinomas of the tongue. Immunohistochemistry detecting the protein expression for *p53* has indicated a comparative lack of expression for *p53* protein in premalignant dysplasias and oral carcinomas of the tongue *(17)*. As noted previously, DMBA application to the buccal mucosa resulted in the overexpression of *p53* protein. The comparison of oral carcinomas induced through the carcinogenic action of DMBA indicates differences in gene and protein expression linked to anatomical site specificity.

4.2.4. PROTO-ONCOGENE *RAS*

Many carcinogens produce mutations in the various codons of the *ras* gene *(64)*. DMBA has been shown to produce an A→T transversion in codon 61 of the Ha-*ras* 1 gene in the mouse skin and rat mammary gland *(64,65)*. The mutations are believed to be dependent on the initiating agent. Wong et al. (1989) first reported the expression of Ki-*ras* mRNA in normal and DMBA-transformed oral keratinocytes derived from the hamster *(66)*. Husain et al. identified the relationship between the amplification of expression of the proto-oncogenes c-erbB and c-Ha-*ras* during DMBA transformation of the buccal mucosa *(67)*. The amplification of c-erbB1 was first recognized following DMBA-induced oral carcinogenesis in studies by Wong *(68)* and Wong and Biswas

(69). Gimenez-Conti et al. established that between human, mouse, and hamster there was a homology of 87.5% for the Ha-*ras* codon 61 *(70).* Conti and colleagues showed that six of 11 carcinomas presented with an A→T transversion in the second position of codon 61, resulting in an amino-acid change from glycine to leucine *(70).* This group indicated that in a study by Robles et al., only three tumors showed an A→T transversion in the second nucleotide of Ha-*ras* codon 61 *(71).* In this study, they also found that this mutation was not sufficient to alter the expression of keratin, as was observed in the mouse skin-tumor model *(71).* Gimenez-Conti and Slaga concluded that approx 60% of the hamster cheek-pouch carcinomas have a mutation in codon 61 of the Ha-*ras* gene. Chang et al. investigated the expression of Ha-*ras* in three of 14 oral carcinomas induced by MBN, and three of eight DMBA-induced oral carcinomas. The Ha-*ras* mutations induced by DMBA formed a mutation "hot spot" A→T transversion *(61).*

In summary, mutations in Ha-*ras* appear to be an early event, and the overexpression of c-erbB and its product the epidermal growth-factor receptor is a later event during DMBA-induced oral carcinogenesis.

4.2.5. PROGRAMMED CELL DEATH

During oral carcinogenesis, a series of anaplastic and pleomorphic changes are observed in the oral keratinocytes treated with DMBA. These histopathologic changes are associated with either the inhibition or promotion of programmed cell death. Notable was the overexpression of *p53* observed early in the process of oral keratinocyte. The overexpression of *p53* has been associated with the induction of programmed cell death. Schwartz showed that tumor-suppressor *p53* overexpression and enhanced mutant *p53* expressions were associated with an increase in the proliferation of the transformed oral keratinocytes during oral carcinogenesis. The initial increase in cells was linked to a percentage of increase of oral carcinoma cells in G_2+ mitosis (34.9%). The percentage of cells decreased in this phase of the cell cycle (26.9%), and 6 wk later an increase in the percentage in G_0/G_1 (29.0 to 42.0%) was found *(14).* These cell-cycle changes and enhanced proliferation-marker expressions (p34cdc2, proliferating-cell nuclear antigen (PCNA), p105, and histone 3) were found in malignant oral keratinocytes that also exhibited increasing levels of nucleosome formation and decreased expression in Bcl-2, an inhibitor of programmed cell death *(14).* Other members of Bcl-2 family that are pro-apoptotic are BAX and BAK. The levels of these markers were elevated in the tongue as compared to the buccal mucosa (Fig. 5). In contrast, nucleosome formation was higher throughout the buccal mucosa, but nucleosome formation was higher in the deeply invasive oral carcinoma cells of the tongue *(17).* One explanation for these observations was that DMBA induction of oral carcinogenesis was the result of a selective process involving programmed cell death. Additional changes in expressions for wild-type and mutant *p53* in the tongue or buccal mucosa was associated with enhanced MDM2 and decreased p21 waf-1 expressions, indicating a complex pathway of *p53*-dependent and independent interactions that resulted in the induction of possible clonal selection.

4.2.6. NEOVASCULARIZATION

During the formation of oral carcinomas induced by DMBA and early in the development of premalignant dysplasias, Shaklar and Schwartz and Schwartz and Shklar

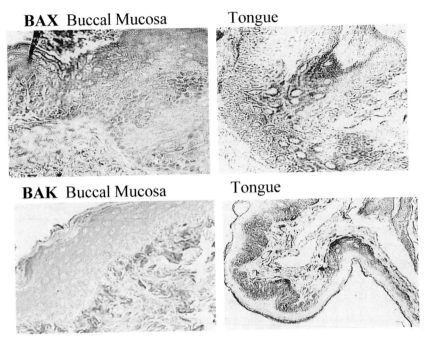

Fig. 5. A Comparison of Proapoptotic Markers in the Tongue and Oral Cancer. Monoclonal antibodies (MAbs) proapoptotic markers BAX and BAK were analyzed as indicated in Fig. 4. The expression/intensity of the antigen-antibody complex was detected in oral carcinomas from the tongue and buccal mucosa. The results show that the tongue oral carcinomas express a higher level for these proapoptotic markers (X200). These observation help to confirm a difference in the process of programmed cell death between the tongue and buccal oral carcinomas induced by DMBA.

have shown that angiogeneisis is an important factor in oral carcinoma growth *(72,73)*. Markers such as factor VIII, transforming growth-factor alpha (TGF-α), vascular endothelial growth factor (UEGF), and basic fibroblast growth factor have been identified in new endothelial-lined vascular spaces. Some of these markers have also been found in the cytoplasm of the oral mucosa *(72,73)*. Figs. 6 and 7 demonstrate the relationships between DNA-adduct 8-OhdG, the stress protein (hsp 70), and glutathione-S-transferase (GST π) expressions and increased neovascular endothelial-lined space growths adjacent to induced oral carcinomas. These results indicated that oxidative stress characterized by hsp 70 and GST π expressions could be associated with the presence of DNA adduct production.

4.2.7. OTHER MARKERS FOR DMBA-INDUCED ORAL CANCER

Other factors have also been examined during DMBA-induced oral carcinogenesis. These have included the transformation marker, γ-glutamyl transpeptidase (GGT). GGT is an enzyme that helps to transport glycine-cysteine residues across the cell membrane. These residues are used to synthesize the cellular antioxidant glutathione, and are associated with the various enzymes of the glutathione pathway (e.g., glutathione reductase, peroxidase, and glutathione-S-transferases) *(74)*. GGT is not normally expressed in the hamster buccal pouch, but GGT becomes expressed 3 d after the first DMBA treatment *(75–76)*. Another glutathione pathway-derived marker is glu-

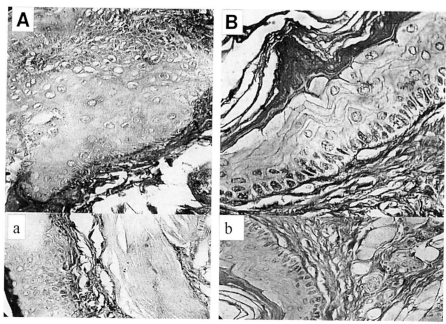

Fig. 6. A Comparison Between the Expression of 8-OhdG in Vitamin E and DMBA and DMBA-Induced Oral Carcinomas. Vitamin E (dl-alpha tocopherol acid succinate) (VES) is fed to hamsters (1.0 mg/0.120 kg) three times a week for 15 wk on days alternate to the application of DMBA (0.5%). The detection of the DNA adduct was identical to methods previously described. A) An oral carcinoma from the VES+DMBA group shows a lack of staining for 8-OhdG. Some cells in the stratum basilis are noted to exhibit a speckled distribution of staining (X200). a) At a higher magnification, a low level of staining for 8-OhdG is found in the proliferative zone adjacent to higher staining of the endothelial-lined vascular spaces. B) DMBA treatment produced high levels of 8-OhdG-positive oral keratinocytes and the number of positive stained adjacent endothelial-lined vascular spaces (X200). b) A higher magnification indicated a diffuse staining of endothelial-lined vascular spaces. The number of vascular spaces was noted to be increased compared to the VES- and DMBA-treated tissues (X400). The histopathology and immuno-histochemistry indicate that the administration of VES reduced the presence of 8-OhdG in the mucosa and in newly formed endothelial-lined vascular space.

tathione-S-transferase (GST), which is required for the synthesis of glutathione. Schwartz showed that during DMBA-induced oral carcinogenesis in early dysplasias, high levels of GST π were expressed, but this level of expression was reduced in the oral carcinoma *(14)* (Fig. 7). Yamamoto et al. reported similar findings, observing that GST p is a useful positive marker for neoplastic lesions, and that a decreased expression occurs with progression of oral carcinomas *(77)*.

After three treatments of DMBA in early dysplasias and in invasive oral carcinomas, the level for the heat-shock protein (hsp) 70 was increased, but only in discrete sites in the mucosa. These sites in the oral carcinomas were areas of invasion into the adjacent connective tissue. Other hsps such as hsp 60 and 25 *(7)* were not expressed in the mucosa, but only in the endothelial lining of vascular spaces undergoing neovascular growth. This level of expression is expected to indicate that oxidative stress products such as diol-expoxide or the DNA adduct,8-OhdG were accumulating at the site of hsp expression. Recent identification of 8-OhdG at these sites has confirmed this localization (Figs. 2–7).

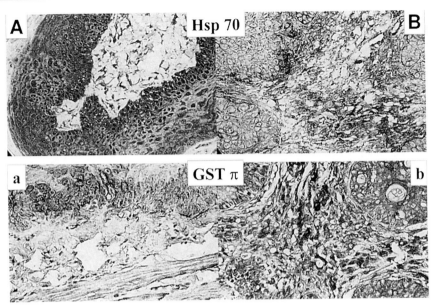

Fig. 7. A Comparison of the Expressions of Hsp 70 and GST π in Vitamin E and DMBA- and DMBA-Treated Buccal Mucosa. A) Vitamin E (VES) and DMBA treatments resulted in high levels of heat-shock protein/stress protein (hsp 70) in the mucosa of developing oral carcinomas, but relatively low levels in the endothelial-lined vascular spaces (X200). a) The level of GST π in contrast was moderately high in the proliferative zone but low in the endothelial-lined vascular spaces (x200). B) DMBA treatment produced a low level of hsp 70 in the mucosa, with only small focal areas of invasive oral-cancer cells deeply stained for expression. The endothelial-lined vascular spaces exhibited high levels of expression (X200). b) DMBA treatment resulted in a lower level of GST π in the mucosa than in the VES + DMBA group, but relatively higher levels were noted in the endothelial-lined vascular spaces (x200). These findings indicated that oxidative/cellular stress was higher in the VES + DMBA-treated oral carcinomas, but GST was produced, increasing possible control of reactive oxygen substances. Hsp 70 was lower in the newly formed vascular spaces, with lower levels of GST also produced.

Keratin formation has been used to determine the level of differentiation following DMBA treatment. Gijare et al. identified keratin, using a protein extraction method and SDS gel elctrophoresis of the mucosa from the buccal pouch after treatment for 1 mo *(37)*. This protocol produced oral carcinoma in only 10–15% of the animals, and therefore the keratin values were predominantly derived from premalignant dysplasias. The analysis of keratins in the untreated buccal pouch showed the presence of eight cytokeratin polypeptides, which included 67, 66, 60, 56, 53, 46, and 43 Kd. In general, the basal cells contain the low mol-wt keratins, and the keratinocytes in the stratum spinosum contain the higher mol-wt keratins, *(37,78)*. Following DMBA treatment, the investigators observed a loss of 67-Kd and a reduction in expression for 66 and 63-Kd cytokeratins. The same pattern was also noted following treatment with DMBA and snuff. The treatment with snuff only produced a loss of the 67-Kd keratin *(37)*. Gimenez Conti et al. *(79)* and Gimenez-Conti and Slaga *(23)* studied the expression of keratins following DMBA treatment of the buccal pouch. They used immunohistochemistry and immunoblotting, and found that the 67-Kd keratin was strongly expressed in hyperplastic lesions, but that dysplastic lesions and carcinomas did not express this protein except for small foci in well-differentiated carcinomas *(23,79)*. A 47-Kd keratin protein was expressed in all stages of DMBA-induced oral carcinogenesis. After 2 wk of treatment with DMBA (six treatments) and the presence of mild dysplasia, a 551-kd keratin protein was expressed throughout the mucosa *(23,79)*. Moderate to severe dysplasias and oral carcinomas also expressed this protein. Schwartz et al. also reported that high mol-wt keratins were lost in moderate, severe dysplasias and oral carcinomas induced by DMBA treatment *(78)*.

Transglutaminase I (TG I), an enzyme required for the formation of a mature cornified envelope of the oral keratinocyte, was examined by Shin et al. (1990) *(80)*. TG I was expressed at limited levels in the stratum basilis of hyperplastic lesions. These levels increased slightly in dysplasias, and were markedly enhanced in oral carcinomas *(80)*.

Putresceine and spermidine, which are required for DNA nucleotide synthesis, dramatically increased after eight (moderate dysplasia) to 16 (oral carcinoma) wk of DMBA treatment *(80)*. Other markers that correlated with DMBA treatment were ornithine decarboxylase and micronuceli levels. Nuclear-organizer region identification was also recognized early in the process of DMBA treatment.

5. IMMUNOLOGIC DIFFERENCES ASSOCIATED WITH CARCINOGEN INDUCTION

Witte et al. studied the ontogeny and function of the thymic (T) lymphocyte in the Syrian hamster *(6,7)*. Immunologic analysis indicated that the hamster had a reduced number of cytotoxic T lymphocytes and a low comparative number of T lymphocytes in the spleen *(6,7)*. There are several unique aspects of the immune system as it relates to chemical carcinogenesis of the hamster buccal pouch. Billingham and Slivers have considered the buccal pouch privileged immunologic site *(81)*. Schwartz et al. has identified various cytotoxic populations in the hamster pouch *(82)*, but the antigen-recognition repertoire of the lymphocyte Ia region is restricted. DMBA treatment does increase the level of cytotoxic and helper populations of T lymphocytes in comparison to the untreated counterpart. In addition, the level of expression for tumor-necrosis factors α and β are also enhanced *(83)*. The cytotoxicity of resident peritoneal macrophages from DMBA-treated hamsters is also reduced *(84)*. The suppression of the immune response is required for the continual growth of oral carcinomas in the buccal pouch. The use of immunosuppressive drugs to produce cortisone- and methotrexate-enhanced oral carcinogenesis was shown in multiple studies by Shklar et al. *(85,86)*. The importance of cell-mediated responses in controlling the growth of DMBA-induced oral carcinomas is found by using anti-lymphocyte serum, as shown in a study by Woods *(87)*, and later, by Giunta and Shklar *(88)*. Immuno-enhancing agents such as bacillus Calmette-Guerin (bCG) as described by Giunta et al. *(89)* and levamisole, as performed by Eisenberg and Shklar *(90)* and Shklar et al., reduced the formation of DMBA-induced carcinomas *(91)*. The movement of the immune-effector populations into and through the buccal pouch is accomplished by a vascular channel, and there is no lymphatic drainage *(8)*.

Schwartz et al. showed that in the oral mucosa of the hamster buccal pouch, the Langerhans cells form a dentritic network that covers much of the surface. In this array, arefocal areas are present, which appear to be antigen-processing centers *(92)*. Following DMBA treatment, the dentritic network is reduced or eliminated, with a dramatic loss of the focal sites *(93)*.

In general, DMBA-induced oral carcinogenesis reduced cytotoxic immune responses that normally target oral cancer cells. In addition, Gould has described the suppression of immune activity in the hamster with DMBA and X-ray treatments *(94)*.

6. IN VIVO/IN VITRO STUDIES

6.1. Proliferation and Growth Characteristics

The hamster buccal-pouch carcinoma induced by DMBA has provided the cell line HCPC-1 *(39)*, and these carcinoma cells can be transplanted directly to the peritoneal cavity of inbred and neonatal hamsters, as described in a study by Merk et al. The transplantable tumors become more anaplastic, and grow more rapidly than primary tumors *(95)*. Meng et al. showed that these transplantable tumors can be re-implanted into the buccal pouch, and can become more anaplastic and aggressive *(96)*.

Schwartz and Shklar studied the oral keratinocytes from the buccal mucosa after they were placed into culture and treated with DMBA. The cells were transformed into malignant oral keratinocytes, using a dose of 5–50 ng/10 mL after 3 wk of treatment *(97)*. Colony formation and thymidine incorporation indicated that the oral keratinocytes were increasing in their growth following repeated treatments (more than three) of DMBA. The continuous treatment by DMBA over a 3-wk period significantly enhanced plating and seeding efficiencies. Cell-cycle analysis using flow cytometry also showed that the continual treatment with DMBA (3 wk) of the oral keratinocytes resulted in an increased percentage of cells in synthesis (S) and G_2 + mitosis *(97)*.

In contrast, the number of cornified cells—a signal for differentiation—was markedly reduced. Another indicator for differentiation—the number of high-molecu-larkeratin-positive cells—was also reduced as the number of oral keratinocytes expressing low-mol-wt keratins increased *(97)*.

6.1.1. Markers for Transformation

In further studies, DMBA treatment of the oral keratinocytes derived from the buccal pouch enhanced the number of GGT positive cells that grew in soft agar in a nonattached manner *(97)*. Changes in GGT expression and growth-pattern changes are believed to be associated with early malignant transformation *(8,75,76)*.

The overexpression of tumor-suppressor *p53*, or the expression of mutant *p53*, is also ascribed to the process of oral malignant transformation. Using flow cytometry, these changes were quantified in the DMBA-treated oral keratinocytes. The injection of the DMBA-treated cells into the buccal pouch and the subsequent histopathologic examination confirmed that DMBA treatment of normal buccal mucosal keratinocytes produced oral carcinoma in four of six recipient hamsters *(97)*.

7. RESPONSES TO THERAPY

7.1. Surgery

The surgical manipulation of the primary oral cancer in the buccal pouch, as described by Safour et al., *can* result in the increased growth of oral carcinomas. Shklar found that manipulation and incision of the developing carcinoma *did not* result in deeper invasion of these lesions or metastatic spread *(98)*. The differences in results may be ascribed to the time of surgical manipulation. Another study conducted by Iida et al. used CO_2 laser surgery and scalpel incisions after initiation with DMBA *(99)*. Using the expression of GST p as a marker for early malignant transformation, the results indicated that *surgery-enhanced promotion* with increased GST expression in hyperplasia and early dysplasia *(99)*, but GST expression is reduced in oral carcinomas.

7.2. Radiation

7.2.1. X-Radiation

Lurie and Cutler investigated the effects of repeated low-dose-rate, high-dose-rate X-radiation of the head and neck on lingual-tumor induction by DMBA in the hamster *(100)*. The hamsters were administered DMBA (0.5%) in acetone to the middle one-third of the tongue for 15 consecutive wk, 20-R X-radiation to the head and neck once a wk for 15 wk, or DMBA and X-radiation for 15 wk. Animals receiving DMBA plus radiation had an excess of benign papillomas compared to animals receiving only DMBA. The DMBA and X-radiation group also produced malignant carcinomas at sites other than the DMBA-treated site. These areas included the lip, gingiva, and floor of the mouth. In a later study, Lurie stated that the timing between DMBA application and X-radiation is also important in the production of oral tumors *(101)*. Lurie et al. investigated the relationship between low-level X-radiation and vascular changes in the hamster buccal pouch *(101)*. It is important to remember that unlike the human oral mucosa, the hamster buccal pouch has no lymphatic drainage—only a vascular path in and out *(8)*. Vascular changes would be of great significance to the development of oral carcinomas in the pouch. X-radiation and/or DMBA application to the mucosa resulted in significant changes in vascular volume over time. DMBA treatments alone resulted in significant changes in vascular permeability over time. In the premalignant stages of oral carcinogenesis, the vascular volumetric changes were similar in the DMBA and the X-radiation groups. The combined treatment of DMBA and X-radiation produced a slower increase in vascular volume, then a gradual decline to levels observed in the radiation-only treatment group during oral carcinoma formation. The reason that DMBA treatments produce a higher level of vascular changes in volume and permeability than radiation treatments is unclear. A possible explanation includes radiation damage to microvascular channels, subsequent inflammatory responses with releases of cytokine or lymphokine factors, connective-tissue effects, and epithelial responses to the released factors. The increase in tumor burden from DMBA and X-radiation would indicate at least an additive effect on the oral keratinocytes, creating more mutation or genomic instability. Inoue and fellow scientists presented proliferation data obtained from the DMBA-treated tongue mucosa 1d and 3d after irradiation by 60Co-gamma ray 20 gy. DMBA induced an increase in vascular proliferation, which was reduced with radiation treatment. The time interval for mitosis in these cells was not affected, but synthesis time will increase 3 d after irradiation *(102)*. Radiation could have a therapeutic effect on DMBA oral carcinogenesis, depending on the dose and time of treatment.

7.2.2. Photodynamic Therapy

Photodynamic therapy has also been studied in the hamster buccal pouch. Burns et al. studied the tumor-localizing and photochemotherapeutic properties of hematopor-phyrin (HPD) derivatives in DMBA-induced oral carcinomas. Oral carcinomas in the hamster injected with HPD (50 µ/g of body wt [av. 0.120 kg]) exhibited a bright salmon-pink fluorescence after exposure to long-wave ultraviolet *(vv)* light 24 h after intraperitoneal (ip) injection. Adjacent tumor-free mucosa did not fluoresce. The histology indicated that the oral carcinomas were edematous and hemorrhagic, with cellular necrosis that progressed with increased time after photochemotherapy. Complete necrosis was observed after 1d *(103)*. Von Glass et al. performed another photodynamic therapy, using hamster oral carcinomas induced with DMBA treatment. This study included aluminum phthalocyanine (AISPc). The therapy produced interstitial bleeding derived from an enhanced vascular leakage. This reaction was also evident in newly formed vessels at the margins of the tumors. The differences in the targets of the photodynamic therapies were apparent, and should be considered *(104)*. To refine the localization and the pharmacokinetics, a laser-induced fluorescence system was employed by Frisoli and colleagues. In this pulsed nitrogen-laser pumped-dye activation system (610 nm) using chloroaluminum sulfonated phthalocyanine (CAISPc), the drug dosimetry was quantified in the hamster pouch *(105)*. In another study, using a Co_2 laser with the hematoporphyrin, Photofrin Kozacko et al. (1996) used in vivo fluorescence to noninvasively identify the timing for oral carcinoma appearance. Primary carcinomas were incised (0–3) 1 wk apart, or three incisions were performed 1 d apart. Another group received the epidermal growth-factor inhibitor, bombesin antagonist (RC-3095) for 4 wk during the time of incision. Laser incisions 1 wk apart enhanced promotion, but incisions 1 d apart did not. RC-3095 inhibited the promotion effect, but when stopped, the promotion effect resumed. The use of inhibitors suppressing selective growth factors appears to be a promising approach for short-term therapy and control of secondary carcinoma growth following surgery *(106)*.

Recent studies have used a second-generation photosensitizer tetra (m-hydroxyphenyl) chlorin (mTHPC). Blant and fellow scientists studied the fluence rate effect in photodynamic therapy in early oral carcinomas induced with DMBA application *(107)*. The fluence rate is a parameter that can influence the therapeutic results. The fluorescent detection is critical for adjusting the level of activation. Two wavelengths were used (652 nm and 514 nm), and the light doses also varied (8–20 J/cm2 and 80 J/cm2 fluences; 15 and 150 mW/cm2 and 25–125 mW/cm2 fluence rates). The higher fluence rates resulted in less tissue damage in tumor and healthy keratinocytes, and lower fluence rates produced slightly less therapeutic selectivity *(107)*. Using this knowledge, the group carried out another study (reported in 1997). Histologic changes in the hamster buccal pouch were described. Two different types of tissue damage were noted. The first type was a nonselective and nonspecific ischemia, producing vascular necrosis. This occurred during the first 48 h after the injection of mTHPC. The second type of change was tissue-specific coagulation necrosis, which occurred more than 3 d after the injection of dye. Initially, mTHPC is relatively nonspecific in distribution between normal mucosa and the formation of early oral carcinomas. Two days after injection, the drug is mainly localized in the endothelial cells of blood vessels. After this period, the dye accumulates in the oral keratinocytes, with a peak level 4 d after injection *(108)*.

Harris and Werkhaven provided a cautionary note concerning the localization of treatment with fluorescence. They stated that in the oral cavity and in oral keratinocytes there is a background of *auto-fluorescence* of bacteria and endogenous porphyrins generated at the site. This background creates a potential for false-positive identification of nonexistent carcinoma *(109)*.

7.3. Detection of Early Premalignant Changes

The detection of early malignant transformation has been an ongoing area of study, using the Hamster buccal pouch. Toluidine blue is a simple staining technique that has been employed in many human clinical patient studies to detect premalignant and malignant changes *(110)*. In the most recent study, using toluidine blue, brush biospy, and computer-assisted analysis, the level of false-negatives and -positives was found to be very low *(111)*. The results in the hamster buccal pouch are less clear. In a study by Miller et al., using turpentine liquid petrolatum (TLP) or DMBA to induce hyperplasia and oral carcinoma, a lack of staining of premalignant lesions and some noncancerous papillomas were stained positive with toluidine blue (5% false-positive result) *(112)*. Martin et al. observed the false-negative findings (42–58%) for moderate to severe dysplasias in the hamster DMBA-treated oral mucosa. These results seem to indicate that the "use of this dye should be restricted to selective cases" *(113)*.

Another detection method using a more sophisticated approach is quantifiable fluorescence (QT). QT imaging has been used to evaluate the development of oral carcinomas in the hamster, as described by Kluftinger et al. Using injection of the porphyrin, porfimer and in vivo fluorescence photometry were used to detect premalignant lesions in the hamster oral-tumor model *(114)*. Malignant transformation resulting from the use of a CO_2 laser was inhibited with a somatostatin RC-160 or bombesin RC-3095 analog *(106)*. The relationship between the number of dysplasias or oral carcinomas detected and those formed was unclear. Light-induced fluorescence spectroscopy and the histologic changes found during DMBA-induced buccal pouch carcinogenesis were examined in a study by Balasubramanian et al. *(115)*. The results suggested the usefulness of this technique for early diagnosis of premalignant change. A correlation of these results to specific genetic and molecular markers has not yet been performed. A comparison between DMBA-induced autofluorescence levels and porfimer-associated fluorescence levels in the DMBA-treated buccal pouch indicated a high level of detection and specificity could be accomplished *(116)*. Another study by Onizawa et al., Dhingra et al., and Chen et al. also confirmed these results, but indicated that the 330-nm excitation wavelength for fluorescence spectroscopy may be useful in the hamster for the detection of oral cancers *(117–119)*. The use of this technique in human patient populations has also been performed, and appears to be a useful technique to distinguish a premalignant from a malignant lesion *(120)*. A correlation with the level of transformation or the detection of transformed clones of cells that do not present with a clinical lesion has not been reported.

8. SIDE EFFECTS (MUCOSITIS)

About 10 separate studies have identified the hamster buccal pouch as an in vivo model for the development of mucositis. Dr. Sonis will present this area of study in Chapter 18

9. CHEMOPREVENTION—A MECHANISM

Several small and large published reviews detail the use of the hamster as a model to study the anti-tumor activities of various nutrient agents. (5, 14, 25, 121–128, 130, 139) (Table 2). The following is a general mechanism for the anti-tumor activities of chemopreventive agents (antioxidant/pro-oxidant [redox] nutrients). It is important to

Table 2
A Selected Survey of Published Chemopreventive Results

Author	Chemopreventive	Year	Hamster cancer site	Effect
Chu	Vitamin A	1965	Oral Cavity/Forestomach	Inhibition
Shklar	13RA	1980	Buccal Mucosa	Inhibition
Shklar	13RA	1980	Tongue Mucosa	Inhibition
Sonis	Vitamin A	1981	Buccal Mucosa	Inhibition
Shklar	Vitamin E	1982	Buccal Mucosa	Inhibition
Burge	Retinyl acetate	1983	Buccal Mucosa	Inhibition
Odukoya	Vitamin E	1984	Buccal Mucosa	Inhibition
Kandarkar	Retinyl acetate	1984	Buccal Mucosa	Inhibition
Schwartz	13RA	1986	Buccal Mucosa/Immune	Inhibition
Suda	β-carotene	1986	Buccal Mucosa	Inhibition
Massedi	Bowman-Birk	1986	Buccal Mucosa	Inhibition
Trickler	Vitamin E	1987	Buccal Mucosa	Inhibition
Schwartz	β-carotene, CAN	1988	Buccal Mucosa	Regression
Schwartz	β-carotene, 13RA CAN, Vitamin E	1989	Buccal Mucosa/Immune	Regression
Schwartz	β-carotene, CAN	1989	Buccal Mucosa/Immune	Inhibition
Gijare	Retinyl palmitate	1990	Buccal Mucosa	Inhibition
Schwartz	β-carotene	1991	Buccal Mucosa	Regression
Schwartz	Glutathione (red)	1996	Buccal Mucosa	Inhibition
Shklar	Vitamin E	1996	Buccal Mucosa	Inhibition
Schwartz	β-carotene	1997	Buccal Mucosa	Inhibition/ Enhancement

The survey indicated 20 studies, which have been published since 1965.

recognize that the *common* biochemical nature of the various families of chemopreventives is their ability to respond to and change the oxygen-state (redox potential) in various cell targets.

9.1. Redox Agent Activation of Immune Effectors

The population of immune effectors found in the hamster oral cavity (e.g., lymphocytes, mast cells, macrophages, eosinophiles, and others) are activated to become modifiers of malignant oral carcinoma development following exposure to a chemical and/or virus. Redox nutrients have been observed to enhance cancer-cell cytotoxicity and to increase the immune surveillance apparatus of the hamster *(131)*. This response is produced at inappropriate moments in the process of oral carcinogenesis (e.g., neovascular proliferation and the formation of fibrin-fibrous capsule), and could also be used to enhance oral cancer growth *(14)*. Various studies have documented the complexity and depth of immune regulation with different redox nutrients in the inhibition and regression of oral carcinoma in the buccal pouch. Taken together, the results indicate an activation in lymphocytes (T and B) and macrophages. This activation results in the production of tumor necrosis factors (alpha and beta) (TNF-α,β) *(139,140)*.

9.1.1. Redox Agent Chemopreventive and Therapy

Another aspect of the anti-tumor activities of redox molecules is their ability to target in a normal, premalignant, or malignant oral keratinocytes of the buccal pouch in a

Table 3
Tumor Burden Responses[1]

Agent	Inhibition CA[a]	Regression of established CA[b]	Induction CA
Carotenoid[2]	yes	yes	yes
Retinoid	yes	yes	yes
Tocopherol	yes	yes	no
Glutathione	yes	yes	no
Ascorbic Acid		no	yes
Mixture	yes	yes	no
DMBA	no	no	yes

[1]=Tumor burden $-4/3 \pi r3$

[2]=Agents were administered (av. 1 mg/0.120 kg) P.O. 3X wk for 16 wk

a=DMBA-induced 0.5% oral cancers applied 3X/wk for 16 wk.

b=Injection of agent in 0.25 mL of phophate buffered saline

The number and sizes of oral carcinomas were counted, and the tumor burden was estimated. Redox agents could inhibit oral carcinogenesis (yes). The regression of established oral carcinomas was also noted, but the induction of oral carcinoma has also been observed.

selective manner. These chemopreventive agents have the positive ability to inhibit the transformation of a normal cell to become a malignant cell. The inhibition of oral carcinogenesis by one redox agent can also be enhanced with the use of mixtures of these agents *(141)* (Table 3). These agents also have the ability to act as chemotherapeutic agents, inducing cell death in carcinoma cells. The capacity to selectively damage malignant and not normal oral keratinocytes is also an important feature of their activity (Tables 3–6).

Unfortunately, depending on the oxygen environment, each agent has the capacity to promote the growth of cancer cells *(14,143)*. This is expected to occur when a strong antioxidant is provided to an established cancer cell. The oral keratinocyte releases oxygen-reactive substances that cause cell damage. The antioxidant quenches the levels of these reactive oxygen molecules. This allows the cancer cell to overcome the damage (e.g., DNA, mRNA) produced during transformation and oxygen metabolic activation, and to maintain an enhanced growth characteristic. The size or type of damage will also determine the form and completeness of repair. Oxidative damage generated by redox agents (e.g., β-carotene) could result in a lack of response to exogenous promotional growth factors (e.g., chemicals, virus, or immune products). The triggering of cell death through the enhanced expression of inducers such as *p53,* FAS/ligand, or pro-apoptotic factors of the Bcl-2 family (e.g., Mcl-1, BAX, BAK, and Bcl-xL) are also evident *(143)* (Fig. 5). The addition of an antioxidant to a normal keratinocyte reduces oxidative damage, reducing the risk for transformation. The redox agent enhances repair of genetic material and resets the cell cycle, and the levels of transcription or programmed regulatory factors (e.g., cyclin regulatory-binding proteins (CRBP), tumor necrosis receptor associated death domain (TRADD), fasassociated death domain (FADD, and others) *(25)*. The enhanced levels of oxidative substances in a cancer cell therefore increase the production of tumorigenic mutations (e.g., *p53*). The inadequate repair and clonal selection through programmed cell-death *p53* and independent and dependent pathways further increases the risk for cancer formation *(17)*.

Table 4
Malignant Oral Keratinocyte Growth Effects

Agent	Differentiation[1]			Cell cycle[2]			
	HMK	LMK[3]	Cornified env[4]	PCNA	p105	p34cdc2[5]	histone 3[6]
Carotenoid3	high	low	high	low	low	low	low
Retinoid	high	low	high	low	low	low	low
Tocopherol	high	low	high	low	low	low	low
Glutathione	high	low	high	low	low	low	low
Ascorbic acid	high	low	high	low	low	low	low
DMBA	low	high	low	high	high	high	high

1=Differentiation-high/low-mol-wt keratin (HMK/LMK) designated by MAbs

4=Cornified envelope microscopic examination

2,5=Cell cycle-proliferating-cell nuclear antigen (PCNA), p105, p34cdc2-designated by MAbs

3=Nutrient agents administered as indicated in Table 3

6=*in situ* hybridization

Redox agent treatments during the inhibition of oral carcinogenesis were found to enhance high mol-wt keratin and a cornified envelope compared to the untreated control. The cell cycle is generally depressed, while in the tumor control, proliferation is increased. The redox agents possibly inhibited carcinogenesis by increasing differentiation and reducing cell growth.

Table 5
Characterization of Cell Processes

Agent	Oncogenes[1]				Apoptosis[2]				Vascular[3]		
	p53wt	p53mut	Ki-ras	Ha-ras	NF	Bcl-2	Bax	Bak	F-8	VEGF	bFGF
Carotenoid[4]	yes	no	no	no	yes	no	yes	yes	no	no	no
Retinoid	yes	no	no	no	yes	no	yes	yes	no	no	no
Tocopherol	yes	no	no	no	yes	no	yes	yes	no	no	no
Glutathione	yes	no	no	no	yes	no	yes	yes	no	no	no
Ascorbic Acid	yes	no	no	no	yes	no	yes	yes	no	no	no
DMBA	yes	yes	yes	yes	yes	yes	yes	yes	yes	yes	yes

1= Oncogenes-*p53* wild-type (wt) and *p53*-mutant (mt) Ki and Ha-*ras* as designated by polyclonal antibodies

2=Apoptosis-nucelosome formation (NF), Bcl-2, Bax, Bak as designated by MAb

3=Vascular-Factor-VIII (F-8), vascular endothelial growth factor (VEGF), basic fibroblast growth factor (bFGF)

During the inhibition of oral carcinogenesis, the redox agents showed an enhanced expression of *p53*, but a reduction in the levels of *ras* compared to the tumor control was noted. Apoptosis was enhanced, with a decrease in vascular angiogenesis. DMBA-induced oral carcinogenesis also enhanced apoptosis, but increased neovascular proliferation.

This relationship between chemopreventive and cancer-cell growth was noted after the treatment of oral carcinoma cells in vitro with high doses of vitamin E acetate *(142)*. In this study, the increased growth of the oral cancer cells was noted. In a hamster oral carcinogenesis study, β-carotene initially inhibited oral carcinogenesis, but with continual treatment β-carotene also enhanced tumor-cell growth in the hamster buccal pouch *(14)* β-carotene and other redox agents, (e.g., Vitamin E) under certain

Table 6
Growth Factor Effects During Oral Carcinogenesis

Agent	Growth factors		
	EGF[1]	TGF-α[2]	TGF-β_1[3]
Carotenoid	no	no	yes
Retinoid	no	no	yes
Tocopherol	no	no	yes
Glutathione	no	no	yes
Ascorbic Acid	no	no	yes
DMBA	yes	yes	yes

1=Epidermal Growth Factor (EGF)

2=Transforming Growth Factor-alpha (TGF-α)

3=Transforming Growth Factor-beta (TGF-β)

Redox agents reduce the expression of some growth factors, while other are enhanced. The level of phosphotyrosine phosphorylation paralleled this pattern of expression. The DMBA tumor control enhanced the expression of these growth factors and their phosphorylation. The administration of the redox agents had a selective effect on growth-factor expression.

high-oxygen conditions, will trigger the expression of reactive oxygen substances *(144,145)*. This state is characterized by the expression of heat-shock proteins (hsps), and the depletion of glutathione-S-transferase *(125,136,144)*. The initial effect upon oral carcinogenesis is a reduction in the number and size of oral carcinomas. Onco-gene-expression analysis indicated an enhanced expression of tumor-suppressor *p53*, while mutant *p53* expression as identified by a monoclonal antibody (MAb) was depressed. This identification has a selective, narrow range for identification of mutant *p53* proteins *(57,73)*. Another study addressed the possible development of new muta-tions in the *p53* gene during the inhibition of oral carcinogenesis, using single-stranded conformational polymorphism (SSCP). The analysis disclosed that β-carotene, retinyl palmitate, canthaxanthin—a carotenoid that does not convert to a retinoid as β-carotene—and alpha tocopherol (vitamin E) induce novel and definitively different mutations, as defined by sequence for each of the redox agent treatments. For example, vitamin E treatments resulted in different, fewer, and smaller base changes than with the retinoid or carotenoid treatments (Figure 8) (Table 1.). This data could indicate that vitamin E has a lower risk to enhance oral carcinogenesis compared to the carotenoids or retinoids. The increased number of *p53* mutations could contribute to enhanced genomic instability, transcriptional abnormalities, and cell-cycle dysregulation. These changes are linked directly or indirectly to the induction of apoptosis. Initial studies conducted for 16 wk of treatment with DMBA and the treatment with the various redox agents inhibited oral carcinogenesis, producing less tumor formation and an accumula-tion of the oral carcinoma cells in G_1 of the cell cycle. During the 16-wk inhibitory period, an enhanced expression of nucleosome formation with a reduction in the apop-tosis inhibitor Bcl-2 was noted. In contrast, continual treatment with β-carotene resulted in a reversal of these markers and more carcinoma growth *(14,145)*.

Specifically, these predominantly hydrophobic agents bind to the cell membrane. The retinoids bind to nuclear receptors (α,β,γ,δ, X) *(146)*, while tocopherol binds to a tocopherol-binding protein *(147)*. The carotenoids most likely use the retinoid recep-

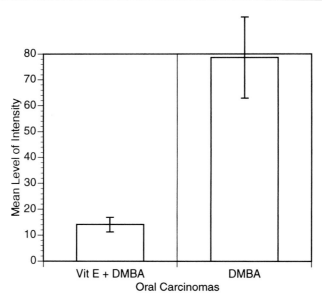

Fig. 8. Quantification of 8-OhdG Expression in Vitamin E and DMBA- and DMBA-Treated Buccal Mucosa. In an identical manner, as described earlier, the level of 8-OhdG expression in the VES + DMBA group compared to the level found in the DMBA group was significantly lower (p<.01).

tors because of their biochemical similarities to retinoids. For example, β-carotenecould can be converted to a retinoid through the action of 15-15′ dioxygenase reductase. The retinoids are metabolized in the liver and the cell to retinol and retinoic acid *(146)*.

The nonretinoid redox agents bind to membrane receptors and enhance the activity of serine-threonine kinases linked to receptors such as epidermal growth factor (EGF) or transforming growth factors α or β *(25)*. Redox-agent binding to the membrane also increases the level of sphingolipids, resulting in an accumulation of ceramide. Ceramide will expectedly induce the expression of the tumor-suppressor *p53,* which has several functions *(148)*. One function is to induce programmed cell death; another is to modify the cell cycle and to modify cell transcription and gene repair. It is believed that chemopreventives such as, tocopherol (vitamin E), in conjunction with ascorbic acid (vitamin C), maintain an antioxidant characteristic. The antioxidant binds to mutant *p53* protein and stabilizes the binding of the protein to DNA by reducing oxidation and adducts formation, and modifies the repair of the *p53* gene to other linked genes. The practical consequence to controlling the mutant *p53* function is to allow wild-type tumor-suppressor *p53* domination to appear. DNA nucleases and polymerases help to stabilize the redox-generated mutations at their binding site. These mutations function as tumor suppressors and support the tumor-suppressor function and induction of programmed cell death (Table 5). During DMBA-induced oral carcinogenesis adducts are produced, but the chemopreventives suppresses their formation (Figure 6). The antioxidant reduces the oxidant-reactive capacity of the adducts modifying mutations (e.g., *p53*) produced (Figure 9). Changes in the transcription capacity of the *p53* gene and the expression of various other proto-oncogenes or oncogenic

P53 Exon 8 (SSCP)

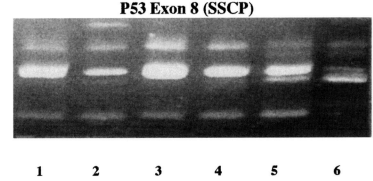

1   2   3   4   5   6

Fig. 9. Single-Strand Conformational Polymorphism Comparison of *p53* Mutations. DNA was extracted and hybridized using polymerase chain reactions (PCR) and hamster-specific primers. Five oral carcinomas from five animals were treated forming the following groups: 1) Untreated (UnRx), 2) DMBA treated (0.5% diss. in mineral oil) applied for 15 wk. 3) β-carotene (1.0 mg/0.120 kg) fed to hamsters on alternate days (three times/wk) to the application of DMBA (three times/wk). 4) Canthaxanthin (CAN) identical dose and time, 5) Retinyl palmitate (RP), identical dose and time, and 6) VES, identical dose and time. Exon 8 of the *p53* gene is shown, and the results are indicative of the general changes noted for each group. Each group produced a mutation profile specific for the group. Mutations in the *p53* gene could be considered a responsive marker for chemopreventive and therapeutic administration.

complexes (e.g., *ras,* AP-1) could also explain changes in differentiation and the cell cycle (Table 4). In response to these genetic changes, there are additional modifications in growth factors (Table 6), which also alters cell-to-cell interactions.

SUMMARY

The hamster oral carcinogenesis model offers a reliable, efficient, and analogous oral carcinoma system for human oral carcinoma development. In addition, the model offers the ability to observe the various stages for oral carcinogenesis both in vivo and in vitro. This model therefore allows the researcher to examine oral cancer formation in vivo in vivo and in vitro, and in vivo, then in vitro followed by further in vivo determinations. The flexibility in this model is significant when there is a need to assess the dynamics of oral carcinogenesis. The hamster-tumor model has also been used to evaluate the chemopreventive and chemotherapeutic aspects of various nutrients during oral carcinogenesis.

REFERENCES

1. Salley JJ. Experimental carcinogenesis in the cheek pouch of the Syrian hamster *J Dent Res* 1954; 33:253–262.
2. Morris AL. Factors influencing experimental carcinogenesis in the hamster cheek pouch. *J Dent Res* 1961; 40:3–15.
3. Shklar G. Metabolic characteristics of experimental hamster pouch carcinoma. *Oral Surg Oral Med Oral Pathol* 1965; 20:336–339.
4. Shklar G. The effect of manipulation and incision on experimental carcinoma of hamster buccal pouch. *Cancer Res* 1968; 28:2180–2182.
5. Shklar G, Schwartz JL. Oral cancer inhibition by micronutrients. The experimental basis for clinical trials. *Oral Oncol Eur J Cancer* 1993; 29:9–16.

6. Witte PL, Streilein JW. Development and ontogeny of hamster T cell subpoluations. *J Immunol* 1986; 137:45–54.

7. Witte PL, Stein-Streilein J, Streilein JW. Description of phenotyically distinct T lymphocyte subsets which mediate helper, DTH and cytotoxic function in the Syrian hamster. *J Immunol* 1985; 134:2908–2915.

8. Giunta JL, Schwartz JL, Antoniades DV. Studies on the vascular drainage system of the hamster buccal carcinogenesis. *J Oral Pathol* 1985; 14:263–267.

9. Slaga TJ, Huberman E, Digiovanni J. The importance of the "Bay Region" diol-epoxide in 7,12-dimethylbenz[a]anthrancene skin tumor initiation and mutagenesis. *Cancer Lett* 1979; 6:213–220.

10. Shklar G, Turbiner S, Siegel W. Chemical carcinogenesis of hamster mucosa. Reactions to dimethyl-sufoxide. *Arch Pathol* 1969; 87:637–642.

11. Slaga TJ, Gleason J, Digiovanni J. Potent tumor initiating activity of the 3,4-dihydrodiol of 7,12-dimethylbenz[a]anthracene in mouse skin. *Cancer Res* 1979; 39:1934–1936.

12. Slaga TJ, Bracken WM. The effects of antioxidants on skin tumor initiation and aryl hydrocarbon hydoxylase. *Cancer Res* 1979; 37:1631–1635.

13. Reiskin AP, Berry RJ. Cell proliferation and carcinogenesis in the hamster cheek pouch. *Cancer Res* 1968; 898–905.

14. Schwartz JL. β-carotene inhibits and enhances oral carcinogenesis. In: Prasad K, Santamaria RM, eds. *Nutrition and Cancer Prevention and Treatment* Humana Press, Totowa, NJ, pp. 121–141.

15. Safour IM, Wood NK, Tsiklakis K, Doemung DB, Joseph G. Incisional biospy and seeding in hamster cheek pouch carcinoma. *J Dent Res* 1984; 63:1116–1120.

16. Santis H, Shklar G, Chauncey HH. Histochemistry of experimentally induced leukoplakia and carcinoma of the hamster buccal pouch. *Oral Surg Oral Med Oral Pathol* 1964; 17:84–95.

17. Schwartz JL, Gu X, Kittles RA, Baptiste A, Shklar G. Experimental oral carcinoma of the tongue and buccal mucosa: possible biologic markers linked to cancers at two anatomic sites. *Eur J Cancer Oral Oncol* 2000; 36:225–235.

18. Schwartz JL and Gu X. Vitamin E models apoptosis in oral keratinocytes and cancer cells, *Cancer Res* 2001; 42:445.

19. Berenblum I. The mechanism of carcinogenesis: a study of the significance of cocarcinogeneic action and related phenomena. *Cancer Res* 1941; 1:807–814.

20. Odukoya O, Shklar G. Initiation and promotion in experimental oral carcinogenesis. *Oral Surg Oral Med Oral Pathol* 1982; 54:547–552.

21. Suda D, Schwartz JL, Shklar G. Inhibition of experimental oral carcinogenesis by topical beta carotene. *Carcinogenesis* 1986; 7:711–715.

22. Odukoya O, Shklar G. Initiation and promotion in experimental oral carcinogenesis. *Oral Surg Oral Med Oral Pathol* 1984; 58:315–320.

23. Gimenez-Conti I, Slaga TJ. The hamster cheek pouch carcinogenesis model. *J Cell Biochem* 1993; 17F:83–90.

24. Rothman K, Keller A. The effect of joint exposure to alcohol and tobacco on risk of cancer of the mouth and pharynx. *J Chronic Dis* 1972; 25:711–719.

25. Schwartz JL. Biomarkers and molecular epidemiology and chemoprevention or oral carcinogenesis. *Crit Rev Oral Biol Med* 2000; 11:92–122.

26. Friedman A, Shklar G. Alcohol and hamster buccal pouch carcinogenesis. *Oral Surg Oral Med Oral Pathol* 1978; 46:774–810.

27. Patel RK, Trivedi AH, Jaju RJ, Adhvaryu SG, Balar DB. Ethanol potentiates the clastogenicity of pan-masula-an in vitro experience. *Carcinogenesis* 1994; 15:2017–2021.

28. Chen YP, Johnson GK, Squier CA. Effects of nicotine and tobacco-specific nitrosamines on hamster cheek pouch and gastric mucosa. *J Oral Pathol Med* 1994; 23:251–255.

29. Moore C, Miller AJ. Effect of cigarette smoke tar on hamster cheek pouch. *Arch Surg* 1958; 76:786–794.

30. Kendrick FJ. Some effects of chemical carcinogen and of cigarette smoke condensate upon hamster cheek pouch mucosa. *Health Sci* 1964; 24:3698–3716.

31. Schwartz JL, Shklar G. Oral pathology: chemical carcinogenesis in the hamster cheek pouch. In: Van Hoosier GL Jr, McPherson CW. Laboratory Hamsters. Amer Coll of Lab Animal Med. Series Academic Press, New York, NY. 1987, pp. 281–299.

32. Hoffman D, Adams JD, Brunnemann KD, Riverson A, Hecht SS. Tobacco specific N-nitrosamines occurrence and bioassays. *IARC Sci Publ* 1982; 41:309–318.

33. Altuwairgi OS, Papageorge MB, Doku HC. The cancer-promoting effect of N-nitrosonornicotine used in combination with a subcarcinogenic dose of 4-nitroquinoline-N-oxide and 7, 12 dimethyl-benz(a)anthracene. *J Oral Maxillofac Surg* 1995; 53:910–913.

34. Jansson T, Romert L, Magnusson J, Jenssen D. Genotoxicity testing of extracts of a Swedish moist snuff. *Mutat Res* 1991; 261:101–115.

35. Park NH, Sapp JP, Herbosa EG. Oral cancer induced in hamsters with herpes simplex infection and simulated snuff dipping. *Oral Surg Oral Med Oral Pathol* 1986; 62:164–168.

36. Grasso P, Mann AH. Smokeless tobacco and oral cancer: an assessment of evidence derived from laboratory animals. *Food Chem Toxicol* 1998; 36:1015–1029.

37. Gijare PS, Rao KV, Bhide SV. Modulatory effects of snuff, retinoic acid, and beta-carotene ED: on DMBA-induced hamster cheek pouch carcinogenesis in relation to keratin expression. *Nutr Cancer* 1990; 14:253–259.

38. Summerlin DJ, Dunipace A, Potter R. Histologic effects of smokeless tobacco and alcohol on the pouch mucosa and organs of the Syrian hamster. *J Oral Pathol Med* 1992; 21:105–108.

39. Odukoya O, Schwartz JL, Weichselbaum R, Shklar G. An epidermoid carcinoma cell line derived from hamster DMBA-induced buccal pouch tumors. *J Natl Cancer Inst* 1983; 71:1253–1264.

40. Muns G, Vishwanatha JK, Rubinstein I. Effects of smokeless tobacco on chemically transformed hmaster oral keratinocytes: role of angiotensin I-converting enzyme. *Carcinogenesis* 1994; 15:1325–1327.

41. Rangan SR, Mukherjee AL, Bang FB. Search for an adenovirus etiology of human oral and pharyngeal tumors, *Int J Cancer* 1968; 3:819–828.

42. Smotkin D, Prokoph H, Wettsteinj FO. Oncogenic and non oncogenic human genital papillomavirus generate the E7 mRNA by different mechanisms. *J Virol* 1989; 63:1441–1447.

43. Shindoh M, Chiba I, Yasuda M, Saito T, Funaoka K, Kohgo T. Detection of human papillomavirus DNA sequences in oral squamous cell carcinoma and their relation to p53 and proliferating cell nuclear antigen expression. *Cancer* 1995; 76:1513–1521.

44. Rajcani J, Ciampor F, Sabo A. Experimental latent herpesvirus infection in rabbits, mice and hmasters: ultrastructure of the virus activation in explanted gasseric ganglia. *Acta Virol* 1975; 19:19–28.

45. Park NH, Herbosa EG, Shklar G. Experimental development of herpes simplex virus infection in hamster buccal pouch. *Oral Surg Oral Med Oral Pathol* 1985; 59:159–166.

46. Park NH, Sapp JP, Herbosa EG. Oral cancer induced in hamsters with herpes simplex infection and simulated snuff dipping. *Oral Surg Oral Med Oral Pathol* 1986; 62:164–168.

47. Stich JE, Li KK, Chun YS, Weiss R, Park NH. Effect of smokeless tobacco on the replication of herpes simples virus in vitro and on production of viral lesions in hamster cheek pouch. *Arch Oral Biol* 1987; 32:291–296.

48. Teale DM, Underwood JC, Potter CW, Rees RC. Therapy of spontaneously metastatic HSV-2 induced hmaster tumours with cortisone acetate administered with or without heparin. *Eur J Cancer Clin Oncol* 1987; 23:93–100.

49. Eskinazi DP, Cantin EM. Monoclonal antibodies to HSV-infection-related antigens cross-react with tumor cell lines and tumor tissue sections. *Oral Surg Oral Med Oral Pathol* 1988; 65:308–315.

50. Cornella FA, Saper CD, Christensen RE, Park NH. Effect of DMBA on oral cancer development with latent HSV-1 infections in trigeminal ganglia. *Oral Surg Oral Med Oral Pathol* 1989; 67:167–171.

51. Park K, Cherrick HM, Min BM, Park NH. Active HSV-1 immunization prevents the cocarcinogenic activity of HSV-1 in the oral cavity of hamsters. *Oral Surg Oral Med Oral Pathol* 1990; 70:186–191.

52. Fujino H, Chino T, Imai T. Experimental production of labial and lingual carcinoma by local application of 4-nitro-quinoline-n-oxide. *J Natl Cancer Inst* 1965; 35:907–918.

53. Dachi SF. Experimental production of carcinomas of the hamster tongue. *J Dent Res* 1967; 46:148–156.

54. Fujita K, Kaku T, Sasaki M, Onoe T. Experimental production of lingual carcinomas in hamsters: tumor characteristics and site of formation. *J Dent Res* 1973; 52:1176–1185.

55. Marefat P, Shklar G. Experimental production of lingual leukoplakia and carcinoma. *Oral Surg Oral Med Oral Pathol* 1977; 44:578–586.

56. Take Y, Umeda M, Teranobu O, Shimada K. Lymph node metastases in hamster tongue cancer induced with 9,10 dimethyl-1,2-benzanthracene: association between histologic findings and the incidence of neck metastases, and the clinical implications for patients with tongue cancer. *Brit J Oral Maxillofac Surg* 1999; 37:29–36.

57. Schwartz JL, Shklar G, Trickler D. p53 in the anticancer mechanism of vitamin E. *Oral Oncol Eur J Cancer* 1993; 29B:313–318.

58. Oreffo VI, Lin HW, Gumerlock PH, Kraegel SA, Witschi H. Mutational analysis of a dominant oncogene (c-Ki-ras-2) and a tumor suppressor gene (p53) in hamster lung tumorigenesis. *Mol Carcinog* 1992; 6:199–202.

59. Oreffo VI, Lin HW, Padmanabhan R, Witschi H. K-ras and p53 point mutations in 4-(methylnitrosamino)-1-(3-pyridyl-1-butanone-induced hamster lung tumors. *Carcinogenesis* 1993; 14:451–455.

60. Chang KW, Mangold KA, Hubchak S, Laconi S, Scarpelli DG. Genomic p53 mutation in a chemically induced hamster pancreatic ductal adenocarcinoma. *Cancer Res.* 1994; 54:3878–3883.

61. Chang KW, Lin SC, Koos S, Pather K, Solt D. p53 and Ha-ras mutations in chemically induced hamster buccal pouch carcinomas. *Carcinogenesis* 1996; 17:595–600.

62. Gimenez-Conti IB, LaBate M, Liu F, Osterndorff E. p53 alterations in chemically induced hamster cheek-pouch lesions. *Mol Carcinog* 1996; 16:197–202.

63. Strauss BS. Silent and multiple mutations in p53 and the question of the hypermutability of tumors. *Carcinogenesis* 1997; 18:1445–1452.

64. Brown K, Buchmann A, Balmain A. Carcinogen-induced mutation in the mouse c-Ha-ras gene provide evidence of multiple pathways for tumor progression. *Proc Natl Acad Sci USA* 1990; 87:538–542.

65. Zarkl H, Sukumar S, Arthur AV, Martin-Zanca D, Barbacid M. Direct mutagenesis of Ha-ras-1 oncogenes by N-nitrosos-N-methylurea during initiation of mammary carcinogenesis in rats. *Nature* 1985; 315:382–385.

66. Wong DTW, Gertz R, Chow P. Detection of Ki-ras mRNA in normal and chemically transformed hamster oral keratinocytes. *Cancer Res* 1989; 49:4562–4567.

67. Husain Z, Fei Y, Roy S, Solt DB, Polverini P, Biswas DK. Sequential expression and cooperation interaction of c-Ha-ras and c-erbB genes in in vivo chemical carcinogenesis. *Proc Natl Acad Sci USA* 1989; 86:1264–1268.

68. Wong DTW. Amplification of c-erbB oncogene in chemically induced oral carcinomas. *Carcinogenesis* 1987; 8:1963–1965.

69. Wong DTW, Biswas DK. Activation of c-erbB oncogene in the hamster cheek pouch during DMBA-induced carcinogenesis. *Oncogene* 1987; 2:67–72.

70. Gimenez-Conti IB, Bianchi AB, Stockman SL, Conti CJ, Slaga TJ. Activating mutation of the Ha-ras in chemically induced tumors of the hamster cheek pouch. *Mol Carcinog* 1992; 5:259–263.

71. Robles AI, Gimenez-Conti IB, Roop D, Slaga TJ, Conti CJ. Low frequency of codon 61 Ha-ras mutations and lack of keratin 13 expression in 7,12 dimethylbenz[a]anthracene-induced hamster skin tumors. *Mol Carcinog* 1993; 7:94–98.

72. Shklar G, Schwartz JL. Vitamin E inhibits experimental carcinogenesis and tumour angiogenesis. *Oral Oncol Eur J Cancer* 1996; 32B:114–119.

73. Schwartz JL, Shklar G. Glutathione inhibits experimental oral carcinogenesis, p53 expression and angiogenesis. *Nutr Cancer* 1996; 26:229–236.

74. Meister A, Anderson ME. Glutathione. *Annu Rev Biochem* 1983; 52:711–760.

75. Solt DB. Localization of gamma-glutamyl transpeptidase in hamster buccal pouch epithelium treated with 7,12-dimethylbenz[a]anthracene. *J Natl Cancer Inst* 1981; 67:193–199.

76. Solt DB, Shklar G. Rapid induction of g-glutamyl transpeptidase rich intraepithelial clones in 7, 12-dimethylbenz[a]anthracene-treated buccal pouch. *Cancer Res* 1982; 42:285–291.

77. Yamamoto K, Kato M, Yoshida K, Kurita K, Tatematsu M. Strong expression of glutathione-S-transferase placental form in early preneoplastic lesions and decrease with progression in hamster buccal pouch carcinogenesis. *Cancer Lett* 1999; 135:129–136.

78. Schwartz JL, West K, Shklar DP, Shklar G. Altered cytopkeratin expression in carcinogenesis inhibition by antioxidant nutrients. *Nutr Cancer* 1995; 24:47–56.

79. Gimenez-Conti IB, Shin DM, Bianchi AB, Roop DR, Hong WK, Conti, CJ, et al. Changes in keratin expression during 7,12 dimethylbenz[a]anthracene-induced hamster cheek pouch carcinogenesis. *Cancer Res* 1990; 50:4441–4445.

80. Shin DM, Gimenez IB, Lee JS, Nishioka K, Wargovich MJ, Thacher S, et al. Expression of epidermal growth factor receptor, polyamine levels, orthnithine decarboxylase, micronuclei and transglutaminase I in a 7, 12 dimethylbenz[a]anthracene-induced hamster buccal pouch carcinogenesis model. *Cancer Res* 1990; 50:2505–2510.

81. Billingham RL, Silvers WK. Syrian hamster and transplantation immunity. *Plast Reconstr Surg* 1964; 34:329–353.

82. Schwartz JL, Sloane D, Shklar G. Prevention and inhibition of oral cancer in the hamster buccal pouch model associated with carotenoid immune enhancement. *Tumor Biology* 1989; 10:297–309.

83. Schwartz JL, Suda D, Light G. Beta carotene is associated with the regression of hamster buccal pouch carcinoma and the induction of tumor necrosis factor in macrophages. *Biochem Biophys Res Commun* 1986; 130:1130–1135.

84. Schwartz JL, Shklar G. A cyanobacteria extract and beta carotene stimulates an antitumor immune response against oral cancer cell line. *Phytotherapy Res* 1989; 3:243–248.

85. Shklar G. Cortisone and hamster pouch carcinogenesis. *Cancer Res* 1966; 26:2461–2463.

86. Shklar G. The effect of cortisone on the induction and development of hamster buccal pouch carcinoma. *Oral Surg Oral Med Oral Pathol* 1965; 20:336–339.

87. Woods DA. Influence of antilymphocyte serum on DMBA induction of oral carcinoma. *Nature* (London) 1969; 224:276–277.

88. Giunta JL, Shklar G. The effect of antilymphocyte serum on experimental hamster buccal pouch carcinogenesis. *Oral Surg Oral Med Oral Pathol* 1971; 31:344–355.

89. Giunta J, Reif AE, Shklar G. Bacillus Calmette-Guerin and antilymphocyte serum in carcinogenesis. *Arch Pathol* 1974; 98:237–240.

90. Eisenberg E, Shklar G. Levamisole and hamster pouch carcinogenesis. *Oral Surg Oral Med Oral Pathol* 1977; 43:562–574.

91. Shklar G, Eisenberg E, Flynn E. Immunoenhancing agents and experimental leukoplakia and carcinoma of the hamster buccal pouch. *Prog Exp Tumor Res* 1979; 24:269–282.

92. Schwartz JL, Solt DB, Pappo J, Weichselbaum R. Distribution of Langerhans cells in normal and carcinogen treated mucosa of buccal pouches of hamsters. *J Dermatol Surg Oncol* 1981; 7:1005–1010.

93. Schwartz JL, Frim SR, Shklar G. RA can alter the distribution of ATPase positive Langerhans cells in the hamster cheek pouch in association with DMBA application. *Nutr Cancer* 1985; 7:77–84.

94. Gould AR. DMBA and immunosuppression in the Syrian golden hamster. *J Dent Res* 1976; Spec. N:D98–102.

95. Merk L, Shklar G, Albright J, Transplantation of hamster buccal pouch carcinoma to neonatal hamsters. *Oral Surg Oral Med Oral Pathol* 1979; 47:533–541.

96. Meng CL, Shklar G, Albright J. A transplanantable anaplastic oral cancer model. *Oral Surg Oral Med Oral Pathol* 1982; 53:179–187.

97. Schwartz JL, Shklar G. Verification in syngeneic hamsters of in vitro transformation of hamster oral mucosa by 7,12 dimethylbenz(a)anthracene. *Eur J Cancer* 1997; 33:431–438.

98. Shklar G. The effect of manipulation and incision on experimental carcinoma of hamster buccal pouch. *Cancer Res* 1968; 28:2180–2182.

99. Ida K, Kato M, Yoshida K, Kurita K, Tatematsu M. Promotional effects of Co2 laser on DMBA-induced hamster buccal pouch carcinogenesis as shown by immunohistochemistry of the placental form of glutathione S transferase. *Lasers Surg Med* 1999; 24:360–367.

100. Lurie AG, Cutler LS. Effects of low-level X radiation on 7,12-dimethylbenz[a]anthracene-induced lingual tumors in Syrian golden hamsters. *J Natl Cancer Inst* 1979; 63:147–152.

101. Lurie AG. Interactions between 7,12-dimethylbenz(a)anthracene (DMBA) and repeated low-level X radiation in hamster cheek pouch carcinogenesis: dependence on the relative timing of DMBA and radiation treatments. *Radiat Res* 1982; 90:155–164.

102. Inoue T, Nasu M, Kai Y, Furumoto K. Change on the cell proliferation kinetics of the central and peripheral regions of DMBA induced hamster tongue cancer following irradiation. *Shigaku* 1989; 77:343–354.

103. Burns RA, Klaunig JE, Shulok JR, Davis WJ, Goldblatt PJ. Tumor-localizing and photosensitizing properties of hematoporphyrin derivative in hamster buccal pouch carcinoma. *Oral Surg Oral Med Oral Pathol* 1986; 61:368–372.

104. Von Glass W, Kasler M, Lang T. Mode of action of photodynamic therapy with sulfonated aluminum phthalocyanine in induced squamous cell carcinomas in animal models. *Eur Arch Oto-rhino-laryngol* 1992; 249:309–312.

105. Frisoli JK, Tudor EG, Flotte TJ, Hasan T, Deutsch TF, Schomacker KT, et al. Tumor-localizing and photosensitizing properties of hematoporphyrin derivative in hamster buccal pouch carcinoma. *Oral Surg Oral Med Oral Pathol* 1986; 61:368–372.

106. Kozacko MF, Mang TS, Schally AV, Priore RL, Liebow C. Bombesin anatagonist prevents CO2 laser-induced promotion of oral cancer. *Proc Natl Acad Sci USA* 1996; 93:2953–2957.

107. Blant SA, Woodtli A, Wagnieres G, Fontolliet C, Van Den Bergh H, Monnier P. In vivo fluence rate effect in photodynamic therapy of early cancers with tetra(m-hydroxyphenyl) chlorin. *Photochem Photobiol* 1996; 64:963–968.

108. Andrejevic-Blant S, Hadjur C, Ballini JP, Wagnieres G, Fontolliet C, Van Den Bergh H, et al. Photodynamic therapy of early squamous cell carcinoma with tetra(m-hydroxyphenyl)chlorin: optimal drug-light interval. *Br J Cancer* 1997; 76:1021–1028.

109. Harris DM, Werkhaven J. Endogenous porphyrin fluorescence in tumors. *Lasers Surg Med* 1987; 7:467–472.

110. Mashberg A, Feldman LJ. Clinical criteria for identifying early oral and oropharyngeal carcinoma: erythroplasia revisited. *Am J Surg* 1988; 156:273–275.

111. Sciubba JJ. Improving detection of precancerous and cancerous oral lesions. *JADA.* 1999; 130:1445–1457.

112. Miller RL, Simms BW, Gould AR. Toluidine blue staining for detection of oral premalignant lesions and carcinomas. *J Oral Pathol* 1988; 17:73–78.

113. Martin IC, Kerawala CJ, Reed M. The application of toluidine blue as a diagnostic adjunct in the detection of epithelial dysplasia. *Oral Surg Oral Med Oral Pathol Oral Radiol Endod* 1998; 85:444–446.

114. Kluftinger AM, Davis NL, Quenville NF, Lam S, Hung J, Palcic B. Detection of squamous cell cancer and pre-cancerous lesions by imaging of tissue autofluorescence in the hamster cheek pouch model. *Surg Oncol* 1992; 1:183–188.

115. Balasubramanian S, Elangovan V, Govindasamy S. Fluorescence spectroscopic identification of 7,12 dimethylbenz[a] anthracene-induced hamster buccal pouch carcinogenesis. *Carcinogenesis* 1995; 16:2461–2465.

116. Crean DH, Liebow C, Penetrante RB, Mang TS. Evaluation of profimer sodium fluorescence for measuring tissue transformation. *Cancer* 1993; 72:3068–3077.

117. Onizawa K, Saginoya H, Furuya Y, Yoshida H. Fluorescence photography as a diagnostic method for oral cancer. *Cancer Lett* 1996; 108:61–66.

118. Dhingra JK, Zhang X, McMillan K, Kabani S, Manoharan R, Itzkan I. Diagnosis of head and neck precancerous lesions in an animal model using fluorescence spectroscopy. *Laryngoscope* 1998; 108:471–475.

119. Chen CT, Wang CY, Kuo YS, Chiang HH, Chow SN, Hsiao IY, et al. Light-induced fluorescence spectroscopy: a potential diagnostic tool for oral neoplasia. *Proc Natl Sci Counc Repub China B* 1996; 20:123–130.

120. Gillenwater A, Jacob R, Gaaneshappa R, Kemp B, El-Naggar AK, Palmer JL, et al. Noninvasive diagnosis of oral neoplasia based on fluorescence spectroscopy and native tissue autofluorescence. *Arch Otolaryngol Head Neck Surg* 1998; 124:1251–1258.

121. Schwartz JL. Nutrition and chemoprevention of head, neck and lung cancers. In: Heber D, Blackburn G, eds. *Nutritional Oncology.* Academic Press. New York, NY, 1999, pp. 421–445.

122. Shklar G. Development of experimental oral carcinogenesis and its impact on current oral cancer research. *J Dent Res* 1999; 78:1768–1772.

123. Schwartz JL. Mechanisms for chemoprevention of cancer. *Cancer Prevent Int* 1997; 3:37–53.

124. Sacks PG. Cell tissue and organ culture as in vitro models to study the biology of squamous cell carcinomas of the head and neck. *Cancer Metastasis Rev* 1996; 15:27–51.

125. Schwartz JL. Molecular and biochemical control of tumor growth following treatment with carotenoids or tocopherols. In: Prasad K, Santamaria L, Williams RM, eds. *Nutrition and Cancer Prevention and Treatment.* Humana Press, Totowa, NJ, 1995, pp. 287–316.

126. Shklar G, Schwartz JL. Ascorbic acid and cancer. In: Harris JR, ed. *Ascorbic acid: Biochemistry, Biomedical and Cell Biology.* Plenum Publ, New York, NY, 1995, pp. 233–247.

127. Shklar G, Schwartz JL. A common pathway for the destruction of cancer cells: experimental evidence and clinical implications (Review). *Int J Oncology* 1994; 4:215–224.

128. Schwartz JL. The clinical control of tumor cell growth through the action of carotenoids, retinoid, and tocopherols. In: Quillian P, ed. *Symposium on Adjuvants and Cancer Treatments.* Cancer Treatment Research Foundation, IL, 1993, 173–233.

129. Schwartz JL, Antoniades DZ, Zhao S. Molecular and biochemical reprogramming of oncogenesis through the activity of antioxidants and prooxidants. *NY Acad Sci* 1992; 686:262–279.

130. Shklar G, Schwartz JL. Effects of Vitamin E on oral cancer carcinogenesis and oral cancer. In: Packer L, ed. The biochemistry and metabolism of vitamin E. Marcel Dekker, New York, NY. 1991; 497–511.

131. Shklar G, Schwartz JL. Prevention of experimental cancer and immunostimulation by vitamin E (immunosurveillance). *J Oral Pathol Med* 1990; 19:123–127.

132. Antoniades DZ, Schwartz JL, Shklar G. The effect of chemically induced oral carcinomas on peritoneal macrophages. *J Clin Lab Immunol* 1984; 14:17–22.

133. Antoniades DZ, Schwartz JL, Niukian K, Shklar G. Effects of smokeless tobacco on the immune system of Syrian hamsters. *J Oral Med* 1984; 39:136–140.

134. Hassan MM, Schwartz JL, Shklar G. Acute effect of DMBA application on Langerhans cells of the hamster buccal pouch mucosa. *Oral Surg Oral Med Oral Pathol* 1984; 58:191–197.

135. Schwartz JL, Odukoya O, Stoufi E, Shklar G. Alpha tocopherol alters the destruction of Langerhans cells in DMBA treated hamster pouch epithelium. *J Dent Res* 1985; 64:117–121.

136. Schwartz JL, Singh R, Teicher B, Wright JE, Trites DH, Shklar G. Induction of a 70 KD protein associated with the selective cytotoxicity of beta carotene in human epidermal carcinoma. *Biophys Biochem Res Commun* 1990; 169:941–946.

137. Schwartz JL, Flynn E, Trickler D, Shklar G. Directed lysis of experimental cancer by beta carotene in liposomes. *Nutr Cancer* 1991; 16:107–124.

138. Flynn EA, Schwartz JL, Shklar G. Sequential mast cell infiltration and degranulation during experimental carcinogenesis. *J Cancer Res Clin Oncol* 1990; 117:115–120.

139. Schwartz JL, Shklar G. The administration of beta carotene to prevent and regress oral carcinoma in the hamster cheek pouch and the associative enhancement of the immune response In: Bendich A, Phillips M, Tengerdy RB, eds. *Advances in Medicine and Biology.* 1988, pp. 77–93.

140. Schwartz JL, Flynn E, Shklar G. The effect of carotenoids on the antitumor immune response in vivo and in vitro with hamster and mouse immune effectors. *NY Acad Sci* 1990; 587:92–109.

141. Shklar G, Schwartz JL, Trickler D, Cheverie SR. The effectiveness of a mixture of b-carotene, a-tocopherol, glutathione, and ascorbic acid for cancer prevention. *Nutr Cancer* 1993; 20:145–151.

142. Odukoya O, Schwartz JL, Shklar G. The effect of vitamin E on the growth of an epidermoid carcinoma cell line in culture. *Nutr Cancer* 1986; 8:101–106.

143. Yang E, Korsmeyer SJ. Molecular thanatopis: a discourse on the Bcl-2 family and cell death. *Blood* 1996; 88:386–401.

144. Schwartz JL, Tanaka J, Khanadekar V, Herman TS, Teicher BA. b-carotene and/or vitamin E as modulattors of alkylating agents in SCC-25 human squamous carcinoma cells. *Cancer Chemother Pharmacol* 1992; 29:207–213.

145. Schwartz JL. The dual roles of nutrients as antioxidants and prooxidants: their effects on tumor cell growth. *J Nutr* 1996; 126:1221–1227.

146. Smith MA, Parkinson DR, Cheson BD, Friedman MA. Retinoids in cancer therapy. *J Clin Oncol* 1992; 10:839–864.

147. Kim HS, Arai H, Arita M, Sato Y, Ogihara T, Inoue K, et al. Effect of a-tocopherol transfers protein expression and its messenger RNA level in rat liver. *Free Radic* 1998; 28:87–92.

148. Verhejj M, Bose R, Lin H, Yao B, Jarvis WD, Grant S, et al. Requirement for ceramide-initiate SDAPK/JNK signaliing in stress induced apoptosis. *Nature* 1996; 380:75–79.

9

Mammary Cancer in Rats

Henry J. Thompson, PhD,
and Michael B. Sporn, MD

1. INTRODUCTION

There is clearly a need for a useful, practical rat model of mammary carcinogenesis, not only to produce invasive, autochthonous tumors that can be used for screening of new agents for treatment of advanced disease, but also for evaluation of new agents for chemoprevention of breast cancer. This latter approach to the control of breast cancer has seen major clinical advances in the past few years, with the demonstration of the clinical efficacy of three agents—namely tamoxifen, raloxifene, and fenretinide—in chemoprevention of breast cancer in selected groups of women at high risk for development of disease (1–3). These experimental clinical trials in chemoprevention have been extremely costly to perform, since they have involved the administration of these drugs to thousands of women over a period of many years. It is therefore of the utmost importance to be certain that there is a strong preclinical rationale for the use of a new chemopreventive agent before it is introduced into clinical trials. We have seen the disaster that has resulted from the large clinical trials that attempted to use β-carotene to prevent cancer before there was any strong evidence that this agent was truly an effective chemopreventive agent in experimental animals. Hopefully, this same mistake will not be repeated in the future with newer agents.

These considerations serve to highlight the importance of a useful rat model of mammary carcinogenesis. It is fortunate that such a model does in fact exist, and that it is easy and relatively inexpensive to set up in the laboratory. It requires only a single dose of a carcinogen, is highly reproducible, and above all, is relevant to human disease. This last criterion has been demonstrated by the experimental data that have shown that all three of the chemopreventive agents that have been found to be clinically effective in preventing breast cancer were first shown to be highly active agents in the animal model (4–6). This model is the one that uses the carcinogen, *N*-nitroso-*N*-methylurea (NMU), as the initiating agent. This chapter describes the use of this model.

From: *Tumor Models in Cancer Research*
Edited by: B. A. Teicher © Humana Press Inc., Totowa, NJ

2. HISTORICAL PERSPECTIVE

Modern studies of mammary carcinogenesis in rats began with the introduction of the use of polynuclear hydrocarbons as carcinogens, most notably in the pioneering work of Huggins and colleagues *(7)*. In a classic paper published in 1961, data were reported on the effective use of 3-methylcholanthrene (3-MC) and 7,12-dimethyl-benz(a)anthracene (DMBA). Both agents were shown to be potent mammary carcinogens when administered orally at appropriate single doses to Sprague-Dawley rats, and a tumor incidence of 100% was readily attained. However, although some of the mammary tumors induced by DMBA are indeed carcinomas, most of the tumors that develop in rats treated with DMBA or 3-MC are benign, and should be classified as fibroadenomas *(8)*. Moreover, the mammary carcinomas induced by these polynuclear hydrocarbons in rats do not metastasize. These important limitations on the usefulness of the DMBA model therefore led to a search for a more effective mammary carcinogen that would induce tumors that are almost exclusively carcinomas. This search culminated with the introduction of NMU in 1975, in a classic paper by Gullino and colleagues *(9)*. Although the model, as presently used, has been modified to make it simpler and easier to use, its basic utility remains unchallenged, and it remains the system of choice at the present time. Unless one is specifically interested in the effects of carcinogenic hydrocarbons on the mammary gland, there is essentially no justification for the continued use of DMBA to induce mammary cancer in rats.

The original system proposed by Gullino and colleagues used three intravenous (iv) injections of NMU, each at a dose of 50 mg/kg, given 4 wk apart, beginning at 50 d of age. Inbred BUF/N rats were the strain of choice (mean latent period, 77 d), although the authors also showed high tumor yields in Sprague-Dawley and F344 rats (mean latent periods, 86 and 94 d, respectively). In marked contrast to the tumors induced by DMBA, all of the 60 tumors from rats treated with NMU that were histologically examined were adenocarcinomas or papillary carcinomas. Rats bearing tumors induced by NMU were hypercalcemic, and bony metastasis was seen in some animals. Tumors were transplantable and sensitive to estrogen. In several hundred animals with primary mammary carcinomas induced by NMU, the authors did not find tumors of other organs growing to a macroscopic size.

The need for a total of three injections of NMU was not evaluated in this initial study. As other investigators became interested in using this model for chemoprevention studies, it became important to shorten the time required for the initiation of carcinogenesis, thus allowing a wider window for evaluation of the antipromoting activity of new agents. One early modification was the elimination of the third iv dosing with NMU, and also to give the second dose 1 wk (rather than 1 mo) after the first *(10)*. Then it was shown that a single iv dose of NMU was just as effective as two doses *(11)*. Finally, to make the model even easier to use, it was shown that an ip injection of NMU was just as effective as iv administration of the carcinogen *(12)*. Thus, it is now possible to give the complete initiating dose of carcinogen to a cohort of 100 rats in only a few hours, with a minimum of technical skill required. Furthermore, the marked instability of NMU in dilute alkaline solution makes this an ideal carcinogen to handle. Finally, the model has been standardized in the readily available Sprague-Dawley rat.

2.1. Induction of Mammary Carcinomas Using NMU

Mammary carcinomas can be induced in female Sprague Dawley rats by administering a single dose of NMU intraperitoneally *(12,13)*. We recommend using this outbred rat strain because it is both readily available and highly susceptible to chemically induced mammary carcinogenesis. The characteristics of the carcinogenic response also are best characterized in this strain. A discussion of the genetic susceptibility of this and other rat strains to chemically induced mammary carcinogenesis can be found in ref. *14*. An extensive description of the technical details by which NMU is prepared, injected, and inactivated has recently been reported *(15)*. A summary of the most critical aspects of this protocol is presented in Table 1.

2.2. Carcinogen Dose and Age of Administration

Currently, there are two additional factors that must be considered in using NMU to induce mammary carcinomas—the dose of carcinogen to be administered and the age at which the carcinogen is injected. The specific research question addressed will, in part, dictate the choices made. The following information should be of value in making these decisions.

A dose-dependent induction of mammary carcinomas is observed in response to NMU. The typical range of doses that has been used is 12.5–50 mg NMU/kg body wt. At the 50-mg/kg dose—the dose most frequently injected—a high incidence and multiplicity of carcinomas is observed, and the latent period is short. Mean time to tumor depends on the age at which NMU is injected. Refs. *12,13,* and *16* provide quantitative information relative to the changes in incidence and multiplicity of palpable mammary carcinomas over time following carcinogen administration at various doses of carcinogen injected at different ages. In general, if the research question simply requires the rapid induction of palpable mammary carcinomas to test a therapeutic agent, or if the research question is best tested when a robust carcinogenic process is induced with a short latency period and the occurrence of carcinomas in essentially all injected animals, then 50 mg NMU/kg is the dose of choice. At the other extreme is the carcinogenic response observed when a dose of 12.5 mg NMU/kg body wt is injected. In general, less than 30% of injected animals are observed with palpable mammary carcinomas after a latency in excess of 6 mo.

The age at which NMU is injected has a significant impact on the rapidity of the carcinogenic response. From the time of the initial report of Huggins *(7)*, the accepted age at which to inject—at least the initial dose of carcinogen if multiple injections were used—was 50 d of age. Clearly, the animal is highly responsive to carcinogenic insult at this age. However, recently reported data have shown that the injection of NMU at ages prior to 50 d results in robust tumor development *(13)*. Most recently, we have reported on the carcinogenic response when rats were injected with 50 mg NMU/kg at 21 d of age *(16)*. Greater than 90% incidence of invasive carcinomas was detected in whole-mount preparations within 35 d postcarcinogen, and at this time greater than 60% of the animals had mammary carcinomas detectable by palpation. This finding is in contrast to the longer latent periods, when NMU was injected at 50 d of age. Moreover, animals can be sacrificed at time-points ranging from 14–35 d postcarcinogen, and a high incidence of premalignant lesions identified and evaluated in mammary-gland whole-mount preparations *(16,17)*. The procedure for preparing whole-mounts is described in detail in ref. *18*.

Table 1
Protocol for the Induction of Mammary Carcinomas Using NMU

Storage and analysis of NMU	• NMU, obtained from a commercial source, is stored on desiccant below $-10°$ C prior to use • A solution of 14 mg/mL dissolved in water is prepared prior to use for the carcinogenesis protocol for spectral analysis to confirm purity of the compound (Use a 1:1000 dilution) • Concentration of NMU can be confirmed by measuring the absorbance at $\lambda_{max} = 231$ nm; the extinction coefficient for NMU is log $\epsilon 3.77$ (in water)
Preparation of NMU for injection	• NMU for animal injection is prepared in 0.9% NaCl acidified to pH ≤ 5.0 using acetic acid • A satisfactory working concentration is 14 mg NMU/mL; more dilute solutions can be prepared, but this increases the injection volume required • Care must be exercised to ensure that NMU is completely dissolved in the saline solution; this is achieved by gentle heating with hot tap water accompanied by vigorous shaking. This process should be carried out in a sealed injection vial • It is usually recommended that NMU be used immediately after preparation. However, spectral analysis indicates that the NMU solution is greater than 95% stable for a period of 8 h at room temperature
Injecting rats with NMU	• NMU is injected intraperitoneally using a 1-mL disposable plastic syringe equipped with a 26-gauge, 3/8″ needle • The amount injected is dictated by carcinogen dose and weight of the animal. There is no need for any type of animal restraining device during the injection procedure • It is helpful to prepare an injection schedule with body wt listed in 5-g increments and the appropriate volume of carcinogen to be injected listed next to the body wt. Animals can be weighed at the time they are injected
Cleanup following injection	• NMU in excess of that used during carcinogen administration should be chemically inactivated in an institutionally designated chemical fume hood. Typically, a saturated solution of sodium carbonate is used for this purpose • A dilute solution of alkali can be used to decontaminate work surfaces • In general, other materials used during carcinogen administration can be disposed of via incineration in compliance with an institution's Biosafety guidelines

Table 2
Advantages of Inducing Mammary Carcinomas Using
A Single Ip Injection of 50 mg NMU/kg Body Wt

Category	Attributes
Induction methodology	• Minimal supplies are needed; readily available • Convenient ip injection protocol requiring minimal manipulation of the animal • NMU has a short half-life in the animal (<2 h); this reduces the management issues and costs associated with containment of carcinogen-treated animals and disposal of animal-related carcinogen waste • Chemical inactivation of NMU is easily accomplished • Overall, the procedures are convenient and economical
Carcinogenic response	• Short latency to tumor emergence • High incidence and multiplicity of mammary carcinomas and low prevalence of benign mammary tumors • Low incidence of tumors at other organ sites • Mammary tumors can be detected by palpation throughout the time-course of an experiment • Rate of tumor growth and/or regression can be monitored via caliper measurements
Experimental design	• Ability to operationally distinguish between carcinogenic initiation and promotion/progression • In general, experimental groups comprised of 25–30 animals provide adequate statistical power • Ability to complete a study in as little time as 5 wk following NMU injection

Based on our experience, if a high incidence of palpable mammary carcinomas with a short latent period is desired, then the model of choice is 50 mg NMU/kg body wt injected at 21 d of age. The added advantage of this model is that it also permits the investigation of the genesis and prevention of premalignant lesions. Whether NMU is injected at 21 or 50 d of age, there are many practical advantages to this method of mammary carcinoma induction. (*see* Table 2).

2.3. Typical Animal Protocols

To facilitate the adaptation of the NMU model for those less experienced in experimental carcinogenesis, we describe two typical experimental protocols.

2.3.1. CHEMOPREVENTION PROTOCOL

In a typical chemoprevention experiment, the effects of a potential chemopreventive agent on the carcinogenic response contrasted to the carcinogenic response observed in a control group of animals that are administered a placebo treatment. The end points of the carcinogenic response that are usually compared are the incidence and multiplicity of carcinoma and the latency to their detection as assessed by palpation. For statistical reasons, we recommend studying the effects of an agent using 30 animals per experimental group. If rats are injected with 50 mg NMU/kg body wt at 21 d of age, the experiment can usually be completed within 7–8 wk if the occurrence of palpable mammary tumors, histopathologically classified, is used as an end point. If the carcinogenic response is assessed in whole-mount preparations, the study can be completed within 5–6 wk of carcinogen treatment. However, this approach incurs more effort and resources and is recommended only if there is an interest in quantifying the occurrence of premalignant as well as malignant mammary-gland lesions. If NMU treatment is delayed until 50 d of age, the typical duration of an experiment is 6 mo., although some investigators have reduced this interval by 1–2 mo. Given that similar information is obtained from both protocols relative to screening a compound for potential chemopreventive activity, the savings in time, effort, and resources can be considerable if the 21 d of age injection protocol is used. Additional information related to the design of experiments and their execution is provided in refs. *15* and *18*.

2.3.2. THERAPEUTIC PROTOCOL

A primary objective of a tumor induction protocol to test a therapeutic agent is to rapidly generate animals bearing palpable mammary tumors of measurable dimensions. It is presumed that the shorter the time period between carcinogen administration and the detection of tumors with measurable dimensions, the more expediently the experiment can be completed. The injection of 21-d-old female Sprague Dawley rats with 50 mg NMU/kg body wt should yield a majority of the animals with palpable tumors within 7–8 wk following carcinogen administration. As reported in *(13)*, it is possible to further shorten latency by injecting up to 75 mg NMU/kg body wt.

What is generally more variable than latency is the time that it takes for palpable mammary tumors to reach dimensions that can be reproducibly measured using vernier calipers. Animals are randomized to treatment regimens as they develop tumors with measurable dimensions. Some investigators who need only a small number of tumor-bearing rats frequently inject only a small number of animals, and at times are disappointed by the failure to rapidly obtain tumors of measurable size. We generally recommend injecting up to twice the number of animals required for a particular experimental protocol, so that animals with tumors of measurable dimensions can be randomized to a treatment protocol over a narrow time frame. We also note that some investigators have not reported tumor yields equivalent to those mentioned here. Our many personal communications with investigators adapting this model system have shown that other than errors in carcinogen preparation or administration, two other factors can impact tumor latency and yield: excessive noise in an animal facility and disruption of the animals' normal routines within an animal room—particularly if such disruptions include frequent transport of animals to different rooms within the facility and/or the frequent administration of anesthesia. Care should also be taken to adjust the light cycle to which animals are exposed; a 12-h light/12-h dark cycle is generally recommended in the animal holding room.

2.4. Biological Characteristic of Mammary Carcinomas Induced by NMU

The biological characteristics of chemically induced mammary carcinomas in rats have been reviewed *(19,20)*, and are briefly summarized in Table 3. Chemically induced mammary carcinomas in the rat originate from ductal mammary epithelial cells, most likely from cells in the terminal end bud. This is important because the

Table 3
Biological Characteristics Similar to the Human Disease Process

Histogenesis	*Ductal epithelial cells*
Pathogenesis	Ductal hyperplasia, ductal carcinoma *in situ,* invasive carcinoma
Histopathology	Carcinoma with cribiform, papillary, and mixed morphology are most common
Ovarian-hormone dependence	Greater than 70% of mammary tumors that reach a palpable size regress in response to ovariectomy
Pregnancy	Full-term pregnancy prior to carcinogenic initiation protects against tumor formation
Metastasis	While infrequent, metastases to the lung have been noted
Pathogenetic characteristics	Altered expression of TGFα, ErbB2, cyclin D1 and gelsolin has been reported

majority of human breast cancers have a ductal histogenesis *(21)*. Moreover, most evidence indicates that these carcinomas have a similar pathogenesis to the human disease—i.e., they progress from ductal hyperplasias without or with atypia, to ductal carcinoma *in situ,* to invasive carcinoma. As ref. *16* indicates, both premalignant and malignant stages of the disease can be studied in animals injected with NMU at 21 d of age. Histologically, the carcinomas induced and their premalignant precursors have many similarities to the human disease, although there are also obvious differences *(21)*. A histological comparison of the lesions induced in this model relative to those observed in the human disease has recently been published *(22)*. Other characteristics of the human disease process reflected in the NMU model are the occurrence of both ovarian hormone-dependent and -independent carcinomas, and the protection against tumor development conferred by a full-term live birth prior to carcinogenic initiation. One characteristic of major concern in the human disease, which is rarely observed in this model, is the occurrence of metastases. The lung appears to be a primary site of occurrence when metastases are observed.

An understanding of the molecular biological characteristics of mammary carcinomas induced by NMU is only beginning to emerge. This topic was recently reviewed *(23)*. To date, it appears that NMU-induced mammary carcinomas, like their human counterparts, have an altered expression of TGFα, ErbB2, cyclin D1, and gelsolin. A *G* to *A* transition mutation in codon 12 of the Ha-*ras* gene is frequently observed in NMU-induced mammary carcinomas, but is rare in human breast cancer *(24)*. Interestingly, NMU-induced mammary carcinomas do not appear to have dysregulated *p53* activity, as is commonly seen in the human disease. Further studies are needed to clarify the pathogenetic basis of the disease process induced in the mammary gland by NMU.

2.5. Value of this Model Relative to Genetically Engineered Models for Mammary Cancer

The advantage of the NMU-induced model is that autochthonous mammary carcinomas can be induced rapidly, reproducibly, and relatively inexpensively. These carcinomas share many characteristics with the human disease, and this model has been shown to have value in identifying agents that are effective in the control and treatment of the human disease process. While the availability of transgenic and knockout models for the study of mammary carcinogenesis clearly provides a new set of tools with which to investigate the genesis, prevention, and treatment of breast cancer, currently none of these models can fully replace the advantages offered in the NMU-induced mammary carcinogenesis model in the rat.

REFERENCES

1. Fisher B, Costantino JP, Wickerham DL, Redmond CK, Kavanah M, Cronin WM, et al. Tamoxifen for prevention of breast cancer: report of the national surgical adjuvant breast and bowel project P-1 study. *J Natl Cancer Inst* 1998; 90:1371–1388.
2. Cummings SR, Eckert S, Krueger KA, Grady D, Powles TJ, Cauley JA, et al. The effect of raloxifene on risk of breast cancer in postmenopausal women: results from the MORE randomized trial. *JAMA* 1999; 281:2189–2197.
3. Veronesi U, De Palo G, Marubini E, Costa A, Formelli F, Mariani L, et al. Randomized trial of fenretinide to prevent second breast malignancy in women with early breast cancer. *J Natl Cancer Inst* 1999; 91:1847–1856.
4. Gottardis MM, Jordan VC. Antitumor actions of keoxifene and tamoxifen in the N-nitrosomethylurea-induced rat mammary carcinoma model. *Cancer Res* 1987; 47:4020–4024.
5. Anzano MA, Peer CW, Smith JM, Muller LT, Shrader MW, Logsdon DL, et al. Chemoprevention of mammary carcinogenesis in the rat: combined use of raloxifene and 9-*cis*-retinoic acid. *J Natl Cancer Inst* 1996; 88:123–125.
6. Moon RC, Thompson HJ, Becci PJ, Grubbs CJ, Gander RJ, Newton DL, et al. 4-Hydroxyphenyl retinamide, a new retinoid for prevention of breast cancer in the rat. *Cancer Res* 1979; 39:1339–1346.
7. Huggins C, Grand LC, Brillantes FP. Mammary cancer induced by a single feeding of polynuclear hydrocarbons, and its suppression. *Nature* 1961; 189:204–207.
8. McCormick GM, Moon RC. Effect of pregnancy and lactation on growth of mammary tumors induced by 7,12-dimethyl-benz(a)anthracene (DMBA). *Br J Cancer* 1965; 19:160–166.
9. Gullino PM, Pettigrew HM, Grantham FH. N-Nitrosomethylurea as mammary gland carcinogen in rats. *J Natl Cancer Inst* 1975; 54:401–414.
10. Moon RC, Grubbs CJ, Sporn MB, Goodman DG. Retinyl acetate inhibits mammary carcinogenesis induced by N-methyl-N-nitrosourea. *Nature* 1977; 267:620–621.
11. McCormick DL, Adamowski CB, Fiks A, Moon RC. Lifetime dose-response relationships for mammary tumor induction by a single administration of N-methyl-N-nitrosourea. *Cancer Res* 1981; 41:1690–1694.
12. Thompson HJ, Adlakha H. Dose-responsive induction of mammary gland carcinomas by the intraperitoneal injection of 1-methyl-1-nitrosourea. *Cancer Res* 1991; 51:3411–3415.
13. Thompson HJ, Adlakha H, Singh M. Effect of carcinogen dose and age at administration on induction of mammary carcinogenesis by 1-methyl-1-nitrosourea. *Carcinogenesis* 1992; 13:1535–1539.
14. Shepel LA, Gould MN. The genetic components of susceptibility to breast cancer in the rat. *Prog Exp Tumor Res* 1999; 35:158–169.
15. Thompson HJ. Methods for the induction of mammary carcinogenesis in the rat using either 7,12 dimethylbenz[α]anthracene or 1-methyl-1-nitrosourea. In: Ip M, Asch B, eds. *Methods in Mammary Gland Biology and Breast Cancer Research*. Kluwer Academic/Plenum Press, 2000; p 19–30.
16. Thompson HJ, McGinley JN, Rothhammer K, Singh M. Rapid induction of mammary intraductal proliferations, ductal carcinoma *in situ* and carcinomas by the injection of sexually immature female rats with 1-methyl-1-nitrosourea. *Carcinogenesis* 1995; 16:2407–2411.
17. Thompson HJ, McGinley JN, Wolfe P, Singh M, Steele VE, Kelloff GJ. Temporal sequence of mammary intraductal proliferations, ductal carcinomas in situ and adenocarcinomas induced by 1-methyl-1-nitrosourea in rats. *Carcinogenesis* 1998; 19:2181–2185.
18. Thompson HJ, Singh M, McGinley JN. A simple method for investigating pre-malignant and malignant stages of mammary carcinogenesis in the rat using 1-methyl-1-nitrosourea. *J Mammary Gland Biology and Neoplasia* 2000; 5:201–210.

19. Welsch CW. Host factors affecting the growth of carcinogen-induced rat mammary carcinomas: a review and tribute to Charles Brenton Huggins. *Cancer Res* 1985; 45:3415–3443.
20. Russo J, Russo IH. Experimentally induced mammary tumors in rats. *Breast Cancer Res Treat* 1996; 39:7–20.
21. Russo J, Gusterson BA, Rogers AE, Russo IH, Wellings SR, van Zwieten MJ. Comparative study of human and rat mammary tumorigenesis. *Lab Investig* 1990; 62:244–278.
22. Singh M, McGinley JN, Thompson HJ. A comparison of the histology of pre-malignant and malignant mammary gland lesions in sexually immature rats with those occurring in the human. *Lab Investig* March 2000; 80:221–231.
23. Medina D, Thompson HJ. A comparison of the salient features of mouse, rat and human mammary tumorigenesis. In: Ip M, Asch B, eds. *Methods in Mammary Gland Biology and Breast Cancer Research.* Kluwer Academic/Plenum Press, 2000; p 31–36.
24. Zhang R, Haag, JD, Gould MN. Reduction in the frequency of activated ras oncogenes in rat mammary carcinomas with increasing N-methyl-N-nitrosourea doses or increasing prolactin levels. *Cancer Res* 1990; 50:4286–4290.

10 Carcinogen-Induced Colon-Cancer Models for Chemoprevention and Nutritional Studies

Bandaru S. Reddy, DVM, PhD

CONTENTS

INTRODUCTION
LABORATORY ANIMAL MODELS FOR COLON CANCER
SUMMARY
REFERENCES

1. INTRODUCTION

In studies of various human diseases, it is critical that reliable animal models are developed that demonstrate similarity to the human disease. The relative rarity of spontaneous epithelial tumors of the colon in experimental animals and the absence of evidence of virally induced large bowel tumors have provided a rationale to develop chemically induced experimental models for colon carcinogenesis. Such animal models have been developed to study the multiple environmental factors involved in the pathogenesis of cancer of the colon. These animal models are:

1. Induction of colon tumors in rats through aromatic amines such as 3,2′-dimethyl-4-Aminobi-phenyl (DMBA);
2. Derivatives and analogs of cycacin, such as methyazoxymethanol (MAM), 1,2-dimethyl-hydrazine (DMH), and azoxymethane (AOM) in rats and mice of selected strains;
3. Direct-acting carcinogens of the type of alkylureas, such as methylnitrosourea (MNU) or N-methyl-N′ nitro-N-nitrosoguanidine (MNNG);
4. Heterocyclic amines such as 2-amino-3-methylimidazo [4,5-*f*] quinoline (IQ) and 2-amino-1-methyl-6-phenylimidazo[4,5-*b*]pyridine (PhIP).

The spectrum of epithelial lesions induced in the colon by these chemical carcinogens is similar to various types of neoplastic lesions observed in the colorectum of humans. Some of the earlier studies tested the carcinogenicity of the agents. Subsequent studies were done to study histogenesis, cell-proliferation kinetics, genetic susceptibilities, effects of dietary components, and the effect of fecal stream, bile acids, and bacterial flora, among other factors. Some recent studies were directed toward inhibition of colon carcinogenesis by nutritional and chemopreventive agents.

From: *Tumor Models in Cancer Research*
Edited by: B. A. Teicher © Humana Press Inc., Totowa, NJ

This chapter examines the carcinogen-induced colon-cancer model to study the relationship between nutritional factors and chemopreventive agents and colon carcinogenesis. Animal models are extremely valuable in our understanding of the human disease, but extreme care must be used in the selection of realistic models. It is essential to be familiar with the limitations of the model system being used to study the human disease. Animal models should bear relevance to human colorectal cancer, with similarities not only in terms of histopathology and in molecular and genetic lesions during early and progression stages of carcinogenesis, but also adequacy of the model for prevention studies. In addition, dysplastic lesions induced in a model should be similar to those seen in humans so that they can be used as a surrogate end points *(1)*. The animal models should reflect the efficacy of both effective and ineffective nutritional and chemopreventive agents that have been evaluated in humans *(1)*. It should also be recognized that extrapolation of data obtained in animal-model systems entail inherent sources of uncertainty that must be considered in predicting human responsiveness. Based on an analysis of the weaknesses and strengths of several models, we found that the AOM model system appears to be an appropriate model because of the similarities of histopathology of adenomas and adenocarcinomas induced in the colon and regional distribution of colon tumors with human large-bowel tumors. Also, the ongoing nutritional and chemoprevention trials in humans are, in part, based on the results generated from this model system.

2. LABORATORY ANIMAL MODELS FOR COLON CANCER

2.1. Aromatic Amines

The carcinogenic action of 32′-dimethyl-4-aminobiphenyl (DMAB) was first recorded by Walpole et al. *(2)*, who described the induction of large-bowel tumors in rats by subcutaneous (sc) administration of this agent. The carcinogenic action of DMBA to induce large-bowel tumors was also evaluated in our laboratory and other laboratories *(3–5)*. Administration of 20 weekly sc injection of DMAB to male F344 rats at a dose rate of 50 mg/kg body wt induced multiple colon tumors in about 26–30% of animals fed a low-fat diet, and 74% of animals fed a high fat-diet. DMAB induced both adenomas and adenocarcinomas, with a yield of approx 1.2–2.7 tumors per tumor-bearing rat. Adenomas of the colon were benign, with mild or moderate epithelial atypism. Adenocarcinomas were frank malignant tumors, showing invasion across the line of muscularis mucosa, and were well-differentiated and poorly differentiated adenocarcinomas. The major weakness of this model is that it requires multiple injections of DMBA to induce colon tumors. On a molar equivalent basis, DMAB is less potent in rodent models than the series of compounds derived from DMH or AOM. Another weakness of this model system is the induction of numerous neoplasms in various other sites of the body, such as adenocarcinomas of mammary glands in female rats, sarcomas of the salivary glands, squamous-cell carcinomas (SCCs) of the ear duct and skin, gastric papillomas, sarcomas and lymphomas, and carcinomas of urinary bladder.

2.2. Alkylnitrosoureido Compounds

MNNG and MNU are direct alkylating agents, which do not require metabolic activation, and thus they are topical and potent carcinogens *(6)*. Intrarectal instillation of NMU or MNNG induced colorectal tumors in rodent models *(7–11)*. In rats and mice, most of the induced colon tumors are sessile or polypoid papillary lesions. Because biochemical activation is not required for these carcinogens, it is an ideal way to induce colon tumors in animals and to study modifying effects during the postinitiation stage of colon carcinogenesis without involving the metabolism of the genotoxic, initiating carcinogen *(11)*. Intrarectal administration of MNNG at a dose rate of 1–3 mg/rat/wk for 20 wk induced colon tumors in 100% of male F344 rats, of which 43% tumors were adenocarcinomas and 57% were adenomas. The neoplasms were all located in the distal colon and rectum, as MNNG and MNU are locally acting carcinogens. The adenocarcinomas were mostly well-differentiated, and exhibited infiltration into the submucosa, whereas some were poorly differentiated adenocarcinomas showing mucous-cell infiltration into the submucosa. Metastatic lesions were not usually observed. Because MNNG and MNU given intrarectally provided the most reliable model for the topical and selective production of tumors of the distal colon and rectum, these models have been widely used. The major weakness of this model is that the technique of intrarectal injection requires a highly skilled technician, and quantification of carcinogens instilled intrarectally is difficult.

2.3. 1,2-Dimethylhydrazine

DMH is an effective carcinogen for the specific induction of tumors of the colon and rectum in rats and mice by systematic sc or intraperitoneal injection *(12–17)*. The usefulness of this organospecific carcinogen, which induces selectively tumors in the colon, was confirmed by several laboratories *(12,16–18)*. Despite the differences in doses, schedules, and animal strains used by different investigators, there is some consistency in their results in using DMH as a colon carcinogen. The SC injection of DMH at a dose rate of 20 mg/kg body wt, once weekly for 20 wk, induces colon adenomas and adenocarcinomas in about 60% of male F344 rats *(11)*. Adenocarcinomas were well-differentiated, invading into the submucosal and muscular layer. Some were signet-ring infiltrating carcinomas, and were prominent in the distal colon. The adenomas were benign neoplasms of the intestinal glandular structure lining with slight or moderate atypical epithelial cells, yet were not invasive into the submucosal layer. Maskens *(19)* demonstrated that the earliest recognizable lesions induced after 15 wk of treatment were small clusters of irregularly shaped glands consisting of poorly differentiated epithelial cells with nuclear atypia. Some of these foci showed clear evidence of invasiveness through muscularis mucosa and, therefore were interpreted as microscopic carcinomas. DMH-induced colon tumors are very close to human colon cancer with regard to morphology, pattern of growth, and clinical manifestations *(12)*. However, the major weakness of this model is that multiple injections of DMH are required to induce colon tumors in laboratory rodents.

2.4. Azoxymethane

Since 1971, we have been involved in the development and usage of animal models for studying various dietary and environmental factors in the pathogenesis of colon cancer. AOM, a metabolite of DMH *(6)*, has been used extensively by many investigators to induce colon tumors and to study the effects of nutritional factors and chemopreventive agents in colon carcinogenesis *(20–25)*.

Studies by Druckrey *(20)*, Ward *(26)*, and Reddy et al. *(22)* have shown that AOM is a potent inducer of carcinomas of the large intestine in various strains of the male and female rats. A dose-response study of AOM in male F344 rats by Ward *(26)* demonstrated that rats given a single sc dose of 3.4 mg (29.6 mg/kg body wt) and 1.7 mg (14.8 mg/kg body wt) per rat developed intestinal tumors in about 80% and 50% of rats, respectively. We have used a two-dose (15 mg/kg body wt, once weekly for 2 wk subcutaneously) method in all our chemoprevention and nutritional studies over the last 15 yr *(21–23,25)*. Our results and those of others indicate that this dose regimen in male F344 rats will induce intestinal tumors in about 80% of animals with mean of 3 tumors/rat after 40–50 wk after the second AOM treatment (Table 1). Endoscopic examination of animals treated with this dose of AOM revealed that the first endoscopically visible colon tumor can be detected 15 wk after the AOM treatment, and the mean latency period of such tumors is approx 20 wk. Over the last several years, several potential chemopreventive and nutritional agents have been evaluated for their anticancer properties, using AOM-colon-cancer models.

The histopathology of colon and small-intestinal tumors induced by AOM has been well-described by Ward et al. *(26)*. Shamsuddin *(27,28)*, and Elwell and McConnel *(29)*. The microscopic features of the tumors were similar to those in humans. Epithelial neoplasms of colon induced by AOM in F344 rats include both adenomas and adenocarcinomas. Based on our past experience with this model, about 70% of colon tumors and 90% of small-intestinal tumors are adenocarcinomas; the rest are adenomas. Induction of adenocarcinomas in this model system depends on the dose of AOM and the length of time that the animals are kept after carcinogen treatment. Histologically, adenomas of the colon and small intestine are benign, with mild or moderate epithelial atypia. The malignant neoplasms of the colon and small intestine (epithelial origin) are the adenocarcinomas, and the majority are well-differentiated, frank malignant tumors showing invasion across the line of the muscularis mucosa. Some of them are poorly differentiated, highly infiltrative, often reach the intestinal wall and the serosa, and may even invade the neighboring organs. Some well-differentiated adenocarcinomas are characterized by well-formed glands containing a varying amount of mucus. A few adenocarcinomas are mucinous colloid type, and are characterized by abundant intracellular and extracellular mucin. These are also seen to invade and metastasize rapidly. Although local invasion is characteristic for adenocarcinomas of the intestine, metastatic lesions are not commonly observed. In our past experience with this model, extension of lesions into the adjacent peritoneal tissues can occur and metastatic lesions, if occur, can be seen in the mesenteric lymph nodes, lung, and liver. Metastatic lesions include the appearance of groups of signet-ring cells and mucinous lakes in the lungs, and liver.

Similar to regional distribution of tumors in human colon, AOM treatment induces colon tumors predominantly in the distal colon *(30)*. AOM treatment also induces *ras* oncogene mutations at codon 12 of K- and H-*ras,* and increases the expression of the *ras* family of proto-oncogenes, which have been causally associated with colon-tumor development *(31,32)*. Enhanced *ras* oncogene expression has been observed in a variety of human colon tumors *(33)*. AOM-induced colon tumors also demonstrate enhanced cyclooxygenase-2 expression similar to human colon tumors *(34,35)*. Mutations in the tumor-suppressor gene, APC, are known to be early events in the colon-

Table 1
AOM-Induced Colon-Tumor Incidence in Male F344 Rats

Dose of azoxymethane	Incidence (% of animals with adenocarcinomas)	Multiplicity (adenocarcinomas/ animal)	Reference
15 mg/kg body wt., weekly for 2 wk	81	1.50	Rao et al., 1995 (21)
"	78	1.35	Reddy et al., 1997 (23)
"	97	3.73	Zeng et al., 1997 (24)
"	85	1.91	Kawamori et al., 1998 (25)

cancer process in humans (36). APC gene mutations have been identified in patients with familial adenomastous polyposis, who have germline mutation in one of the APC alleles, and in sporadic colorectal cancer (37,38). Evidence in humans thus implicates the APC-suppressor gene as causal in large-bowel carcinogenesis. A recent study by Caderni et al. (39) indicates the presence of APC mutation in AOM-induced colon tumors in F344 rats. Studies conducted by Maltzman et al. (40) also demonstrate that APC protein is aberrant in AOM-induced mouse colon adenomas and adenocarcinomas, which is consistent with the results of human colon carcinogenesis. These studies indicate that APC is involved in chemically induced rodent colon-cancer models, strengthening the concept that these models are appropriate for human colon-cancer studies. These are some of several similarities between human colon tumors and AOM-induced colon tumors in rodents.

Of all the model systems, the use of rats—especially Fischer (F344) rats—and AOM seem to be appropriate because the rat colon has light- and electron-microscopic morphology as well as histochemical properties that are quite similar to that of humans, and biological behaviors of AOM-induced rat-colon carcinomas are very similar to those of the human colon carcinomas. AOM-induced carcinomas metastasize to regional lymph nodes and liver, and these carcinomas are transplantable (27).

Attention has recently been drawn to use of surrogate end point biomarkers for purposes of determining the usefulness of potential colon-cancer inhibitors (41). Aberrant crypt foci (ACF), which are recognized as early preneoplastic lesions, have consistently been observed in AOM-treated rat colon visualized by the application of methylene blue staining in either fresh or fixed colonic tissue (42). The ACF can be visualized under light-microscope 4 wk after AOM treatment (15 mg/kg body wt, once weekly for 2 wk). Pretlow et al. (43) have also shown that these lesions are present in the colonic mucosa of patients with colon cancer, and have suggested that aberrant crypts are putative precursor lesions from which adenomas and carcinomas may develop in the colon. ACF contain elements of dysplasia and express mutation in the *apc* gene and *ras* oncogene, which suggests that they are part of the most commonly hypothesized pathway leading to colon cancer (41,44). There is evidence that several inhibitors of ACF formation reduce the incidence of colon tumors in laboratory animals (41), suggesting that ACF induction can be used to evaluate novel agents for their potential chemopreventive properties against colon carcinogenesis.

2.5 Heterocyclic Amines

The formation of mutagens upon broiling fish and meat was first discovered by Sugimura et al. IQ, a heterocyclic aromatic amine produced from food pyrolysis, was first isolated from broiled fish *(37)*. Subsequently, it was isolated from a variety of broiled or cooked fish and meat *(45,46)*. IQ is a strong mutagen in *S. typhimurium*, and also induces mutations in Chinese hamster lung cells and hepatocellular carcinomas in rodents and nonhuman primates *(47,48)*. Other cooked food mutagens, which are heterocyclic aromatic amines, include IQ, 2-amino-3, 8-dimethylimidazo[4,5-*f*]quinoxaline, 2-amino-3,4-dimethylimidazo[4,5-f]quinoline, and 2-amino-1-methyl-6-phenylimidazo[4,5-*b*]pyridine. Among a number of heterocyclic amines that have been demonstrated to be highly mutagenic and tumorigenic in rodent models, IQ and PhIP have attracted a lot of attention because they demonstrate a multitarget organospecificity, with specific cancer induction in Zymbal gland, skin, colon, oral cavity, and mammary gland of rodents *(48,49)*. The precursors of IQ-type heterocyclic amines are creatinine, amino acids, and sugars in meat and fish *(50)*. It has been shown that IQ requires metabolic activation by liver microsomes for conversion to its ultimate carcinogen, and forms high levels of DNA adducts in a number of organs *(51,52)*. Although it is not clear whether these heterocyclic amines may contribute to human cancer development, it is certain that these compounds are present in cooked foods, and pose a credible risk to humans.

Ito et al. *(53)* and Hasegawa et al. *(54)* induced colon tumors in male F344 rats by administering PhIP daily in the diet at 100 and 400 ppm for 52 wk and 104 wk. Although the colon-tumor incidences were about 43% and 55% in animals given PhIP at 100 and 400 ppm, respectively, severe toxicity resulted from PhIP.

We have also utilized heterocyclic amines such as 2-amino-3-methylimidazo[4,5-*f*]quinoline (IQ) or 2-amino-1-methyl-6-phenylimidazo[4,5-*b*]pyridine (PhIP) to induce colon tumors. The results of these studies from our laboratory indicate that the tumor incidence is very low, ranging from 5–28% when these agents were administered daily in the diet for 52 wk *(55)*. Most of the tumors were localized in the small intestine (20%), and very few tumors were identified in the colon (8%). In another study, when PhIP was administered by gavage daily for 3 wk and kept the animals for 58 wk, none of the animals developed intestinal tumors (unpublished results). Although the heterocyclic amines may be very important with regard to human colon-cancer development, these factors discouraged the use of aromatic heterocyclic amines to induce colon carcinogenesis in the animal model systems and to investigate the chemopreventive activity of potential agents against colon carcinogenesis.

SUMMARY

Every animal model has its strengths and weaknesses. However, some of these models have proven useful in evaluating hereditary factors, whereas other models were found to be useful in understanding the relationship between nutritional factors and colon cancer. We believe that the results obtained by these models will contribute to the understanding of genetic and nutritional factors as they relate to colon carcinogenesis.

REFERENCES

1. Kensler TW, Tsuda H, Wogan GN. United States-Japan *Epidemiol* workshop on new rodent models for the analysis and prevention of carcinogenesis. *Cancer Epidemiol Biomark Prev* 1999; 8:1033–1037.

2. Walpole AL, Williams MHC, Robert DC. The carcinogenic action of 4-aminobiphenyl and 3,2'-dimethyl-4-aminobiphenyl. *Br J Ind Med* 1952; 9:255.

3. Reddy BS, Mori H. Effect of dietary wheat bran and dehydrated citrus fiber on 3,2'-dimethyl-4-amino-biphenyl-induced intestinal carcinogenesis in F344 rats. *Carcinogenesis* 1981; 2:21.

4. Reddy BS, Ohmori T. Effect of intestinal microflora and dietary fat on 3,2'-dimethyl-4-aminobiphenyl-induced colon carcinogenesis in F344 rats. *Cancer Res* 1981; 41:1363.

5. Spjut HJ, Noal MW. Experimental induction of tumors of the large bowel of rats. A review of the experience with 3,2' dimethyl-4-animobiphenyl. *Cancer* 1971; 28:29.

6. Weisburger JH, Fiala ES. Experimental colon carcinogenesis and their mode of action. In: Autrup H, Williams GM, eds. *Experimental Colon Carcinogenesis.* CRC Press, Boca Raton, FI, 1983, p. 27.

7. Druckery H, Preussmann R, Matzkies F, Ivankovic S. Selective induction of intestinal cancer in rats by 1,2-dimethylhydrazine [in German]. *Naturwisenschanften* 1976; 54:291.

8. Narisawa T, Magadia NE, Weisburger JH, Wynder EL. Promoting effect of bile acid on colon carcinogenesis after intrarectal instillation of N-methyl-N'-nitro-N-nitrosoguanidine in rats. *J Natl Cancer Inst* 1974; 55:1093.

9. Narisawa T, Sato T, Hayakawa M, Sakuma A, Nakano H. Carcinoma of the colon and rectum of rats by rectal infusion of N-methyl-N'-nitro-N-nitrosoguanidine. *Gann* 1971; 68:231.

10. Narisawa T, Weisburger JH. Colon cancer induction in mice by intrarectal instillation of N-methylnitrosourea. *Proc Soc Exp Biol Med* 1975; 148:166.

11. Reddy BS, Narisawa T, Maronpot R, Weisburger J. Animal models for the study of dietary factors and cancer of the large bowel. *Cancer Res* 1975; 35:3421.

12. Pozharisski KM. Tumors of the intestines. In: Turuso V, Mohr U, eds. *Pathology of Tumors in Laboratory Animals,* vol. 1. Tumors of the Rat, IARC Scientific Publication No. 99, Lyon, France, 1990, p. 159.

13. Enker WE, Jocobitz JL. Experimental carcinoma of the colon induced by 1,2-dimethylhydrazine-diHCl: value as a model of human disease. *J Surg Res* 1976; 21:291.

14. Pozharisski KM, Likhachev AJ, Klimashevski VF, Shaposhinkov JD. Experimental intestinal cancer research with special reference to human pathology. *Adv Cancer Res* 1979; 30:165.

15. Pozharisski KM. Intestinal tumors induced in rats by 1,2-dimethylhydrazine [in Russian]. *Vopr Onkol* 1972; 18:64.

16. Reddy BS, Wantanabe K, Weisburger JH. Effect of high-fat diet on colon carinogenesis in F344 rats treated with 1,2-dimethylhydrazine, methylazoxymethanol acetate, or methylnitrosourea. *Cancer Res* 1997; 37:4156.

17. Reddy BS, Weisburger JH, Wynder EL. Effects of dietary fat level and dimethylhydrazine on fecal acid and neutral sterol excretion and colon carcinogenesis in rats. *J Natl Cancer Inst* 1974; 52:507.

18. Rogers AE, Newberne PM. Dietary enhancement of intestinal carcinogenesis by dimethylhydrazine in rats. *Nature* 1973; 246:491.

19. Maskens AP. Histogenesis and growth pattern of 1,2-dimethylhydrazine-induced rat colon adenocarcinomas. *Cancer Res* 1976; 36:1585.

20. Druckrey H. Production of colonic carcinomas by 1,2-dilkylhydrazines and azoxyalkanes. In: Burdette WJ, ed. *Carcinoma of the Colon and Antecedent Epithelium.* Charles C. Thomas, Springfield, IL, 1970, p. 267.

21. Rao CV, Rivenson A, Simi B, Zang E, Kelloff G, Steele V, et al. Chemoprevention of colon carcinogenesis by sulindac, a non-steroidal antiinflammatory agent. *Cancer Res* 1995; 55:1464.

22. Reddy BS, Maruyama H. Effect of different levels of dietary corn oil and lard during the initiation phase of colon carcinogenesis in F344 rats. *J Natl Cancer Inst* 1986; 77:815.

23. Reddy BS, Wang C-X, Samaha H, Lubet R, Steele V, Kelloff G, et al. Chemoprevention of colon carcinogenesis by dietary perillyl alcohol. *Cancer Res* 1997; 57:420.

24. Zeng Y, Kramer P, Olsen G, Lubet RA, Steele VE, Kelloff GJ, et al. Prevention by retinoids of azoxymethane-induced tumors and aberrant crypt foci and their modulation of cell proliferation in the colon of rats. *Carcinogenesis* 1997; 18:2119.

25. Kawamori T, Rao CV, Siebert K, Reddy BS. Chemopreventive activity of celecoxib, a specific cyclooxygenase-2 inhibitor, against colon carcinogenesis. *Cancer Res* 1998; 58:409.

26. Ward JM. Morphogenesis of chemically induced neoplasms of the colon and small intestine in rats. *Lab Investig* 1974; 30:505.

27. Shamsuddin AKM. Comparative studies of primary, metastatic and transplanted adenocarcinomas of Fischer 344 rats. *J Submicrosc Cytol* 1984; 16:697.

28. Shamsuddin AKM. Mucinous colloid adenocarcinoma of colon in Fisher-344 rats. Light microscopy, histochemistry and ultrastructure. *J Submicrosc Cytol* 1984; 16:327.

29. Elwell MR, McConnell ES: Small and large intestine. In: Boorman GA, Eustis SL, Wlwell MR, Montgomer CA, Mackenzie, eds. *Pathology of Fischer Rat.* Academic Press, San Diego, CA, 1990, p. 43.

30. Holt PR, Mokuolu AO, Distler P, Liu T, Reddy BS. Regional distribution of carcinogen-induced colon neoplasia in the rat. *Nutr Cancer* 1996; 25:129.

31. Singh J, Kulkarni N, Kelloff G, Reddy BS. Modulation of azoxymethane-induced mutational activation of *ras* protooncogenes by chemopreventive agents in colon carcinogenesis. *Carcinogenesis* 1994; 15:1317.

32. Singh J, Rivenson A, Tomita M, Shimamura S, Ishibasi N, Reddy BS. *Bifidobacterium longum,* a lactic acid-producing intestinal bacteriuminhibits colon cancer and modulates the intermediate biomarkers of colon carcinogenesis. *Carcinogenesis* 1997; 18:833.

33. Forrester K, Almoguera C, Han K, et al. Detection of high incidence of K-*ras* oncogenes during human colon tumorigenesis. *Nature* 1987; 327:298.

34. Dubois RN, Radhika A, Reddy BS, Entingh AJ. Increased cycloozygenase-2 levels in carcinogen-induced rat colonic tumors. *Gastroenterology* 1996; 110:1259.

35. Singh J, Hamid R, Reddy BS. Dietary fat and colon cancer: modulation of cyclooxygenase-2 by types and amount of dietary fat during the postinitiation stage of colon carcinogenesis. *Cancer Res* 1997; 57:3465.

36. Fearon ER, Vogelstein B. A genetic model for colorectal tumorigenesis. *Cell* 1990; 61:759.

37. Kasai H, Nishimura S, Wakabayashi K. Chemical synthesis of 2-amino-3-methylmidazo[4,5-*f*]quinoline (IQ), a potent mutagen isolated from broiled fish. *Proc Jpn Acad* 1980; 56B:382.

38. Powel SM, Zilz N, Beazer-Barclay Y, Bryan TM, Hamilton SR, Thibadeau SN, et al. APC mutations occur early during colorectal tumorigenesis. *Nature* 1992; 359:235.

39. Caderni G, De Fillippo D, Luceri C. APC mutations in aberrant crypt foci and colonic tumors induced by azoxymethane in rats. In: Pusztay HM, ed. American Association for Cancer Research. AACR, San Diego, CA, vol. 38, 1997, p. 467.

40. Maltzman T, Whittington J, Drigers L, Stephens J, Ahnen D. AOM-induced mouse colon tumors do not express full-length APC protein. *Carcinogenesis* 1997; 18:2435.

41. Wargovich MJ, Chen C-D, Jimenez A, Steele VE, Velasco M, Stephens LC, et al. Aberrant crypts as biomarker for colon cancer: evaluation of potential chemopreventive agents in the rat. *Cancer Epidemiol Biomark Prev* 1996; 5:355–360.

42. Bird RP. Observation and quantification of aberrancty crypts in the murine colon treated with a colon carcinogen: preliminary finding. *Cancer Lett* 1987; 37:147–151.

43. Pretlow TP, Oriordan MA, Pretlwo TG, Stellato TA. Aberrant crypts in human colonic mucosa: putative preneoplastic lesions. *J Cell Biochem* 1992; 16G:55–62.

44. Vivona AA, Shpitz B, Medline A, Bruce WR, Hay K, Ward MA, et al. K-ras mutation in aberrant crypt foci, adenomas and adenocarcinomas during azoxymethane-induced colon carcinogenesis. *Carcinogenesis* 1993; 14:1777–1781.

45. Barnes WS, Maher JC, Weisburger JH. High pressure liquid chromatographic method for the analysis of 2-amino-3-methylimidazo[4,5-*f*]quinoline, a mutagen formed from the cooking of food. *J Agric Food Chem* 1983; 31:883.

46. Felton JS, Knize MG, Wood C, Wuebbles BJ, Healy SK, Stuermer DH, et al. Isolation and characterization of new mutagens from fried ground beef. *Carcinogenesis* 1984; 5:95.

47. Adamson RH, Thoregirsson UP, Synderwine EG, et al. Carcinogenicity of 2-amino-3-methylimidazo[4,5-*f*]quinoline in nonhuman primates: induction of tumors in three macaques. *Jpn J Cancer Res* 1990; 81:10.

48. Sugimura T, Wakabayashi K, Ohgaki H. Heterocyclic amines produced in cooked food: unavailable xenobiotics. In: Ernster L, ed. *Xenobiotics and Cancer.* Tokyo, Japan Scientific Societies Press, 1991, p. 279.

49. Ito N, Hasegawa R, Imaida K, et al. Carcinogenicity of 2-amino-1-methyl-6-phenylimidazo[4,5-*f*]pyridine (PhIP) in the rat. *Mutation Res* 1997; 376:107.

50. Griva S, Nyhammar T, Olsson K, et al. Isolation and identification of food mutagens IQ and MeIQx from a heated model system of creatinine, glycine, and fructose. *Food Chem* 1986; 20:127.

51. Kato R. Metabolic activation of mutagenic heterocyclic aromatic amines for aromatic amines from protein prolysates. *CRC Crit Rev Toxicol* 1988; 16:307.

52. Schut HAJ, Putman KL, Randerath K. DNA adduct formation of the carcinogen 2-amino-3-methylim-idazo[4,5-*f*]quinoline in the target tissues of F344 rats. *Cancer Lett* 1988; 41:345.
53. Ito N, Hasegawa R, Sano S, Tamano S, Esumi H, Takayama S, et al. A new colon and mammary car-cinogen in cooked food, 2-amino-1-methyl-6-phenylimidazo-[4,5-*b*]pyridine (PhIP). *Carcinogenesis* 1991; 12:1503.
54. Hasegawa R, Sano M, Tamano S, Imaida K, Shirai T, Nagao M, et al. Dose-dependence of 2-amino-1-methyl-6-phenylimidazo[4,5-*b*]pyridine (PhIP) carcinogenesis in rats. *Carcinogenesis* 1993; 14:2553.
55. Reddy BS, Rivenson A. Inhibitory effect of *Bifidobacterium longum* on colon, mammary, and liver carcinogenesis induced by 2-amino-3-methylimidazo[4,5-*f*]quinoline, a food mutagen. *Cancer Res* 1993; 53:3914.

V

MUTANT, TRANSGENIC, AND KNOCKOUT MOUSE MODELS

11 Cancer Models

Manipulating the Transforming Growth Factor-β Pathway in Mice

John J. Letterio, MD

CONTENTS

1. INTRODUCTION

Among the variety of functions regulated by TGF-β pathways and their involvement in disease pathogenesis, it is perhaps their role in the suppression of malignant transformation and tumorigenesis that has gained the most attention. There are now several connections between the disruption of the cellular components of this pathway and human cancer. Mutations in the type II TGF-β receptor gene were the first to be described, and occur frequently in hereditary forms of nonpolyposis colorectal cancer with a phenotype of microsatellite instability *(1,2)*. The downstream effectors of TGF-β signals are now also recognized as frequent molecular targets. Mutations in the Smad4 gene are common in familial juvenile polyposis and in pancreatic carcinomas, and are also found in other forms of epithelial cancers, while novel cytoplasmic oncoproteins that directly interact with and inhibit receptor-activated Smad proteins have been found in leukemias *(2–7)*. In addition, many studies of cultured primary-tumor cells, cell lines, and established in vivo tumor models have described the now prototypical alterations in cancer-cell production and responsiveness to TGF-β that are widely recognized as important events. The recently established mouse models that explore these features and probe their relationship to the pathogenesis of human malignancy are of great significance, and represent the focus of this chapter.

From: *Tumor Models in Cancer Research*
Edited by: B. A. Teicher © Humana Press Inc., Totowa, NJ

1.1. The Transforming Growth Factors-β

The transforming growth factors-β (TGF-β) were first identified in culture supernatants of Moloney MuSV-transformed mouse fibroblasts as the factor responsible for supporting the anchorage-independent growth of a responder-cell line in a standard transformation assay (8), reflecting how the name was established. Following the purification and characterization of TGF-β as a 25-kDa homodimeric signaling molecule, the relationship between this peptide and a family of structurally related but functionally distinct regulatory proteins was quickly established (9–13). The recognition of a much larger family of peptide-signaling molecules carrying structural similarity to TGF-β established the outlines of a TGF-β superfamily, and membership has grown from roughly 17 molecules in 1990 to over 45 at present (Fig. 1). New members are classically identified by landmarks within the mature carboxy-terminal segment of 110–140 amino acids (14), including the nearly invariant seven cysteine residues. Members with the most highly related sequences are grouped into distinct subfamilies, including the activins, the homologs of the *Drosophila* genes *decapentaplegic* and *60A* (mainly the bone morphogenetic proteins, or BMPs), and the TGF-βs. Such apparent gene duplications resulting in alternate forms of a peptide growth factor also exist within the PDGF, NGF, and EGF families, and likely represent the evolutionary conservation of structurally important characteristics (15). Indeed, it is intriguing that while the latter gene families have little amino-acid sequence similarity to the TGF-βs, they do share a common three-dimensional conformation and a similar cysteine-knot motif (14). It has been suggested that this structural motif may have provided stability in a variety of extracellular environments, and may ultimately have served as the basis for further diversification (16).

1.2. Diversity of Functional Roles in Multiple Tissues

During the decade following the isolation and purification of TGF-β, the repertoire of activity described for TGF-β was extended well beyond that associated with the induction of a transformed phenotype in mesenchymal cells (13,17). We now know that this effect results directly from the induction of adhesion molecules by TGF-β. More important, the concept that TGF-β is a proximal effector of transformation has largely been supplanted by one that defines this ligand, its cognate receptors, and signaling intermediates as components of a tumor-suppressor pathway.

In vitro studies conducted during the 1980s and early 1990s suggested a broad range of activities and potentially overlapping functions—not only for closely related members of subfamilies, such as the individual TGF-β isoforms (TGF-β1, β2, -β3), but also between the TGF-βs and their more distant relatives. For example, TGF-β, inhibin, activin, and BMPs have all been shown to modulate chemotaxis in both human and murine monocytes, neutrophils, and lymphocytes (18–21). BMP, TGF-β, and activin each induce growth arrest and apoptosis of B cells and T cells (22–24), while TGF-β1 and BMP2 have been shown to have similar effects on odontoblast differentiation in vitro (25,26). The BMP relative GDF-5 and TGF-β each possess angiogenic activity (27,28), and multiple family members regulate mesoderm induction and dorsoventral patterning during Xenopus development, including Vg1, activin, the nodal-related proteins Xnr1 and Xnr2, TGF-β; and BMP (29–31). Thus, the high degree of similarity that exists at the structural level is accompanied by a significant overlap in function, as

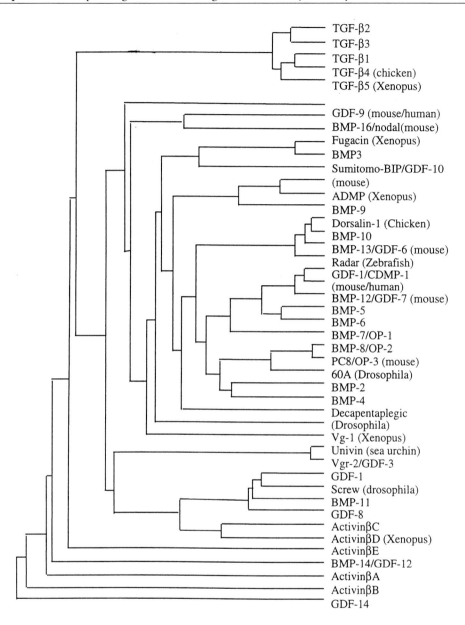

Fig. 1. The TGF-β Superfamily.

defined by many in vitro model systems and by in vivo systems involving the administration either of exogenous ligand or of ligand-specific blocking antibodies.

1.3. Receptor-Activated Smads Orchestrate Context-Specific TGF-β Responses

In many ways, the high degree of structural similarity and functional overlap of ligands within the immediate and extended TGF-β family telegraphed the existence of a complex signaling system. In particular, one would have predicted the existence of a pathway capable of conferring both context- and ligand-specificity to ligand-receptor interactions in cells of multiple lineages. The backbone of this signaling system has been elucidated with the cloning of the signaling receptors for TGF-β and the identification of a family of cytoplasmic signaling intermediates (now referred to as Smads), representing two major advances in the TGF-β field during the 1990s (reviewed in *32*). All family members signal via a set of membrane-bound serine/threonine-kinase receptors (receptors type I, or TβRI, and type II, or TβRII). Ligand binding to TβRII initiates assembly of a receptor complex, in which the activation of the TβRI kinase is achieved by a conformational change. In this process, TβRII is responsible for the phosphorylation of a site known as the (GS)-region (a conserved stretch of glycerine and serine residues) in TβRI, thereby disrupting its interaction with the TβRI kinase domain. The active type I receptor kinase propagates the signal via the Smad family of receptor substrates, which assemble into multi-subunit complexes that effect gene responses to the specific ligands (reviewed in *33*).

There are a number of combinatorial events that lead to both the diversity and specificity of responses to ligands within this family. For example, each type I receptor will designate a particular set of Smad proteins, with the TβRI of either activin or TGF-β activating Smad2 and Smad3, while BMP and GDF type I receptors are known to recognize either Smad1, Smad5, or Smad8. The target gene response is further specified by the context-dependent association of the Smad complex with specific DNA-binding cofactors (reviewed in *34*). In addition to this receptor-activated class of Smad proteins, there is also a group of inhibitory Smads that block ligand-induced signaling, designated as Smad6 and Smad7. These inhibitory Smads lack the region normally phosphorylated by TβRI, and can effect the autocrine-feedback inhibition of this pathway, and mediate environmental signals that dictate a downregulation of this pathway *(35,36)*. We are only now beginning to learn about the exact processes through which Smad complexes activate or suppress transcriptional events in response to different signals. However, it is clear that through their ability to recruit distinct sets of transcriptional co-activators and corepressors, they are able to orchestrate ligand-specific and context-specific responses, and to mediate cross-communication between ligands within the TGF-β family and those, for example, that signal via tyrosine-kinase receptors *(37,38)*.

As noted previously, the function of the signaling components of this pathway as "tumor suppressors" has been promoted by a number of observations in human cancers. The fact that nearly every cell can produce and respond to TGF-β—and that it acts as a potent inhibitor of proliferation in epithelial, hematopoietic, and endothelial cell types—suggest a central role for this cytokine in a homeostatic regulation of cell growth and differentiation. It is now clear that this activity is effected by Smad-dependent events that lead to suppressed production of important cell-cycle regulatory proteins, such as the cyclin-dependent kinases cdk2 and cdk4 and cyclins A and E, and to enhanced production of inhibitory proteins such as *p15* and *p21*[Cip1]. In most instances, the mutations in the TGF-β pathway that have been described confer resistance to growth inhibition through TGF-β by interfering with the production or function of these critical downstream targets, and ultimately the phosphorylation of the retinoblastoma (Rb) protein, thus allowing uncontrolled proliferation of cancer cells. These cell-autonomous events are independent of the local effects of TGF-β on vasculature and stroma that may be critical to tumor progression. Mutations in genes encoding both TβRII and TβRI, and Smad2 and Smad4, have chiefly been described in epithelial malignancies, and invariably lead either to impaired function or decreased expression of these proteins *(39)*. Somatic mutations have been described in 30% of colorectal cancers, and Smad4 (also known as *DPC4* for deleted in pancreatic cancer) is now known to be mutated in as many as 50% of pancreatic cancers and 30% of colorectal cancers *(40,41)*. Similar mutations have not been found in hematopoietic malignances, but the expression of oncoproteins that interfere with the function of specific Smads has been described *(42)*. For example, the expression of Evi-1, a zinc-finger protein, confers TGF-β resistance to myeloid leukemic cells by direct interaction with Smad3 and disruption of transcriptional activity *(43,44)*. Mouse models involving the disruption of either the function or expression of genes encoding specific TGF-β signaling intermediates have been developed, and largely substantiate the role of these mutations in the pathogenesis of human cancer. Several of these murine models are discussed in detail in subsequent sections.

1.4. Downregulation of TGF-β Receptors: A Common Event in Neoplasia

The inactivation or downregulation of either of the two transmembrane serine/threonine TGF-β receptors are perhaps the most common alterations in the TGF-β pathway. A correlation between loss of plasma-membrane receptors and insensitivity to TGF-β was initially described for squamous-cell carcinoma (SCC) *(45)* and Rb cell lines *(46)*, and is now considered a frequent event in many forms of cancer. A variety of deregulatory mechanisms affecting TGF-β receptors have been demonstrated. These include abnormalities in transcriptional regulation of TβRII *(47)* and structural defects of the RII gene, such as deletions *(48)*, mutations within the kinase domain *(49,50)* and mutations uniquely associated with the microsatellite instability phenotype *(51–53)*. Recent evidence that transcriptional repression of the receptor contributes directly to tumorigenesis has come from studies of primitive neuroectodermal tumors or Ewing's sarcoma. The tumor-specific gene rearrangements translocate the *EWS* gene from 22q-12 to sites that result in a fusion with *FLI1* and other *ets* transcription factors that bind through the conserved ETS domain (reviewed in *53*). These tumors express nearly undetectable levels of the type II receptor. An introduction of the *EWS-FLI1* fusion protein into normal cells suppresses the expression of TβRII *(54,55)*. A relatively newer mechanism, invoking the loss of wild-type receptors on the cell surface caused by defects in trafficking *(56,57)* provides an explanation for the reduced cell-surface expression of TβRI and TβRII observed in the absence of mutations. Not surprisingly, global disruption of the expression of TβRI or TβRII genes in mice is uniformly associated with embryonic lethality. However, approaches that interfere with receptor function by overexpression of dominant-negative-acting receptors have been useful in creating models that explore the role of receptor function in the suppression of tumorigenesis. These and other murine models focused on the conditional and lineage-specific mutation of these receptors are discussed here.

1.5. Pleiotropic Activity Predicts Complex Roles in Carcinogenesis

Unlike their signaling intermediates, the TGF-βligands play a much more complex role in disease pathogenesis, and their effects on stroma, vasculature, and immune cells all contribute to the ultimate development, growth, and metastasis of a tumor cell. Although cancer cells exhibit a selective loss of sensitivity to the growth-inhibitory effects of TGF-β, they also frequently acquire the ability to produce and secrete the ligand in an active state.

1.5.1. TGF-β Effects on Stroma and Angiogenesis Impact Tumor Growth and Metastasis

TGF-β production by tumor cells may theoretically enhance their survival by enhancing the production of matrix and stroma required for tumor-cell attachment, growth, and ultimately invasion through basement-membrane barriers. Evidence from several murine models supports the hypothesis that TGF-β production by tumor cells contributes directly to the processes of invasion and metastasis. These include studies documenting the ability of the immunosuppressive agent cyclosporine to induce autocrine TGF-β activity in tumor cells, thereby promoting invasiveness by a cell-autonomous mechanism (58). Paracrine effects of tumor-derived TGF-β on surrounding normal cells are known to decrease the production of collagenase, stromelysin, and other enzymes that degrade extracellular matrix, while providing a chemotactic and inductive signal to fibroblasts and promoting the deposition of fibronectin, collagen, and the expression of integrins. Indeed, studies have shown that TGF-β can enhance the metastatic potential of mammary tumors by controlling their ability to destroy and invade basement-membrane barriers (59).

TGF-β is also a potent stimulator of angiogenesis, a role highlighted by the defects in angiogenesis associated with mutations in genes encoding the TGF-β receptors endoglin and ALK1, the molecular targets in hereditary hemorrhagic telangiectasias (HHT) type I and type II, respectively. The importance of this angiogenic activity in tumor progression has been implicated in several tumor models, including studies of chemotherapy-resistant variants of the EMT-6 mammary carcinoma, which produce active TGF-β and have increased numbers of intratumoral vessels (60–61). Most recently, Schwarte-Waldhoff and colleagues have shown that restoration of Smad4 to TGF-β-resistant human pancreatic carcinoma cells suppressed tumor formation in vivo by influencing angiogenesis, leading to decreased expression of vascular endothelial growth factor (VEGF) and increasing expression of thrombospondin-1 (62). Interestingly, it did not restore sensitivity of the tumor cell to TGF-β. Rather, Smad4 restoration created variants that induced only small nonprogressive tumors with reduced vascular density. These data have been interpreted to demonstrate an angiogenic switch as an alternative mechanism for tumor suppression by Smad4, while clearly demonstrating a role for the angiogenic mediators *VEGF* and thrombospondin-1 as key Smad4 target genes.

1.5.2. TGF-β Effects on Immune Cells Suppress Anti-Tumor Responses

TGF-β-mediated mechanisms for tumor-induced immunosuppression are also quite complex. Early studies demonstrated that TGF-β1 suppressed macrophage-tumor cytocidal activity in vitro (63), and later in vivo studies confirmed these findings (64–66). Studies of xenotransplants in athymic mice have shown that production of TGF-β by both colonic and breast carcinoma suppresses cytotoxicity of activated monocytes and natural killer (NK) cells (67). This effect is reversed by systemic administration of blocking antibodies to TGF-β which inhibits development of primary tumors and distant metastases (68). T-cell-mediated immunity is also generally impaired in hosts bearing TGF-β producing tumors. The suppression of CD4+ T-cell function associated with the growth of the MH134 hepatoma in vivo can be reversed by systemic administration of anti-TGF-β antibodies (69). Immune dysfunction is a hallmark of mice with plasmacytomas. These mice have substantial levels of active TGF-β present in ascites fluid, as do supernatants of cultured plasmacytoma cells *(70)*. In an interesting set of experiments, treatment of plasmacytoma-bearing mice with a low dose of the alkylating agent melphalan resulted in a drop in the circulating TGF-β levels and an induction of tumor-specific cytolytic T cells *(71)*. In transfection experiments, stable expression of TGF-β1 in a highly immunogenic fibrosarcoma completely impairs the ability of the tumor to elicit cytotoxic T-lymphocyte (CTL) responses, and results in a tumorigenic phenotype *(72)*. Less is known about effects of TGF-β on presentation of tumor antigens by antigen presenting cells (APCs), but this is also an area of great interest. Studies of EL-4 tumor bearing mice reveal a link between TGF-β production and increased IL-10 expression, producing a bias toward Th2 responses, possibly through inhibitory effects on APCs *(65)*. Recent studies of modified tumor vaccines document the ability of IL-10 to prevent APC from obtaining access to tumor antigens. Other studies have suggested that introduction of TGF-β antisense expression vectors into TGF-β-producing tumors converted their phenotype to highly immunogenic, and rendered these cells effective as CTL-inducing whole-tumor-cell vaccines *(73,74)*. Remarkably, similar results have been obtained in a rat model of prostatic carcinoma *(75)*. These studies must be reproduced in more stringent models, but do suggest the potential benefits of manipulating local TGF-β production in the process of generating tumor-specific responses.

2. DISRUPTION OF GENES ENCODING THE TGF-βs IN MICE

2.1. Targeted Disruption of Gene Expression Defines Isoform-Specificity

Because of the vast array of activities that have been ascribed to members of the TGF-β family, the accurate prediction of phenotypes that may result from the disruption of a specific isoform have been difficult at best. The wide distribution of expression of each isoform during embryogenesis seems to indicate that the absence of a single TGF-β gene would not be compatible with normal development. Indeed, the observation that 50% of mice lacking the *Tgf-β1* gene were viable, with limited postnatal survival, prompted suggestions of redundancy *(76)*. Moreover, the possibility that expression of TGF-β2 or TGF-β3 may compensate for the loss of TGF-β1 led to questions regarding the utility of gene-knockout studies in mice. With the benefit of more extensive study of the individual null models, we can now confidently state that these genes do not merely serve a redundant function, as more than 30 nonoverlapping phenotypes have been described for these mouse models to date *(77)*.

Indeed, the more thorough analysis and utilization of these models for more specific in vivo tests of function are teaching us how to discern the relevant and critical activities that often exist in the absence of an overt phenotype. Several studies, including those involving mice heterozygous for the individual null mutations, are providing insight into the nature of the critical autocrine activity of these molecules, the potential importance of maternal sources of these proteins, and the existence of relevant gene-dosage effects *(78,79)*. Many of these functions have been revealed in studies focused on the response to environmental or pathologic events, such as wounding or exposure to chemical carcinogens. The creative pursuit of these models has established their utility in defining the role of these ligands in tumorigenesis.

2.2. The Tgf-β1⁻/⁻ Mouse as a Model of Neoplasia

Since the original publication of the phenotype of the TGF-β1-null mouse in 1992, this model has been one of the most extensively studied, and has been responsible for providing significant insight into the major biological functions of this isoform. The embryonic phenotypes and extensive immune pathologies associated with deletion of the *Tgf-β1* gene have been extensively reviewed, and are not presented here. More recent studies focused on this model have aimed to define the role of this ligand in the suppression of tumorigenesis.

It is noteworthy that enhanced susceptibility to spontaneous tumor formation in humans has thus far not been associated with inactivating mutations in any of the genes encoding the TGF-β ligands. As noted here, this may reflect the rather complex role that these ligands play in the processes of initiation, progression, and metastasis of the tumor cell. In mice, the embryonic and inflammatory phenotypes that accompany global disruption of the *Tgf-β1* gene expression are problematic when trying to discern the contribution of this deletion to tumor susceptibility. However, enhanced survival of the *Tgf-β1⁻/⁻* mouse in the absence of a competent immune system has allowed for longitudinal assessment of tumor susceptibility, by obviating the associated immune pathology in *Tgf-β1⁻/⁻* progeny. Evaluation of the *Tgf-β1⁻/⁻* mouse in the severe combined immunodeficiency (SCID) background has revealed an increased susceptibility to invasive tumors in the region of the cecum in the large bowel *(80)*. In this study, all *Tgf-β1⁺/⁺* and *Tgf-β1⁻/⁻* mice in the SCID background developed a proliferative epithelial phenotype and inflammation in the intestinal mucosa, but invasive lesions typical of adenocarcinoma were only noted in mice null for TGF-β1. Similar observations have been made in the *Tgf-β1⁻/⁻* mouse on a background that lacks the gene for the inhibitor of cyclin-dependent kinases (cdk) *p21^Cip1*. This cdk inhibitor is highly expressed in activated immune cells, and the absence of *p21^Cip1* expression has allowed for an extended survival of the *Tgf-β1⁻/⁻* mouse (unpublished observation). In this instance, mice are noted to be free of the intestinal pathogen, *Helicobacter pylori*, which is often associated with proliferative colitis in mice. *Tgf-β1⁻/⁻; p21^Cip1⁻/⁻* mice exhibit invasive lesions at several sites within the gastrointestinal tract that are not associated with an underlying inflammatory process. These studies support the importance of TGF-β1 in the homeostasis of intestinal epithelia, and of this pathway in general as a suppressor of colon-cancer formation. Interestingly, while deletion of specific intracellular signaling intermediates of the TGF-β pathway have been associated with a metastatic colon-cancer phenotype in mice *(81–84)*, tumors of the TGF-β1-null mouse are not metastatic, perhaps indicating a role for the ligand in promoting dissemination beyond the intestinal wall.

The TGF-β1-null mouse model has also been utilized to study multistage carcinogenesis using v-*ras^Ha*-initiated *Tgf-β1⁻/⁻* keratinocytes *(85)*. Mutations in the c-*ras^Ha* gene are known to occur following exposure of the epidermis to specific carcinogens, but other events controlling the early stages of premalignant progression are less defined. Interestingly, the v-*ras^Ha*-initiated *Tgf-β1⁻/⁻* keratinocytes progressed rapidly to multifocal SCC within dysplastic papillomas, while similarly initiated control keratinocytes formed only well-differentiated papillomas. The carcinomas arising from v-*ras^Ha*-initiated *Tgf-β1⁻/⁻* keratinocytes retained sensitivity to TGF-β1 in culture, and did not develop mutations in the *p53* gene or the c-*ras^Ha* gene.

The functional significance of this observation has been demonstrated through more recent studies of v-ras^{Ha}-retrovirus transduced primary wild-type mouse keratinocytes, which display a hyperproliferative phase followed by a TGF-β1-dependent G1 growth arrest and senescence. The arrest phase is accompanied by a 15-fold increase in total secreted TGF-β1, and a fourfold increase in secreted active TGF-β1. However, v-ras^{Ha}-retroviral transduction of keratinocytes from *Tgf-β1$^{-/-}$* mice, or from those expressing a dominant negative TβRII, is not associated with G1 growth arrest or followed by senescence. This resistance was found to be associated with low expression of $p15^{ink4b}$ and $p16^{ink4a}$, constitutive Rb phosphorylation, and high levels of cdk4 and cdk2 kinase activity *(86)*. Most importantly, the inactivation of TGF-β1 secretion or response was sufficient to block the senescence program, demonstrating that disruption in TGF-β signaling accelerates malignant progression in this instance by overcoming oncogene-induced replicative senescence.

Studies in this model system have also served well to highlight the unique and sometimes opposing effects of autocrine and paracrine sources of TGF-β. This was clearly demonstrated by the observation that the tumor-cell labeling index was lower when the v-ras^{Ha}-initiated *Tgf-β1$^{-/-}$* keratinocytes were grafted together with *Tgf-β1$^{-/-}$* fibroblasts than when they were grafted with wild-type fibroblasts. Furthermore, evidence of TGF-β1 protein within grafts of uninitiated *Tgf-β1$^{-/-}$* keratinocytes also documented the ability of normal, nontransformed cells to localize paracrine-derived TGF-β1, an effect that was not observed in tumor cells within initiated skin grafts. The results can be viewed in a broader context when considering the evidence for immunolocalization of TGF-β1 protein in the tissues of the TGF-β1 null fetus (progeny of *Tgf-β1$^{+/-}$* females) *(78)*. The latter finding suggests that maternal sources of this protein can contribute to normal development of the null embryo, and together these observations serve to highlight the potential importance of both endocrine and paracrine functions of this molecule.

2.3. Haploinsufficiency of the TGF-β1 Tumor-Suppressor Function

As noted in the previous section, the early lethality associated with each of the null mutations of the TGF-β ligands in mice initially hampered the ability to discern the role of these models in carcinogenesis. One consideration that again proved important in the analysis of the tumor-suppressor function of the TGF-β1 ligand is whether a relevant gene-dosage effect for tumor suppression might be detected in *Tgf-β1$^{+/-}$* mice when compared to wild-type litter mates. This hypothesis was tested in studies of carcinogen-induced tumor formation, with *Tgf-β1$^{+/-}$* mice demonstrating an increased rate of tumor formation and malignant progression, and tumors continued to express TGF-β1 from the retained normal TGF-β1 allele *(79)*. Indeed, *in situ* analysis of *Tgf-β1* gene expression in hepatic and lung carcinomas suggested that the tumor cells have enhanced production of the TGF-β1 ligand, indicating that there is a selective advantage to retaining TGF-β1 expression. This also represented the first evidence for a tumor-suppressor gene that functions with haploinsufficiency, as opposed to the classical tumor suppressor that requires inactivation of both alleles before expression of the malignant phenotype. Haploinsufficiency has since been suggested for the TGF-β type II receptor in a model of pituitary tumorigenesis. All *TβRII$^{+/-}$* mice subjected to chronic estrogen exposure using estradiol pellets developed pituitary adenomas, as compared with an incidence of only one in 10 wild-type mice subjected to similar treatment (87). Interestingly, many genes believed to function as classic tumor-suppressor genes according to the Knudson two-hit model have since been found to show a similar haploinsufficient tumor-suppressor function, including bax, *p53,* and the cdk inhibitor *p27*[Kip1] (88,89).

2.4. *Tgf-β3 Gene Deletion and Effects on Tumorigenesis*

The outcome of experiments involving the disruption of the other TGF-β isoforms, TGF-β2 and TGF-β3, were more predictable based on preceding work documenting the very prominent temporal and spatial regulation of the expression of these isoforms during development. The type 2 isoform was believed to play critical roles in multiple developmental processes, a presumption supported by the rather broad range of congenital defects associated with this single gene deletion (90). Many of the defects in TGF-β2-null mice appear to be strain-dependent. These include several phenotypes exhibiting a high level of penetrance on a mixed C57BL/6 × SV129 background, such as ventricular septal defects, lung abnormalities, and skeletal defects such as spina bifida, along with several other phenotypes that are only partially penetrant. The fact that many of the affected tissues have contributions from cells of neural crest origin is consistent with the predominant expression of TGF-β2 in neural tissues of the spinal cord and peripheral nervous system during development. TGF-β2 is also normally strongly expressed in chondrocytes and osteocytes, and disrupted expression results in numerous defects in the craniofacial, axial, and appendicular skeleton. Although the mechanisms leading to this array of malformations are unclear, it is likely that loss of the effects of TGF-β2 on matrix production and tissue remodeling, and on epithelial-mesenchymal interactions, are the cause of the diversity of the observed defects.

It is important, to note that the phenotypes associated with the *Tgf-β2*-null mutation are completely nonoverlapping with any of the phenotypes of the *Tgf-β2*-null mouse, and are also quite distinct from that of the *Tgf-β3*-null mutants. The latter exhibit an incompletely penetrant failure of the palatal shelves to fuse, with a resultant cleft palate (91,92). Again, in vitro studies neatly predicted a role for TGF-β3 in fusion of the palatal shelves, and *Tgf-β3* null mice appears to suffer from defective adhesion of the apposing medial-edge epithelia on the palatal shelves. The absence of craniofacial abnormalities distinguishes this mouse model from other mutants with cleft palate, and supports the idea that the failure of palatal fusion results from an intrinsic defect and is therefore not secondary to skeletal abnormalities.

Although *Tgf-β3*[−/−] mice survive to term, the defective palatogenesis together with delayed pulmonary maturation are incompatible with postnatal survival. However, the *Tgf-β3*-null mouse model has been successfully used to study the role of this isoform in maintenance of epithelial homeostasis and in susceptibility to carcinogenesis of the skin (93). While the development of full-thickness grafts of wild-type, *Tgf-β1*[−/−], and *Tgf-β3*[−/−] mice all developed normally, exposure to the tumor promoter 12-O-tetradecanoly phorbol-13-acetate (TPA) yielded very disparate responses. Consistent with studies of v-*ras*[Ha]-initiated *Tgf-β3*[−/−] keratinocytes, full-thickness grafts of *Tgf-β1*[−/−] mice displayed a hyperplastic response to TPA, but in striking contrast, extensive keratinocyte death was observed in full-thickness grafts of *Tgf-β3*[−/−] mice. The observation was associated with a significant reduction in c-Jun N-terminal kinase activity in TPA exposed *Tgf-β3*[−/−] keratinocytes, and highlights the isoform-specific activities of

TGF-βs in the suppression of tumorigenesis and cell. At present, no developmental phenotypes have been associated with heterozygosity for either the TGF-β2 or TGF-β3 gene. However, further study of the adult heterozygotes in assays designed to evaluate their response to environmental stimuli, including carcinogens, may shed additional light on the roles of these isoforms in adult tissues.

3. DISRUPTION OF TGF-β SIGNALING IN THE MOUSE

3.1. Tissue-Specific Expression of Dominant-Negative TGF-β Receptors

Transgenic mice provide a powerful model to explore mechanisms of gene expression as well as the regulation of cellular and physiological processes. Targeted expression of a protein can be achieved in different cell types and specific tissues, can affect multiple internal targets, and can be achieved in a controlled fashion by expressing the corresponding gene either ectopically, ubiquitously, or in a tissue-specific manner through the use of its own promoter. When evaluating the function of the TGF-β signaling pathway, this approach has been used either to overexpress a specific isoform, or to interfere with signaling in a target tissue by overexpression of a mutant cell-surface receptor. These are capable of acting in a dominant negative fashion to the endogenously expressed receptor proteins, and thereby preclude signaling via any of the isoforms.

As noted here, each TGF-β isoform signals through the same heteromeric receptor complex of type I and type II serine/threonine kinases. The type II receptor (TβRII) is necessary for ligand binding and subsequent growth suppression by TGF-β. Multiple studies with several kinase receptors known to function in multimeric complexes have demonstrated that expression of receptors carrying deletions in their cytoplasmic domains interferes with signaling via intact receptor proteins, effectively creating kinase-dead complexes. This strategy has successfully been applied in transgenic models to disrupt all TGF-β signaling in a tissue-specific manner.

As a target organ, the skin is a site where each TGF-β isoform exhibits some level of expression, and has some effect on normal physiology and response to events such as wounding and exposure to carcinogens. Studies demonstrating higher frequencies of malignant transformation in isolated keratinocytes of the *Tgf-β1⁻/⁻* mouse are corroborated by studies in mouse keratinocytes expressing a dominant negative TβRII. The latter leads to disruption of TGF-β signaling and is followed by rapid changes in cell ploidy, implicating a major role for this pathway in maintaining genomic stability *(85,94,95)*. In vivo, overexpression of a dominant negative TβRII in the epidermis blocks TGF-β signaling and results in a significant increase in the DNA-labeling index in the skin *(96)*. These mice have thickened, wrinkled skin that is markedly hyperplastic and hyperkeratotic, and is severe enough to result in restricted movement and perinatal lethality in the homozygous F1 generations. Transgenic mice expressing a dominant negative TβRII in the epidermis on a truncated loricrin promoter have been tested for their response to TPA *(97)*. These mice developed papillomas at twice the rate of control mice, and the papillomas progressed to carcinomas despite withdrawal of TPA. Similar results were observed in response to tumor promotion in mice expressing a dominant negative TβRII in the basal-cell compartment and follicular cells of the skin *(98)*, although disruption of TGF-β signaling in follicular cells did not disturb tissue homeostasis.

The mammary gland represents a second target organ in which the multiple TGF-β isoforms have been implicated in normal physiology, particularly TGF-β1 and TGF-β3, as they are expressed at high levels during quiescence and at all stages of development, with the exception of lactation. Using the mouse mammary-tumor virus *(MMTV)* promoter/enhancer, expression of a dominant negative TβRII was localized to the epithelial cells of terminal ducts and alveolar buds *(99)*. Virgin female transgenic mice displayed varying degrees of epithelial hyperplasia, and exhibited alveolar development and milk-protein expression. The phenotype suggests that TGF-βs normally act to suppress epithelial proliferation, as well as alveolar development and differentiation in the mammary gland. In a similar model, use of the MMTV-long-terminal repeat to drive expression of the dominant negative TβRII results in a marked increase in lateral side branching of ductal epithelium in older nulliparous females, with high levels of expression of the transgene *(100)*. Moreover, these mice exhibit a significant increase in the incidence and multiplicity of tumor formation following exposure to the carcinogen 7,12-dimethylbenz[a]anthracene *(DMBA)*, supporting a role for this pathway in the suppression of tumorigenesis. In a model designed to test the effects of TGF-β resistance in mammary stroma, expression of a dominant negative TβRII under the control of a metallothionein-derived promoter resulted in increases in lateral branching of ductal epithelium *(101)*. The result highlights the existence of stromal-epithelial interactions that are under regulation of the TGF-βs, and their importance in homeostasis of the mammary gland.

Another model has been recently developed to address similar issues with respect to the role of TGF-β in the prostate *(102)*. A transgenic system in which epithelial cells of the ventral prostate are made insensitive to the actions of TGF-β by virtue of a prostate-specific promoter, C3(1), driving the expression of the dominant-negative TβRII. The prostates of transgenic mice exhibited an abnormal morphology characterized by multiple layers of epithelial cells lining the proximal ducts, in contrast to the simple cuboidal mono-layer of cells seen in the normal prostate. There was an associated reduction in baseline rates of apoptosis in the prostatic epilthelial tissue, a factor presumed to underlie the abnormal growth. This model also promises to be a valuable experimental tool to study the role of TGF-β in prostatic growth and tumorigenesis.

Several other models have yielded phenotypes in skeletal tissues—where expression of the kinase-defective TβRII in the periosteum/perichondrium, syno-vium, and articular cartilage promotes terminal chondrocyte differentiation and osteoarthritis, suggesting a role for the TGF-βs in the maintenance of synovial joints *(103)*—and expression driven by the osteocalcin promoter has led to diminished bone remodeling *(104)*. These osteocalcin-TβRII mice exhibited an age-dependent increase in bone mass as a result of the loss of osteoblast responsiveness to TGF-β. Models based on expression of a dominant negative TβRII have also shown that disruption of TGF-β signaling in the exocrine pancreas results in increased proliferation of acinar cells and perturbed acinar differentiation *(105)*. The abnormalities are associated with pancreatic fibrosis, neoangiogenesis, macrophage infiltration, and marked upregulation of TGF-β expression within the acinar cells. The latter effect may initiate the observed abnormalities in the surrounding stroma, and provides a clue to the mechanisms by which loss of responsiveness to TGF-βs may promote the process of carcinogenesis. More recent observations suggest that TGF-β may be important in controlling the local immune response in the pancreas, and that loss of responsiveness to TGF-β may contribute to the development of pancreatitis. Inactivation of TGF-β signaling in the mouse pancreas by the expression of a dominant negative mutant form of the TGF-β type II receptor has been accomplished by using the pS2 mouse trefoil peptide promoter for pancreas-specific gene expression. pS2-dnRII transgenic mice showed marked increases in major histo-compatibility complex (MHC) class II molecules and matrix metalloproteinase (MMP) expression in pancreatic acinar cells. These mice also showed increased susceptibility to cerulein-induced pancreatitis, with severe pancreatic edema, inflammatory-cell infiltration, and T- and B-cell hyperactivation, immunoglobulin (IgG) type autoantibodies against pancreatic acinar cells, and IgM-type autoantibodies against pancreatic-ductal-epithelial cells *(106)*. These observations suggest that TGF-β signaling may be essential to maintain local immune homeostasis and to preserve the integrity of pancreatic acinar of TGF-β in maintaining tolerance in T cells, and that maintenance of B-cell tolerance to self-antigens is dependent on normal TGF-β signaling in T cells.

Overall, the strategy of expression of a kinase-defective TβRII has been highly successful in unveiling the function of this pathway in many tissues and physiological processes. More importantly, these results have demonstrated the therapeutic potential of systems aiming to deliver kinase-defective TβRII for blocking the deleterious effects of TGF-β. Indeed, adenoviral expression of a soluble truncated TβRII has been useful for preventing liver fibrosis and dysfunction in dimethylnitrosamine-exposed rats *(109,110)*. These studies suggest the potential utility of strategies that can achieve significant levels of inhibition of TGF-β signaling in vivo, and are a strong argument for their continued development.

3.2. Disrupting the TGF-β Pathway Through Conditional Mutagenesis

The popularity of the approach utilizing dominant-negative acting transgenes may be diminished by the availability of the Cre/loxP system providing for cell type-specific mutagenesis *(111,112)*. The fact that embryonic lethality is almost invariably associated with inactivation of genes encoding either the TGF-β ligands, receptors, or their downstream Smad intermediates begs the use of such conditional strategies for gene disruption. Several laboratories are currently developing models that utilize this strategy. At present, the only published example that concerns such an approach in the TGF-β system is the B-cell-specific deletion of the type II receptor through use of CD19cre mice *(113,114)*. It provides a genetic model in which the B-cell-specific function of TGF-β can be determined in a cell-autonomous manner. The results suggest that TGF-β plays a critical role in regulating B-cell homeostasis. The mice exhibited a reduced life span of conventional B cells, expansion of peritoneal B-1 cells, B-cell hyperplasia in Peyer's patches, elevated serum immunoglobulin, B-cell hyperresponsiveness, and a serum IgA deficiency.

Although a tumor phenotype was not described in this study, the results suggest that this model will allow investigators to explore the relationship between loss of TGF-β responsiveness and susceptiblity to malignant transformation in B cells. Picomolar concentrations of TGF-β inhibit the proliferation of normal, activated human tonsillar and peripheral blood B cells in a dose-dependent manner *(115)*. By contrast, the non-mitotic, resting peripheral-blood B cells *(116)* and fully mature murine plasma cells *(117)* each have been shown to undergo apoptosis upon exposure to TGF-β. Activated B lymphocytes also secrete biologically active TGF-β in vitro, and studies in human B-cell (chronic lymphocytic leukemia [CLL]) also strongly implicate a role for this cytokine in an autocrine negative feedback loop controlling the expansion of these cells *(118)*. TGF-β-insensitivity has been described in some B-cell lymphomas exhibiting loss of TGF-β receptor expression *(119)*, including primary tumor cells isolated from several patients with advanced CLL *(57)*. Our studies conducted in the murine plasmacytoma model revealed a complete and consistent absence of cell-surface TGF-β receptors *(117)*. More importantly, this phenotype is not linked to mutational inactivation or transcriptional downregulation of the receptors, but rather to a novel mechanism that links autocrine production of active TGF-β to receptor downmodulation *(120)*. These data all support the hypotheses that:

1. TGF-β is an important negative regulator of B cells and mature plasma cells
2. acquired resistance to TGF-β may be an important step in the progression of lymphoid malignancies
3. activation of ligand by the tumor cell can lead to a cytosolic ligand-receptor interaction that precludes signaling

The model created by Cazac and Roes will be an important tool in studies that test the hypothesis that disruption of TGF-β signaling contributes to tumorigenesis in B cells.

3.3. Tumor Phenotypes Associated With Disruption of SMAD Genes Mice

In a manner similar to what has been observed following targeted disruption of TGF-β ligand and receptor genes in mice, global disruption of the expression of genes encoding members of the Smad family have documented the critical importance of their function during embryogenesis. With the exception of the mutational inactivation of Smad3, disruption of Smad gene expression uniformly leads to embryonic lethality in mice, and these developmental phenotypes are not considered here *(121–127)*. Three distinct models in which the *SMAD3* gene is deleted have been described *(127–129)*, and one model is distinguished by the frequent development of a metastatic colon tumor, with 100% frequency on a pure SV129 background *(129)*. The results have been considered surprising by most investigators, as mutations in this gene have not been associated with human intestinal tumorigenesis, and because they are at odds with phenotype Smad3 mutants produced by two other laboratories, which are phenotypic replicates. It has been suggested that the fact that this mutant allele gives rise to colon carcinomas may suggest that it represents a hypomorphic or neomorphic allele, but this possibility has not yet been tested *(130)*.

Although embryonic lethality of the Smad4 mutation obviates the assessment of tumor-suppressor function, Smad4 heterozygotes are phenotypically normal, and have been useful for this purpose *(81,131)*. Taketo and Takaku have shown that as Smad4 heterozygotes age, these mice develop multiple polyps within the stomach and duodenum. These polyps have abundant stroma and eosinophilic infiltrates—features that are also characteristic of the human juvenile polyposis syndrome—in kindreds that carry germline mutations in the *SMAD4* gene. More importantly, loss of heterozygosity (LOH) for the *SMAD4* gene occurred in 100% of polyps of 18-mo-old heterozygotes, indicating LOH for SMAD4 as an early event in polyp formation. Taketo and Takaku have also created a mouse model of the human familial adenomatous polyposis syndrome by introducing the Smad4 mutation into the Apc$^{\Delta716}$-knockout mouse *(132)*. Their sophisticated in vivo genetic analysis utilized meiotic recombination to create compound heterozygotes carrying both mutations on mouse chromosome 18 *(83,84)*.

When compared to the Apc$^{\Delta716}$-knockout mouse, the compound heterozygotes develop tumors that are highly malignant and invasive in phenotype. This model verifies the importance of Smad4 as a suppressor of colon tumorigenesis, and creates a valuable tool to further define the role of this pathway in the homeostasis of intestinal epithelia, and for testing new strategies for the management and prevention of the gastrointestinal cancers linked to these mutations. It also creates the opportunity for investigators in the field to identify loci that may modify disease expression, and for developing novel chemopreventive strategies.

4. TISSUE-SPECIFIC OVEREXPRESSION OF TGF-β IN THE MOUSE

4.1. Effects of TGF-β1 Transgenes on Skin Development and Carcinogenesis

TGF-β1 protein is expressed by the basal cells of the normal epidermis. Studies of transgenic mice with targeted overexpression of TGF-β1 to the epidermis *(133)*, and of keratinocytes derived from *Tgf-β1$^{-/-}$* mice *(95,134)* indicate that TGF-β1 acts as an endogenous negative regulator of basal-cell proliferation and suppresses genomic instability. As with other tumors, SCCs of the skin acquire resistance to the inhibitory effects of TGF-β1 in later stages of progression, and typically do not express TGF-β. Yet while these malignant epithelial cells may not produce TGF-β1, this protein is highly expressed in the stroma of mouse and human skin tumors *(136–137)*, and in the dermis and epidermis after treatment of mouse skin with tumor promoters. Indeed, the observation that SC injection of TGF-β1 enhances skin-tumor promotion suggests distinct roles for stroma-derived paracrine and autocrine epithelial TGF-β1 in the maintenance of epithelial homeostasis *(138)*.

Several models using keratin promoters have been created to address this question directly. Sellheyer et al. made a transgenic model in which TGF-β1 expression was targeted to the epidermis of transgenic mice using an epidermal-specific vector derived from the regulatory sequences of the human keratin 1 (HK1) gene that is not expressed until d 15 of development, to avoid embryonic lethality *(135)*. Transgenic mice had litters of pups with rigid bodies and restricted ability to move and breathe. The size of the body was slightly smaller, as were their appendages, such as paws and ears. The skin appeared shiny and tautly stretched, and did not show a normal dermatoglyphic pattern. In addition, a slightly thinner interfollicular epidermis and a more compact ortho-hyperkeratosis were observed. The other prominent phenotype was a significant reduction in the number of hair follicles. These results clearly demonstrate that constitutive overexpression of TGF-β1 suppresses epidermal-cell proliferation and adversely affects skin development, and that regulation of the expression of active forms of TGF-β1 in the epidermis may be beneficial in the treatment of hyperproliferative diseases of the skin.

Cui et al. also generated and characterized a number of keratin-promoter TGF-β1 transgenic lines, which express recombinant TGF-β1 and are viable in the homozygous state *(138)*. These models have helped to examine the influence of TGF-β1 on the induction and progression of skin tumors in vivo. Five homozygous TGF-β1 transgenic lines were utilized for chemical carcinogenesis studies. Line H is transgenic for a construct driving constitutive expression of activated simian TGF-β1 (sTGF-β1^{act}) in suprabasal keratinocytes of the skin on a bovine keratin promoter (corresponding to human K10 gene promoter). M2 and M5 lines drive expression of sTGF-β1^{act} in suprabasal keratinocytes, but utilize an inducible keratin promoter, KIV (corresponding to human K6), which is only expressed in the hyperplastic state, following application of TPA or in hyperplastic keratinocytes of papillomas and carcinomas. Additional lines, designated D and F, were transgenic for the inducible K6 promoter driving expression of native, latent TGF-β1. A biphasic effect of TGF-β1 was noticed during multistage skin carcinogenesis, acting early as a tumor suppressor and later enhancing the malignant phenotype. The actions of TGF-β1 in enhancing malignant progression may mimic its proposed function in modulating epithelial-cell plasticity during embryonic development. The malignant conversion rate in these transgenics was vastly increased, yet they showed resistance to induction of benign skin tumors. There was also a higher incidence of spindle-cell carcinomas expressing high levels of endogenous TGF-β3, suggesting that TGF-β1 can elicit an epithelial-mesenchymal transition in vivo, and that TGF-β3 may be involved in maintenance of the spindle-cell phenotype.

Fowlis et al. used a truncated inducible bovine KIV keratin gene promoter to target expression of latent or activated TGF-β1 to keratinocytes in transgenic mice *(139)*. This short (2.2-kb) K6 promoter was generally silent in untreated animals, but was induced in vivo in response to the hyperplasia that follows topical application of the tumor promoter, TPA. Relative to controls, the K6-TGF-β1 transgenic line showed attenuation of basal keratinocyte proliferation in response to TPA, while one of the six lines showed constitutive transgene expression at low levels in the skin, with a two- to three-fold increase in the epidermal DNA-labeling index over control mice. This model has shown that TGF-β1 can act as either a positive or negative regulator of keratinocyte proliferation in vivo. It may also induce apoptosis in vivo, as elevated basal-cell DNA synthesis does not lead to hyperplasia in lines with low levels of expression and increased basal proliferation.

Blessings et al. have shown that an expression vector based on the bovine cytokeratin IV gene, corresponding to the human cytokeratin 6 gene (expressed in interfollicular epidermis), is also inducible by TPA *(140,141)*. In order to evaluate the role of polypeptide growth factors in chemically induced carcinogenesis, the authors used transgenic mice expressing cDNA for BMP4 under the control of regulatory elements of the cytokeratin IV gene. In control litter mates, TPA induced epidermal hyperproliferation and atypia with dark cells and dermal inflammation, followed by papillomas and SCCs in 13 of 26 control animals. In BMP4 transgenic mice, TPA-induced expression of the BMP4 transgene in the interfollicular epidermis was associated with minimal inflammation, epidermal thickening, or hyperproliferation. The mitotic index was significantly lower after 9 mo of TPA treatment relative to controls. In addition, none of the BMP4-overexpressing animals developed papillomas or SCCs. This promoter was also used by the same investigators to study the role of BMP2 and BMP4 in the development of hair and whiskers. BMP2 and BMP4 are closely related proteins that have been shown to elicit quantitatively identical effects, both in cartilage and bone formation and in the specification of posterior mesoderm in Xenopus. BMP2 and BMP4 cDNA coupled to the cytokeratin IV promoter were expressed in squamous and glandular epithelia. In mature hair follicles, BMP-2 transcripts were normally seen only in precortex cells at the base of the hair shaft, while in the BMP4 transgenic mice, the transgene was ectopically expressed in the outer root sheath of hair and whisker follicles. In response to transgene expression, both outer-root sheath cells below the stem-cell compartment and hair matrix cells around the dermal papilla cease to proliferate. The complete absence of DNA synthesis in these compartments results in complete deficiency of hair growth after the first growth cycle in transgenic BMP4 mice, leading to progressive balding. The follicles were grossly aberrant, with size and production rate both greatly reduced. The dermis of these animals is much thinner than normal, and the mice are generally lean and growth-retarded. In addition, the whiskers of transgenic mice are underdeveloped and produce only rudimentary shafts.

In the normal, quiescent mouse epidermis, expression levels of the TGF-β type II receptor are very low, but—like TGF-β1—they are induced in association with TPA-stimulated hyperplasia. In another transgenic animal model using the keratin 10 gene promoter to drive constitutive expression of TGF-β1 in the suprabasal keratinocyte compartment, induction of the receptor correlates with keratinocyte acquisition of sensitivity to the growth-inhibitory effects of recombinant TGF-β1. Thus, keratinocyte growth responsiveness to TGF-β1 in vivo appears to be determined by the levels of expression of TβRII. In contrast, the TGF-β type I receptor levels are not substantially altered by perturbation of epidermal homeostasis. These mice also have an increased epidermal DNA-labeling index, suggesting that, in vivo, quiescent basal keratinocytes are refractile to negative growth regulation by TGF-β1. It appears that ectopic TGF-β1 expression, either directly or indirectly, downregulates the already low levels of TβRII expression, with a resultant further reduction in TGF-β sensitivity, and a corresponding increase in the DNA-labeling index. This phenomenon does not lead to epidermal hyperplasia in transgenic animals. Therefore, there may be an induction of positive growth-regulatory molecules, such as TGF-α, kerotinocyte growth factor, and growth-promoting extracellular matrix components, either in the epidermis or dermis by the forced transgenic expression of TGF-β1. Synthesis of TGF-β1 protein in the epidermis and secretion into the dermal layers is likely responsible for such paracrine effects. This elevated basal level of cell proliferation may be linked to increased keratinocyte turnover in the transgenic epidermis. A role for TGF-β1 in keratinocyte turnover would be supported by the predominant immunolocalization of TβRII to suprabasal cells seen during the differentiative phase following TPA treatment. Thus, in vivo, TGF-β1 may have more complex actions than those revealed from in vitro studies. True to its plieotropic behavior in other systems, TGF-β may act as regulator of both keratinocyte proliferation and turnover, to maintain homeostatic equilibrium within the epidermis.

4.2. Transgenic Expression of TGF-β and Mammary-Gland Carcinogenesis

The distribution of the various TGF-β isoforms in the mammary gland is consistent with their major role in many aspects of the normal biology of this gland, but particularly in the regulation of epithelial-cell proliferation. In mice, there is intense staining for TGF-β1 and TGF-β3 in the extracellular matrix surrounding quiescent ducts, but no staining in ductal end buds or small lateral branches where active proliferation is occurring *(142,143)*. The *Tgf-β* null mouse models have provided limited information regarding the role of the individual isoforms in breast function because of the severe embryonic phenotypes that limit viability of the *Tgf-β2*- and *Tgf-β3*-null mice, and by the autoimmune manifestations and short survival of the TGF-β1-null mouse. Furthermore, although the latter have been able to survive in immunodeficient backgrounds, female TGF-β1-null mice still exhibit difficulty completing a normal gestation. However, in at least one *Tgf-β1⁻/⁻* female that has delivered live-born offspring, we have been able to detect mature, milk-protein-containing glands (unpublished observations). As in the skin, it has been proposed that the TGF-βs would function as anti-promoters in breast epithelium in the setting of carcinogenesis. Thus, transgenic models designed to target expression of the TGF-βs to the mammary gland have been pursued to study their roles in development and tumorigenesis.

Jhappan et al. derived a transgenic mouse model harboring a fusion transgene consisting of the porcine TGF-β1 cDNA inserted into the first exon of the mammary-specific, pregnancy responsive, whey-acidic protein (WAP) gene *(144)*. The authors intended to evaluate the in vivo influence of TGF-β1 on the development of the lactating mammary gland. Transgenic expression over the course of pregnancy was greatly enhanced at later stages and was coincident with an inhibition of alveolar development and lactogenesis, resulting in a failure to lactate. Alveolar structures in mammary tissue from 15–19-d pregnant transgenic mice were relatively sparse and organized in small clusters, but nevertheless were capable of producing WAP and casein protein. While ductal development was generally not impaired, the defect in milk production and a general lactation-deficient phenotype were linked to the significant induction of transgene expression at mid pregnancy. TGF-β1 protein was localized to numerous alveoli and to the periductal extracellular matrix in the mammary gland of transgenic females late in pregnancy. Epithelial cells from cultured transgenic mammary glandular tissue were unable to produce fully differentiated lobular outgrowths. These studies confirm that phenotypic changes in lobulo-alveolar development associated with expression of the WAP-TGF-β1 transgene are intrinsic to the transgenic epithelial-cell population.

Kordon et al. performed reciprocal transplants of mammary tissue between normal and WAP/-TGF-β1 transgenic hosts to examine whether ectopic TGF-β1 affects the transgenic epithelium either directly or indirectly through trans (paracrine) mechanisms *(145)*. Reciprocal transplantation of mammary tissues between normal and transgenic hosts resulted in the development of the respective phenotypes of the transplants within the same mammary fat pad. When isolated mammary epithelial cells from both were mixed before implantation so that transgenic and normal epithelium would develop together in greater proximity, both phenotypes were simultaneously observed in the resultant chimeric mammary outgrowths, and no trans effect was detectable. During pregnancy, early expression of the transgene resulted in compromised development of lobular progenitor cells through an apparent "intracrine" mechanism. Transplantation of the WAP-TGF-β1 mammary gland into a nonpregnant host revealed that transgenic implants, even those from young postpubertal virgin females, had a diminished ability to repopulate epithelium-free mammary fat pads. Therefore, WAP-TGF-β1 not only impairs lobular progenitors, but also promotes an early senescence and reduction in the regenerative capacity of the mammary ductal epithelium.

Pierce et al. derived transgenic mice expressing TGF-β1 under the control of the complete, hormone-inducible, MMTV-long-terminal repeat (LTR) promoter/enhancer *(146)*. This simian MMTV-TGF-β1[act] also encodes a cDNA for active TGF-β1, by mutating those sites that allow interaction with the processed latency-associated peptide (LAP) protein. In this model, a resulting reduction in total ductal-tree volume is observed soon after the estrous cycle begins, and is most apparent at 13 wk, when ductal growth in the normal mammary gland declines. There is formation of alveolar outgrowths from the hypoplastic ductal tree, and one of the most striking features is the virtual absence of lateral branching. This may result from a difference in biological effectiveness of exogenously administered TGF-β1 vs that produced endogenously, with the latter being more effective. It is possible that the expression of the transgene does not specifically affect one population, but causes a general retardation of ductal-tree development so that lateral branching does not occur. Although evidence of lactation was detected, lactating mammary tissue from transgenic animals frequently was more flattened and somewhat atrophic. The MMTV-TGF-β1 transgene caused conditional hypoplasia of the mammary ductal tree, and there was no increase in spontaneous mammary-tumor formation.

In another unique and important model, Pierce et al. examined offspring generated by cross-breeding experiments involving the production of mice carrying both the MMTV-TGF-β1 and TGF-α transgenes *(147)*. Transgenic mice in which a human TGF-α cDNA is expressed under the control of the MMTV enhancer/promoter exhibit overexpression of TGF-α in the mammary epithelium, as confirmed by *in situ* hybridization and immunohistochemistry. This expression is associated with hyperplasia of alveoli and terminal ducts in virgin female and pregnant transgenic mice. Hyperplasia is associated with a range of morphologic abnormalities, including lobular hyperplasia, cystic hyperplasia, adenoma, and adenocarcinoma, all seen in the mammary tissue of transgenic females. TGF-α can therefore act as an oncogene in vivo, and appears to predispose mammary epithelium to neoplasia and carcinoma. In mice expressing both the MMTV-TGF-β1 and TGF-α transgenes, there is marked suppression of mammary-tumor formation, and the MMTV-TGF-β1 transgenic mice are resistant to DMBA-induced mammary-tumor formation, demonstrating that overexpression of TGF-β1 in vivo can markedly suppress mammary-tumor development. However, it should be remembered that TGF-β1 can have bifunctional effects in the process of carcinogenesis. While in normal epithelia TGF-β inhibits proliferation and suppresses the early stages of carcinoma development, once carcinoma cells have progressed to a state in which TGF-β can no longer inhibit proliferation in an autocrine manner, increased expression of TGF-β may then exert predominantly paracrine effects on the host. These include suppression of immune surveillance or alterations in tumor stroma formation and angiogenesis that favor tumor growth and spread.

4.3. Acceleration of Hepatocarcinogenesis by TGF-β1 Transgenes

Several recently established models have demonstrated the pathologic consequences of chronic exposure to TGF-β, either systemic or local, in the kidneys and liver. The evaluation of several fibrotic disorders affecting these organs predicted that TGF-β may be a primary effector of these clinical syndromes. Clouthier et al. generated a transgenic mouse model that led to the overexpression of TGF-β1 in liver, kidney, and white (WAT) and brown (BAT) adipose tissue by using a regulatory sequence of the rat phosphoenol pyruvate carboxykinase gene (PEPCK) *(148)*. The goal of this study was to discern the ability of TGF-β1 to regulate cell proliferation and differentiation in vivo and to evaluate its role in the pathogenesis of fibrosis. Indeed, these mice develop a fibrotic disorder with varying degrees of severity, depending on the level of TGF-β1 expression. The hepatic phenotype includes hemorrhage, thrombosis, hepatocyte apoptosis, and a mild increase in hepatic mass. The importance of TGF-β1 in this phenotype is corroborated by the studies of Sanderson et al. in their transgenic mouse model containing a fusion gene (Alb-TGF-β1) consisting of a modified porcine TGF-β1 cDNA under the control of regulatory elements of the mouse albumin gene *(149)*. The TGF-β1 cDNA in this model contained conversions of cys 223 and cys 225 in the TGF-β propeptide to serine residues, allowing for expression of a fully mature TGF-β1 selectively in hepatocytes and for the direct evaluation of the role of TGF-β1 in hepatic fibrosis. All transgenic lines expressing high levels of the transgene have an increased hepatic mitotic index, apoptosis, and fibrosis, along with elevated TGF-β1 plasma levels (to >10-fold above wild-type control mice).

The Alb-TGF-β1 transgenic model has been used to study the role of TGF-β1 in liver carcinogenesis. As in other organ systems, loss of sensitivity to growth inhibition by TGF-β is believed to contribute to the pathogenesis of malignancy in the liver. Several studies have shown that TGF-β1 expression also increases in the liver during carcinogenesis *(150)*. Factor and colleagues have shown that hepatocellular tumors develop spontaneously in 59% of Alb-TGF-β1 transgenic mice by 16–18 mo of age. They further demonstrated that co-expression of a c-*myc* transgene accelerated hepatic tumor growth in both the presence and absence of carcinogen, and a high rate of malignant conversion in double transgenics with dethylnitrosamine-initiated tumors *(151)*. These mice also exhibit increased sensitivity to the carcinogenic effects of thioacetamide and N-OH-acetylaminofluorene *(152)*. In a manner similar to what has been described for cell lines established from hepatic tumors, DEN-induced tumors of double transgenics had a characteristic reduction or loss of expression of the TGF-β type II receptor.

Each of these models also demonstrates the important endocrine and paracrine effects of TGF-β1, expressed either locally or in distant organs. In the PEPCK-TGF-β1 transgenic mice, kidneys develop fibrosis and glomerular disease, eventually leading to complete loss of renal function. Similar kidney lesions evolve in Alb-TGF-β1 transgenics, primarily involving the glomeruli, but interstitial fibrosis and vacuolation of proximal tubular epithelial cells were also detected *(151,153)*. Vascular lesions were detected in small- to medium-sized arteries in both the kidney and heart, including severe inflammatory reactions involving all layers of the vessel, as seen in polyarteritis nodosa. In the heart, myocarditis, endocarditis, and/or myocardial fibrosis resulted in sudden death in some transgenic lines. The important observation here is that the diffuse glomerulonephritis, hypercellularity, and fibrosis within the kidney and cardiac manifestations each result from expression of the TGF-β1 transgene in the liver, demonstrating that these lesions are caused by paracrine and endocrine effects of the TGF-β1.

Lastly, these models create a valuable tool for investigating the potential of TGF-β antagonists for combating the effects of chronic expression of TGF-β in disease states. In the Alb- TGF-β1 transgenic model, Bottinger et al. have shown that the systemic administration of the LAP of the TGF-β precursor can successfully block the antiproliferative effects of active TGF-β1 during liver regeneration *(154)*. LAP is known to target latent TGF-β1 complexes to cell-surface receptors, such as the mannose-6-phosphate/insulin-like growth-factor receptor, that have been implicated in the activation of latent TGF-β1 in vitro. Thus, LAP could conceivably contribute to enhanced TGF-β activity. In the Bottinger study, LAP inhibits TGF-β activity, suggesting that the in vivo reconstituted latent complex does not direct TGF-β to sites of activation. The results also indicate that LAP is a potent antagonist of the growth inhibitory and gene-inducing activities of exogenous TGF-β, and of paracrine TGF-β in vitro. Similar antagonists of TGF-β may form the basis of important and novel future approaches for the treatment of a large spectrum of chronic conditions with fibrotic and immune-mediated complications linked to the overproduction of TGF-β.

SUMMARY AND CONCLUSIONS

Viewed in a historical perspective, this large body of work focusing on the function and biology of the members of the TGF-β superfamily provides a number of important lessons. The efforts required for the somewhat incredible large-scale column purification required to provide sufficient biological material for early studies now seem indeed remarkable when one considers how new family members are almost routinely identified today. Determining the multiple functions of TGF-β through a large array of in vitro tests of function largely defined this factor as the prototypical pleiotropic cytokine, but also created the challenge of identifying the critical or essential roles of the various isoforms in the course of normal physiological events. In many instances, in vivo tests of function were focused on the effects of exogenous, pharmacologic doses of the cytokine, and were supportive of functions predicted by many in vitro studies. However, this approach has suffered from the limitations that arise with trying to adequately deliver small, biologically active peptides to systemic targets. Moreover, these studies lack the ability to discern the role of a factor in host responses to environmental stimuli, particularly when the activities are broadly known to be context-dependent.

The evolution of more sophisticated in vivo genetic tests of function has proven invaluable in their ability to explore the mechanisms governing the activity of the members of the TGF-β family. The studies outlined in this chapter are not important merely for their ability to support our hypotheses regarding the activities of TGF-β that we have come to appreciate from the preceding decade of studies. More importantly, these models are raising new questions regarding the role of each ligand in processes such as wound healing and the immune response, and identifying previously unappreciated activities. As these approaches continue to evolve and allow us to study cytokine activity in a more cell- and time-dependent manner, we will better understand the biology of this class of secreted signaling molecules, and gain valuable insights for designing approaches for targeting the complex cellular pathways mediating their responses. As we move into the next decade, the goal for this field will necessarily move toward the application of this knowledge to the treatment of disease processes.

REFERENCES

1. Markowitz S, Wang J, Myeroff L, Parsons R, Sun L, Lutterbaugh J, et al. Inactivation of the type II TGF-beta receptor in colon cancer cells with microsatellite instability. *Science* 1995; 268:1336–1338.
2. Markowitz SD, Roberts AB. Tumor suppressor activity of the TGF-beta pathway in human cancers. *Cytokine Growth Factor Rev* 1996; 7:93–102.
3. Bresalier RS. Tumor progression in the intestine: smad about you. *Gastroenterology* 1998; 115:1598–1599.
4. Lange D, Persson U, Wollina U, ten Dijke P, Castelli E, Heldin CH, et al. Expression of TGF-beta related Smad proteins in human epithelial skin tumors. *Int J Oncol* 1999; 14:1049–1056.
5. Le Dai J, Turnacioglu KK, Schutte M, Sugar AY, Kern SE. Dpc4 transcriptional activation and dysfunction in cancer cells. *Cancer Res* 1998; 58:4592–4597.
6. Luo K, Stroschein SL, Wang W, Chen D, Martens E, Zhou S, et al. The Ski oncoprotein interacts with the Smad proteins to repress TGFbeta signaling. *Genes Dev* 9-1-1999; 13:2196–2206.

7. Schutte M. DPC4/SMAD4 gene alterations in human cancer, and their functional implications. *Ann Oncol* 1999; 10(Suppl 4):56–59.

8. de Larco JE, Todaro GJ. Growth factors from murine sarcoma virus-transformed cells. *Proc Natl Acad Sci USA* 1978; 75:4001–4005.

9. Frolik CA, Dart LL, Meyers CA, Smith DM, Sporn MB. Purification and initial characterization of a type beta transforming growth factor from human placenta. *Proc Natl Acad Sci USA* 1983; 80:3676–3680.

10. Roberts AB, Frolik CA, Anzano MA, Assoian RK, Sporn MB. Purification of type beta transforming growth factors from nonneoplastic tissues. In: Methods for preparation of media, supplements, and substrata for serum-free animal cell culture. Alan R. Liss, Publisher. New York, NY. 1984; 181–194.

11. Assoian RK, Komoriya A, Meyers CA, Miller DM, Sporn MB. Transforming growth factor-beta in human platelets. Identification of a major storage site, purification, and characterization. *J Biol Chem* 1983; 258:7155–7160.

12. Roberts AB, Anzano MA, Meyers CA, Wideman J, Blacher R, Pan YC, et al. Purification and properties of a type beta transforming growth factor from bovine kidney. *Biochemistry* 1983; 22:5692–5698.

13. Roberts AB, Lamb LC, Newton DL, Sporn MB, de Larco JE, Todaro GJ. Transforming growth factors: isolation of polypeptides from virally and chemically transformed cells by acid/ethanol extraction. *Proc Natl Acad Sci USA* 1980; 77:3494–3498.

14. Kingsley DM. The TGF-beta superfamily: new members, new receptors, and new genetic tests of function in different organisms *Genes Dev* 1994; 8:133–146.

15. Roberts AB, Sporn MB. The transforming growth factors-β. 1990; 95:419–472.

16. McDonald NQ, Hendrickson WA. A structural superfamily of growth factors containing a cystine knot motif. *Cell* 1993; 73:421–424.

17. Shipley GD, Tucker RF, Moses HL. Type beta transforming growth factor/growth inhibitor stimulates entry of monolayer cultures of AKR-2B cells into S phase after a prolonged prereplicative interval. *Proc Natl Acad Sci USA* 1985; 82:4147–4151.

18. Petraglia F, Sacerdote P, Cossarizza A, Angioni S, Genazzani AD, Franceschi C, et al. Inhibin and activin modulate human monocyte chemotaxis and human lymphocyte interferon-gamma production. *J Clin Endocrinol Metab* 1991; 72:496–502.

19. Cunningham NS, Paralkar V, Reddi AH. Osteogenin and recombinant bone morphogenetic protein 2B are chemotactic for human monocytes and stimulate transforming growth factor beta 1 mRNA expression. *Proc Natl Acad Sci USA* 1992; 89:11,740–11,744.

20. Postlethwaite AE, Seyer JM. Identification of a chemotactic epitope in human transforming growth factor-beta 1 spanning amino acid residues 368–374. *J Cell Physiol* 1995; 164:587–592.

21. Adams DH, Hathaway M, Shaw J, Burnett D, Elias E, Strain AJ. Transforming growth factor-beta induces human T lymphocyte migration in vitro. *J Immunol* 1991; 147:609–612.

22. Ishisaki A, Yamato K, Hashimoto S, Nakao A, Tamaki K, Nonaka K, et al. Differential inhibition of smad6 and smad7 on bone morphogenetic protein- and activin-mediated growth arrest and apoptosis in B cells. *J Biol Chem* 5-7-1999; 274:13,637–13,642.

23. Weller M, Constam DB, Malipiero U, Fontana A. Transforming growth factor-beta 2 induces apoptosis of murine T cell clones without down-regulating bcl-2 mRNA expression. *Eur J Immunol* 1994; 24:1293–1300.

24. Nishihara T, Okahashi N, Ueda N. Activin A induces apoptotic cell death. *Biochem Biophys Res Commun* 1993; 197:985–991.

25. Begue-Kirn C, Smith AJ, Loriot M, Kupferle C, Ruch JV, Lesot H. Comparative analysis of TGF beta s, BMPs, IGF1, msxs, fibronectin, osteonectin and bone sialoprotein gene expression during normal and in vitro-induced odontoblast differentiation. *Int J Dev Biol* 1994; 38:405–420.

26. Begue-Kirn C, Smith AJ, Ruch JV, Wozney JM, Purchio A, Hartmann D, et al. Effects of dentin proteins, transforming growth factor beta 1 (TGF beta 1) and bone morphogenetic protein 2 (BMP2) on the differentiation of odontoblast in vitro. *Int J Dev Biol* 1992; 36:491–503.

27. Yamashita H, Shimizu A, Kato M, Nishitoh H, Ichijo H, Hanyu A, et al. Growth/differentiation factor-5 induces angiogenesis in vivo. *Exp Cell Res* 1997; 235:218–226.

28. Pepper MS, Vassalli JD, Orci L, Montesano R. Biphasic effect of transforming growth factor-beta 1 on in vitro angiogenesis. *Exp Cell Res* 1993; 204:356–363.

29. Thomsen GH. Antagonism within and around the organizer: BMP inhibitors in vertebrate body patterning. *Trends Genet* 1997; 13:209–211.

30. Thomsen GH. Xenopus mothers against decapentaplegic is an embryonic ventralizing agent that acts downstream of the BMP-2/4 receptor. *Development* 1996; 122:2359–2366.
31. Dosch R, Gawantka V, Delius H, Blumenstock C, Niehrs C. Bmp-4 acts as a morphogen in dorsoventral mesoderm patterning in Xenopus. *Development* 1997; 124:2325–2334.
32. Massague J, Chen YG. Controlling TGF-beta signaling. *Genes Dev* 3-15-2000; 14:627–644.
33. Massague J. TGF-beta signal transduction. *Annu Rev Biochem* 1998; 67:753–791.
34. Massague J, Wotton D. Transcriptional control by the TGF-beta/Smad signaling system. *EMBO J* 4-17-2000; 19:1745–1754.
35. Ulloa L, Doody J, Massague J. Inhibition of transforming growth factor-beta/SMAD signalling by the interferon-gamma/STAT pathway. *Nature* 1999; 397:710–713.
36. Bitzer M, von Gersdorff G, Liang D, Dominguez-Rosales A, Beg AA, Rojkind M, et al. E.P.A mechanism of suppression of TGF-beta/SMAD signaling by NF-kappa B/RelA. *Genes Dev* 2000; 14:187–197.
37. Piek E, Heldin CH, ten Dijke P. Specificity, diversity, and regulation in TGF-beta superfamily signaling. *FASEB J* 1999; 13:2105–2124.
38. de Caestecker MP, Piek E, Roberts AB. Role of Transforming Growth Factor-beta Signaling in Cancer. *J Natl Cancer Inst* 2000; 92:1388–1402.
39. Blobe GC, Schiemann WP, Lodish HF. Role of transforming growth factor beta in human disease. *N Engl J Med* 2000; 342:1350–1358.
40. Hahn SA, Schutte M, Hoque AT, Moskaluk CA, da Costa LT, Rozenblum E, et al. DPC4, a candidate tumor suppressor gene at human chromosome 18q21.1. *Science* 1996; 271:350–353.
41. Howe JR, Roth S, Ringold JC, Summers RW, Jarvinen HJ, Sistonen P, et al. Mutations in the SMAD4/DPC4 gene in juvenile polyposis. *Science* 1998; 280:1086–1088.
42. Vogel G. A new blocker for the TGF-beta pathway. *Science* 1999; 286:665.
43. Kurokawa M, Mitani K, Irie K, Matsuyama T, Takahashi T, Chiba S, et al. The oncoprotein Evi-1 represses TGF-beta signalling by inhibiting Smad3. *Nature* 1998; 394:92–96.
44. Kurokawa M, Mitani K, Imai Y, Ogawa S, Yazaki Y, Hirai H. The t(3;21) fusion product, AML1/Evi-1, interacts with Smad3 and blocks transforming growth factor-beta-mediated growth inhibition of myeloid cells. *Blood* 1998; 92:4003–4012.
45. Shipley GD, Pittelkow MR, Wille JJ, Jr, Scott RE, Moses HL. Reversible inhibition of normal human prokeratinocyte proliferation by type beta transforming growth factor-growth inhibitor in serum-free medium. *Cancer Res* 1986; 46:2068–2071.
46. Kimchi A, Wang XF, Weinberg RA, Cheifetz S, Massague J. Absence of TGF-beta receptors and growth inhibitory responses in retinoblastoma cells. *Science* 1988; 240:196–199.
47. Yang HK, Kang SH, Kim YS, Won K, Bang YJ, Kim SJ. Truncation of the TGF-beta type II receptor gene results in insensitivity to TGF-beta in human gastric cancer cells. *Oncogene* 1999; 18:2213–2219.
48. Park K, Kim SJ, Bang YJ, Park JG, Kim NK, Roberts AB, et al. Genetic changes in the transforming growth factor beta (TGF-beta) type II receptor gene in human gastric cancer cells: correlation with sensitivity to growth inhibition by TGF-beta. *Proc Natl Acad Sci USA* 1994; 91:8772–8776.
49. Chen T, Carter D, Garrigue-Antar L, Reiss M. Transforming growth factor beta type I receptor kinase mutant associated with metastatic breast cancer. *Cancer Res* 11-1-1998; 58:4805–4810.
50. Takenoshita S, Tani M, Nagashima M, Hagiwara K, Bennett WP, Yokota J, et al. Mutation analysis of coding sequences of the entire transforming growth factor beta type II receptor gene in sporadic human colon cancer using genomic DNA and intron primers. *Oncogene* 1997; 14:1255–1258.
51. Markowitz S, Wang J, Myeroff L, Parsons R, Sun L, Lutterbaugh J, et al. Inactivation of the type II TGF-beta receptor in colon cancer cells with microsatellite instability. *Science* 1995; 268:1336–1338.
52. Grady WM, Rajput A, Myeroff L, Liu DF, Kwon K, Willis J, et al. Mutation of the type II transforming growth factor-beta receptor is coincident with the transformation of human colon adenomas to malignant carcinomas. *Cancer Res* 1998; 58:3101–3104.
53. Kim SJ, Im YH, Markowitz SD, Bang YJ. Molecular mechanisms of inactivation of TGF-beta receptors during carcinogenesis. *Cytokine Growth Factor Rev* 2000; 11:159–168.
54. Im YH, Kim HT, Lee C, Poulin D, Welford S, Sorensen PH, et al. EWS-FLI1, EWS-ERG, and EWS-ETV1 oncoproteins of Ewing tumor family all suppress transcription of transforming growth factor beta type II receptor gene. *Cancer Res* 2000; 60:1536–1540.

55. Hahm KB, Cho K, Lee C, Im YH, Chang J, Choi SG, et al. Repression of the gene encoding the TGF-beta type II receptor is a major target of the EWS-FLI1 oncoprotein. *Nat Genet* 1999; 23:222–227.

56. DeCoteau JF, Knaus PI, Yankelev H, Reis MD, Lowsky R, Lodish HF, et al. Loss of functional cell surface transforming growth factor beta (TGF-beta) type 1 receptor correlates with insensitivity to TGF-beta in chronic lymphocytic leukemia. *Proc Natl Acad Sci USA* 1997; 94:5877–5881.

57. Capocasale RJ, Lamb RJ, Vonderheid EC, Fox FE, Rook AH, Nowell PC, et al. Reduced surface expression of transforming growth factor beta receptor type II in mitogen-activated T cells from Sezary patients. *Proc Natl Acad Sci USA* 1995; 92:5501–5505.

58. Hojo M, Morimoto T, Maluccio M, Asano T, Morimoto K, Lagman M, et al. Cyclosporine induces cancer progression by a cell-autonomous mechanism. *Nature* 1999; 397:530–534.

59. Welch DR, Fabra A, Nakajima M. Transforming growth factor beta stimulates mammary adenocarcinoma cell invasion and metastatic potential. *Proc Natl Acad Sci USA* 1990; 87:7678–7682.

60. Teicher BA, Maehara Y, Kakeji Y, Ara G, Keyes SR, Wong J, et al. Reversal of in vivo drug resistance by the transforming growth factor-beta inhibitor decorin. *Int J Cancer* 1997; 71:49–58.

61. Teicher BA, Ikebe M, Ara G, Keyes SR, Herbst RS. Transforming growth factor-beta 1 overexpression produces drug resistance in vivo: reversal by decorin. *In Vivo* 1997; 11:463–472.

62. Schwarte-Waldhoff I, Volpert, OV, Bouck NP, Sipos B, Hahn SA, et al. Smad4yDPC4-mediated tumor suppression through suppression of angiogenesis. *Proc Nat Acad Sci USA* 2000; 97(17):9624–9629.

63. Haak-Frendscho M, Wynn TA, Czuprynski CJ, Paulnock D. Transforming growth factor-beta 1 inhibits activation of macrophage cell line RAW 264.7 for cell killing. *Clin Exp Immunol* 1990; 82:404–410.

64. Alleva DG, Burger CJ, Elgert KD. Tumor-induced regulation of suppressor macrophage nitric oxide and TNF-alpha production. Role of tumor-derived IL-10, TGF-beta, and prostaglandin E2. *J Immunol* 1994; 153:1674–1686.

65. Maeda H, Tsuru S, Shiraishi A. Improvement of macrophage dysfunction by administration of anti-transforming growth factor-beta antibody in EL4-bearing hosts. *Jpn J Cancer Res* 1994; 85:1137–1143.

66. Alleva DG, Walker TM, Elgert KD. Induction of macrophage suppressor activity by fibrosarcoma-derived transforming growth factor-beta 1: contrasting effects on resting and activated macrophages. *J Leukoc Biol* 1995; 57:919–928.

67. Hoefer M, Anderer FA. Anti-(transforming growth factor beta) antibodies with predefined specificity inhibit metastasis of highly tumorigenic human xenotransplants in nu/nu mice. *Cancer Immunol Immunother* 1995; 41:302–308.

68. Arteaga CL, Hurd SD, Winnier AR, Johnson MD, Fendly BM, Forbes JT. Anti-transforming growth factor (TGF)-beta antibodies inhibit breast cancer cell tumorigenicity and increase mouse spleen natural killer cell activity. Implications for a possible role of tumor cell/host TGF-beta interactions in human breast cancer progression. *J Clin Investig* 1993; 92:2569–2576.

69. Tada T, Ohzeki S, Utsumi K, Takiuchi H, Muramatsu M, Li XF, et al. Transforming growth factor-beta-induced inhibition of T cell function. Susceptibility difference in T cells of various phenotypes and functions and its relevance to immunosuppression in the tumor-bearing state. *J Immunol* 1991; 146:1077–1082.

70. Berg DJ, Lynch RG. Immune dysfunction in mice with plasmacytomas. I. Evidence that transforming growth factor-beta contributes to the altered expression of activation receptors on host B lymphocytes. *J Immunol* 1991; 146:2865–2872.

71. Weiskirch LM, Bar-Dagan Y, Mokyr MB. Transforming growth factor-beta-mediated down-regulation of antitumor cytotoxicity of spleen cells from MOPC-315 tumor-bearing mice engaged in tumor eradication following low-dose melphalan therapy. *Cancer Immunol Immunother* 1994; 38:215–224.

72. Torre-Amione G, Beauchamp RD, Koeppen H, Park BH, Schreiber H, Moses HL, et al. A highly immunogenic tumor transfected with a murine transforming growth factor type beta 1 cDNA escapes immune surveillance. *Proc Natl Acad Sci USA* 1990; 87:1486–1490.

73. Dorigo O, Shawler DL, Royston I, Sobol RE, Berek JS, Fakhrai H. Combination of transforming growth factor beta antisense and interleukin-2 gene therapy in the murine ovarian teratoma model. *Gynecol Oncol* 1998; 71:204–210.

74. Liau LM, Fakhrai H, Black KL. Prolonged survival of rats with intracranial C6 gliomas by treatment with TGF-beta antisense gene. *Neurol Res* 1998; 20:742–747.

75. Matthews E, Yang T, Janulis L, Goodwin S, Kundu SD, Karpus WJ, et al. Down-regulation of TGF-beta1 production restores immunogenicity in prostate cancer cells. *Br J Cancer* 2000; 83:519–525.
76. Erickson HP. Gene knockouts of c-src, transforming growth factor beta 1, and tenascin suggest superfluous, nonfunctional expression of proteins. *J Cell Biol* 1993; 120:1079–1081.
77. Doetschman T. Interpretation of phenotype in genetically engineered mice. *Lab Anim Sci* 1999; 49:137–143.
78. Letterio JJ, Geiser AG, Kulkarni AB, Roche NS, Sporn MB, Roberts AB. Maternal rescue of transforming growth factor-beta 1 null mice. *Science* 1994; 264:1936–1938.
79. Tang B, Bottinger EP, Jakowlew SB, Bagnall KM, Mariano J, Anver MR, et al. Transforming growth factor-beta1 is a new form of tumor suppressor with true haploid insufficiency. *Nat Med* 1998; 4:802–807.
80. Engle SJ, Hoying JB, Boivin GP, Ormsby I, Gartside PS, Doetschman T. Transforming growth factor beta1 suppresses nonmetastatic colon cancer at an early stage of tumorigenesis. *Cancer Res* 7–15–1999; 59:3379–3386.
81. Takaku K, Miyoshi H, Matsunaga A, Oshima M, Sasaki N, Taketo MM. Gastric and duodenal polyps in Smad4 (Dpc4) knockout mice. *Cancer Res* 1999; 59:6113–6117.
82. Zhu Y, Richardson JA, Parada LF, Graff JM. Smad3 mutant mice develop metastatic colorectal cancer. *Cell* 1998; 94:703–714.
83. Takaku K, Oshima M, Miyoshi H, Matsui M, Seldin MF, Taketo MM. Intestinal tumorigenesis in compound mutant mice of both Dpc4 (Smad4) and Apc genes. *Cell* 1998; 92:645–656.
84. Taketo MM, Takaku K. Gastro-intestinal tumorigenesis in Smad4 mutant mice. *Cytokine Growth Factor Rev* 2000; 11:147–157.
85. Glick A, Popescu N, Alexander V, Ueno H, Bottinger E, Yuspa SH. Defects in transforming growth factor-beta signaling cooperate with a ras oncogene to cause rapid aneuploidy and malignant transformation of mouse. *Proc Natl Acad Sci USA* 1999; 96:14,949–14,954.
86. Tremain R, Marko M, Kinnimulki V, Ueno H, Bottinger E, Glick A. Defects in TGF-beta signaling overcome senescence of mouse keratinocytes expressing v-Ha-ras. *Oncogene* 3-23-2000; 19:1698–1709.
87. Shida N, Ikeda H, Yoshimoto T, Oshima M, Taketo MM, Miyoshi I. Estrogen-induced tumorigenesis in the pituitary gland of TGF-beta(+/–) knockout mice. *Biochim Biophys Acta* 1998; 1407:79–83.
88. Shibata MA, Liu ML, Knudson MC, Shibata E, Yoshidome K, Bandey T, et al. Haploid loss of bax leads to accelerated mammary tumor development in C3(1)/SV40-TAg transgenic mice: reduction in protective apoptotic response at the preneoplastic stage. *EMBO J* 1999; 18:2692–2701.
89. Fero ML, Randel E, Gurley KE, Roberts JM, Kemp CJ. The murine gene p27Kip1 is haplo-insufficient for tumour suppression. *Nature* 1998; 396:177–180.
90. Sanford LP, Ormsby I, Gittenberger-de Groot AC, Sariola H, Friedman R, Boivin GP, et al. TGFbeta2 knockout mice have multiple developmental defects that are non-overlapping with other TGFbeta knockout phenotypes. *Development* 1997; 124:2659–2670.
91. Kaartinen V, Voncken JW, Shuler C, Warburton D, Bu D, Heisterkamp N, et al. Abnormal lung development and cleft palate in mice lacking TGF-beta 3 indicates defects of epithelial-mesenchymal interaction. *Nat Genet* 1995; 11:415–421.
92. Proetzel G, Pawlowski SA, Wiles MV, Yin M, Boivin GP, Howles PN, et al. Transforming growth factor-beta 3 is required for secondary palate fusion. *Nat Genet* 1995; 11:409–414.
93. Li J, Foitzik K, Calautti E, Baden H, Doetschman T, Dotto GP. TGF-beta3, but not TGF-beta1, protects keratinocytes against 12-O-tetradecanoylphorbol-13-acetate-induced cell death in vitro and in vivo. *J Biol Chem* 1999; 274:4213–4219.
94. Glick AB, Kulkarni AB, Tennenbaum T, Hennings H, Flanders KC, O'Reilly M. Loss of expression of transforming growth factor beta in skin and skin tumors is associated with hyperproliferation and a high risk for malignant conversion. *Proc Natl Acad Sci USA* 1993; 90:6076–6080.
95. Glick AB, Lee MM, Darwiche N, Kulkarni AB, Karlsson S, Yuspa SH. Targeted deletion of the TGF-beta 1 gene causes rapid progression to squamous cell carcinoma. *Genes Dev* 1994; 8:2429–2440.
96. Wang XJ, Greenhalgh DA, Bickenbach JR, Jiang A, Bundman DS, Krieg T, et al. Expression of a dominant-negative type II transforming growth factor beta (TGF-beta) receptor in the epidermis of transgenic mice blocks TGF-beta-mediated growth inhibition. *Proc Natl Acad Sci USA* 1997; 94:2386–2391.

97. Go C, Li P, Wang XJ. Blocking transforming growth factor beta signaling in transgenic epidermis accelerates chemical carcinogenesis: a mechanism associated with increased angiogenesis. *Cancer Res* 1999; 59:2861–2868.

98. Amendt C, Schirmacher P, Weber H, Blessing M. Expression of a dominant negative type II TGF-beta receptor in mouse skin results in an increase in carcinoma incidence and an acceleration of carcinoma development. *Oncogene* 1998; 17:25–34.

99. Gorska AE, Joseph H, Derynck R, Moses HL, Serra R. Dominant-negative interference of the transforming growth factor beta type II receptor in mammary gland epithelium results in alveolar hyperplasia and differentiation in virgin mice. *Cell Growth Differ* 1998; 9:229–238.

100. Bottinger EP, Jakubczak JL, Haines DC, Bagnall K, Wakefield LM. Transgenic mice overexpressing a dominant-negative mutant type II transforming growth factor beta receptor show enhanced tumorigenesis in the mammary gland and lung in response to the carcinogen 7,12-dimethylbenz-[a]-anthracene. *Cancer Res* 1997; 57:5564–5570.

101. Joseph H, Gorska AE, Sohn P, Moses HL, Serra R. Overexpression of a kinase-deficient transforming growth factor-beta type II receptor in mouse mammary stroma results in increased epithelial branching. *Mol Biol Cell* 1999; 10:1221–1234.

102. Kundu SD, Kim IY, Yang T, Doglio L, Lang S, Zhang X, et al. Absence of proximal duct apoptosis in the ventral prostate of transgenic mice carrying the C3(1)-TGF-beta type II dominant negative receptor. *Prostate* 2000; 43:118–124.

103. Serra R, Johnson M, Filvaroff EH, LaBorde J, Sheehan DM, Derynck R, et al. Expression of a truncated, kinase-defective TGF-beta type II receptor in mouse skeletal tissue promotes terminal chondrocyte differentiation and osteoarthritis. *J Cell Biol* 1997; 139:541–552.

104. Filvaroff E, Erlebacher A, Ye J, Gitelman SE, Lotz J, Heillman M, et al. Inhibition of TGF-beta receptor signaling in osteoblasts leads to decreased bone remodeling and increased trabecular bone mass. *Development* 1999; 126:4267–4279.

105. Bottinger EP, Jakubczak JL, Roberts IS, Mumy M, Hemmati P, Bagnall K, et al. Expression of a dominant-negative mutant TGF-beta type II receptor in transgenic mice reveals essential roles for TGF-beta in regulation of growth and differentiation in the exocrine pancreas. *EMBO J* 1997; 16:2621–2633.

106. Hahm KB, Im YH, Lee C, Parks WT, Bang YJ, Green JE, et al. Loss of TGF-beta signaling contributes to autoimmune pancreatitis. *J Clin Investig* 2000; 105:1057–1065.

107. Lucas PJ, Kim SJ, Melby SJ, Gress RE. Disruption of T cell homeostasis in mice expressing a T cell-specific dominant negative transforming growth factor beta II receptor. *J Exp Med* 2000; 191:1187–1196.

108. Gorelik I, Flavell RA. Abrogation of TGFbeta signaling in T cells leads to spontaneous T cell differentiation and autoimmune disease. *Immunity* 2000; 12:171–181.

109. Qi Z, Atsuchi N, Ooshima A, Takeshita A, Ueno H. Blockade of type beta transforming growth factor signaling prevents liver fibrosis and dysfunction in the rat. *Proc Natl Acad Sci USA* 1999; 96:2345–2349.

110. Ueno H, Sakamoto T, Nakamura T, Qi Z, Astuchi N, Takeshita A, et al. A soluble transforming growth factor beta receptor expressed in muscle prevents liver fibrogenesis and dysfunction in rats. *Hum Gene Ther* 2000; 11:33–42.

111. Le Y, Sauer B. Conditional gene knockout using cre recombinase. *Methods Mol Biol* 2000; 136:477–485.

112. Sauer B. Inducible gene targeting in mice using the Cre/lox system. *Methods* 1998; 14:381–392.

113. Rickert RC, Rajewsky K, Roes J. Impairment of T-cell-dependent B-cell responses and B-1 cell development in CD19-deficient mice. *Nature* 1995; 376:352–355.

114. Cazac BB, Roes J. TGF-beta receptor controls B cell responsiveness and induction of IgA in vivo. *Immunity* 2000; 13:443–451.

115. Smeland EB, Blomhoff HK, Holte H, Ruud E, Beiske K, Funderud S, et al. Transforming growth factor type beta (TGF beta) inhibits G1 to S transition, but not activation of human B lymphocytes. *Exp Cell Res* 1987; 171:213–222.

116. Lomo J, Blomhoff HK, Beiske K, Stokke T, Smeland EB. TGF-beta 1 and cyclic AMP promote apoptosis in resting human B lymphocytes. *J Immunol* 1995; 154:1634–1643.

117. Amoroso SR, Huang N, Roberts AB, Potter M, Letterio JJ. Consistent loss of functional transforming growth factor beta receptor expression in murine plasmacytomas. *Proc Natl Acad Sci USA* 1998; 95:189–194.

118. Lotz M, Ranheim E, Kipps TJ. Transforming growth factor beta as endogenous growth inhibitor of chronic lymphocytic leukemia B cells. *J Exp Med* 1994; 179:999–1004.

119. Kumar A, Rogers T, Maizel A, Sharma S. Loss of transforming growth factor beta 1 receptors and its effects on the growth of EBV-transformed human B cells. *J Immunol* 1991; 147:998–1006.

120. Fernandez TM, Amoroso SR, Potter M, Letterio J. Acquired TGF-beta receptor trafficking defect in murine plasmacytomagenesis. *Proc Am Assoc Canc Res* 2000; 41:358–359.

121. Weinstein M, Yang X, Deng C. Functions of mammalian Smad genes as revealed by targeted gene disruption in mice. *Cytokine Growth Factor Rev* 2000; 11:49–58.

122. Chang H, Huylebroeck D, Verschueren K, Guo Q, Matzuk MM, Zwijsen A. Smad5 knockout mice die at mid-gestation due to multiple embryonic and extraembryonic defects. *Development* 1999; 126:1631–1642.

123. Chang H, Zwijsen A, Vogel H, Huylebroeck D, Matzuk MM. Smad5 is essential for left-right asymmetry in mice. *Dev Biol* 2000; 219:71–78.

124. Weinstein M, Yang X, Li C, Xu X, Gotay J, Deng CX. Failure of egg cylinder elongation and mesoderm induction in mouse embryos lacking the tumor suppressor smad2. *Proc Natl Acad Sci USA* 1998; 95:9378–9383.

125. Yang X, Castilla LH, Xu X, Li C, Gotay J, Weinstein M, et al. Angiogenesis defects and mesenchymal apoptosis in mice lacking SMAD5. *Development* 1999; 126:1571–1580.

126. Yang X, Li C, Xu X, Deng C. The tumor suppressor SMAD4/DPC4 is essential for epiblast proliferation and mesoderm induction in mice. *Proc Natl Acad Sci USA* 1998; 95:3667–3672.

127. Yang X, Letterio JJ, Lechleider RJ, Chen L, Hayman R, Gu H, et al. Targeted disruption of SMAD3 results in impaired mucosal immunity and diminished T cell responsiveness to TGF-beta. *EMBO J* 1999; 18:1280–1291.

128. Datto MB, Frederick JP, Pan L, Borton AJ, Zhuang Y, Wang XF. Targeted disruption of smad3 reveals an essential role in transforming growth factor beta-mediated signal transduction. *Mol Cell Biol* 1999; 19:2495–2504.

129. Zhu Y, Richardson JA, Parada LF, Graff JM. Smad3 mutant mice develop metastatic colorectal cancer. *Cell* 1998; 94:703–714.

130. Datto M, Wang X. The Smads: transcriptional regulation and mouse models. *Cytokine Growth Factor Rev* 2000; 11:37–48.

131. Xu X, Brodie SG, Yang X, Im YH, Parks WT, Chen L, et al. Haploid loss of the tumor suppressor Smad4/Dpc4 initiates gastric polyposis and cancer in mice. *Oncogene* 2000; 19:1868–1874.

132. Oshima H, Oshima M, Kobayashi M, Tsutsumi M, Taketo MM. Morphological and molecular processes of polyp formation in Apc(delta716) knockout mice. *Cancer Res* 1997; 57:1644–1649.

133. Sellheyer K, Bickenbach JR, Rothnagel JA, Bundman D, Longley MA, Krieg T. Inhibition of skin development by overexpression of transforming growth factor beta 1 in the epidermis of transgenic mice. *Proc Natl Acad Sci USA* 1993; 90:5237–5241.

134. Glick AB, Weinberg WC, Wu IH, Quan W, Yuspa SH. Transforming growth factor beta 1 suppresses genomic instability independent of a G1 arrest, p53, and Rb. *Cancer Res* 1996; 56:3645–3650.

135. Fowlis DJ, Flanders KC, Duffie E, Balmain A, Akhurst RJ. Discordant transforming growth factor beta 1 RNA and protein localization during chemical carcinogenesis of the skin. *Cell Growth Differ* 1992; 3:81–91.

136. Stamp GW, Nasim M, Cardillo M, Sudhindra SG, Lalani EN, Pignatelli M. Transforming growth factor-beta distribution in basal cell carcinomas: relationship to proliferation index. *Br J Dermatol* 1993; 129:57–64.

137. Furstenberger G, Rogers M, Schnapke R, Bauer G, Hofler P, Marks F. Stimulatory role of transforming growth factors in multistage skin carcinogenesis: possible explanation for the tumor-inducing effect of wounding in initiated NMRI mouse skin. *Int J Cancer* 1989; 43:915–921.

138. Cui W, Fowlis DJ, Bryson S, Duffie E, Ireland H, Balmain A, et al. TGFbeta1 inhibits the formation of benign skin tumors, but enhances progression to invasive spindle carcinomas in transgenic mice. *Cell* 1996; 86:531–542.

139. Fowlis DJ, Cui W, Johnson SA, Balmain A, Akhurst RJ. Altered epidermal cell growth control in vivo by inducible expression of transforming growth factor beta 1 in the skin of transgenic mice. *Cell Growth Differ* 1996; 7:679–687.

140. Blessing M, Nanney LB, King LE, Hogan BL. Chemical skin carcinogenesis is prevented in mice by the induced expression of a TGF-beta related transgene. *Teratog Carcinog Mutagen* 1995; 15:11–21.

141. Blessing M, Nanney LB, King LE, Jones CM, Hogan BL. Transgenic mice as a model to study the role of TGF-beta-related molecules in hair follicles. *Genes Dev* 1993; 7:204–215.

142. Robinson SD, Silberstein GB, Roberts AB, Flanders KC, Daniel CW. Regulated expression and growth inhibitory effects of transforming growth factor-beta isoforms in mouse mammary gland development. *Development* 1991; 113:867–878.

143. Silberstein GB, Flanders KC, Roberts AB, Daniel CW. Regulation of mammary morphogenesis: evidence for extracellular matrix-mediated inhibition of ductal budding by transforming growth factor-beta 1. *Dev Biol* 1992; 152:354–362.

144. Jhappan C, Geiser AG, Kordon EC, Bagheri D, Hennighausen L, Roberts AB, et al. Targeting expression of a transforming growth factor beta 1 transgene to the pregnant mammary gland inhibits alveolar development and lactation. *EMBO J* 1993; 12:1835–1845.

145. Kordon EC, McKnight RA, Jhappan C, Hennighausen L, Merlino G, Smith GH. Ectopic TGF beta 1 expression in the secretory mammary epithelium induces early senescence of the epithelial stem cell population. *Dev Biol* 1995; 168:47–61.

146. Pierce DF, Jr, Johnson MD, Matsui Y, Robinson SD, Gold LI, Purchio AF, et al. Inhibition of mammary duct development but not alveolar outgrowth during pregnancy in transgenic mice expressing active TGF-beta 1. *Genes Dev* 1993; 7:2308–2317.

147. Pierce DF, Jr, Gorska AE, Chytil A, Meise KS, Page DL, Coffey RJ, Jr, et al. Mammary tumor suppression by transforming growth factor beta 1 transgene expression. *Proc Natl Acad Sci USA* 1995; 92:4254–4258.

148. Clouthier DE, Comerford SA, Hammer RE. Hepatic fibrosis, glomerulosclerosis, and a lipodystrophy-like syndrome in PEPCK-TGF-beta1 transgenic mice. *J Clin Investig* 1997; 100:2697–2713.

149. Sanderson N, Factor V, Nagy P, Kopp J, Kondaiah P, Wakefield L, et al. Hepatic expression of mature transforming growth factor beta 1 in transgenic mice results in multiple tissue lesions. *Proc Natl Acad Sci USA* 1995; 92:2572–2576.

150. Braun L, Gruppuso P, Mikumo R, Fausto N. Transforming growth factor beta 1 in liver carcinogenesis: messenger RNA expression and growth effects. *Cell Growth Differ* 1990; 1:103–111.

151. Factor VM, Kao CY, Santoni-Rugiu E, Woitach JT, Jensen MR, Thorgeirsson SS. Constitutive expression of mature transforming growth factor beta1 in the liver accelerates hepatocarcinogenesis in transgenic mice. *Cancer Res* 1997; 57:2089–2095.

152. Schnur J, Nagy P, Sebestyen A, Schaff Z, Thorgeirsson SS. Chemical hepatocarcinogenesis in transgenic mice overexpressing mature TGF beta-1 in liver. *Eur J Cancer* 1999; 35:1842–1845.

153. Kopp JB, Factor VM, Mozes M, Nagy P, Sanderson N, Bottinger EP, et al. Transgenic mice with increased plasma levels of TGF-beta 1 develop progressive renal disease. *Lab Investig* 1996; 74:991–1003.

154. Bottinger EP, Factor VM, Tsang ML, Weatherbee JA, Kopp JB, Qian SW, et al. The recombinant proregion of transforming growth factor beta1 (latency-associated peptide) inhibits active transforming growth factor beta1 in transgenic mice. *Proc Natl Acad Sci USA* 1996; 93:5877–5882.

12 Cyclin D1 Transgenic Mouse Models

Oliver G. Opitz, MD,
Hiroshi Nakagawa, MD, PhD,
and Anil K. Rustgi, MD

CONTENTS

1. CYCLIN D1 AND THE CELL CYCLE

G1 cyclins influence whether initiation of a new cell cycle occurs. Expression of these cyclins is cell-cycle-phase dependent and regulated transcriptionally, post-transcriptionally and post-translationally *(1–4)*. In addition, distinct human cyclin-dependent kinases—cdks—have been identified that associate with cyclins and share extensive amino-acid sequence identity with p34cdc2 (cdk). Thus, each cyclin is believed to regulate the cell cycle at its designated time-point by binding to and activating the cdks *(1–4)*.

Human cyclin D1, also called PRAD1 and mapped to chromosome 11q13, was first isolated in human parathyroid adenomas as a gene rearranged by translocation to the parathyroid hormone locus at 11p15 *(5)*. Subsequently, cyclin D1 has been found to be overexpressed in a variety of human tumors, including breast carcinomas, B-cell lymphomas, and squamous-cell carcinomas (SCC) derived from the oral cavity, larynx, and esophagus *(4)*. Two other human D-type cyclin genes, cyclins D2 and D3, have been cloned. All three human D-type cyclin genes encode small (33–34-kDa) proteins that share an average of 57% identity over the entire coding region, and 78% in the cyclin box

From: *Tumor Models in Cancer Research*
Edited by: B. A. Teicher © Humana Press Inc., Totowa, NJ

(region of cyclins that interacts with cdks). Cyclin D2 has been mapped to chromosome 12p13, and cyclin D3 to chromosome 6p21. The RNA transcripts corresponding to the cyclin D1 gene are 4.8 Kb and 1.7 Kb; 7.4 Kb for cyclin D2; and 2.2 Kb for cyclin D3.

There is compelling evidence for a role of cyclin D1 in G1 phase progression in the cell cycle. Microinjection of cyclin D1 antibodies or an antisense cyclin D1 plasmid blocks cells from entering the S phase *(6)*. Overexpression of cyclin D1 shortens the G1 phase in the cell cycle *(7,8)*. Cyclin D1 also rescues G1 cyclin-defective *Saccharomyces cerevisiae*. In mid-G1 phase, cyclin D1 is associated with one of several cdks, especially cdk4 or cdk6. This is part of a larger complex including proliferating-cell nuclear antigen (PCNA), a 36-kDa protein involved in DNA replication and repair, and also *p21*, a 21-kDa protein variably called Cip1 or WAF1, which negatively regulates the synthesis of the cdks, and *p16 (9,10)*. p21 or WAF1/Cip1 is known to be transcriptionally activated by wild-type *p53,* but not by mutant *p53 (11)*. p16 is a tumor-suppressor gene on chromosome 9p21–22, and encodes a protein called *p16,* which is an inhibitor of cdk4. Notably, *p19* is generated by an alternative reading frame of the INK4a tumor-suppressor-gene locus *(7)*. Investigations indicate that the retinoblastoma (Rb) tumor-suppressor gene product, pRB, a negative regulator of cell progression from late G1 phase to S phase, interacts with cyclin D1 in vitro and in vivo *(12,13)*. Cyclin D1, in association with cdk4 or cdk6, increases phosphorylation of pRb and pRb-related proteins *(p107, p130)* and contributes to progression through G1 phase. In contrast, it is the hypophosphorylated form of pRB that negatively regulates cell growth by binding cellular proteins, e.g., E2F *(14,15)*.

By the same token, the effects of cyclin D1 may also be independent of cdk. For example, ectopic expression of cyclin D1 can stimulate the transcriptional activity of the estrogen receptor (EB) in the absence of estradiol, and this activity can be inhibited by 4-hydroxytamoxifen and ICI 182,780 *(16)*. Cyclin D1 can form a specific complex with the ER. Stimulation of the ER by cyclin D1 is independent of cyclin-dependent kinase 4 activation.

2. CYCLIN D1 TRANSGENIC MOUSE MODELS

A number of studies have shown that cyclin D1 is frequently overexpressed through gene amplification in *SCCs* and breast cancers, and translocated in mantle-cell lymphomas. The association of cyclin D1 with cancer has led to the investigation of its oncogenic properties in vitro and in vivo. Cyclin D1 can cooperate with either the *ras* oncogene to transform cultured cells or complement a defective adenovirus *E1a* oncogene to contribute to cell transformation *(17)*.

In order to investigate the functional consequences of cyclin D1 in vivo, both physiologically and by overexpression, a number of cyclin D1 transgenic mouse models as well as models in which cyclin D1 has been disrupted in mouse embryonic stem (ES) cells through homologous recombination have been generated. These have provided insights into the biology of cyclin D1 in different cell lineages, but it is also clear that the functions of cyclin D1 may vary in a cell-type-specific fashion.

3. CYCLIN D1 AND LYMPHOID TISSUES

Chromosomal translocation t (11:14) involving cyclin D1 is associated with human lymphoma that affect centrocytic B cells. As a result, the cyclin D1 gene is juxtaposed to the immunoglobulin heavy-chain enhancer E *mu*. The notion that cyclin D1 is activated in this context is supported by observations in transgenic mice that carry cyclin D1 under the transcriptional control of the E *mu* element. E *mu* cyclin D1 transgenic mice display cell-cycle abnormalities in their B lymphocytes in contrast to their wild-type mice litter mates, and also without any lymphoma *(18)*. However, when E *mu* transcriptionally activates cyclin D1 with either N-*myc* or L-*myc* in double transgenic mice, the onset of clonal pre-B and B-cell lymphomas occurs. This study was independently noted as well by Bodrug et al. *(19)*. The immunoglobulin enhancer, when linked to cyclin D1, resulted in transgenic mice with normal cell-cycle kinetics in their lymphocytes and normal response to mitogens. However, there was a diminution in mature B cells and T cells. The development of lymphoma was very rapid in transgenic mice that co-expressed both cyclin D1 and *myc*. It should also be noted that targeting of myc alone to the B cells of transgenic mice results in enhanced expression of endogenous cyclin D1. Taken together, these studies support the notion that cyclin D1 and *myc* cooperate in the development and progression of lymphoma.

4. CYCLIN D1 AND BREAST CARCINOGENESIS

A number of studies have established the association of cyclin D1 and breast carcinogenesis. This was addressed by overexpression of cyclin D1 in the mammary tissues of transgenic mice. This resulted in abnormal cell proliferation, accompanied by mammary hyperplasia and carcinomas and a critical demonstration of the important role of cyclin D1 as an oncogene in vivo *(20)*. It is conceivable that cyclin D1 may act as an oncogene in breast cancer through physical interaction with the ER and also activation of the receptor's transcription, as this receptor is an important regulator of growth and differentiation of breast epithelium. It is also known that the ER has a leucine-rich motif, which constitutes a ligand-regulated binding site for steroid-receptor co-activators (SRCs). It has been demonstrated that cyclin D1 also interacts in a ligand-independent fashion with co-activators of the SRC-1 family through a motif that resembles the leucine-rich coactivator-binding motif of nuclear receptors *(21)*. By acting as a bridging factor between the ER and SRCs, cyclin D1 can recruit SRC-family co-activators to ER in the absence of ligand. These data indicate that cyclin D1 contributes significantly to ER activation in breast cancers in which the protein is overexpressed through two different mechanisms: direct interaction and co-activator recruitment to ER.

5. CYCLIN D1 AND ONCOGENESIS IN SQUAMOUS EPITHELIAL TISSUES

The squamous epithelium represents a model system in which to study key cellular processes such as proliferation, differentiation, senescence, and apoptosis. The stratified squamous epithelium is present in the skin, oral cavity, pharynx, esophagus, bronchus, and anogenital tract. Here, proliferating basal cells migrate toward the luminal surface, undergoing am exquisite program of differentiation accompanied by morphological, biochemical, and genetic changes. Eventually, cells desquamate, and the process is renewed.

To investigate the role of cyclin D1 in the squamous epithelium of the skin, the keratin 5 promoter, which is active in basal cells, was used to target cyclin D1 in transgenic mice *(22)*. Squamous epithelia of the skin, oral mucosa, trachea, and the vagina expressed abnormal levels of cyclin D1, with evidence of basal-cell hyperplasia and epithelial hyperproliferation. Interestingly, differentiation was not impaired, as newborn mouse primary keratinocytes were induced to growth arrest by the addition of high extracellular calcium. Additionally, transgenic mice developed a severe thymic hyperplasia with increased thymic weight that caused premature death. The hyperplastic thymi had normal T cells and normal thymus cortex and medulla. It was suggested that proliferation and differentiation are not coordinately regulated, at least by cyclin D1. Notably, epithelial and thymic tumors were not found in the transgenic mice.

Our own group has sought to understand the role of cyclin D1 in oral and esophageal SCC. Although no oral-esophageal specific promoter had been reported, we were able to demonstrate that the Epstein-Barr virus (EBV) ED-L2 promoter, which regulates two short eopen reading frames located 5′ to the late membrane protein-1 (LMP-1) gene, was specifically active in human oral and esophageal cell lines, but inactive in cell lines of other origin, through the interplay of relatively tissue-specific transcription factors *(23–26)*. This led us to utilize the EBV ED-L2 promoter in a construct to target human cyclin D1 in transgenic mice *(27)*. Expression studies indicated the unique expression of the cyclin D1 transgene product in oral, esophageal, and forestomach epithelia (the forestomach is squamous and nonglandular). The resulting phenotype was one of mild dysplasia by 6–8 mo, with progression to moderate-severe dysplasia by 16–18 mo, yet, without evidence of cancer. Secondary alterations included increased cell proliferation, enhanced epidermal growth-factor-receptor expression, increased cdk4 expression, and occasional increased *p53* expression, the latter suggestive of *p53* mutation *(28)*. It is conceivable that the cdk4 overexpression parallels cyclin D1 overexpression. In order to develop a model of oral-esophageal cancer, we initially treated EBV ED-L2 cyclin D1 transgenic mice with N-nitrosomethylbenzylamine (NMBA) which led to the temporal acceleration of dysplasia and abnormal cell proliferation *(29)*. Because *p53* mutation is frequent in oral and esophageal cancers, we have subsequently crossbred the cyclin D1 mice with *p53* knockout mice. The resulting compound mice have histologic evidence of oral and esophageal cancer (Opitz, Suliman and Rustgi, unpublished observations). This suggests that the combination of cyclin D1 overexpression and *p53* inactivation is sufficient to induce cancer in the oral cavity and esophagus.

Our findings, and those of others, suggest that apart from breast epithelium, cyclin D1 requires cofactors to cause malignant transformation. The topical application of 12-O-tetradecanoyl-phorbol 13-acetate (TPA) is a well-accepted approach to induce synchronized proliferation in the skin. The combination of TPA and cyclin D1 overexpression in the skin in the keratin 5-cyclin D1 transgenic mice leads to increased proliferation in the epidermis *(30)*. In contrast to wild-type mice, the labeling index remained high in transgenic mice. In addition, cyclin D1/cyclin-dependent kinase (cdk) complex formation increased in the transgenic mice, and was correlated with elevated cdk4 and cdk6 kinase activities. However, the increased cdk activities were not sufficient to effect mouse skin-tumor development *(30)*.

6. CYCLIN D1 AND THE HEART

Transgenic mice that overexpress cyclin D1 in the heart were produced to determine if D-type cyclin deregulation would alter myocardial development. Cyclin D1 overexpression resulted in a concomitant increase in cdk4 levels in the adult myocardium, as well as modest increases in proliferating-cell nuclear antigen (PCNA) and cdk2 levels *(31)*. Flow cytometric and morphologic analyses of dispersed cell preparations indicated that the adult transgenic cardiomyocytes had abnormal patterns of multinucleation. Histochemical analyses confirmed a marked increase in number of cardiomyocyte nuclei in sections prepared from the transgenic mice, as compared with those from control animals. Tritiated thymidine incorporation analyses revealed sustained cardiomyocyte DNA synthesis in adult transgenic hearts.

7. COOPERATION WITH OTHER ONCOGENES

Cooperation of cyclin D1 with c-*myc* has been established in lymphocytes and for cyclin D1 and mutant *p53,* as noted previously. This cooperation also extends to cyclin D1 and the *ras* oncogene in the skin. Several lines of evidence have shown that the cell-cycle machinery—specifically cyclin D1/cdk 4 and 6p16pRb—lies downstream of *ras.* In particular, *ras* mutations have been well-characterized in the mouse skin two-stage carcinogenesis model, and a large body of literature has indicated that initiation with the genotoxic carcinogen 7,12-dimethylbenz[a]anthracene (DMBA) induces a specific point mutation in Ha-*ras* gene in this model. It has been demonstrated that cyclin D1 is a critical target of oncogenic *ras* in mouse-skin carcinogenesis *(32)*. The cooperation of cyclin D1 and *ras* is further underscored by studies in cyclin D1-mutant mice, where evidence is provided that *ras*-mediated tumorigenesis depends on signaling pathways that act preferentially through cyclin D1 *(33)*. Cyclin D1 expression and the activity of its associated kinase are upregulated in keratinocytes in response to oncogenic *ras.* Furthermore, cyclin D1 deficiency results in a significant decrease in frequency of squamous tumors generated through grafting of retroviral *ras*-transduced keratinocytes, phorbol ester treatment of *ras* transgenic mice, or two-stage carcinogenesis models *(33)*.

CDC37 is a gene that encodes a 50-kDa protein that targets unstable kinases, such as cdk4, Raf-1, and v-src to the molecular chaperone Hsp90, which is believed to be essential for some signaling pathways. CDC37 is co-expressed with cyclin D1 in proliferative zones during mouse development. CDC37 may be critical for cell proliferation during development, but also in oncogene-induced abnormal cell proliferation. It has been reported that mouse mammary-tumor virus (MMTV)-CDC37 transgenic mice develop mammary-gland tumors in a manner similar to that observed in MMTV-cyclin D1 mice *(34)*. Moreover, CDC37 was noted to cooperate with cyclin D1 to transform the mammary gland. These data are consistent with the notion that CDC37 can function as an oncogene in mice, and the signal pathways are initiated with subsequent upregulation of cyclin D1.

8. CYCLIN D1 MUTANT MICE

Mice lacking cyclin D1 have been generated by gene targeting in ES cells. Sicinski et al. *(35)* showed that cyclin D1-deficient mice develop to term, but have diminished body size, decreased viability, and neurological compromise. Their retinas have a reduction in cell number because of impaired proliferation during embryogenesis, whereas in wild-type mice there is a special dependence on cyclin D1. The breast epithelium does not witness prominent proliferation in the setting of pregnancy in cyclin D1-mutant mice, despite adequate ovarian steroid levels—again underscoring the importance of the cooperation between steroids and cyclin D1.

Fantl et al. *(36)* generated cyclin D1-deficient mice, which were found to be viable and fertile, but smaller compared to heterozygous or wild-type litter mates. These mice also harbored evidence of retinopathy because of developmental impairment of the retina, as well as reduced mammary acinar development during pregnancy, with resulting lactation failure. About one-half of cyclin D1-deficient mice had jaw malformations. However, mouse embryo fibroblasts (MEFs) from 14d null, heterozygous, or wild-type embryos had similar cell-cycle and growth features, suggesting that cyclin D1 is dispensable for most cell lineages and tissues. It has been shown that knockin of cyclin E in cyclin D1-deficient mice can rescue abnormal phenotypes, and in this context, the restoration of cell-cycle progression is important in retinal and breast epithelial-cell homeostasis *(37)*.

The retinopathy observed in cyclin D1-deficient mice, which has been further investigated was associated with reduced retinal-cell proliferation and photoreceptor cell death. The latter was initially noted in scattered clusters of retinal cells, but then spread to the photoreceptor layer *(38)*. Holes in the photoreceptor layer were replete with with interneurons from the inner nuclear layer. This defect could not be rescued by bcl-2 transgene expression.

9. THE RELATIONSHIP OF D-TYPE CYCLINS

The three D-type cyclins, which share structural and functional properties, are expressed in similar and seemingly redundant fashion in proliferating tissues. To explore this further, mice harboring a disrupted cyclin D2 gene by using gene targeting in ES cells were generated. Cyclin D2-deficient female mice are not fertile, which is attributable to the lack of response to follicle-stimulating hormone (FSH) by ovarian granulosa cells *(39)*. Cyclin D2-deficient males show evidence of hypoplastic testes. It was postulated that cyclin D2 was especially critical for ovarian and testicular proliferation, and indeed, cyclin D2 mRNA is overexpressed in human ovarian and testicular tumors. In the context of another cell type, B cells from cyclin D2-deficient mice displayed a requirement for cyclin D2 in BCR- but not CD40- or lipopolysaccharide-induced proliferation *(40)*. Although B-cell development is normal in cyclin D2-mutant mice, the CD5 B-cell compartment is markedly reduced.

SUMMARY AND FUTURE DIRECTIONS

Cyclin D1 plays a critical role in progression of the cell through the G1 phase of the cell cycle. This is caused by complex formation with either cdk4 or cdk6, which in turn phosphorylates pRb and related proteins. Other substrates exist that may be important in a cell-specific context. Overexpression of cyclin D1 in cancer can occur through a variety of mechanisms, including gene amplification, mitogen-mediated transcriptional activation, post-transcriptional stabilization of cyclin D1 mRNA, and post-translational modifications. The recapitulation of the role of cyclin D1 as an oncogene has been made possible through transgenic mouse models, and some themes have emerged. Cyclin D1 alone appears to be sufficient for inducing cancer in the breast epithelium. However, in lymphocytes, squamous epithelia and the thymus, cofactor(s) are needed—e.g., an activated oncogene such as c-*myc* or *ras*. Gene ablation approaches in mice have underscored the role of cyclin D1 in development and differentiation in the breast and retina, but also have indicated that it is dispensible for embryogenesis, perhaps because of the compensatory roles of cyclin D2 and D3. Future experiments in mice will be aimed at understanding how cyclin D1 functions differently in a tissue-specific context—identification of cellular substrates, tissue-specific roles of cdk4 and cdk6 *(41)*, and ultimately, the employment of approaches to downregulate cyclin D1 in vivo.

ACKNOWLEDGMENTS

This work was supported by NIH grants R01 DK53377 P01 DE12467, N01, and the Abraman Family Cancer Research Institute.

REFERENCES

1. Sherr CJ. Mammalian G1 cyclins. *Cell* 1993; 73:1059–1065.
2. Sherr CJ. D-type cylins. *Trends Biochem Sci* 1994; 20:187–190.
3. Sherr CJ. G1 phase progression: cycling on cue. *Cell* 1994; 79:551–555.
4. Sherr CJ. The Pezcoller lecture: cancer cell cycles revisited. *Cancer Res* 2000; 60:3689–3695.
5. Motokura T, Bloom T, Kim HG, Juppner H, Ruderman JV, Kronenberg HM, et al. A novel cyclin encoded by a bcll-linked candidate oncogene. *Nature* 1991; 350:512–515.
6. Baldin V, Lukas J, Marcote MJ, Pagano M, Draetta G. Cyclin D1 is a nuclear protein required for cell cycle progression in G1. *Genes Dev* 1993; 7:812–821.
7. Quelle DE, Ashmun RA, Shurtleff SA, Kato JY, Bar-Sagi D, Roussel MF, et al. Overexpression of mouse D-type cyclins accelerates G1 phase in rodent fibroblasts. *Genes Dev* 1993; 7:1559–1571.
8. Sauter ER, Nesbit M, Litwin S, Klein-Szanto AJ, Cheffetz S, Herlyn M. Antisense cyclin D1 induces apoptosis and tumor shrinkage in human squamous carcinomas. *Cancer Res* 1999; 59:4876–4881.
9. Harper JW, Adami GR, Wei N, Keyomarsi K, Elledge SJ. The p21 CDK-interacting protein cip1 is a potent inhibitor of G1 cyclin-dependent kinases. *Cell* 1993; 75:805–808.
10. Waga S, Hannon GJ, Beach D, Stillman B. The p21 inhibitor of cyclin-dependent kinases controls DNA replication by interaction with PCNA. *Nature* 1994; 369:574–578.
11. El-Deiry WS, Tokino T, Velculescu VE, Levy DB, Parsons R, Trent JM, et al. WAF1, a potential mediator of p53 tumor suppression. *Cell* 1993; 75:817–825.
12. Hinds PW, Mitttnacht S, Dulic V, Arnold A, Reed SI, Weinberg RA. Regulation of retinoblastoma protein functions by ectopic expression of human cyclins. *Cell* 1992; 70:993–1006.
13. Weinberg RA. The retinoblastoma protein and cell cycle control. *Cell* 1995; 248:76–79.
14. Dynlacht BD, Flores O, Lees JA, Harlow E. Differential regulation of E2F transactivation by cyclin/cdk2 complexes. *Genes Dev* 1994; 8:1772–1786.
15. Lundberg AS, Weinberg RA. Control of the cell cycle and apoptosis. *Eur J Cancer* 1999; 35:1886–1894.
16. Neuman E, Ladha MH, Lin N, Upton TM, Miller SJ, DiRenzo J, et al. Cyclin D1 stimulation of estrogen receptor transcriptional activity independent of cdk4. *Mol Cell Biol* 1997; 17:5338–5347.
17. Hinds PW, Dowdy SF, Eaton EN, Arnold A, Weinberg RA. Function of a human cyclin gene as an oncogene. *Proc Natl Acad Sci USA* 1994; 91:709–713.
18. Lovec H, Grzeschiczek A, Kowalski MB, Moroy T. Cyclin D1/bcl-1 cooperates with myc genes in the generation of B-cell lymphoma in transgenic mice. *EMBO J* 1994; 13:3487–3495.
19. Bodrug SE, Warner BJ, Bath ML, Linderman GJ, Harris AW, Adams JM. Cyclin D1 transgene impedes lymphocyte maturation and collaborates in lymphomagenesis with the myc gene. *EMBO J* 1994; 13:2124–2130.
20. Wang TC, Cardiff RD, Zukerberg L, Lees E, Arnold A, Schmidt EV. Mammary hyperplasia and carcinoma in MMTV-cyclin D1 transgenic mice. *Nature* 1994; 369:669–671.
21. Zwijsen RM, Buckle RS, Hijmans EM, Loomans CJ, Bernards R. Ligand-independent recruitment of steroid receptor coactivators to estrogen receptor by cyclin D1. *Genes Dev* 1998; 12:3488–3498.
22. Robles AI, Larcher F, Whalin RB, Murillas R, Richie E, Gimenez-Conti IB, et al. Expression of cyclin D1 in epithelial tissues of transgenic mice results in epidermal hyperproliferation and severe thymic hyperplasia. *Proc Natl Acad Sci USA* 1996; 93:7634–7638.
23. Nakagawa H, Inomoto T, Rustgi AK. A CACCC box like *cis*-regulatory element of the Epstein-Barr virus ED-L2 promoter interacts with a nuclear transcriptional factor in tissue-specific squamous epithelia. *J Biol Chem* 1997 (a); 272:16,688–16,699.

24. Jenkins TD, Nakagawa H, Rustgi AK. The keratinocyte specific Epstein-Barr Virus ED-L2 promoter is regulated by phorbol 12-myristate 13-acetate through two *cis*-regulatory elements containing E-box and Krüppel-like factor motifs. *J Biol Chem* 1997; 272:24,433–24,442.

25. Jenkins TD, Opitz OG, Okano JI, Rustgi AK. Transactivation of the human keratin 4 and Epstein-Barr virus ED-L2 promoters by gut-enriched Krüppel-like factor. *J Biol Chem* 1998; 273:10,747–10,754.

26. Opitz OG, Jenkins TD, Rustgi AK. Transcriptional regulation of the differentiation-linked human keratin 4 promoter is dependent upon esophageal-specific nuclear factors. *J Biol Chem* 1998; 273:23,912–23,921.

27. Nakagawa H, Wang TC, Zukerberg L, Odze R, Togawa K, May GHW, et al. The targeting of the cyclin D1 oncogene by an Epstein-Barr virus promoter in transgenic mice causes dysplasia in the tongue, esophagus and forestomach. *Oncogene* 1997(b); 14:1185–1190.

28. Mueller A, Odze R, Jenkins TD, Shahsesfaei A, Nakagawa H, Inomoto T, et al. A transgenic mouse model with cyclin D1 overexpression results in cell cycle, epidermal growth factor receptor and p53 abnormalities. *Cancer Res* 1997; 57:5542–5549.

29. Jenkins TD, Mueller A, Odze R, Shahsafaei A, Zukerberg LR, Kent R. Cyclin D1 overexpression combined with N-nitrosomethylbenzylamine increases dysplasia and cellular proliferation in murine esophageal squamous epithelium. *Oncogene* 1999; 18:59–66.

30. Rodriguez-Puebla ML, LaCava M, Conti CJ. Cyclin D1 overexpression in mouse epidermis increases cyclin-dependent kinase activity and cell proliferation in vivo but does not affect skin tumor development. *Cell Growth Differ* 1999(a); 10:467–472.

31. Soonpaa MH, Koh GY, Pajak L, Jing S, Wang H, Franklin MT, et al. Cyclin D1 overexpression promotes cardiomyocyte DNA synthesis and multinucleation in transgenic mice. *Clin Investig* 1997; 99:2644–2654.

32. Rodriguez-Puebla ML, Robles AI, Conti CJ. ras activity and cyclin D1 expression: an essential mechanism of mouse skin tumor development. *Mol Carcinog* 1999(b); 24:1–6.

33. Robles AI, Rodriguez-Puebla ML, Glick AB, Trempus C, Hansen L, Sicinski P, et al. Reduced skin tumor development in cyclin D1-deficient mice highlights the oncogenic ras pathway in vivo. *Genes Dev* 1998; 12:2469–2474.

34 Stepanova L, Finegold M, DeMayo F, Schmidt EV, Harper JW. The oncoprotein kinase chaperone CDC37 functions as an oncogene in mice and collaborates with both c-myc and cyclin D1 in transformation of multiple tissues. *Mol Cell Biol* 2000; 20:4462–4473.

35. Sicinski P, Donaher JL, Parker SB, Li T, Fazeli A, Gardner H, et al. Cyclin D1 provides a link between development and oncogenesis in the retina and breast. *Cell* 1995; 82:621–630.

36. Fantl V, Stamp G, Andrews A, Rosewell I, Dickson C. Mice lacking cyclin D1 are small and show defects in eye and mammary gland development. *Genes Dev* 1995; 9:2364–2372.

37. Geng Y, Whoriskey W, Park MY, Bronson RT, Medema RH, Li T, et al. Rescue of cyclin D1 deficiency by knockin cyclin E. *Cell* 2000; 97:767–777.

38. Ma C, Papermaster D, Cepko CL. A unique pattern of photoreceptor degeneration in cyclin D1 mutant mice. *Proc Natl Acad Sci USA* 1998; 95:9938–9943.

39. Sicinski P, Donaher JL, Geng Y, Parker SB, Gardner H, Park MY, et al. Cyclin D2 is an FSH-responsive gene involved in gonadal cell proliferation and oncogenesis. *Nature* 1996; 384:470–474.

40. Solvason N, Wu WW, Parry D, Mahony D, Lam EW, Glassford J, et al. Cyclin D2 is essential for BCR-mediated proliferation and CD5 B cell development. *Int Immunol* 2000; 12:631–638.

41 Timmerman S, Hinds P, Münger K. Elevated activity of cyclin-dependent kinase 6 in human squamous cell carcinoma lines. *Cell Growth Diff* 1997; 8:361–370.

13

Mice Expressing the Human Carcinoembryonic Antigen

An Experimental Model of Immunotherapy Directed at a Self, Tumor Antigen

John W. Greiner, PhD

CONTENTS

1. INTRODUCTION

A series of important studies have led to a relaxation in the paradigms overseeing self/nonself immunity. Antigens which are oncofetal and/or serve as markers of cellular differentiation that are overexpressed or ectopically expressed by malignant cells were believed not to be targets for immunotherapy because of host immune tolerance. That conclusion has been challenged in recent years by a series of studies indicating that antigenic determinants of self have not induced absolute immune tolerance. Thus, under specific immunological conditions, specific peptides from those antigens can be processed by the antigen-presenting machinery, bound in MHC groove and serve as targets for immune intervention *(1–4)*. Those actions, in turn, offer the possibility that differentiation antigens, oncogenes and tumor-suppressor genes that are found in tumor cells may be considered targets for attack by the immune system *(5–8)*. One of the tissue-specific, tumor-associated antigens that shows much higher expression levels on tumors than on corresponding normal epithelial is carcinoembryonic antigen (CEA). This chapter reviews recent data that offers convincing evidence that CEA can indeed be a target for vaccine-mediated therapy of human cancers. The first part briefly introduces the CEA gene family and the use of CEA as an indicator for tumor diagnosis and patient management. More in-depth examinations of those subjects have been published elsewhere *(9,10)*. The second part introduces an experimental transgenic mouse model that expresses CEA as a self, tumor antigen. The major focus of the chapter is

From: *Tumor Models in Cancer Research*
Edited by: B. A. Teicher © Humana Press Inc., Totowa, NJ

the development of an experimental model that can provide some important insights into CEA-based vaccine strategies. The final section summarizes some of the early clinical results in which CEA is the immunotherapeutic target.

2. CEA GENE FAMILY

CEA was first described in 1965 *(11)*, and approx 25 yr later the *CEA* gene was isolated and characterized *(12)*. CEA is one member of a family that consists of approx 30 genes, 17 of which are transcriptionally active *(13)*. The gene family is tightly clustered on the long arm of human chromosome 19, and all are part of the larger immunoglobulin (Ig) supergene family *(14)*. Two main subgroups within the CEA gene family have been identified: the first is comprised of CEA, the well-known nonspecific cross-reacting antigen (NCA) and the biliary glycoproteins (BGP). Those antigens are further divided according to structural characteristics, specifically those (CEA, NCA, and others) that are attached to the outer membrane by a glycosyl phosphatidylinositol linkage *(15)* and those (BGP splice variants) that have both transmembrane and cytoplasmic domains. The second CEA subgroup consists of 11 genes encoding the secreted pregnancy-specific glycoproteins of unknown function *(16)*.

3. CEA EXPRESSION

CEA is one of the most studied of the human tumor markers. It is a M_r 180,000–200,000 oncofetal antigen whose expression is found on normal epithelial tissues as well as on a high percentage of adenocarcinomas, particularly those of the colon, pancreas, breast, and lung *(17–20)*. The identification of CEA as a member of the Ig superfamily provided the initial indication of its potential function. Since all Ig-like molecules are capable of interacting with other molecules, it came as no surprise that one function of CEA was that of a molecule involved in intercellular adhesion *(21,22)*. Others have argued that the location of CEA at the tips of the microvilli in the colonic mucosa was inconsistent with that function. Other studies have described an interaction between the bacterial fimbriae of the and lectins the carbohydrates on CEA and other family members *(23)*, and concluded that the adhesive qualities of CEA may be integral in the cell-surface recognition by bacteria. This function seems feasible in the gut for either bacterial colonization and its regulation by CEA shedding or for protection against infection by pathogenic bacteria. A third possible function of CEA has been as an accessory molecule for collagen type I binding *(24)*, a property that may be useful for cells involved in metastatic spread *(25)*.

The use of CEA in patient management is well-established *(20)*. The monitoring of serum CEA levels has been routinely used for the staging and follow-up of patients with solid tumors. While the CEA serum assay is not reliable for cancer diagnosis because of low sensitivity, the probability of malignancy increases directly with CEA serum concentration. Therefore, at the present time, the primary clinical applications of the measurement of serum CEA levels are prognosis, early diagnosis of recurrence, and patient follow-up. For instance, presurgical CEA serum levels are a well-established prognostic indicator in colorectal, breast, and lung cancer. Patients that present with increased pre-operative CEA serum levels experience a shorter disease-free interval and lower overall survival than patients with normal serum CEA levels. With the diagnosis of early recurrence, serum CEA was elevated in >70% of patients diagnosed with colorectal and approx 50% of breast-cancer patients. A recent report (26) compared CEA quantitative levels in tissues and sera samples from patients diagnosed with colorectal cancer, benign colonic disease, and healthy donors. Interestingly, no correlations were found between the CEA tissue levels and either the stage of disease or the presence of serum CEA levels. However, there was a positive correlation between CEA tissue levels and the degree of tumor differentiation. The lack of correlation between serum and tumor CEA expression levels may have important implications if CEA is to be used as a target for immunotherapy protocols. This finding indicates that tumor-tissue CEA expression, not serum CEA levels, should be the criteria for the selection of immune-based clinical protocols for patients. Finally, previous studies have exploited CEA expression as a target for passive immunodetection and therapy. Specifically, CEA-specific radioimmunoconjugates are being used to target human tumors for oncologic imaging and/or from the identification of occult tumor when used in conjunction with an intra-operative hand-held probe (27,28).

4. CEA TRANSGENIC (CEA.Tg) MICE

CEA gene families have been characterized in rodents. Despite homology, it has proven difficult to determine rodent counterparts for individual human genes through sequence comparison. Surprisingly, no CEA homolog has been identified. In fact, no rodent CEA-related molecules containing a glycosyl phosphatidylinositol anchor have yet to be characterized. The renewed interest in utilizing CEA as an immunotherapeutic target is one reason for an experimental rodent model expressing CEA. The development of such a model would provide an experimental setting to examine host factors that may influence CEA-based tumor vaccines. Mice expressing human CEA as a transgene have been developed in three laboratories (29–31). In one model, CEA expression was found in all tissues (29). In the model used in the present study (31), the spaciotemporal pattern of CEA expression correlated well with that of humans. Those CEA-transgenic mice were generated with a cosmid clone containing the complete coding region of the *CEA* gene, including 3.3 kb of the 5′-flanking region and 5 kb of the 3′-flanking sequences. Inclusion of a 424-basepair region, upstream from the translational start site, allowed for cell-type-specific expression of the *CEA* gene. Expression of CEA was confined primarily to the gastrointestinal tract, and other sites of ectopic CEA expression—such as the trachea, esophagus, small intestine, and lung—were found to exist (31). Quantitative CEA measurements revealed high antigen levels in the colonic tissues, feces, and sera of the CEA.Tg mice when compared with humans (Table 1). Concomitant with the development of CEA.Tg mice was the generation of a murine colon adenocarcinoma cell MC-38 ($H-2^b$) that also expressed CEA. MC-38 tumor cells were stably transduced with a human CEA cDNA using the retroviral expression vector pBNC (32), and the resulting CEA-expressing tumor cell was designated MC-38-CEA-2. The cell line was cloned, routinely examined for stable CEA expression by the cell-surface reactivity using an anti-CEA monoclonal antibody, and grew rapidly as a subcutaneous (SC) tumor in the CEA.Tg mice. Moreover, immunohistochemical staining and RIA examination of the SC tumors taken at different time intervals demonstrated stable CEA expression within the tumors for up to 2 mo.

Therefore, the CEA.Tg mice offered an opportunity to study the generation of an immune response against a tissue-specific self antigen. The CEA-expressing MC-

Table 1
CEA Expression Levels in Colonic Tissue, Feces,
and Serum of CEA-Transgenic Mice and Humans

	CEA Concentration		
Species	Colonic tissue (ng/mg protein)	Feces (ng/mg protein)	Serum (ng/mL)
CEA. Tg mice[a]	1,350–1,800	28,400–57,200	14.0–30.5
Humans (ref. 30)	108 ± 38	13,800 ± 12,400	1.5

[a] Individual mice were sacrificed and tissues, feces, and serum samples were taken and CEA levels quantitated in protein extracts using a solid-phase, double-determinant ELISA kit (AMDL, Inc. Tustin, CA).

32-CEA-2 tumor cells will provide additional information as to whether the anti-CEA host immunity can translate into antitumor immunity. If the concentration of the self antigen impacts the development of an immune response (i.e., breaking tolerance), then the higher level of CEA expression in these CEA.Tg mice might make the generation of an anti-CEA immune response more arduous. Finally, the expression of CEA in the gastrointestinal tract should provide some insight into the balance between antitumor and autoimmunity in the host.

Although the CEA.Tg mice should provide some interesting insights, it is important to recognize that their use has limitations. For example, it remains unclear how a transgenic murine model reflects the human in terms of degree of gene expression during embryonic development and the expression levels of the antigen in normal tissues. It remains difficult to predict the relative immunogenicity or the ability to break tolerance to a self antigen in the human based solely on the findings from a transgenic model. Nonetheless, mice expressing a human transgene can be used to help predict the broad principles of generating immunity to a self, tumor antigen. Furthermore, these experimental models may provide additional insights into the approaches that are needed to translate immunogenicity into antitumor immunity by implementing defined approaches to augment the antitumor immune response.

For the studies summarized here and in a previous publication (33), several questions were addressed to define and understand the experimental CEA.Tg mouse model system:

- Are CEA.Tg mice immune tolerant to CEA?
- Is there a difference in CEA-specific immunity in CEA.Tg vs wild-type B6 mice?
- Can antitumor immunity be generated in the CEA.Tg mice?
- Does antitumor immunity involve CEA-expressing normal tissues?

4.1. Are CEA-Transgenic Mice Immune Tolerant to CEA?

The elevated CEA levels found in the colonic tissues, feces, and serum could be considered a danger signal (1) to the immune system and result in the development of low levels of CEA immunity in the naive CEA.Tg mice. In order to test that hypothesis, naive mice were initially analyzed for the presence of anti-CEA serum antibodies. As shown in Table 2, no measurable anti-CEA (IgM) or IgG antibody titers were detected in the sera of naive CEA.Tg mice. Thus, CEA overexpression by the colonic tissue or the presence of elevated CEA levels in the feces and serum seems to be

Table 2
CEA Serum Ig Titers in Naive and Immunized CEA.Tg and CEA-Negative Littermate Mice[a]

Mice	Immunogen + adjuvant	Serum Ab titers[b] (OD=0.5 @ A_{490nm})					
		CEA			OVA		
		IgM	IgG		IgM	IgG	
CEA-transgenic	none	<100	<100		<100	<100	
	CEA/OVA + detox-PC	200–300	<100		4000–8000	5000–6000	
CEA-negative littermate	none	<100	<100		<100	<100	
	CEA/OVA + detox-PC	2500–4500	6000–7500		5000–6500	4500–7200	

[a] Mice were administered 20 μg of CEA and OVA mixed with Detox-PC adjuvant at the base of the tail 2× at biweekly intervals. Naive mice received HBSS. Two weeks after the second injection, mice were bled and serum tested for the presence of anti-CEA and -OVA IgGs by ELISA.

[b] Data are the ranges of Ig titers for 4–5 mice/group. Ab titers were defined as 1/serum dilution that results in an A_{490nm} of 0.5, with 100 being the lower limit of ab detection.

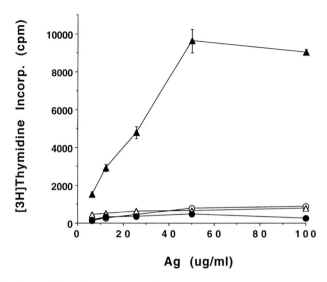

Fig. 1. Splenic CD4+ proliferative responses following a prime and a boost immunization of CEA.Tg with CEA and OVA in adjuvant. CEA.Tg mice (solid symbols) were immunized at biweekly intervals by injecting a mixture of 100 μg CEA/OVA in adjuvant s.c. at the base of the tail. Untreated CEA.Tg mice received HBSS (open symbols). Four weeks after the second immunization, mice were sacrificed, splenic T cells were isolated from each group and pooled. A 5-d lymphoproliferative assay was carried out in the presence of soluble CEA (circles) and OVA (triangles) and freshly prepared APC. ^{3}H-Thymidine was added during the final 24 h. Each data point represents the mean ± SEM for the amount of [3H]thymidine incorporated from triplicate wells. Some error bars are covered by the symbol.

physiological in the CEA.Tg mice and does not generate a humoral response to CEA. Another study *(31)* reported that CEA.Tg mice implanted with CEA-positive SC tumors did not develop detectable serum CEA antibody titers. In subsequent studies, the CEA.Tg and their CEA-negative littermate mice were administered CEA and ovalbumin (OVA) proteins mixed with adjuvant (Detox-PC, RIBI ImmunoChem Research, Inc., Hamilton, MT). Following two injections of these immunogens, serum samples from individual mice were analyzed for the presence of anti-CEA or anti-OVA IgG titers. As expected, the CEA-negative littermate mice development strong humoral responses to both CEA and OVA, both of which are foreign antigens (Table 2). In contrast, the CEA.Tg mice injected with CEA/OVA in adjuvant developed significant anti-OVA IgG serum titers, but only a weak IgM (serum titer = 200–300) response to CEA. Those results indicate that CEA.Tg mice are fully immune-competent and can mount a robust humoral response to foreign antigens. Secondly, the CEA.Tg mice seem to remain immunologically silent to CEA, providing additional evidence for their tolerance to this self antigen.

To further define immune tolerance to CEA in the CEA.Tg mice, further studies have investigated whether cellular responses to CEA could be generated in either the naive or immune CEA.Tg mice. When splenic T cells isolated from naive CEA.Tg mice were grown in vitro for 5 d in the presence of exogenous CEA protein, no significant cellular proliferation, as measured by ^{3}H-thymidine incorporation, was observed (Fig. 1). Analysis of splenic T cells isolated from CEA.Tg mice immunized with

CEA/OVA in adjuvant revealed the presence of a strong anti-OVA proliferative response and, for the most part, no measurable cellular immune response to CEA (Fig. 1). Therefore, the CEA.Tg mice presents a workable experimental model in which to study the generation of immunity directed at CEA, which functions in those mice as a self, tumor antigen.

4.2. Is There a Difference in CEA-Specific Immunity in CEA.Tg vs Wild-Type B6 Mice?

Replication-competent recombinant poxvirus (i.e., vaccinia) vaccines engineered to express a foreign gene are excellent candidates to induce antigen-specific active immunization against a self antigen, such as CEA. Vaccinia can accept large inserts of a foreign gene and express it within a wide host range, and the copresentation of a weakly immunogenic gene product with the highly immunogenic vaccinia proteins often boosts the immune response to the inserted gene product (34–36). A recombinant vaccinia virus expressing CEA (rV-CEA) was produced by homologous recombination of a plasmid containing a human CEA cDNA inserted into the Hind III M site of the Wyeth strain of vaccinia virus. A complete description of the design and generation of the rV-CEA construct has been published (37,38). Quantitative and Western blot analyses were used to check the fidelity and amount of CEA produced from cells infected with the recombinant vaccinia virus. Further indications for using a recombinant poxvirus expressing a self, tumor antigen are revealed by the findings from previous studies that have suggested that the unresponsiveness of lymphocytes may not be determined solely by the self and non-self nature of the antigen. In fact, specific conditions in which the antigen—in this case, CEA—is presented to the immune system—i.e., antigen dose, type of antigen-presenting cell, or the use of an heterokaryon of dendritic and tumor cells—have all been shown to generate host immunity directed at self antigens (2–4,39). The recombinant vaccinia virus expressing CEA combines some of those same conditions—i.e., local inflammation—with high production levels of a weak immunogen that might contribute to the generation of a CEA-specific host immunity in the CEA.Tg mouse model. Studies were carried out to examine whether presentation of CEA in a recombinant vaccinia virus could induce a CEA-specific humoral response in CEA.Tg mice, which might be the first indication of breaking immune tolerance to CEA. Furthermore, the corresponding CEA-negative littermate mice were also immunized with rV-CEA to directly compare the relative strengths of CEA-specific humoral immunity generated in different host in which CEA is self vs non-self. Other mice received multiple immunizations (via tail scarification) of a control vaccinia virus, referred to as V-Wyeth. Sera samples were analyzed for the presence of anti-CEA antibodies. Not surprising was the robust humoral response to CEA that was observed in the CEA-negative littermate mice after a single administration of rV-CEA. By comparison, after a single immunization with rV-CEA, measurable anti-CEA IgG levels were observed in the sera of 70–80% the CEA.Tg mice (30). Upon subsequent rV-CEA immunization, all of the CEA.Tg mice developed anti-CEA IgG serum antibody titers. Fig. 2 summarizes the relative anti-CEA serum IgG titers generated in the CEA.Tg and CEA-negative littermate mice after three immunizations with rV-CEA. Clearly, although anti-CEA IgG titers were present in all CEA.Tg mice tested, the relative strengths of the humoral response to CEA was approx 40-fold less than that measured in the CEA-negative littermate mice.

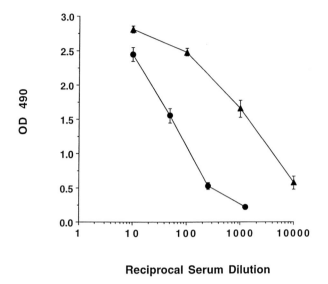

Reciprocal Serum Dilution

Fig. 2. Comparison of anti-CEA IgG responses in CEA.Tg (circles) and CEA-negative littermate mice (triangles). All mice were immunized 3× with 10^7 pfu rV-CEA at 2-wk intervals. Serum samples were collected from individual mice 2 wk after the final immunization and the presence of anti-CEA serum IgG was assayed by ELISA. Results are the mean ± SEM of the 4–6 mice/group.

Despite the apparent blunting of the anti-CEA humoral response in the CEA.Tg mice immunized with rV-CEA, further analysis uncovered switching in Ig class subtypes as evidenced by IgG1, IgG2a, and IgG2b anti-CEA antibody responses *(33)*. Ig class switching is known to indicate an underlying presence of a cellular immune response. Therefore, experiments were carried out to examine whether immunization of the CEA.Tg mice with rV-CEA also generated CEA-specific cellular host immunity. Splenic T cells were isolated from the CEA.Tg mice immunized 1–3× with rV-CEA and evaluated for the ability to proliferate in the presence of exogenous CEA and antigen-presenting cells. As summarized in Table 3, significant levels of ^{3}H-thymidine incorporation were achieved by splenic T cells from CEA.Tg mice following a single vaccination with rV-CEA. In prime and boost immunization protocols, CEA.Tg mice could be administered rV-CEA twice, which resulted in an augmentation of the CEA-specific lymphoproliferative response. However, a third injection of rV-CEA led to no further increase in the CEA-specific CD4+ response, perhaps because of the generation of neutralizing anti-vaccinia antibody titers.

There remained a possibility that immune tolerance to CEA in the CEA.Tg mice was not broken following immunization with rV-CEA. The CEA-specific humoral and cell-mediated immunity were both generated against an epitope(s) expressed on the CEA produced by the recombinant vaccinia virus and the exogenous CEA used in the immunoassays. The assumption was that those same antigenic epitope(s) were expressed by the endogenous CEA expressed in the CEA.Tg mice. An approach was designed that would directly answer the question of whether immunization of the CEA.Tg mice with rV-CEA did, indeed, overcome tolerance and induce immunity against the endogenous CEA. Feces were collected from a group of CEA.Tg mice,

Table 3
CEA-Specific Splenic T-Cell Proliferation from rV-CEA-Immunized CEA-Transgenic Mice[a]

Antigen	[3H]Thymidine Incorp. (delta cpm)		
	1×	2×	3×
CEA, 100	$5,811 \pm 667$[b]	$12,712 \pm 1132$[c]	$10,998 \pm 450$
50	$4,266 \pm 932$	$10,221 \pm 876$[c]	$8,445 \pm 213$
25	$2,713 \pm 253$	$7,645 \pm 444$[c]	$7,112 \pm 914$
12.5	$2,007 \pm 791$	$5,489 \pm 567$[c]	$5,309 \pm 634$
6.25	$2,167 \pm 567$	$4,788 \pm 234$[c]	$3,214 \pm 222$
V-Wyeth, 2×10^7 pfu	56,108	79,112[c]	98,414
ovalbumin, 100 µg/ml	1,044	2,045	1,604
Con A, 2.0 µg/ml	101,673	98,889	101,223

[a] CEA.Tg mice (2–3/group) were administered 10^7 pfu of rV-CEA or V-Wyeth tail scarification (10 µl) 3× at biweekly intervals. Two-4 weeks after the third immunization, mice were sacrificed, splenic T cells isolated and pooled according to treatment group. T-cell proliferative responses to soluble CEA, OVA, and UV-inactivated V-Wyeth were measured in a 5-d. ^{3}H-thymidine incorporation assay. T-cell response to Con A was performed in a 72-h proliferative assay.

[b] Data are presented as the mean ± SEM. For V-Wyeth, oval butenin Con A-stimulated cells, the average cpm are shown (SEM <10%).

[c] $p < 0.05$ (vs 1× rV-CEA).

and endogenous CEA was isolated using an anti-CEA MAb affinity column. The anti-CEA MAb-reactive products were analyzed by Western blot, which revealed predominate bands at 180–200 kDa as well as numerous other smaller immunoreactive mol-wt moieties of 50–150 kDa. The most probable explanation is that the 180–200 kDa bands correspond to intact CEA, and the smaller bands represent several uncharacterized metabolic breakdown products of fecal CEA. Radioimmunoassays were used to approximate the amount of immunoreactive, CEA-related fecal material isolated. CEA.Tg mice were immunized 2x with rV-CEA, V-Wyeth or whole CEA protein in Detox-PC adjuvant. The stimulation indices (SI), i.e., ^{3}H-thymidine incorporation) were calculated and compared for each immunized group of CEA.Tg mice. As summarized in Fig. 3, multiple immunizations with whole CEA protein in Detox-PC adjuvant did not induce significant CEA-specific cellular immunity in the CEA.Tg mice. The CEA-specific T-cell proliferation measured in CEA.Tg mice administered whole CEA in adjuvant was not significantly higher from that for splenic T cells from naive CEA.Tg mice. CEA.Tg mice immunized twice with rV-CEA developed a strong CEA-specific T-cell proliferative response that was significantly higher (p <0.05) than that of CEA.Tg mice treated with V-Wyeth or whole CEA. More importantly, the addition of the endogenous CEA isolated from the feces to the lymphoproliferative assays with purified splenocytes from rV-CEA-immunized CEA.Tg mice resulted in significant amounts of [3H]thymidine incorporation (Fig. 3, dashed line). The ability to stimulate cellular immune responses directed at the endogenous CEA, provides additional evidence that rV-CEA immunization had broken immune tolerance which resulted in the development of CEA-specific cellular immunity in the CEA.Tg mice.

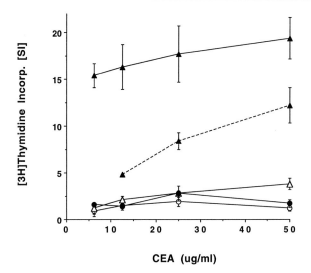

Fig. 3. CD4+ proliferative responses in CEA.Tg mice following a prime and boost immunization. CEA.Tg mice (2–3/group) were immunized 2× with 100 μg CEA in adjuvant (open triangles), 10^7 pfu rV-CEA (closed triangles) or V-Wyeth (closed circles). Untreated CEA.Tg mice received HBSS (open circles). Four weeks after the second immunization, mice were sacrificed, splenic T cells isolated and the proliferative responses to soluble CEA (50–6.25 μg/mL) as outlined for Fig. 1. The dashed line represents the data generated from incubating the isolated splenic T cells from the rV-CEA-immunized mice in the presence of endogenous CEA isolated from mice feces. Data represent the stimulation index calculated as follows as follows: [cpm (cells from immunized mice)]/[cpm (cells from naive mice)].

Functionally specific subsets of CD4+ T cells produce and secrete selective sets of cytokines in response to antigen. IFN-γ, IL-2 and TNF-α are produced in a type 1 response and promote cell-mediated immunity, whereas IL-4, IL-5, and IL-10 production promote a type 2 or humoral immunity. Supernatant was collected from splenic T cells isolated from either untreated mice or CEA.Tg mice treated with rV-CEA, V-Wyeth, or whole CEA protein in adjuvant, and subsequently stimulated in vitro in the presence or absence of soluble CEA. Measurement of IFN-γ and IL-4 production was used to indicate the presence of either a type 1 or type 2 response, respectively. Splenocytes from CEA.Tg mice immunized 2x with rV-CEA produced substantial quantities of IFN-γ when cultured in the presence of CEA (Table 4). These same cells also produce low but detectable levels of IL-4. In contrast, splenic T cells from CEA.Tg mice treated with whole CEA in adjuvant produced no detectable IFN-γ (Table 4). Interestingly, those T cells produced low but measurable levels of IL-4. No appreciable amounts of either cytokine were detected following the incubation of splenic T cells from unimmunized or V-Wyeth-immunized CEA.Tg mice in the presence of CEA. No measurable levels of IL-10 were found in any of the cultures.

Subsequent studies were carried out to determine whether rV-CEA immunization of CEA.Tg mice could also generate CEA-specific cell-mediated cytotoxicity. Attempts to measure primary CTL activity from lymph nodes or spleens of rV-CEA-immunized mice were, for the most part, unsuccessful. A series (>50) of CEA peptides were

Table 4
Cytokine Release and CEA Peptide-Specific Lysis by T Cells Isolated
from rV-CEA-Immunized CEA. Tg Mice[a]

Immunogen	Cytokine release[b] (ng/10^5 cells/48 h)		CTL activity (lytic units)[c]
	Gamma-IFN	IL-4	
HBSS	<0.01	<0.01	neg
CEA protein + Detox-PC	<0.01	6.8 ± 0.8	neg
rV-CEA	776.3 ± 85.3	0.9 ± 0.4	7.9 ± 0.9
V-Wyeth	<0.01	<0.01	neg

[a] CEA.Tg mice (2–3 mice/group) were immunized with HBSS, CEA protein in adjuvant, V-Wyeth or rV-CEA 2× every other wk. Mice were sacrificed 2 wk after the final immunization, and spleens were pooled and T-cells isolated.

[b] For cytokine measurement, the isolated splenic T cells were incubated in the presence of irradiated APCs and 50 μg CEA for 48 h. Results are the mean from triplicate wells (SEM ± 15%) from a representative experiment, repeated with similar results. No measurable amounts of either IFN-γ or IL-4 were found in wells containing splenic T cells grown in the absence of CEA or in the presence of an irrelevant antigen (i.e., OVA). Con A-stimulated splenic T cells from each group produced approx 5–10 μg IFN-γ and 200–300 ng IL-4/10^5 cells during the same time period.

[c] Approximately 2 wk after the second immunization, spleens from 2–3 mice/group were pooled as single-cell suspensions, and a total of 25×10^6 splenocytes were added in 10 mL to T-25 flasks along with 10 μg/mL of the CEA 8-mer peptide (referred to as CEA peptide) corresponding to amino-acid positions 526–533 (EAQNTTYL). T-cell cultures were restimulated 6 d later in 24-well plates. Two hundred thousand T-cells were added along with 5×10^6 irradiated syngeneic splenocytes, 1 μg CEA peptide/mL and 10 U/mL recombinant human IL-2 (Proleukin, Chiron Corp., Emeryville, CA). Cytolytic activity was assessed 6 d later using EL-4, a murine lymphoma cell line pulsed with 0.2 μg CEA peptide or a control peptide (i.e., gp 100). Lytic units were calculated as follows: (# effectors [25% lysis] × # targets)/10^5 cells. Data are the mean ± SEM from a representative experiment. Three separate experiments were performed with similar results.

screened for their ability to bind H-2b antigens and to lyse peptide-pulsed EL-4 cells in a primary CTL using splenic T cells isolated from rV-CEA-immunized wild-type B6 mice. A single CEA 8-mer peptide corresponding to amino-acid positions 526–533 (EAQNTTYL) was selected, and has been routinely used for in vitro stimulation of splenic T cells isolated from immunized CEA.Tg mice. In the initial study, CEA.Tg mice were immunized twice with rV-CEA, V-Wyeth, CEA protein in adjuvant or Hank's Balanced Salt Solution (HBSS), and the splenic T cells were isolated and grown in vitro in the presence of CEA peptide and IL-2 of two rounds of stimulation. Only those T cells that were originally isolated from rV-CEA-immunized mice were capable of inducing lysis of CEA peptide-pulsed target cells (i.e., EL-4) (Table 4). More recently, accompanying additional in vitro stimulations of splenic T cells from immune CEA.Tg mice have generated a CEA peptide-specific CD8+ CTL line. The line is being characterized for its T-cell receptor repertoire and its ability to recognize and lyse the MC-38-CEA-2 tumor-cell line.

4.3. Does Antitumor Immunity Involve CEA-Expressing Normal Tissues?

The previous results present a convincing argument that immunization of CEA-transgenic mice with a vaccinia-CEA recombinant virus generates anti-CEA host immunity that consists of both humoral, anti-CEA IgG titers, and cell-mediated, T_H1

type CEA-specific CD4$^+$ response, and CEA peptide-specific cytotoxicity. The next question is whether that anti-CEA directed immunity could elicit antitumor immunity. CEA.Tg and CEA-negative littermate mice were immunized with rV-CEA or V-Wyeth three times every 2 wk. Fourteen days after the third immunization, each mouse received a tumor burden of MC-38-CEA-2 cells. CEA.Tg mice treated with (HBSS) or immunized with the control virus, V-Wyeth, developed progressively growing tumors and, by wk 7, 80–90% of those mice had been sacrificed (Fig. 4). Approximately 50% of the rV-CEA-immunized CEA.Tg mice were protected against tumor growth and remained tumor-free at wk 7. Of the five rV-CEA-immunized CEA.Tg mice that developed tumors, the time of tumor appearance and the subsequent growth rates were significantly delayed when compared with the HBSS-treated or V-Wyeth-immunized CEA.Tg mice ($p < 0.05$) (Fig. 4). Immunization of the CEA-negative littermate mice with rV-CEA protected 80% (8 of 10) from tumor growth. No protection was afforded CEA-negative littermate mice treated with HBSS or V-Wyeth.

All the CEA.Tg mice immunized with rV-CEA or V-Wyeth were routinely monitored for overt signs of toxicity (i.e., weight loss, diarrhea, feeding abnormalities, basic neurological parameters, or changes in fur coloration). All appeared healthy, and weight was maintained when compared with CEA-negative littermates. Blood chemistries were performed on CEA.Tg mice and CEA-negative littermates immunized with rV-CEA or V-Wyeth 1 mo after tumor challenge, a time at which CEA immunity should still be active. Elevations in creatinine phosphokinase and amylase were noted in CEA.Tg and the CEA-negative littermate mice immunized with either rV-CEA or V-Wyeth. The significance of elevated amylase levels—particularly in mice immunized with vaccinia virus—is unknown (33). Normal tissues (intestinal tract, kidneys, esophagus/stomach, liver) from rV-CEA-immunized CEA.Tg mice were analyzed for histological indicators for the presence of autoimmunity and possible changes in the relative levels of CEA expression. No major changes in tissue/cellular architecture in rV-CEA-immunized mice were observed. Immunohistochemical analysis confirmed CEA expression in the intestinal tract and esophagus/stomach of the CEA.Tg mice, and no substantial alterations in CEA staining were observed in rV-CEA-immunized CEA.Tg mice that had rejected the CEA-expressing tumor.

5. FUTURE DIRECTIONS: IMMUNOGENICITY OF CEA IN HUMANS

The question of whether CEA is immunogenic in humans and could be a target for active immunization has been re-examined. Previously, healthy individuals and cancer patients were considered unresponsive to CEA, since most of the experimental data was, by and large, equivocal (40–42). More recent reports have, for the most part, assuaged the idea that humans are tolerant to CEA. In vitro studies reported the generation of human anti-CEA antibodies (43) and proliferation of tumor-infiltrating lymphocytes from patients diagnosed with colorectal cancer and administered an anti-CEA anti-idiotypic antibody (44,45). A wide range of immunogens, including CEA (45), have induced CEA-specific CTL, T-cell proliferative and anti-CEA antibody responses in humans (8,46–48). Most of the current interest seems focused on developing immu-

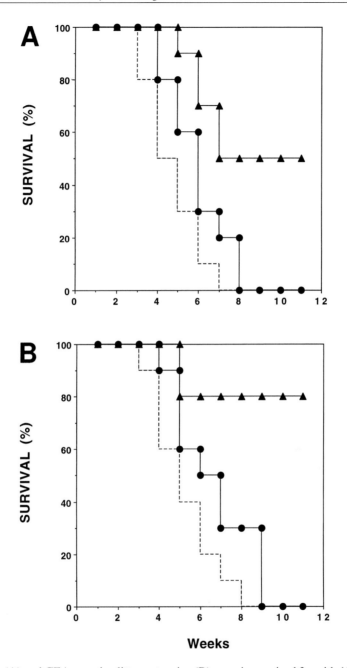

Fig. 4. CEA.Tg (A) and CEA negative littermate mice (B) were immunized 3× with 10^7 pfu rV-CEA (solid triangles) or V-Wyeth (solid circles) every 2 wk. Control mice (dashed line) received an equal volume of HBSS. All mice were challenged with CEA-expressing tumor cells 2 wks after the final immunization.

nization strategies involving recombinant poxvirus vectors expressing CEA. Although early clinical studies established that rV-CEA was well-tolerated in patients and was capable of inducing CEA-specific CTL activity, most of the subsequent interest has turned to evaluate replication-deficient poxviruses in order to circumvent the anti-vaccinia immunity that exists in much of the population. These studies with canarypox- and fowlpox-recombinant viruses expressing CEA, have also induced CEA-specific CTL responses capable of lysing CEA-peptide-pulsed T2, C1R-A2, and autologous B cells, as well as CEA-expressing allogeneic and/or autologous tumor cells *(49–51)*. CEA-specific lysis was MHC-restricted, indicating the ability of human colorectal tumors to process and present immunologically relevant peptides to their cell surface. Despite these early successes, evidence that the ability of generating anti-CEA immunity in patients translates into CEA-specific antitumor immunity has been, at best, anecdotal. It is not known whether the inability of patients to mount a robust anti-CEA response results from the presence of cancer at an advanced stage, the blunting of the immune response because CEA is a self, tumor antigen, a combination of both, or because of other unexplained reasons. It appears that at this juncture, experimental data generated in the CEA.Tg mice closely parallels that seen in the clinical studies. In both situations, subsequent CEA vaccine strategies will include molecules that can augment CEA-specific immunity in preclinical studies. Through the use of cytokines such as granulocyte-macrophage colony-stimulating factor (GM-CSF), interleukin-2, and/or by engineering costimulatory molecules such as B7-1, LFA-3, and ICAM-1, as part of the recombinant poxvirus vaccine, increases in humoral and cell-mediated responses to CEA and other experimental antigens have been reported *(52,53)*. It is hoped that utilization of those biological vaccine adjuvants will boost the immune response to CEA to include antitumor therapy.

REFERENCES

1. Matzinger P. Tolerance, danger, and the extended family. *Annu Rev Immunol* 1994; 12:991–1045.
2. Sarzotti M, Robbins DS, Hoffman PM. Induction of protective CTL responses in newborn mice by a murine retrovirus. *Science* 1996; 271:1726–1728.
3. Forsthuber T, Yip HC, Lehmann PV. Induction of T_H1 and T_H2 immunity in neonatal mice. *Science* 1996; 271:1728–1730.
4. Ridge JP, Fuchs E, Matzinger P. Neonatal tolerance revisited: turning on newborn T cells with dendritic cells. *Science* 1996; 271:1723–1726.
5. Van der Bruggen P, Traversari C, Chomez P, Lurquin C, De Plaen E, Van den Eynde B, et al. A gene encoding an antigen recognized by cytotoxic T lymphocytes on a human melanoma. *Science* 1991; 254:1643–1647.
6. Houbiers JGA, Nij HW, van der Burg SH, Drijhout JW, Kenemans P, van de Velde CJH, et al. *In vitro* induction of human cytotoxic T lymphocyte responses against peptides of mutant and wild-type p53. *Eur J Immunol* 1993; 23:2072–2077.
7. Peoples GE, Goedegebuure PS, Smith R, Linehan DC, Yoshino I, Eberlein TJ. Breast and ovarian cancer-specific cytotoxic T lymphocytes recognize the same HER2/neu-derived peptide. *Proc Natl Acad Sci USA* 1995; 92:432–436.
8. Tsang KY, Zaremba S, Nieroda CA, Zhu MZ, Hamilton JM, Schlom J. Generation of human cytotoxic T cells specific for human carcinoembryonic antigen epitopes from patients immunized with recombinant vaccinia-CEA vaccine. *J Natl Cancer Inst* 1995; 87:982–990.
9. Thompson J, Zimmermann W. The carcinoembryonic antigen gene family: structure, expression and evolution. *Tumor Biol* 1988; 9:63–83.
10. Gold P, Goldenberg NA. The carcinoembryonic antigen (CEA): past, present and future. *McGill J Med* 1997; 3:46–66.
11. Gold P, Freedman SO. Demonstration of tumor-specific antigens in human colonic carcinomata by immunological tolerance and absorption techniques. *J Exp Med* 1965; 121:439–462.
12. Schrewe H, Thompson J, Bona M, Hefta LJF, Maruya A, Hassauer M, et al. Cloning of the complete gene for the carcinoembryonic antigen: analysis of its promoter indicates a region conveying cell-type specific expression. *Mol Cell Biol* 1990; 10:2738–2748.

13. Thompson JA. Molecular cloning and expression of carcinoembryonic antigen gene family members. *Tumor Biol* 1995; 16:10–16.

14. Tynan K, Olsen A, Trask B, de Jong P, Thompson J, Zimmermann W, et al. Assembly and analysis of cosmid contigs in the CEA-gene family region of human chromosome 19. *Nucleic Acids Res* 1992; 20:1629–1636.

15. Hefta SA, Hefta LJF, Lee TD, Paxton RJ, Shively JE. Carcinoembryonic antigen is anchored to membranes by covalent attachment to a glycosyl-phosphatidylinositol moiety: identification of the ethanolamine linkage site. *Proc Natl Acad Sci USA* 1988; 85:4648–4652.

16. Watanabe H, Chou JY. Human pregnancy-specific β1-glycoprotein: a new member of the carcinoembryonic antigen gene family. *Biochem Biophys Res Commun* 1998; 152:762–768.

17. Shuster J, Thomson DMP, Fuks A, Gold P. Immunologic approaches to diagnosis of malignancy. *Prog Exp Tumor Res* 1980; 25:89–139.

18. Thompson JA, Grunert F, Zimmermann W. Carcinoembryonic antigen gene family: molecular biology and clinical perspectives. *J Lab Clin Anal* 1991; 5:344–366.

19. Shively JE, Beatty JD. CEA-related antigens: molecular biology and clinical significance. *Crit Rev Oncol Hematol* 1985; 2:355–399.

20. Ballesta A, Molina R, Filella X, Jo J, Gimenez N. Carcinoembryonic antigen in staging and followup of patients with solid tumors. *Tumor Biol* 1995; 16:32–41.

21. Hammarstrom S, Olsen A, Teglund S, Baranov V. The nature and expression of the human CEA family. In: Stanners CP, ed. *Cell Adhesion and Communication Mediated by the CEA Family,* (C.P. Stanners, ed.) Cell Adhesion and Communication Book Series, Harwood Academic Publishers, Amsterdam, pp. 289–302.

22. Benchimol S, Fuks A, Jothy S, Beauchemin N, Shirota K, Stanners CP. Carcinoembryonic antigen, a human tumor marker, functions as an intracellular adhesion molecule. *Cell* 1989; 57:327–334.

23. Leusch H-G, Hefta SA, Drzeniek Z, Hummel K, Markos-Pusztai Z, Wagener C. *Escherichia coli* of human origin binds to carcinoembryonic antigen (CEA) and non-specific crossreacting antigen (NCA). *FEBS Lett* 1990; 261:405–409.

24. Pignatelli M, Durbin H, Bodmer WF. Carcinoembryonic antigen functions as an accessory adhesion molecule mediating colon epithelial cell-collagen interactions. *Proc Natl Acad Sci USA* 1990; 87:1541–1545.

25. Hostetter RB, Augustus LB, Mankarious R, Chi K, Fan D, Toth C, et al. Carcinoembryonic antigen as a selective enhancer of colorectal cancer metastasis. *J Natl Cancer Inst* 1990; 82:380–385.

26. Guadagni F, Roselli M, Cosimelli M, Spila A, Cavaliere F, Arcuri R, et al. Quantitative analysis of CEA expression in colorectal adenocarcinoma and serum: lack of correlation. *Int J Cancer* 1997; 72:949–954.

27. Goldenberg DM, Kim EE, Deland FH, Bennett S, Primus FJ. Radioimmunodetection of cancer with radioactive antibodies to carcinoembryonic antigen. *Cancer Res* 1980; 40:2984–2992.

28. Behr TM, Sharkey RM, Juweid ME, Dunn RM, Vagg RC, Ying Z, et al. Phase I/II clinical radioimmunotherapy with an iodine-131-labeled anti-carcinoembryonic antigen murine monoclonal antibody IgG. *J Nucl Med* 1997; 38:858–870.

29. Hasegawa T, Isobe K, Tsuchiya Y, Oikawa S, Nakazato H, Ikezawa H, et al. Establishment and characterization of human carcinoembryonic antigen transgenic mice. *Br J Cancer* 1991; 64:710–714.

30. Eades-Perner A-M, van der Putten H, Hirth A, Thompson J, Neumaier M, von Kleist S, et al. Mice transgenic for the human carcinoembryonic antigen gene maintain its spatiotemporal expression pattern. *Cancer Res* 1994; 54:4169–4176.

31. Clarke P, Mann J, Simpson JF, Rickard-Dickson K, Primus FJ. Mice transgenic for human carcinoembryonic antigen as a model for immunotherapy. *Cancer Res* 1998; 58:1469–1477.

32. Robbins PF, Kantor J, Salgaller M, Horan Hand P, Fernsten PD, Schlom J. Transduction and expression of the human carcinoembryonic antigen (CEA) gene in a murine colon carcinoma cell line. *Cancer Res* 1991; 51:3757–3762.

33. Kass E, Schlom J, Thompson J, Guadagni F, Graziano P, Greiner J. Induction of protective host immunity to carcinoembryonic antigen (CEA), a self antigen in CEA transgenic mice, by immunizing with a recombinant vaccinia-CEA virus. *Cancer Res* 1999; 59:676–683.

34. Coupar BEH, Andrew ME, Boyle DB. A general method for the construction of recombinant vaccinia viruses expressing multiple foreign genes. *Gene* 1988; 68:1–10.

35. Smith GL, Moss B. Infectious poxvirus vectors have capacity for at least 25,000 base pairs of foreign DNA. *Gene* 1983; 25:21–28.

36. Stephens EB, Compans RW, Earle P, Moss B. Surface expression of viral glycoproteins is polarized in epithelial cells infected with recombinant vaccinia viral vectors. *EMBO J* 1986; 5:237–245.

37. Kaufman H, Schlom J, Kantor J. A recombinant vaccinia virus expressing human carcinoembryonic antigen (CEA). *Int J Cancer* 1991; 48:900–907.

38. Kantor J, Irvine K, Abrams S, Kaufman H, DiPietro J, Schlom J. Antitumor activity and immune response induced by a recombinant carcinoembryonic antigen-vaccinia virus vaccine. *J Natl Cancer Inst* 1992; 84:1084–1091.

39. Gong J, Chen D, Kashiwaba M, Li Y, Chen L, Takeuchi H, et al. Reversal of tolerance to human MUC1 antigen in MUC1 transgenic mice immunized with fusions of dendritic and carcinoma cells. *Proc Natl Acad Sci USA* 1998; 95:6279–6283.

40. Kapsopoulou-Dominos K, Anderer FA. Circulating carcinoembryonic antigen immune complexes in sera of patients with carcinomata of the gastrointestinal tract. *Clin Exp Immunol* 1979; 35:190–195.

41. Lejtenyi CM, Freedman SO, Gold P. Response of lymphocytes from patients with gastrointestinal cancer to the carcinoembryonic antigen of the digestive system. *Cancer* 1971; 28:115–120.

42. Orefice S, Fossati E, Pietrojusti E, Bonfanti G. Delayed cutaneous hypersensitivity reaction to carcinoembryonic antigen in patients. *Tumori* 1982; 68:473–475.

43. Koda J, Glass MC, Chang HR. Generation of human monoclonal antibodies against colon cancer. *Arch Surg* 1990; 125:1591–1597.

44. Durrant LG, Denton GWL, Jacobs E, Mee M, Moss R, Austin EB, et al. An idiotypic replica of carcinoembryonic antigen inducing cellular and humoral responses directed against human colorectal tumours. *Int J Cancer* 1992; 50:811–816.

45. Foon KA, Chakraborty M, John WJ, Sherratt A, Kohler H, Bhattacharya-Chatterjee M. Immune response to the carcinoembryonic antigen in patients treated with an anti-idiotype antibody vaccine. *J Clin Investig* 1995; 96:334–342.

46. Samanci A, Yi Q, Fagerberg J, Strigard K, Smith G, Ruden U, et al. Pharmacological administration of granulocyte/macrophage-colony-stimulating factor is of significant importance for the induction of a strong humoral and cellular response in patients immunized with recombinant carcinoembryonic antigen. *Cancer Immunol Immunother* 1998; 47:131–142.

47. Nair SK, Boczkowski D, Morse M, Cumming RI, Lyerly HK, Gilboa E. Induction of primary carcinoembryonic antigen (CEA)-specific cytotoxic T lymphocytes in vitro using human dendritic cells transfected with RNA. *Nature Biotech* 1998; 16:364–369.

48. Conry RM, Khazaeli MB, Saleh MN, Allen KO, Barlow DL, Moore SE, et al. Phase I trial of a recombinant vaccinia virus encoding carcinoembryonic antigen in metastatic adenocarcinoma: comparison of intradermal *versus* subcutaneous administration. *Clin Cancer Res* 1999; 5:2330–2337.

49. Marshall JL, Hawkins MJ, Tsang KY, Richmond E, Pedicano JE, Zhu M-Z, Phase I study in cancer patients of a replication-defective avipox recombinant vaccine that expresses human carcinoembryonic antigen. *J Clin Oncol* 1999; 17:332–337.

50. Zhu MZ, Marshall J, Cole D, Schlom J, Tsang KY. Specific cytolytic T-cell responses to human carcinoembryonic antigen from patients immunized with recombinant canarypox (ALVAC)-CEA vaccine. *Clin Cancer Res* 2000; 6:24–33.

51. Von Mehren M, Arlen P, Tsang KY, Rogatko A, Cooper HS, Davey M, et al. Pilot study of a dual gene recombinant Avipox vaccine containing both CEA and B7.1 transgenes, in patients with recurrent CEA expressing adenocarcinomas. *Clin Cancer Res* 6, 2219–2228.

52. McLaughlin JP, Schlom J, Kantor JA, Greiner JW. Improved immunotherapy of a recombinant CEA vaccinia vaccine when given in combination with interleukin-2. *Cancer Res* 1996; 56:2361–2367.

53. Hodge JW, Sabzevari H, Yafal AG, Gritz L, Lorenz MG, Schlom J. A triad of costimulatory molecules synergize to amplify T-cell activation. *Cancer Res* 1999; 59:5800–5807.

14 The *p53*-Deficient Mouse as a Cancer Model

Sundaresan Venkatachalam, Stuart Tyner, and Lawrence A. Donehower, PhD

CONTENTS

INTRODUCTION
TUMOR INCIDENCE AND SPECTRUM IN *p53*-DEFICIENT MICE
EFFECTS OF GENETIC BACKGROUND ON TUMORIGENESIS
BIOLOGICAL AND GENETIC ATTRIBUTES OF *p53*-DEFICIENT
    TUMORS
INFORMATIVE CROSSES USING THE *p53*-DEFICIENT MICE
EFFECTS OF CARCINOGENS ON TUMORIGENESIS
    IN *p53*-DEFICIENT MICE
FUTURE DIRECTIONS
ACKNOWLEDGMENTS
REFERENCES

1. INTRODUCTION

Among the various tumor-suppressor mouse models that have been generated since 1992 *(1)*, the *p53*-knockout mouse has been the most widely used for cancer studies for a number of reasons. The *p53* tumor-suppressor gene is mutated in over 50% of all human cancers, and it has been estimated that over 80% of all cancers have disruptions in *p53* signaling pathways *(2,3)*. Because loss or mutation of *p53* is such a central event in the progression of human tumors, it has become perhaps the most intensively studied cancer-associated gene. Moreover, both heterozygous and nullizygous *p53*-deficient mice display an accelerated tumorigenesis phenotype in comparison to their wild-type *p53*-containing litter mates *(4–7)*. Because of the increased sensitivity of the heterozygous *p53*-deficient mice to a variety of carcinogens, they are considered by the U.S. Food and Drug Administration as one of the rodent models which can be utilized in carcinogenicity assays of candidate pharmaceuticals *(8)*. Use of the *p53*-deficient mice has provided important insights into *p53* function in cell-cycle control, regulation of apoptosis, response to DNA damage, hypoxia, oncogenic stimuli, embryonic development, cancer biology, molecular biology, treatment, and prevention *(9–13)*. The focus

From: *Tumor Models in Cancer Research*
Edited by: B. A. Teicher © Humana Press Inc., Totowa, NJ

of this chapter is on the insights provided by the *p53*-deficient mice in cancer-related studies at the organismal level. Further discussion of the biology of *p53*-deficient mice is also available *(9–13)*.

Since 1989, *p53* has been known to be a critical tumor suppressor *(14,15)*. Aside from its frequent mutation and loss in somatically arising human tumors *(16)*, germline lesions in *p53* have been linked to a familial cancer predisposition called Li-Fraumeni syndrome *(17,18)*. Affected Li-Fraumeni family members have a 50% likelihood of developing cancer by age 30. The *p53* gene, when transduced into tumor cells or normal cells, has been shown to suppress growth in a variety of assays *(14,15,19)*. The *p53* protein is a transcriptional regulatory protein that responds to a variety of cell stresses, including DNA damage, hypoxia, activated oncogenes, ribonucleotide depletion, and alterations in cell adhesion *(20,21)*. These stressors induce phosphorylation of *p53* and cause it to assume an activated conformation that allows it to transcriptionally activate or repress genes that regulate cell-cycle control pathways or apoptotic pathways. Thus, activated *p53* can initiate a program of cellular apoptosis or cell-cycle arrest. Either program will prevent the cell from replicating damaged DNA or from dividing in response to illegitimate growth signaling *(20,21)*. The end result is that the organism is protected from the outgrowth of nascent cancer cells. The *p53*-deficient mice have provided a particularly valuable tool in testing some of the mechanisms by which *p53* prevents cancer.

2. TUMOR INCIDENCE AND SPECTRUM IN *P53*-DEFICIENT MICE

The development of mouse embryonic stem (ES) cell gene targeting methods provided the technological breakthrough that facilitated studies of tumor-suppressor function in mammalian systems *(22,23)*. The first germline inactivation of a tumor-suppressor gene through gene-targeting techniques was reported by our laboratory—in collaboration with Allan Bradley—in 1992, with the successful targeting of the murine *p53* gene *(4)*. The mouse that resulted from our targeting strategy contained a deletion in *p53* exon 5, accompanied by an insertion of a selectable marker cassette. Other mice generated by the Jacks and Clarke laboratories contained more extensive deletions of *p53* exons 2–6 *(6,7)*. Regardless of targeting strategy, all three lines of mice were shown to be null for *p53* function by the absence of detectable *p53* protein in nullizygous cells. Intercrossing of *p53* heterozygotes resulted in *p53*-nullizygous offspring in almost the expected Mendelian proportion of 25% *(4)*. However, subsequent studies showed that a small fraction of null embryos—all females—developed exencephaly, a perinatal lethal condition resulting from a failure of neural-tube closure during midgestation *(24,25)*.

The first cohorts of *p53*-deficient mice were of mixed inbred C57BL/6 (75%) and 129/Sv background and were monitored for tumor susceptibility *(4,5)*. Roughly 75% of the nullizygous *p53* mice developed tumors by 6 mo of age, and all had succumbed to cancer by 10 mo of age (Fig. 1). Tumor incidences in the *p53*-null lines from the Jacks and Clarke laboratories were similar to our line, although higher proportions had developed tumors by 6 mo of age *(6,7)*. The predominant tumor type observed in all three null mouse lines was a thymic lymphoma (Fig. 2). Other tumor types included lymphomas of B-cell origin, as well as soft-tissue sarcomas (particularly hemangiosarcomas). Carcinomas were relatively rare. The lymphomas tended to be

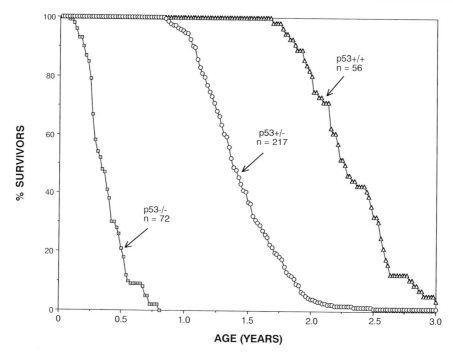

Fig. 1. Tumor-free survival in *p53*-deficient mice and their wild-type litter mates. *p53–/–, p53+/–,* and *p53+/+* mice of mixed C57BL/6 X 129/Sv genetic background were monitored for tumors over a period of 3 yr. The number of animals monitored for each genotype is indicated. Moribund animals were sacrificed and subjected to necropsy. Over 90% of *p53–/–* mice, over 80% of *p53+/–* mice, and approx 50% of *p53+/+* mice developed overt tumors. The remainder died of other diseases or natural causes, or died without a necropsy.

monoclonal in origin, indicating that loss of both *p53* alleles was insufficient for tumor formation, and that other cooperating genetic alterations were necessary for malignancy *(26)*.

Compared to the *p53–/–* mice, the *p53+/–* animals had a relatively delayed onset of tumors *(5,9,26)*. The heterozygotes did not develop tumors until roughly 9 mo of age. By 1 yr, about 5% of the *p53+/–* mice had developed tumors and by 2 yr of age, over 95% had died or were sacrificed because of cancer (Fig. 1). The tumor spectrum of the *p53+/–* mice was markedly different from that of the *p53–/–* mice. Most of the *p53+/–* tumors were evenly distributed among B-cell lymphomas, osteosarcomas, and soft-tissue sarcomas, although significant numbers of carcinomas were also noted *(5,9,26)* (Fig. 2). The differences in tumor spectrum between *p53+/–* and *p53–/–* mice have been commented on, and may relate to the vulnerability of thymic compartments early in life to *p53* nullizygosity, which then predisposes to thymic lymphomas *(10)*. This early thymic lymphoma incidence in the *p53–/–* mice precludes the observation of the other tumor types that do appear in the *p53+/–* animals. In *p53+/–* mice, thymic involution occurs before appreciable numbers of thymocytes lose the remaining wild-type *p53* allele, and thus, tumors are much less likely to arise in this compartment.

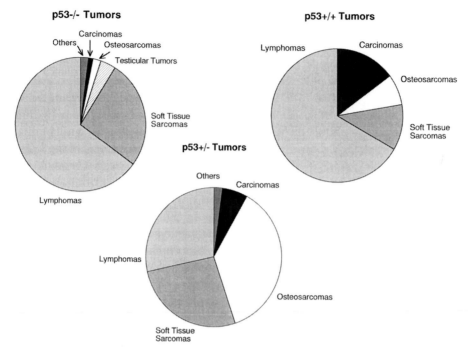

Fig. 2. Tumor spectra of *p53–/–*, *p53+/–*, and *p53+/+* mice. The relative frequency of each tumor type is indicated by the size of the pie slice.

One of the goals in developing the *p53+/–* mice was to provide a mouse model for the cognate human familial-cancer predisposition Li-Fraumeni syndrome. As previously noted, the *p53+/–* mice and affected Li-Fraumeni individuals (*p53+/–* humans) exhibit a number of similarities in their susceptibility to cancer *(9)*. Roughly one-half of affected Li-Fraumeni individuals and *p53+/–* mice develop tumors by midlife. In addition, the tumor spectra between *p53+/–* mice and humans share certain tumor types including lymphoid neoplasms, soft-tissue sarcomas, and osteosarcomas. There are differences in spectra—brain tumors and breast tumors are frequently observed in Li-Fraumeni patients, but infrequently in the *p53+/–* mice. However, such differences in spectra may be more a result of the genetic background of the predominantly C57BL/6 mice rather than any inherent species differences.

The *p53+/–* litter mates of the *p53+/–* and *p53–/–* animals have also been monitored for tumors for over 3 yr. Roughly 50% of the wild-type C57BL/6-129/Sv mice develop overt, life-threatening tumors, while most of the remainder may die of covert tumors or other natural causes. The vast majority of the wild-type mice develop tumors or die between 2 and 3 yr of age (Fig. 1), which is consistent with historical reports of longevity for C57BL strains *(27)*. The tumor types observed in the *p53+/+* mice were primarily lymphomas of B-cell origin, although sarcomas and carcinomas were occasionally observed. Overall, median survival for *p53–/–*, *p53+/–*, and *p53+/+* mice of mixed C57BL/6-129/Sv background was 17.5, 71.5, and 118 wk, respectively. Clearly, loss of *p53* function promotes early tumor formation in a dosage-dependent manner.

3. EFFECTS OF GENETIC BACKGROUND ON TUMORIGENESIS

The use of inbred strains for studying inherited tumor-suppressor gene lesions is likely to influence the resulting tumor incidence and spectrum. Different strains are known to exhibit different types of naturally occurring tumors, and such differences may affect tumor rates and types in their *p53*-deficient counterparts *(27)*. Since the *p53*-deficient mice have been developed in the C57BL/6-129/Sv background, the Jackson Laboratory and individual investigators have been backcrossing the *p53* mutations into other inbred backgrounds. In our own early experiments, we generated two lines of *p53*-deficient mice—C57BL/6-129/Sv mixed inbred mice and pure 129/Sv mice. Interestingly, while the 129/Sv-null mice still developed a high percentage of lymphomas and soft-tissue sarcomas, as observed in the C57BL/6-129/Sv mice, one-half of the *p53–/–* 129/Sv males developed testicular tumors, particularly teratomas *(26,28)*. 129/Sv mice have been previously noted to exhibit a modest predisposition to teratomas (1–2% of males) *(29)*, and it is clear that *p53* loss greatly accentuated this predisposition. Moreover, the rate of tumor incidence was accelerated in the null and heterozygous 129/Sv mice compared to their mixed-background counterparts *(26)*. These genetic-background-dependent differences in tumor incidence and spectrum are likely to be the result of genetic-modifier loci inherent in each strain.

In another study, the *p53* mutation was also crossed into the VM inbred strain, and the VM *p53–/–* mice exhibited significantly earlier lymphoma development than the C57BL/6-129/Sv-null mice. The lymphomas in the VM mice were more often poorly differentiated and confined to the thymus than those observed in the C57BL/6 lines *(30)*. Such differences again suggest the presence of strain-specific modifers affecting the onset of lymphomagenesis.

Finally, Jerry, Medina, and colleagues have backcrossed the *p53* mutation for 10 generations into the mammary-tumor-susceptible Balb/c inbred background *(31)*. Balb/c p53+/– congenic mice display a markedly increased susceptibility to mammary tumors compared to the C57BL/6-129/Sv and 129/Sv heterozygotes, in addition to the lymphomas, osteosarcomas, and soft-tissue sarcomas observed in all p53+/– strains studied to date. Moreover, transplantation of Balb/c *p53*-null mammary glands into Balb/c p53+/+ mice resulted in dramatically increased rates of mammary-tumor incidence in the transplanted hosts *(32)*. The higher incidence of mammary carcinomas in the p53+/– Balb/c lines increases the similarity in the tumor spectrum of the *p53*+/– mouse to that of the affected Li-Fraumeni families, who exhibit a high rate of breast-cancer incidence.

4. BIOLOGICAL AND GENETIC ATTRIBUTES OF *P53*-DEFICIENT TUMORS

A number of reports have shown that normal cells derived from various tissues of *p53*-null mice have increased proliferative potential in vitro *(9)*. Moreover, cells from *p53–/–* mice exhibit increased levels of genomic instability and resistance to apoptosis following apoptotic stimuli, both in vitro and in vivo. All of these attributes may contribute to the increased susceptibility of *p53–/–* cells to early tumorigenesis, particularly in those tissues with a high mitotic compartment such as the lymphoid organs. We have compared the tumors arising in *p53–/–*, *p53+/–*, and *p53+/+* mice of similar genetic background. Not surprisingly, as *p53* dosage is decreased, tumors of many types appear less differentiated and more anaplastic in morphology *(33,34)*. Moreover, decreased *p53* dosage also correlates with an increase in the percentages of tumor cells that are in S phase and mitosis, indicating increased rates of proliferation. Surprisingly, although *p53* is an important pro-apoptotic factor, apoptosis levels in the tumor cells appear to be independent of *p53* status *(34)*. Moreover, levels of tumor angiogenesis and metastases also appear to be relatively unaffected by *p53* genotype *(34)*. Perhaps the dysregulation of angiogenic and apoptotic pathways occurs much earlier in the *p53*-deficient tumors, and the lack of *p53* accelerates these changes without increasing the quantitative levels of angiogenesis and apoptosis in the end-stage tumors. This is consistent with mathematical modeling studies on tumor incidence in *p53*-deficient mice performed by Wheldon and colleagues *(35)*, who hypothesized that *p53* loss accelerates tumorigenesis by increasing the probability of occurrence of a viable cellular mutant by a factor of about 10. Presumably, some of these viable cellular mutants would include genes with dysregulated apoptotic and angiogenic responses.

The importance of *p53* as a caretaker gene—i.e. a gene that maintains genomic integrity—has been well-established by a number of studies. Loss of *p53* leads to polyploidy, aneuploidy, gene amplification, abnormal centrosome duplication, and other markers of genomic instability *(36)*. Studies have shown that even normal tissues of *p53*-deficient mice have higher percentages of cells with abnormal karyotypes and centrosome numbers than in wild-type mice *(37,38)*. We have examined tumors arising in the *p53*-deficient mice by comparative genomic hybridization (CGH), a technique that measures DNA copy-number gains or losses in each chromosome of the cell *(39)*. Tumor cells with chromosome losses or gains are readily identified by this technique. CGH analysis of 35 *p53*+/– and *p53*–/– tumors (mostly lymphomas and osteosarcomas) showed that *p53*–/– tumors had higher levels of mean chromosomal instability than *p53*+/– tumors *(40)*. Moreover, the pattern of chromosomal losses and gains was partially nonrandom in that each tumor type showed specific chromosomal regions that were frequently altered in copy number. For example, the majority of osteosarcomas exhibited loss of chromosome 12 sequences, while lymphomas often showed copy-number gains on chromosomes 14 and 15 *(40)*. These results suggest that specific tumor suppressors and oncogenes may be altered in specific tumor types and collaborate with *p53* in the induction of tumorigenesis.

Genetic analysis of *p53* status in the *p53*+/– tumors revealed that while almost one-half of the tumors did lose the entire wild-type copy of *p53* during tumorigenesis, the majority of these tumors appeared to retain the wild-type allele *(40)*. Sequence analysis revealed that the wild-type *p53* gene in this latter category of *p53*+/– tumors had not incurred a point mutation. A number of *p53* functional assays were performed on the *p53*+/– tumors that retained wild-type *p53*. All showed functional *p53*, and the tumors that lost *p53* were missing functional *p53* activity *(40)*. This result was surprising, in that the "two-hit" hypothesis for tumor suppressors, first formulated by Knudson *(41)*, holds that tumor suppressors are recessive and that both alleles must be lost or mutated as a prerequisite for tumor formation. Our hypothesis is that *p53* may be an exception to the two-hit rule, and that mere reduction of *p53* dosage may be sufficient to promote tumor formation. Thus, *p53* may be haploinsufficient for tumor suppression.

Recently, in an attempt to generate a mouse with a germline point mutation in *p53*, Lozano and colleagues have produced a mouse with a codon 172 Arg → His mutation *(42)*. This particular mutation is identical to a "hot spot" mutation in human tumors (codon 175), and it was hypothesized that such a lesion would produce a protein with a gain-of-function activity in tumorigenesis. While the mutation was successfully introduced into the mouse germline, the codon 172 mutation was accompanied by a splice-junction mutation that resulted in aberrant splicing of the mutant allele so that only a fraction of the full-length mutant *p53* mRNA was produced. Nevertheless, mutant *p53* protein was detected at roughly the same level as wild-type protein because of its increased stabilization. Interestingly, while the mice homozygous for this mutant allele did not exhibit accelerated tumorigenesis compared to *p53*-null mice, they did display a greatly elevated level of metastases, indicating that point-mutant forms of *p53* could have gain-of-function activity not observed in the *p53*-null mice *(42)*.

5. INFORMATIVE CROSSES USING THE *P53*-DEFICIENT MICE

Many mutant mouse strains have been mated to *p53*-deficient mice in an attempt to determine whether a particular genetic alteration, in conjunction with *p53,* can alter either the tumor phenotype or incidence in the double-mutant offspring. If such offspring do show differences from the parental phenotypes, then cooperativity is said to have occurred. Cooperativity also implies that the two genes affect different oncogenic pathways rather than the same pathway. However, this interpretation may be complicated by the fact that *p53* may affect tumorigenesis by globally accelerating the rate at which other oncogenic lesions occur, as proposed by Wheldon and colleagues *(35)*. Thus, if the latter interpretation is correct, it is likely that the vast majority of tumor-susceptible mutant mice crossed to *p53*-deficient mice will exhibit some level of enhanced tumorigenesis in their double-mutant offspring because of the *p53*-dependent accelerated rate of *de novo* oncogenic mutations. With a few exceptions, this is what has been observed in the literature. Moreover, in some cases, the tumor spectrum is altered in comparison to the tumor-susceptible parental mice. Such crosses have provided important new insights into *p53* function in tumor suppression. Representative examples are discussed in the following sections.

5.1. Crosses to Immunodeficient Mice

The high level of lymphomas in *p53*-deficient mice was initially hypothesized by us to be a result of the C57BL/6 genetic background *(4)*. Normal C57BL/6 mice have a relatively high lymphoma incidence in old age *(27)*. However, lymphomas occur in high numbers in virtually every strain background into which the mutant *p53* allele is crossed *(10)*. Thus, subsequent models postulated that the early lymphomas in *p53*-deficient mice may be a result of aberrant checkpoint control during V(D)J recombination in the lymphoid precursor cells. The *p53* protein may play a role in induction of apoptosis in cells with abnormal V(D)J recombination events. In the absence of *p53,* those cells with aberrant V(D)J recombinations would not be eliminated and a fraction of such defective cells may become lymphomas. To test this model, tumorigenesis, lymphoid-cell differentiation, and V(D)J recombination has been assessed in mice crossed to *scid* (severe combined immunodeficiency) mice. *Scid* mice have a defect in the DNA-dependent protein kinase (DNA-PK), which results in defective end processing during V(D)J recombination and defective B- and T-cell differentiation. In the absence of *p53, scid* mice exhibit enhanced B-cell lymphomagenesis compared to *p53*-null parental mice, as well as partial rescue of T-cell differentiation, suggesting the possibility that the tumorigenic enhancement was related to V(D)J recombination *(43–45)*.

If V(D)J recombination is a critical cause of lymphomagenesis in *p53*-deficient mice, then *p53*-deficient mice incapable of initiating V(D)J recombination should show delayed or reduced levels of lymphomas. In fact, *p53*-null mice missing *Rag-1* or *Rag-2* (which are required to form the cleavage products at the beginning of V(D)J recombination) displayed accelerated or equivalent lymphomagenesis, respectively, compared to *p53*-null animals *(46,47)*. These results indicated that events other than V(D)J recombination are responsible for lymphomagenesis in *p53*-null mice.

5.2 Crosses to Oncogene-Containing Transgenic Mice

A large number of oncogene-containing transgenic lines have been crossed to *p53*-deficient mice. Most (but not all) of the transgenic offspring showed an enhanced tumorigenesis in the absence of *p53*. In some cases, such as the MMTV-*c-H-ras* transgenic mice, synergistic effects were observed in increased salivary-gland tumors rather than mammary tumors *(48)*. Likewise, MMTV-*c-myc, p53*-deficient mice showed enhancement of T-cell lymphomagenesis rather than mammary tumors *(49)*. In most cases, however, the expected synergistic effect was noted. *Wnt-1, c-myc,* and *Scl* oncogenes all behaved synergistically with *p53*—not a surprising result since it is unlikely that the pathways regulated by these oncogenes overlap completely with those of *p53 (33,50,51)*.

Two crosses in which the transgene pathways were likely to overlap with *p53* were performed by our laboratory. The first cross was between a mouse with a globally expressed mutant murine *p53* transgene (codon 135 ala→val) and the *p53*-deficient mice *(52)*. This particular cross was of interest because of the evidence that intact mutant forms of *p53* have gain-of-function activity. Would the mutant *p53* transgene show accelerated tumorigenesis in the absence of wild-type *p53?* In fact, the *p53*-null mice with the mutant transgene developed tumors at the same rate as *p53*-null mice, arguing against a gain-of-function activity for this particular mutant *p53* in vivo. Interestingly, *p53*+/– mice with the mutant *p53* transgene showed an earlier tumor incidence than *p53*+/– mice, indicating that the mutant *p53* did possess dominant negative function (the ability to suppress wild-type *p53* function), if not gain-of-function activity *(52)*. The second overlapping cross was between an mdm2 transgenic mouse (resulting in global expression of Mdm2 protein) and the *p53*-deficient mice *(53)*. Mdm2 protein interacts with wild-type *p53* and mediates its degradation *(54)*. Thus, Mdm2 overexpression is likely to be functionally equivalent to *p53* inactivation. In fact, *mdm2* transgenic mice develop tumors at a rate roughly equivalent to that of the *p53*+/– mice, with a similar tumor spectrum (sarcomas and lymphomas) *(53)*. *Mdm2* transgenic *p53*–/– mice developed tumors at the same rate as *p53*–/– mice, though the incidence of sarcomas was increased in the mdm2 transgenic *p53*-null mice *(53)*. This altered sarcomagenesis result indicates that mdm2 does have a *p53*-independent role in mesenchymal tissues, but its nature remains unclear.

5.3. Crosses to Tumor-Suppressor-Deficient Mice

Crosses of *p53*-deficient mice to other tumor-suppressor-deficient mice usually resulted in offspring with enhanced susceptibility to cancer. Moreover, the doubly deficient mice often displayed novel tumor types not observed in either singly deficient parent. An example is the *p53* crosses performed by our laboratory and the Jacks laboratory with mice deficient in the retinoblastoma *(Rb)* susceptibility locus *(55,56)*. Humans with germline *RB* mutations are susceptible to childhood retinoblastomas, but mouse *Rb* heterozygotes (Rb–/– mice display embryonic lethality) are susceptible primarily to pituitary adenomas rather than retinoblastomas. Mice heterozygous for both *p53* and *Rb* showed a mean survival of 9 mo vs 11 mo for *Rb*+/– mice and 16 mo for *p53*+/– mice. The double heterozygotes also displayed novel endocrine tumors (pancreatic islet-cell carcinomas, pinealoblastomas, and medullary thryroid carcinomas) not observed in the *p53*+/– or *Rb*+/– parents.

In other tumor-suppressor-deficient mouse crosses, mice deficient for *Apc* and *p53* exhibited either novel pancreatic tumors or desmoid fibromas *(57,58)*. Germline APC mutations in humans confer susceptibility to intestinal polyps, and *Apc*-mutant mice exhibit a strong predisposition to early intestinal tumors *(59)*. In one case, enhancement of intestinal tumor incidence was noted in the absence of *p53* (58), while in another instance, intestinal tumor incidence in the doubly deficient mice was similar to that of the *Apc*-mutant parental mice *(57)*. The contrast in intestinal tumor enhancement was ascribed to genetic background differences *(58)*.

Another interesting interaction has been observed between *Brca1* and *p53* in these types of crosses. In humans, *BRCA1* mutations predispose to breast and ovarian cancers, and up to 90% of these tumors have a *p53* mutation *(60)*. However, *Brca1* heterozygosity in mice does not predispose the animals to early mammary cancers *(1)*. Following crosses of *p53*-deficient and *Brca1*-deficient mice, *p53*–/– *Brca1*+/– mice had a modestly increased mammary-tumor incidence compared to *p53*–/– mice *(61)*. Moreover, irradiated *p53*+/– *Brca1*+/– mice showed a slight increase in mammary-tumor formation compared to irradiated *p53*+/– mice. Encouraging as this result was, a more definitive experiment was performed by Xu et al. *(62)* when they generated a conditional allele of *Brca1* in mice that could be partially deleted specifically in the mammary gland following crossing to a mouse with expression of the mammary-gland-specific Cre recombinase. When both alleles of *Brca1* were excised in the mammary gland of the offspring, they developed mammary tumors after a long latency period. However, in the absence of *p53* and the presence of mammary-gland-specific Cre, these mice homozygous for the mutant *Brca1* conditional allele developed mammary tumors much sooner *(62)*.

5.4. Crosses to DNA Repair Gene-Deficient Mice

Mice deficient in a variety of DNA repair genes have been crossed to *p53*-deficient mice, and the offspring have almost uniformly shown increased susceptibility to early cancers *(10)*. *Atm*-null mice deficient for the ataxia telangiectasia gene develop lymphomas (like their human counterparts) that can be accelerated by introduction of mutant *p53* *(63)*. ATM is a kinase involved in maintaining genome stability, in part through its phosphorylation of *p53* following DNA damage. The cooperativity indicates that the oncogenic role of *Atm* deficiency is not only a result of its interactions with *p53*. In another example, mice with defects in the mismatch repair gene *Msh2* and the nucleotide excision-repair gene *Xpc* exhibit accelerated tumorigenesis in a *p53*-mutant background *(64)*. A number of other DNA repair genes also cooperate with *p53* in enhancing tumorigenesis. These data indicate that the absence of different proteins active in maintaining genomic stability through different mechanisms can synergize and enhance tumor susceptibility.

6. EFFECTS OF CARCINOGENS ON TUMORIGENESIS IN *P53*-DEFICIENT MICE

A critical function of *p53* is in its response to DNA damage. Genotoxic agents frequently produce increased levels of activated and stabilized *p53* protein, which can induce either a growth arrest or apoptosis. Cells without *p53* are more likely to survive and propagate the induced DNA damage in the form of mutations. Moreover, such mutagenized *p53*-deficient cells appear to be more likely to acquire subsequent genomic alterations, which may accelerate the tumorigenic process. The *p53*-deficient mice have provided a useful tool for assessing *p53* function in response to DNA-damaging agents and carcinogens. In particular, there has been a great deal of interest from the toxicology community in validating the *p53*+/– mice as testing vehicles for suspected carcinogens *(8,65,66)*. Current 2-y rodent bioassays for carcinogenicity are time-consuming and expensive. More sensitive testing models should reduce testing time, animal numbers, labor, and expense. Currently, 6-mo carcinogenicity assays on *p53*+/– mice are being evaluated as a substitute for the longer 2-y carcinogenicity assay on wild-type mice and rats *(8,65,66)*. The *p53*+/– mice may have significant advantages over wild-type mice for carcinogenicity assays for a number of reasons *(1)*. Aside from enhanced tumor susceptibility, they are completely normal, and similar to *p53*+/+ mice in virtually every measurable way *(2)*. They are susceptible to a broad range of tumor types *(3)*. They rarely develop tumors until about 9 mo of age, providing a useful low background of spontaneous tumors *(4)*. *p53* mutations frequently arise in human somatic tumors, making this particular mouse a more genetically relevant model for human tumors *(5)*. The retention of the wild-type *p53* allele in some *p53*+/– tumors indicates that *p53* loss of heterozygosity *(LOH)* is not a prerequisite for tumor formation *(40)*, and thus a suspected carcinogen need not directly target the *p53* gene to induce tumors *(6)*. Finally, a wide array of physical and chemical carcinogens have been shown to accelerate tumors in the *p53*+/– mice compared to wild-type mice *(8, 65, 66)*.

Scores of published papers have now described the effects of mutagens on tumorigenesis on *p53*-deficient mice. Using appropriate marker animals, we and others have found that *p53* deficiency does not necessarily increase point mutation rates in mutagenized animals *(67–69)*. Instead, *p53* deficiency may promote tumorigenesis through its inability to eliminate cells that do acquire oncogenic mutations. It has been well-established that *p53*-deficient mice have deficiencies in apoptosis following irradiation and other DNA-damage events *(70,71)*. Moreover, the reduction in cell-cycle checkpoint control and consequent chromosomal instability arising from increased cell-cycle progression may increase the likelihood that these cells will acquire further oncogenic lesions. Indirect support for this idea has come from Sukata et al. *(72)*, who demonstrated that *p53*-deficient mice treated with several different carcinogens showed increased rates of cell proliferation in a variety of target organs compared to wild-type mice, particularly in those organs that have been shown to be highly susceptible to carcinogen-induced tumorigenesis.

Several tentative conclusions can be drawn from the carcinogen treatment studies. Early studies have indicated that *p53*-deficient heterozygous mice are more susceptible to genotoxic carcinogens and insensitive to nongenotoxic carcinogens *(73,74)*. In fact, 6-mo carcinogenicity assays on *p53*+/– mice have demonstrated increased tumorigenesis for 13 of 16 genotoxic carcinogens and 0 of 11 nongenotoxic carcinogens (J. French, personal communication). This result is consistent with the role of *p53* in DNA damage response. In those cases where *p53*-null mice are used, they usually show enhanced tumorigenesis. However, because *p53*–/– mice have such a high rate of early spontaneous tumor formation, they may not be particularly useful in the development of new rodent carcinogen bioassays.

When *p53*+/– animals are treated with carcinogens, enhanced tumorigenesis does not invariably result. Some organs appear to be highly susceptible to accelerated carcinogenesis while others are not noticeably affected. Organs that appear highly susceptible are the skin, lymphoid organs, connective tissue, bladder, and stomach. Less sensitive organs appear to include the liver, lung, and mammary glands. However, recent studies have shown that carcinogen sensitivity in the mammary gland can be greatly augmented by changing the genetic background from C57BL/6 to Balb/c *(31,32)*. Given the mixed sensitivity of the *p53*+/– mice to carcinogens, it is clear that further testing must be performed in order to clarify which organs and carcinogens will be likely to generate an accelerated response. In addition, it may be useful to assess strains of mice other than C57BL/6 for carcinogen-induced tumor susceptibility in the context of *p53* deficiency. Nevertheless, despite the potential limitations of the model, it is likely to provide important new insights into carcinogenesis and a useful tool to complement current rodent carcinogenicity assays.

7. FUTURE DIRECTIONS

Most of the emphasis in this chapter has been on the first-generation *p53*-mutant mice that were null mutations. However, as the point-mutant *p53* mouse described by the Lozano lab has indicated *(42)*, new second-generation *p53*-mutant mice are in development and are providing important conceptual advances. Other mice with point mutations similar to those observed in human tumors or in Li-Fraumeni lineages are being generated and should provide more genetically accurate replicas of human tumor models. In addition to generating oncogenic mutations in *p53* alleles, mutations to identify defined functional domains in *p53* are being engineered. These should provide new insights into *p53* function in vivo. Another approach will be the generation of conditional mutant alleles of *p53*, to inactivate it only in specific spatial or temporal contexts within the organism. The Cre-LoxP targeting strategies will allow the generation of inactivated *p53* alleles only in select tissues. Recently, such a mouse with a germline *p53* allele flanked by excisable loxP sites has been described *(75)*. These mice will circumvent the limitations associated with early lymphomas in the current models, which prevent the visualization of tumors in other *p53*-deficient tissues. The development and progression of the new gene-targeting technologies will usher in a host of new and exciting mouse models for *p53*, which will not only facilitate our understanding of the role of *p53* in tumor prevention, but its role in a number of other biological processes, including development, differentiation, and aging.

ACKNOWLEDGMENTS

This work was supported by grants to L.A.D. from the National Cancer Institute, the National Institute of Environmental Health Sciences, and the U.S. Army Breast Cancer Program. S.T. and S.V. were supported by a Viral Oncology training grant from the National Cancer Institute.

REFERENCES

1. Ghebranious N, Donehower LA. Mouse models in tumor suppression. *Oncogene* 1998; 17:3385–3400.
2. Levine AJ. p53, the cellular gatekeeper for growth and division. *Cell* 1997; 88:323–331.
3. Lozano G, Elledge SJ. p53 sends nucleotides to repair DNA. Nature 404:23–25.
4. Donehower LA, Harvey M, Slagle BL, McArthur MJ, Montgomery CA Jr, Butel JS, et al. Mice deficient for p53 are developmentally normal but susceptible to spontaneous tumours. *Nature* 1992; 356:215–221.
5. Harvey M, McArthur MJ, Montgomery CA Jr, Butel JS, Bradley A, Donehower LA. Spontaneous and carcinogen-induced tumorigenesis in p53-deficient mice. *Nat Genet* 1993; 5:225–229.
6. Jacks T, Remington L, Williams BO, Schmitt EM, Halachmi S, Bronson RT, et al. Tumor spectrum analysis in p53-mutant mice. *Curr Biol* 1994; 4:1–7.
7. Purdie CA, Harrison DJ, Peter A, Dobbie L, White S, Howie SEM, et al. Tumour incidence, spectrum and ploidy in mice with a large deletion in the p53 gene. *Oncogene* 1994; 9:603–609.
8. Contrera JF, DeGeorge JJ. In vivo transgenic bioassays and assessment of the carcinogenic potential of pharmaceuticals. *Environ Health Perspect* 1998; 106 (Suppl. 1):71–80.
9. Donehower LA. The p53-deficient mouse: a model for basic and applied cancer studies. *Semin Cancer Biol* 1996; 7:269–278.
10. Attardi LD, Jacks T. The role of p53 in tumour suppression: lessons from mouse models. *Cell Mol Life Sci* 1999; 55:48–63.
11. Jacks T. Lessons from the p53 mutant mouse. *J Cancer Res Clin Oncol* 1996; 122:319–327.
12. Donehower LA. Effects of p53 mutation on tumor progression: recent insights from mouse tumor models. *Biochim Biophys Acta* 1996; 1242:171–176.
13. Lozano G, Liu G. Mouse models dissect the role of p53 in cancer and development. *Semin Cancer Biol* 1998; 8:337–344.
14. Finlay CA, Hinds PW, Levine AJ. The p53 proto-oncogene can act as a suppressor of transformation. *Cell* 1989; 57:1083–1093.
15. Eliyahu D, Michalovitz D, Eliyahu S, Pinhasi-Kimhi O, Oren M. Wild-type p53 can inhibit oncogene-mediated focus formation. *Proc Natl Acad Sci USA* 1989; 86:8763–8767.
16. Nigro JM, Baker SJ, Preisinger AC, Jessup JM, Hostetter R, Cleary K, et al. Mutations in the p53 gene occur in diverse human tumour types. *Nature* 1989; 342:705–708.
17. Malkin D, Li FP, Strong LC, Fraumeni JF Jr, Nelson CE, Kim DH, et al. Germ line p53 mutations in a familial syndrome of breast cancer, sarcomas, and other neoplasms. *Science* 1990; 250:1233–1238.
18. Srivastava S, Zou ZQ, Pirollo K, Blattner W, Chang EH. Germ-line transmission of a mutated p53 gene in a cancer-prone family with Li-Fraumeni syndrome. *Nature* 1990; 348:747–749.
19. Baker SJ, Markowitz S, Fearon ER, Willson JK, Vogelstein B. Suppression of human colorectal carcinoma cell growth by wild-type p53. *Science* 1990; 249:912–915.
20. Giaccia AJ, Kastan MB. The complexity of p53 modulation: emerging patterns from divergent signals. *Genes Dev* 1998; 12:m2973–2983.
21. Steele RJ, Thompson AM, Hall PA, Lane DP. The p53 tumour suppressor gene. *Br J Surg* 1998; 85:1460–1467.
22. Bradley A, Zheng B, Liu P. Thirteen years of manipulating the mouse genome: a personal history. *Int J Dev Biol* 1998; 42:943–950.
23. Kumar TR, Donehower LA, Bradley A, Matzuk MM. Transgenic mouse models for tumour-suppressor genes. *J Intern Med* 1995; 238:233–238.
24. Sah VP, Attardi LD, Mulligan GJ, Williams BO, Bronson RT, Jacks T. A subset of p53-deficient embryos exhibit exencephaly. *Nat Genet* 1995; 10:175–180.
25. Armstrong JF, Kaufman MH, Harrison DJ, Clarke AR. High-frequency developmental abnormalities in p53-deficient mice. *Curr Biol* 1995; 5:931–936.
26. Donehower LA, Harvey M, Vogel H, McArthur MJ, Montgomery CA Jr, Park SH, et al. Effects of genetic background on tumorigenesis in p53-deficient mice. *Mol Carcinog* 1995; 14:16–22.
27. Altman PL, Katz DD. Biological Handbooks III: inbred and genetically defined strains of laboratory animals. Part 1: mouse and rat. *FASEB J.* Bethesda, MD, 1979.
28. Harvey M, McArthur MJ, Montgomery CA Jr, Bradley A, Donehower LA. Genetic background alters the spectrum of tumors that develop in p53-deficient mice. *FASEB J* 1993 Jul;7(10):938–943.
29. Stevens LC, Little CC. Spontaneous testicular teratomas in an inbred strain of mice. *Proc Natl Acad Sci USA* 1954; 40:1080–1087.

30. van Meyel DJ, Sanchez-Sweatman OH, Kerkvliet N, Stitt L, Ramsay DA, Khokha R, et al. Genetic background influences timing, morphology and dissemination of lymphomas in p53-deficient mice. *Int J Oncol* 1998; 13:917–922.

31. Kuperwasser C, Hurlbut GD, Kittrell FS, Dickinson ES, Laucirica R, Medina D, Naber SP, Jerry DJ. Development of spontaneous mammary tumors in BALB/c p53 heterozygous mice: A model for Li-fraumeni syndrome. *Am J Pathol.* 2000; 157:2151–2159.

32. Jerry DJ, Kittrell FS, Kuperwasser C, Laucirica R, Dickinson ES, Bonilla PJ, et al. A mammary-specific model demonstrates the role of the p53 tumor suppressor gene in tumor development. *Oncogene* 2000; 19:1052–1058.

33. Donehower LA, Godley LA, Aldaz CM, Pyle R, Shi YP, Pinkel D, et al. Deficiency of p53 accelerates mammary tumorigenesis in Wnt-1 transgenic mice and promotes chromosomal instability. *Genes Dev* 1995; 9:882–895.

34. Tyner SD, Choi J, Laucirica R, Ford RJ, Donehower LA. Increased tumor cell proliferation in murine tumors with decreasing dosage of wild-type p53. *Mol Carcinog* 1999; 24:197–208.

35. Mao JH, Lindsay KA, Balmain A, Wheldon TE. Stochastic modelling of tumorigenesis in p53 deficient mice. *Br J Cancer* 1998; 77:243–352.

36. Wahl GM, Linke SP, Paulson TG, Huang LC. Maintaining genetic stability through TP53 mediated checkpoint control. *Cancer Surv* 1997; 29:183–219.

37. Cross SM, Sanchez CA, Morgan CA, Schimke MK, Ramel S, Idzerda RL, et al. A p53-dependent mouse spindle checkpoint. *Science* 1995; 267:1353–1356.

38. Fukasawa K, Wiener F, Vande Woude GF, Mai S. Genomic instability and apoptosis are frequent in p53 deficient young mice. *Oncogene* 1997; 15:1295–1302.

39. Kallioniemi OP, Kallioniemi A, Sudar D, Rutovitz D, Gray JW, Waldman F, et al. Comparative genomic hybridization: a rapid new method for detecting and mapping DNA amplification in tumors. *Semin Cancer Biol* 1993; 4:41–46.

40. Venkatachalam S, Shi YP, Jones SN, Vogel H, Bradley A, Pinkel D, et al. Retention of wild-type p53 in tumors from p53 heterozygous mice: reduction of p53 dosage can promote cancer formation *EMBO J* 1998; 17:4657–4667.

41. Knudson AG Jr. Mutation and cancer: statistical study of retinoblastoma. *Proc Natl Acad Sci USA* 1971; 68:820–823.

42. Liu G, McDonnell TJ, Montes de Oca Luna R, Kapoor M, Mims B, El-Naggar AK, et al. High metastatic potential in mice inheriting a targeted p53 missense mutation. *Proc Natl Acad Sci USA* 2000; 97:4174–4179.

43. Bogue MA, Zhu C, Aguilar-Cordova E, Donehower LA, Roth DB. p53 is required for both radiation-induced differentiation and rescue of V(D)J rearrangement in scid mouse thymocytes. *Genes Dev* 1996; 10:553–565.

44. Nacht M, Strasser A, Chan YR, Harris AW, Schlissel M, Bronson RT, et al. Mutations in the p53 and SCID genes cooperate in tumorigenesis. *Genes Dev* 1996; 10:2055–2066.

45. Guidos CJ, Williams CJ, Grandal I, Knowles G, Huang MT, Danska JS. V(D)J recombination activates a p53-dependent DNA damage checkpoint in scid lymphocyte precursors. *Genes Dev* 1996; 10:2038–2054.

46. Nacht M, Jacks T. V(D)J recombination is not required for the development of lymphoma in p53-deficient mice. *Cell Growth Differ* 1998; 9:131–138.

47. Liao MJ, Zhang XX, Hill R, Gao J, Qumsiyeh MB, Nichols W, et al. No requirement for V(D)J recombination in p53-deficient thymic lymphoma. *Mol Cell Biol* 1998; 18:3495–3501.

48. Hundley JE, Koester SK, Troyer DA, Hilsenbeck SG, Subler MA, Windle JJ. Increased tumor proliferation and genomic instability without decreased apoptosis in MMTV-ras mice deficient in p53. *Mol Cell Biol* 1997; 17:723–731.

49. Elson A, Deng C, Campos-Torres J, Donehower LA, Leder P. The MMTV/c-myc transgene and p53 null alleles collaborate to induce T-cell lymphomas, but not mammary carcinomas in transgenic mice. *Oncogene* 1995; 11:181–190.

50. Blyth K, Terry A, O'Hara M, Baxter EW, Campbell M, Stewart M, et al. Synergy between a human c-myc transgene and p53 null genotype in murine thymic lymphomas: contrasting effects of homozygous and heterozygous p53 loss. *Oncogene* 1995; 10:1717–1723.

51. Condorelli GL, Facchiano F, Valtieri M, Proietti E, Vitelli L, Lulli V, et al. T-cell-directed TAL-1 expression induces T-cell malignancies in transgenic mice. *Cancer Res* 1996; 56:5113–5119.

52. Harvey M, Vogel H, Morris D, Bradley A, Bernstein A, Donehower LA. A mutant p53 transgene accelerates tumour development in heterozygous but not nullizygous p53-deficient mice. *Nat Genet* 1995; 9:305–311.

53. Jones SN, Hancock AR, Vogel H, Donehower LA, Bradley A. Overexpression of Mdm2 in mice reveals a p53-independent role for Mdm2 in tumorigenesis. *Proc Natl Acad Sci USA* 1998; 95:15,608–15,612.

54. Freedman DA, Wu L, Levine AJ. Functions of the MDM2 oncoprotein. *Cell Mol Life Sci* 1999; 55:96–107.

55. Williams BO, Remington L, Albert DM, Mukai S, Bronson RT, Jacks T. Cooperative tumorigenic effects of germline mutations in Rb and p53. *Nat Genet* 1994; 7:480–484.

56. Harvey M, Vogel H, Lee EY, Bradley A, Donehower LA. Mice deficient in both p53 and Rb develop tumors primarily of endocrine origin. *Cancer Res* 1995; 55:1146–1151.

57. Clarke AR, Cummings MC, Harrison DJ. Interaction between murine germline mutations in p53 and APC predisposes to pancreatic neoplasia but not to increased intestinal malignancy. *Oncogene* 1995; 11:1913–1920.

58. Halberg RB, Katzung DS, Hoff PD, Moser AR, Cole CE, Lubet RA, et al. Tumorigenesis in the multiple intestinal neoplasia mouse: redundancy of negative regulators and specificity of modifiers. *Proc Natl Acad Sci USA* 2000; 97:3461–3466.

59. Bilger A, Shoemaker AR, Gould KA, Dove WF. Manipulation of the mouse germline in the study of Min-induced neoplasia. *Semin Cancer Biol* 1996; 7:249–260.

60. Schuyer M, Berns EM. Is TP53 dysfunction required for BRCA1-associated carcinogenesis? *Mol Cell Endocrinol* 1999; 155:143–152.

61. Cressman VL, Backlund DC, Hicks EM, Gowen LC, Godfrey V, Koller BH. Mammary tumor formation in p53- and BRCA1-deficient mice. *Cell Growth Differ* 1999; 10:1–10.

62. Xu X, Wagner KU, Larson D, Weaver Z, Li C, Ried T, et al. Conditional mutation of Brca1 in mammary epithelial cells results in blunted ductal morphogenesis and tumour formation. *Nat Genet* 1999; 22:37–43.

63. Westphal CH, Rowan S, Schmaltz C, Elson A, Fisher DE, Leder P. Atm and p53 cooperate in apoptosis and suppression of tumorigenesis, but not in resistance to acute radiation toxicity. *Nat Genet* 1997; 16:397–401.

64. Cheo DL, Meira LB, Hammer RE, Burns DK, Doughty AT, Friedberg EC. Synergistic interactions between XPC and p53 mutations in double-mutant mice: neural tube abnormalities and accelerated UV radiation-induced skin cancer. *Curr Biol* 1996; 6:1691–1694.

65. Robinson D. The International Life Sciences Institute's role in the evaluation of alternative methodologies for the assessment of carcinogenic risk. *Toxicol Pathol* 1998; 26:474–475.

66. Tennant RW, Stasiewicz S, Mennear J, French JE, Spalding JW. Genetically altered mouse models for identifying carcinogens. *IARC Sci Publ* 1999; (146):123–150.

67. Sands AT, Suraokar MB, Sanchez A, Marth JE, Donehower LA, Bradley A. p53 deficiency does not affect the accumulation of point mutations in a transgene target. *Proc Natl Acad Sci USA* 1995; 92:8517–8521.

68. Nishino H, Knoll A, Buettner VL, Frisk CS, Maruta Y, Haavik J, et al. p53 wild-type and p53 nullizygous Big Blue transgenic mice have similar frequencies and patterns of observed mutation in liver, spleen and brain. *Oncogene* 1995; 11:263–270.

69. Buettner VL, Nishino H, Haavik J, Knoll A, Hill K, Sommer SS. Spontaneous mutation frequencies and spectra in p53 (+/+) and p53 (–/–) mice: a test of the guardian of the hypothesis in the Big Blue transgenic mouse mutation detection system. *Mutat Res* 1997; 379:13–20.

70. Bates S, Vousden KH. Mechanisms of p53-mediated apoptosis. *Cell Mol Life Sci* 1999; 55:28–37.

71. Lowe SW, Schmitt EM, Smith SW, Osborne BA, Jacks T. p53 is required for radiation-induced apoptosis in mouse thymocytes. *Nature* 1993; 362:847–849.

72. Sukata T, Ozaki K, Uwagawa S, Seki T, Wanibuchi H, Yamamoto S, et al. Organ-specific, carcinogen-induced increases in cell proliferation in p53-deficient mice. *Cancer Res* 2000; 60:74–79.

73. Tennant RW, Spalding J, French JE. Evaluation of transgenic mouse bioassays for identifying carcinogens and noncarcinogens. *Mutat Res* 1996; 365:119–127.

74. Spalding JW, French JE, Stasiewicz S, Furedi-Machacek M, Conner F, Tice RR, et al. Responses of transgenic mouse lines p53(+/–) and Tg.AC to agents tested in conventional carcinogenicity bioassays. *Toxicol Sci* 2000; 53:213–223.

75. Marino S, Vooijs M, van Der Gulden H, Jonkers J, Berns A. Induction of medulloblastomas in p53-null mutant mice by somatic inactivation of Rb in the external granular layer cells of the cerebellum. *Genes Dev* 2000; 15;14:994–1004.
76. Kemp CJ, Donehower LA, Bradley A, Balmain A. Reduction of p53 gene dosage does not increase initiation or promotion but enhances malignant progression of chemically induced skin tumors. *Cell* 1993; 74:813–822.
77. Tennant RW, French JE, Spalding JW. Identifying chemical carcinogens and assessing potential risk in short-term bioassays using transgenic mouse models. *Environ Health Perspect* 1995; 103:942–950.
78. Jerry DJ, Butel JS, Donehower LA, Paulson EJ, Cochran C, Wiseman RW, et al. Infrequent p53 mutations in 7,12-dimethylbenz[a]anthracene-induced mammary tumors in Balb/c and p53 hemizygous mice. *Mol Carcinog* 1994; 9: 175–183.
79. Jerry DJ, Kittrell FS, Kuperwasser C, Laucirica R, Dickinson ES, Bonilla PJ, et al. A mammary-specific model demonstrates the role of the p53 tumor suppressor gene in tumor development. *Oncogene* 2000; 21:1052–1058.
80. Kemp CJ. Hepatocarcinogenesis in p53-deficient mice. *Mol. Carcinog* 1995; 12:132–136.
81. Matzinger SA, Crist KA, Stoner GD, Anderson MW, Pereira MA, Steele VE, et al. K-ras mutations in lung tumors from A/J and A/J x TSG-p53 F1 mice treated 4-(methylnitrosamino)-1-(3-pyridyl)-1-butanone and phenethyl isothiocyanate. *Carcinogenesis* 1995; 16:2487–2492.
82. Dunnick JK, Hardisty JF, Herbert RA, Seely JC, Furedi-Machacek EM, Foley JF, et al. Lacks GD, Stasiewicz S, French JE. Phenolphthalein induces thymic lymphomas accompanied by loss of the p53 wild type allele in heterozygous p53-deficient (+/–) mice. *Toxicol Pathol* 1997; 25:533–540.
83. Yamamoto S, Min W, Lee CC, Salim EI, Wanibuchi H, Sukata T, et al. Enhancement of urinary bladder carcinogenesis in nullizygous p53-deficient mice by N-butyl-N-(4-hydroxybutyl)nitrosamine. *Cancer Lett* 1999; 135:137–144.
84. Dass SB, Bucci TJ, Heflich RH, Casciano DA. Evaluation of the transgenic p53+/– mouse for detecting genotoxic liver carcinogens in a short-term bioassay. *Cancer Lett* 1999; 143:81–85.
85. Kemp CJ, Wheldon T, Balmain A. p53-deficient mice are extremely susceptible to radiation-induced tumorigenesis. *Nat Genet* 1994; 8:66–69.
86. Park CB, Kim DJ, Uehara N, Takasuka N, Hiroyasu BT, Tsuda H. Heterozygous p53-deficient mice are not susceptible to 2-amino-3,8-dimethylimidazo[4,5-f] quinoxaline (MeIQx) carcinogenicity. *Cancer Lett* 1999; 139:177–182.
87. Li G, Tron V, HoV. Induction of squamous cell carcinoma in p53-deficient mice after ultraviolet irradiation. *J Invest Dermatol* 1998; 110:72–75.
88. Boley SE, Anderson EE, French JE, Donehower LA, Walker DB, Recio L. Loss of p53 in benzene-induced thymic lymphomas in p53+/– mice: evidence of homologous recombination. *Cancer Res* 2000; 60:2831–2835.
89. Ohgaki H, Fukuda M, Tohma Y, Huang, H, Stoica G, Tatematsu M, et al. Effect of intragastric application of N-Methylnitrosourea (MNU) in p53 knockout mice. *Mol Carcinog* 28, 97–101.
90. Finch GL, March TH, Hahn FF, Barr EB, Belinsky SA, Hoover MD, et al. Carcinogenic responses of transgenic heterozygous p53 knockout mice to inhaled 239PuO2 or metallic beryllium. *Toxicol Pathol* 1998; 26:484–491.

15 The Utility of Transgenic Mouse Models for Cancer Prevention Research

Stephen D. Hursting, PhD, MPH
and Ronald A. Lubet, PhD

CONTENTS

1. INTRODUCTION

Humans are exposed to a wide variety of carcinogenic insults, including chemicals, radiation, physical agents, and viruses. Animal models have contributed significantly to our understanding of the carcinogenesis process and ways to interfere with that process. The major stages of carcinogenesis (Fig. 1), deduced primarily from chemically induced tumor studies in mice and rats over the past fifty years, are termed initiation, promotion, and progression (1). Tumor initiation begins in cells with DNA damage, resulting from exposure of that cell's genetic material to exogenous or endogenous carcinogens. Unless repaired, DNA damage results in genetic mutations that can alter the responsiveness of the mutated cells to their microenvironment, eventually providing them with a growth advantage relative to normal cells. The tumor-promotion stage is characterized by clonal expansion of initiated cells caused by alterations in the expression of genes whose products are associated with hyperproliferation, apoptosis, tissue remodeling, and inflammation (2). During the tumor-progression stage, preneoplastic cells develop into invasive tumors through further clonal expansion, usually associated with altered gene expression and additional genetic damage caused by progressive genomic instability (3).

From: *Tumor Models in Cancer Research*
Edited by: B. A. Teicher © Humana Press Inc., Totowa, NJ

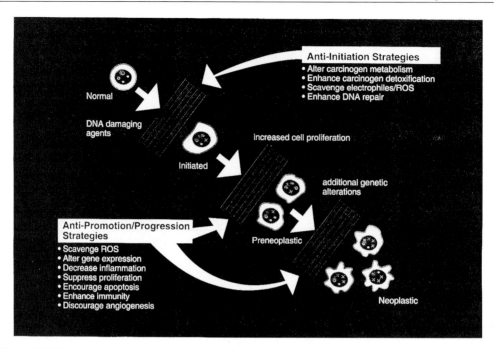

Fig. 1. Multistage carcinogenesis: Processes and prevention strategies. Schematic presentation of the stages in experimental carcinogenesis and potential targets for prevention. The initiation stage is depicted as the conversion of a normal cell to an initiated cell in response to DNA damaging agents, with the genetic damage indicated by an X. The promotion stage is depicted as the transformation of an initiated cell into a preneoplastic cell caused by alterations in gene expression and cell proliferation. The progression stage is shown as the transformation of a preneoplastic cell to a neoplastic cell as a result of additional genetic alterations (indicated by additional X's). Stage-specific strategies for preventing these processes are depicted as brick-walls along the pathway.

The classic view of experimental carcinogenesis, in which tumor initiation is followed by tumor promotion and progression in a sequential fashion, remains conceptually important. However, many of the processes involved in each stage of experimental carcinogenesis also appear to be involved in human carcinogenesis *(4),* and the temporal nature of initiation, promotion, and progression events in the natural world is complex. For instance, we know from the work of Vogelstein and others that multiple mutational events are involved in the formation of a tumor *(5).* Humans are generally exposed to mixtures of agents that can simultaneously act at different stages of the carcinogenesis process. It has become clear that promotional events, which frequently lead to enhanced cellular proliferation and/or decreased apoptosis, can influence subsequent initiation events *(6).*

Thus, rather than three discrete stages occurring in a predictable order, human carcinogenesis is best characterized as an accumulation of alterations in genes regulating cellular homeostasis—such as oncogenes, tumor-suppressor genes, apoptotic-regulating genes, and DNA repair genes *(7).* Most animal models used in carcinogenesis research were developed prior to: the identification of the major cancer-related genes; the recognition of the importance of host susceptibility to a carcinogenic insult; or the elucidation of mitogenesis **and** apoptosis as balanced regulatory components of normal cell homeostasis. The major goal in the development of these carcinogen-induced tumor models was the rapid generation of neoplasia to provide investigators with sufficient material in a timely fashion for studying the biology of the tumors. Although some models are based on low-dose carcinogen exposure, most generally involve high-dose regimens of a single genotoxic carcinogen—often with no apparent relationship to the etiology of human cancer, such as dimethylbenz(a)anthracene (DMBA)—which can induce large-scale genetic damage in a random fashion *(8)*. Although some molecular alterations have been identified in the commonly employed models, the types of alterations caused by high-dose chemical exposures do not generally reflect the gene-environment interactions underlying the pathogenesis of cancer in humans. Furthermore, the interpretation of the activity of preventive compounds being evaluated in these models can often be confounded by the effects of those compounds on the metabolic activation or detoxification specific to high doses of a particular carcinogen, which may be less relevant to typical chronic, low-level human exposures to mixtures of exogenous or endogenous carcinogens.

Future progress in cancer prevention research may be facilitated by the use of animals with specific genetic susceptibilities for tumor development *(9)*. The recent development of mouse strains with carcinogenesis-related genes overexpressed or inactivated provides investigators with new models for studying the carcinogenesis process, and for testing preventive strategies that can offset specific and highly relevant genetic susceptibilities to cancer in humans. Thus far, prevention studies in genetically altered mice have predominantly focused on alterations in a limited number of specific genes implicated in human cancer, particularly: 1) the *p53* tumor-suppressor gene; 2) the adenomatous polyposis coli *(APC)* gene; and 3) human papillomavirus (HPV) early genes (e.g., E6 and E7). The purpose of this chapter is to provide a summary of the studies to date that have used these models for cancer prevention studies, and to introduce several emerging models that may be useful for prevention research.

2. *P53*-KNOCKOUT MICE AND GERMLINE *P53*-MUTANT MICE

Mutation of the *p53* tumor-suppressor gene is the most frequently observed genetic lesion in human cancer; over 50% of all human tumors examined to date have identifiable *p53* gene point-mutations or deletions *(9)*. Donehower et al. *(10)* first reported in 1992 that homozygous *p53*-knockout (*p53–/–*) mice were viable but highly susceptible to spontaneous tumorigenesis (particularly lymphomas) at an early age. The *p53–/–* mice have been useful tools for studying the role of *p53* in carcinogenesis. For example, in response to the two-stage skin-carcinogenesis protocol, *p53–/–* mice, relative to wild-type (*p53+/+*) mice, showed no difference in benign papilloma formation, but did display greatly accelerated progression to malignant carcinomas *(11)*. Furthermore, the carcinomas formed in the *p53–/–* mice showed higher indices of malignancy as measured by histopathology, further confirming the importance of *p53* loss in acceleration of tumor progression.

The *p53–/–* mice also provide an attractive and potentially relevant tumorigenesis model for studying cancer-prevention strategies, given the frequency of *p53* mutations in human tumors and the rapidity with which spontaneous tumors develop in these mice. Hursting et al. *(12–15)* have evaluated the ability of several dietary and chemopreventive interventions to offset the increased susceptibility of *p53–/–* mice to spontaneous tumorigenesis. Calorie restriction reduces cell proliferation in most tissues studied *(16,17)*. This decreased rate of DNA replication in normal cells in response to calorie restriction may make those cells less susceptible to mutations induced by carcinogens, and may suppress the progression of preneoplastic cells. In *p53–/–* mice, Calorie restriction (60% of the control group's intake of carbohydrate calories) increased the latency of spontaneous tumor development (mostly lymphomas) by approx 75%, and significantly slowed thymocyte and splenocyte cell-cycle traverse *(12)*. The time to tumor onset in these mice is *p53*-dependent, and the majority of *p53–/–* mice develop and die from spontaneous tumors by approx 6 mo of age compared to nearly 2 yr for *p53+/+* mice. However, the highly statistically significant tumor-delaying effect of calorie restriction, relative to *ad libitum* feeding, was similar in both *p53–/–* and wild-type (*p53+/+*) mice, indicating that the mechanisms underlying calorie restriction may be *p53*-independent *(13)*. In addition, the chemopreventive steroid dehydroepiandrosterone (DHEA; 0.3% in the diet) significantly delayed spontaneous tumorigenesis in *p53–/–* mice, and in particular, suppressed lymphoma development *(14)*. Furthermore, the DHEA analog 16-α-fluoro-5-androsten-17-one (fluasterone; 0.15% in the diet) also suppressed spontaneous lymphoma development and extended survival in *p53–/–* mice *(15a)*. Taken together, these findings clearly demonstrate that the increased susceptibility to cancer as a result of a genetic lesion, such as loss of *p53* tumor-suppressor function, may be offset, at least in part, by preventive approaches.

The use of *p53–/–* mice has helped to elucidate the mechanism of action underlying the tumor-inhibitory effects of calorie restriction and the chemopreventive steroids. For example, the antitumor effect of DHEA (or its fluorinated analog fluasterone) in *p53–/–* mice is independent of its effects on food intake or on nucleotide pool levels *(15a)*, as has been previously suggested in other models *(18)*. Wang et al. *(19)* showed that both calorie restriction and DHEA decreased thymocyte proliferative rates, and Poetschke et al. *(20)* showed that calorie restriction, DHEA, and fluasterone each blocked thymocyte development and induced apoptosis in the lymphoma-susceptible subpopulation of immature thymocytes. The apoptosis-inducing effects of the chemopreventive steroids appeared to be mediated by decreased *Bcl-2* gene expression. In addition, Mei et al. showed that calorie restriction, DHEA, and fluasterone each suppressed nitric oxide levels and downregulated nitric oxide synthetase expression *(21)*.

Heterozygous *p53*-knockout (*p53+/–*) mice, with only one *p53* allele inactivated, are analogous to humans susceptible to heritable forms of cancer caused by decreased *p53* gene dosage, such as individuals with Li-Fraumeni Syndrome *(22)*. The spontaneous tumors that occur most frequently in *p53+/–* mice (hematopoietic neoplasias and osteosarcomas) are similarly observed in humans with Li-Fraumeni syndrome. However, the two most common epithelial tumors observed in Li-Fraumeni patients (lung tumors in males and breast tumors in females) are infrequent in the mice. While *p53+/–* mice have low rates of spontaneous tumorigenesis for up to 12 mo of age *(23)*, they do display increased susceptibility to chemically induced tumor development relative to wild-type mice. *p*-Cresidine-induced bladder tumors *(22)*, dimethylnitrosamine-induced liver tumors *(23)*, nitrosomethylurea-induced lymphomas (S.Perkins, S, Hursting, manuscript in preparation), azoxymethane-induced aberrant crypt foci and colon tumors *(24)*, and radiation-induced lymphomas and sarcomas *(25)* all appear significantly earlier in *p53+/–* mice than in similarly treated *p53+/+* mice. As mentioned previously, malignant progression of DMBA-initiated, 12-O-tetradecanoyl phorbol 13-acetate (TPA)-promoted skin papillomas occur much faster in *p53+/–* mice than in *p53+/+* mice *(11)*. These findings suggest that *p53+/–* mice exhibit an increased sensitivity to several classes of mutagenic carcinogens when compared to *p53+/+* mice, and appear to be susceptible to at least some low-dose, chronic carcinogen regimens that more closely mimic human exposures. Thus, these mice have tremendous potential for the development of models facilitating the study of gene-environment interactions relevant to human cancer prevention.

A rapid *p53*+/– mouse mammary-tumor model has also been developed by crossing *p53*+/– mice with mouse mammary tumor virus (MMTV)-*Wnt-1* transgenic mice *(26)*. In these mice, calorie restriction, a 1-d/wk fast, the synthetic retinoid fenretinide, the chemopreventive steroid fluasterone, and a high-soy diet each delay spontaneous mammary-tumor development *(27,28)*. Mammary tumors from these mice are estrogen-receptor (ER) positive, overexpress cyclooxygenase-2 (COX-2), and show reduced BRCA-1 expression, suggesting that this model, which involves alterations in two critical carcinogeneis pathways, may be highly relevant for the development of breast-cancer prevention strategies.

A transgenic model expressing a dominant negative *p53* mutation (rather than a germline *p53*-knockout) has also recently been developed and characterized *(29)*. Like the p53-knockout mice, these dominant-negative *p53*-mutant mice spontaneously develop a variety of hematopoietic neoplasias and sarcomas. However, they also demonstrate an increased incidence of lung adenomas (a common Li-Fraumeni syndrome tumor), possibly caused by their mixed FVB background (the *p53*-knockout mice described here are on a C57BL/6 background). Inbred FVB mice with normal *p53* display a low but reproducible incidence of lung adenomas. Mice with the (A/J × FVB) F1 background with the dominant negative *p53* mutation show increased numbers of and size of lung adenomas following challenge with various carcinogens, including two tobacco-related carcinogens—benzo(a)pyrene and 4-methylnitrosoamino-1(3)-pyridyl-1-butanone (NNK) *(30)*. Tumors from these mice display K-*ras* mutations. These findings imply that the *p53* mutation affects both tumor initiation (increased numbers of adenomas) and tumor growth (increased size of the tumors). This model also involves mutations in two of the most commonly altered genes (*p53* and K-*ras*) associated with human lung cancer. Employing this tumor model, these investigators showed that two distinct chemopreventive regimens, specifically dexamethasone (plus myo-inositol) and green tea, were equally effective as chemopreventives in mice with or without *p53* mutations *(30)*. In a subsequent experiment, the effects of the carcinogen 1,2-dimethylhydrazine (DMH) was also examined in these mice. Mice with the dominant negative *p53* mutation on a (B6 × FVB) F1 displayed increased levels of colon, uterine, hepatic, and lung tumors when compared with similar F1 mice with two wild-type *p53* alleles *(31)*. The non-steroidal anti-inflammatory drug (NSAID) piroxicam effectively inhibited colon-tumor formation in mice with or without *p53* mutation, but had no effect on the incidence or multiplicity of liver, uterine, or lung tumors *(32)*.

Taken together, these studies show that mice with a knockout or mutation in the *p53* tumor-suppressor gene provides relevant and rapid spontaneous or chemically induced tumor models that may be useful for testing nutritional, chemopreventive, or other strategies to offset cancer susceptibility caused by alterations in this so-called "guardian of the genome." Studies thus far with several preventive interventions (i.e., calorie restriction, DHEA, fluasterone, NSAIDs, and glucocorticoids) suggest that these interventions are similarly effective against certain types of neoplasias in mice with or without alterations in *p53*. This contrasts with results from therapeutic trials, in which mutations in *p53* often decrease the responsiveness of tumors to therapy *(33)*. In addition, these mice are highly susceptible to various carcinogens, and serve as useful models for testing potential etiologic agents. Furthermore, using these mice in conjunction with highly relevant human carcinogens, or crossing them with other relevant transgenic strains, may provide important models for studying gene-environment interactions.

3. MIN MICE AND APC-KNOCKOUT MICE

As reviewed by Dove et al. *(34)*, mutation of the *APC* gene may be a common denominator of most human colon cancers, including polypoid and nonpolypoid familial colon cancers as well as sporadic occurrences. Thus, an animal model with an alteration in this gene should be highly relevant for testing prevention strategies. The Min (multiple intestinal neoplasia) mouse, which carries a fully penetrant dominant mutation converting codon 850 of the murine *Apc* gene from a leucine to a stop codon, was first reported in 1990 *(35)*. The Min mutation was discovered by phenotypic screening after random germline mutagenesis with the point mutagen ethylnitrosourea. Min/Min homozygous mice are not viable, but mice heterozygous for the Min mutation develop scores of grossly detectable adenomas throughout the small intestine (rarely in the colon) in 1–3 mo *(35)*. Interestingly, the phenotypic expression of an *Apc* mutation in the Min mouse is markedly different from that of humans with familial adenomatous polyposis, in which adenomas are found exclusively in the colon and duodenum *(34)*. Despite this potential limitation, the Min mouse model should facilitate the study of carcinogenesis and anticarcinogenesis related to *APC* in intestinal neoplasia. *Apc*-knockout mice strains have also been developed *(36,37)*. Oshima et al. *(36)* used gene targeting techniques to introduce a truncation mutation at codon 716 of the mouse *Apc* gene. Like the Min mice, the homozygous $Apc^{\Delta 716}$ knockout mice are not viable, but the heterozygotes develop numerous intestinal polyps at an early age.

Several studies report that NSAIDs reduce spontaneous adenoma formation in Min mice *(38–40)*, and Oshima et al. *(41)* reported that the absence of COX-2 in *Apc*-knockout mice, accomplished by crossing $Apc^{\Delta 716}$-knockout mice with COX-2-knockout mice, dramatically reduced the number and size of intestinal polyps resulting from decreased *Apc*-gene dosage. In addition, treating the $Apc^{\Delta 716}$ mice with the NSAIDs sulindac or the selective COX-2 inhibitor MF tricyclic reduced the polyp number relative to the untreated controls *(41)*. Furthermore, MF tricyclic reduced the polyp number more significantly than sulindac (which inhibits both COX-1 and COX-2). These studies provided strong evidence that COX-2 plays a key role in *APC*-related tumorigenesis, and suggested that selective COX-2 inhibitors have great promise as colon-cancer chemopreventives. Subsequent studies with the selective COX-2 inhibitors nimesulide *(42)* and Celecoxib® (R. Jacoby and R. Lubet, unpublished observations) in Min mice indeed demonstrate striking efficacy against intestinal tumorigenesis. Findings from these studies helped support human trials of Celecoxib® in individuals with familial adenomatous polyposis (FAP, a hereditary syndrome in which individuals develop hundreds of adenomatous polyps), examining the effects on pre-existing lesions and the development of new lesions. The small-scale human trials that showed efficacy in the FAP patients *(43)*, in combination with the results from the Min and *Apc*-knockout mice studies, encouraged the Food and Drug Administration (FDA)'s decision to employ this class of agent in patients with FAP. This is a striking example of a rapid translation of preclinical findings in a relevant genetically altered mouse model to clinical application.

Patients with FAP develop a second form of cancer called desmoids—outgrowths of fibroblasts that cause significant morbidity although they are benign *(44)*. These lesions, like the polyps in persons with FAP and like most human sporadic colon cancers, are associated with an initiating or germline mutation in *APC*, although the *Apc* mutation alone in Min mice is not sufficient to cause desmoid tumors. However, Min mice crossed with *p53*-knockout mice develop desmoid tumors rapidly and at a high frequency *(45)*. Despite the fact that the intestinal polyps in Min × *p53*-knockout mice are responsive to prevention by the NSAID piroxicam and the ornithine decarboxylase suicide inhibitor DFMO, the desmoid tumors show minimal response *(45)*. Thus, by generating a bitransgenic mouse model with alterations in two genetic pathways that are highly relevant to human carcinogenesis (i.e., *Apc* and *p53*), the genetics and histopathology of the resulting tumors may be more similar to human disease. In addition, even with the same common mutations—including *Apc*, which is absolutely necessary for cancer formation—one form of cancer (intestinal) is sensitive to NSAIDs and DFMO, and the second form of cancer (desmoids) is not.

4. HPV-16 TRANSGENIC MICE

The models discussed thus far involve knockouts or mutations of critical carcinogenesis-related genes in the germline. While the majority of human cancers are believed to occur as a result of the accumulation of genetic alterations in critical genes such as *p53*, APC, and several others, as previously mentioned, a significant number of human cancers are associated with exogenous infectious agents, including H. pylori in stomach cancer, hepatitis B and C in liver cancer, and HPV in cervical, anal, and certain skin cancers in immunosuppressed individuals *(46)*. Arbeit et al. *(47)* developed a model in which the early genes of HPV16 were placed under the control of a keratin-14 promoter. The resulting animals have developed spontaneous skin tumors and anal lesions, as well as cervical cancer following stimulation with exogenous estradiol *(47)*. Chemopreventive studies in these mice have demonstrated that DFMO was extremely effective in inhibiting tumor formation and even reversing pre-existing skin lesions *(48)*. Initial studies in the cervical-cancer model with three different preventive agents (indole 3-carbinol, DFMO, and 9-*cis*-retinoic acid) have all demonstrated some efficacy in the cervical model although to a lesser extent than DFMO in the skin model *(49)*. Nevertheless, these mice appear to provide a very promising model for studying HPV-related carcinogenesis, as well as a more generalized method for modeling cancers with an underlying infectious etiology.

5. OTHER TRANSGENIC MODELS WITH POTENTIAL FOR CANCER PREVENTION STUDIES

Numerous mouse models with cancer-related genes (other than *Apc, p53,* or HPV early genes) overexpressed or inactivated have been developed in recent years. Many of these transgenic and knockout strains are catalogued in online databases, such as the Induced Mutation Registry Database maintained by the Jackson Laboratory *(http://www.jax.org/resources/documents/imr)* and the Mouse Knockout and Mutation Database accessible through Biomednet (http://www.research.bmn.com/mkmd). As reviewed *(50)*, many of these models have been effectively used in studies focusing on toxicology and carcinogenesis. In addition, some models have already been utilized in chemoprevention studies. For example, ethylnitrosourea-induced T-cell lymphomas in *pim-1*-transgenic mice—which overexpress the *pim*-1 oncogene in their lymphoid compartments, and are susceptible to genotoxic carcinogens targeting the lymphoid system—are delayed by the synthetic retinoid fenretinide *(51)*. In addition, spontaneous neurofibromatoses in transgenic mice overexpressing part of the human T-lymphotrophic virus genome were delayed by the administration of diet supplemented with red-wine solids rich in catechin, a polyphenolic compound with potent antioxidant activity *(52)*. These studies further support the utility of genetic susceptibility models for cancer-prevention studies.

Progress in prostate cancer prevention has been significantly impeded by the lack of relevant animal models of this disease, which is the most prevalent noncutaneous cancer in males in the United States. Several models have recently been developed based on the overexpression of oncogenes in the prostate *(53–56)*, usually with various promoters that target the Simian virus (SV)-40 large T-antigen (which can bind to and inactivate the *p53* tumor-suppressor protein and the retinoblastoma (Rb) tumor-suppressor protein) to the prostate. Two of these SV40 T-antigen transgenic models have employed probascin as the promoter *(53–54)*, and the third used a hormone-binding protein (C31) expressed in the prostate *(55)*. Although the transgene (SV40 T-antigen) driving the tumorigenic process in these mice is not involved in human prostate cancer, these models each display sufficient histopathologic and molecular similarities to human prostate-tumor progression to warrant the evaluation of their response to preventive interventions. Initial chemoprevention studies in the Greenberg model have shown protective effects with both *R*-flurbiprofen (the enatiomer of flurbiprofen with no direct COX-inhibitory activity) and DFMO *(57)*. An additional transgenic model utilizing a keratin-5 promoter to drive prostatic overexpression of insulin-like growth factor-1, (IGF-1), resulting in a high rate of spontaneous prostatic tumors, has been recently reported *(56)*. These mice may provide a particularly relevant prostate-tumor model for prevention studies, given the recent epidemiologic links between elevated plasma IGF-1 levels and increased prostate-cancer risk *(58)*.

As discussed here, alterations in genes encoding carcinogen-metabolizing or detoxification enzymes, DNA-repair enzymes, and the major factors involved in the epigenetic events associated with tumor promotion and progression can greatly influence cancer development. As recently reviewed, there is a rapidly expanding list of transgenic and knockout mouse models already generated with alterations in genes related to carcinogen metabolism, DNA repair, inflammation, or cell signaling *(50,59)*. Most of these genetically altered mice do not display a tumor phenotype on their own, and thus do not generally represent tumorigenesis models that mimic human cancer. However, they may be extremely useful for studying specific gene-environment interactions on their own, or when used in combination with other models of genetic susceptibility. For example, Min mice crossed with *MSH2*-knockout mice, which are deficient in a critical mismatch-repair gene, displayed a greater number of adenomas at a much earlier age than Min mice with normal *MSH2* function *(60)*.

SUMMARY

As illustrated in Fig. 1, experimental models of carcinogen-induced cancer have been crucial to advancing our understanding of the neoplastic process. Recent progress

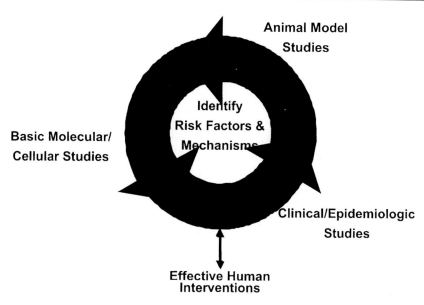

Animal Model Studies

Basic Molecular/ Cellular Studies

Identify Risk Factors & Mechanisms

Clinical/Epidemiologic Studies

Effective Human Interventions

Fig. 2. The role of animal models in cancer prevention research. Schematic presentation of the central role of animal models in contemporary cancer prevention research. One of the major goals of cancer prevention research is the development of effective human interventions to inhibit the carcinogenesis process prior to the development of a clinical tumor. Successful attainment of this goal requires the identification of modulatable risk factors and the determination of underlying mechanisms that will reveal specific targets for intervention. This will be facilitated by the integration of cutting-edge research at various levels, including the development of important leads from clinical and epidemiologic studies and the elucidation of basic mechanisms from studies at the molecular and cellular level. Animal model studies can effectively serve as bridges between these levels of research, and it is therefore critical that the animal models employed be as relevant as possible to the human carcinogenesis process.

in the field of molecular carcinogenesis has revealed multiple targets for the nutritional modulation and chemoprevention of cancer. We must now fully utilize this knowledge base—and capitalize on the availability of new tools such as transgenic mice—to identify critical, modulatable targets and make important progress toward one of the major goals in contemporary cancer-prevention research: the development of effective mechanism-based strategies for preventing human cancer. Successful attainment of this goal will require the integration of the very best science from multiple levels of investigation, including clinical and epidemiologic research, animal studies, and basic molecular and cellular biologic research. All three levels of investigation are essential in this effort, although in our view animal-model studies play a critical central role (Fig. 2). For instance, animal studies are required to confirm (under controlled experimental conditions) potential leads from human studies showing associations between certain risk factors (both protective and harmful) and cancer risk. In addition, preclinical studies are critical in translating basic mechanistic findings from the bench to the clinic. Thus, the availability of highly relevant animal models may greatly facilitate future progress in cancer-prevention research. In this chapter, examples of cancer prevention studies that have utilized genetically altered mouse models are discussed. Taken together, these examples clearly indicate that mice with specific (and human-like) genetic susceptibilities for cancer provide powerful new tools for testing agents that may inhibit the process of carcinogenesis in humans.

REFERENCES

1. Yuspa SH, Shields PG. Etiology of cancer: Chemical factors. In: Devita VT, Hellman SH, Rosenberg SA, eds. *Cancer: Principles and Practices of Oncology,* 5th ed. Lippincott-Raven, Philadelphia, *PA,* 1997, pp. 185–202.
2. Slaga TJ. Mechanisms involved in two-stage carcinogenesis in mouse skin. In: Slaga TJ, ed. *Mechanisms of Tumor Promotion.* CRC Press, Inc., Boca Ratons FL, 1984, pp. 1–93.
3. Pitot HC. Progression: the terminal stage in carcinogenesis. *Jpn J Cancer Res* 1989; 80:599–607.
4. Yuspa SH, Poirier MC. Chemical carcinogenesis: from animal models to molecular models in one decade. *Adv Cancer Res* 1988; 50:25–70.
5. Fearon ER, Vogelstein B. A genetic model of human colorectal tumorigenesis. *Cell* 1990; 61:759–767.
6. Sugimura T. Multistep carcinogenesis: a 1992 perspective. *Science* 1992; 258:603–607.
7. Stanley LA. Molecular aspects of chemical carcinogenesis: the roles of oncogenes and tumor suppressor genes. *Toxicology* 1995; 96:173–194.
8. Huggins CB. Selective induction of hormone-dependent mammary adenocarcinomas in the rat. *J Lab Clin Med* 1987; 109:262–266.
9. Hursting SD, Slaga TJ, Fischer SM, DiGiovanni J, Phang JM. Mechanism-based cancer prevention approaches: targets, examples and the use of transgenic mice. *J Natl Cancer Inst* 1999; 91:215–225.
10. Hollstein, M, Sidransky, D, Vogelstein B, Harris, CC. p53 mutations in human cancers. *Science* 1991; 253:49–53.
11. Donehower LA, Harvey M, Slagle BL, McArthur MJ, Montgomery CA, Butel J, et al. Mice deficient for p53 are developmentally normal but susceptible to spontaneous tumors. *Nature* (London) 1992; 356:215–221.
12. Kemp CJ, Donehower LA, Bradley A, Balmain A. Reduction of p53 gene dosage does not increase initiation or promotion but enhances malignant progression of chemically induced skin tumors. *Cell* 1993; 74:813–822.
13. Hursting SD, Perkins SN, Phang JM. Calorie restriction delays spontaneous tumorigenesis in p53-knockout transgenic mice. *Proc Natl Acad Sci USA* 1994; 91:7036–7040.
14. Hursting SD, Perkins SN, Brown CC, Haines DC, Phang JM. Calorie restriction induces a p53-independent delay of spontaneous carcinogenesis in p53-deficient and wild-type mice. *Cancer Res* 1997; 57:2843–2846.
15. Hursting SD, Perkins SN, Ward J, Haines D, Phang JM. Chemoprevention of spontaneous tumorigenesis in p53-knockout mice. *Cancer Res* 1995; 55:3949–3953.
15a. Perkins SN, Hursting SD, Haines DC, James SJ, Phang JM. Chemoprevention of spontaneous tumorigenesis in nullizygous p53-deficient mice by dehydroepiandro-sterone and its analog, 16-α-fluoro-5-androsten-17-one. *Carcinogenesis* 1997; 18:101–106.
16. Hursting SD, Kari FW. The anti-carcinogenic effects of dietary restriction: mechanisms and future directions. *Mutat Res* 1999; 443:235–249.
17. Weindruch R, Walford RL, eds. *The Retardation of Aging and Disease by Dietary Restriction.* C. Thomas, Springfield, 1988, pp. 1–291.
18. Schwartz AG, Pashko LL. Mechanism of cancer preventive action of DHEA. Role of glucose 6-phosphate dehydrogenase. *Ann NY Acad Sci USA* 1995; 774:180–186.
19. Wang TTY, Hursting SD, Perkins SN, Phang JM. Effects of dehydroepiandrosterone and calorie restriction on the Bcl-2/Bax-mediated apoptotic pathway in p53-deficient mice. *Cancer Lett* 1997; 116:61–69.
20. Poetschke HL, Klug DB, Perkins SN, Wang TTY, Richie ER, Hursting SD. The effects of calorie restriction on thymocyte growth, death and maturation. *Carcinogenesis* 2000; 21:1959–1964.
21. Mei JM, Hursting SD, Perkins SN, Phang JM. p53-independent inhibition of nitric oxide generation by cancer preventive interventions in ex vivo mouse peritoneal macrophages. *Cancer Lett* 1998; 129:191–197.
22. Tennant RW, French JE, Spalding JW. Identifying chemical carcinogens and assessing potential risk in short-term bioassays using transgenic mice. *Environ Health Perspect* 1995; 103:942–950.
23. Harvey M, McArthur MJ, Montgomery CA, et al. Spontaneous and carcinogen-induced tumorigenesis in p53-deficient mice. *Nat Gen* 1993; 4:225–229.

24. Hursting S, Purewal M, Woods C, Velasco M, Wargovich M. Chemoprevention of azoxymethane-induced aberrant crypt foci and colon tumors in p53-deficient mice by sulindac. *Cancer Epideniol Biol Prev* 1998; 7:176.

25. Kemp CJ, Wheldon T, Balmain A. p53-deficient mice are extremely susceptible to radiation-induced tumorigenesis. *Nat Gen* 1994; 8:66–69.

26. Jones JM, Attardi L, Godley LA, Laucirica R, Medina D, Jacks T, et al. Absence of p53 in a mouse mammary tumor model promotes tumor cell proliferation without affecting apoptosis. *Cell Growth Differ* 1997; 8:829–838.

27. Perkins SN, Davis BJ, Donehower LA, DeLa Cerda J, Baum L, Hursting SD. Effects of dietary restriction on spontaneous mammary tumorigenesis in p53-deficient Wnt-1 transgenic mice. *Proc Am Assoc Cancer Res* 2000; 41:A531.

28. Hursting SD, Perkins SN, Donehower LA, Fuchs-Young, R, Clinton S, Baum L, et al. Chemoprevention of spontaneous mammary tumorigenesis in p53-deficient Wnt-1 transgenic mice. *Proc Am Assoc Cancer Res* 2000; 41:A528.

29. Laviguer A, Maltby V, Mock D, Rossant J, Pawson T, Bernstein A. High incidence of lung, bone and lymphoid tumors in transgenic mice overexpressing mutant alleles of the p53 oncogene. *Mol Cell Biol* 1989; 9:3982–3991.

30. Zhang Z, Liu Q, Lantry LE, Wang Y, Kelloff GJ, Anderson MW, et al. A germ-line p53 mutation accelerates pulmonary tumorigenesis: p53-independnet efficacy of chemopreventive agents green tea or dexamethasone/myo-inositol and chemotherapeutic agents taxol and adriamycin. *Cancer Res* 2000; 60:901–907.

31. Zhang Z, Lantry LE, Wang Y, Wiseman RW, Grubbs CH, Lubet RA, et al. Organ-specific effect of a germline p53 mutation on chemical carcinogenesis in mice: a new model for cancer intervention. *Proc Am Assoc Cancer Res* 2000; 41:A2617.

32. Lubet RA, Fischer SM, Conti C, Kelloff GJ, Zhang Z, You M. Chemopreventive efficacy of NSAIDS in tumor models with mutations in the p53 tumor suppressor gene. *Proc Am Assoc Cancer Res* 2000; 41:A2617.

33. Brown J, Wouters BG. Apoptosis, p53 and tumor cell sensitivity to anticancer agents. *Cancer Res* 1999; 59:1391–1399.

34. Dove WF, Gould KA, Luongo C, Moser AR, Shoemaker AR. Emergent issues in the genetics of intestinal neoplasia. *Cancer Surv* 1995; 25:335–355.

35. Moser AR, Pitot HC, Dove WF. A dominant mutation that predisposes to multiple intestinal neoplasia in the mouse. *Science* 1990; 247:322–324.

36. Oshima M, Takahashi M, Oshima H, Tsutsumi M, Yazawa K, Sugimura T, et al. Effects of docosa-hexaenoic acid on intestinal polyp development in APC knockout mice. *Carcinogenesis* 1995; 16:2605–2607.

37. Fodde R, Edelmann W, Yang K. A targeted chain-termination mutation in the mouse Apc gene results in multiple intestinal tumors. *Proc Natl Acad Sci USA* 1994; 91:8969–8973.

38. Jacoby RF, Marshall DJ, Newton MA, Nocakovic K, Tutsch K, Cole CE, et al. Chemoprevention of spontaneous intestinal adenomas in the APC min mouse model by the non-steroidal anti-inflammatory drug piroxicam. *Cancer Res* 1996; 56:710–714.

39. Boolbol SK, Dannenberg AJ, Chadburn A, Martucci C, Guo X, Ramonetti JT, et al. Cyclooxygenase-2 overexpression and tumor formation are blocked by sulindac in a murine model of familial adenomatous polyposis. *Cancer Res* 1996; 56:2556–2560.

40. Beazer-Barclay Y, Levy DB, Moser AR, Dove WF, Hamilton SR, Vogelstein B, et al. Sulindac suppresses tumorigenesis in the Min mouse. *Carcinogenesis* 1996; 17:1757–1760.

41. Oshima M, Dinchuk J, Kargman S, Oshima H, Hancock B, Kwong E, et al. Suppression of intestinal polyposis in APC-knockout mice by inhibition of cyclooxygenase 2 (COX-2). *Cell* 1996; 87:803–809.

42. Nakatsugi S, Fukutake M, Takahashi M, Fukuda K, Isoi T, Taniguchi Y, et al. Suppression of intestinal polyp development by nimesulide, a selective cyclooxygenase-2 inhibitor, in Min mice. *Jpn J Cancer Res* 1997 Dec 88:1117–1120.

43. Steinbach G, Lynch PM, Phillips R. Effects of celecoxib on colorectal polyps in patients with familial adenomatous polyposis (FAP). *Proc Am Coll Gastroenterology* 1999; A51.

44. Middleton SB, Frayling IM, Phillips RK. Desmoids in familial adenomatous polyposis are monoclonal proliferations. *Br J Cancer* 2000; 82:827–832.

45. Halberg RB, Katzung DS, Hoff PD, Moser AR, Cole CE, Lubet RA, et al. Tumorigenesis in the multiple intestinal neoplasia mouse: redundancy of negative regulators and specificity of modifiers. *Proc Natl Acad Sci USA* 2000; 97:3461–3466.

46. Butel J. Viral carcinogenesis: revelation of molecular mechanisms and etiology of human disease. *Carcinogenesis* 2000; 21:405–426.

47. Arbeit JM, Howley PH, Hanahan D. Chronic estrogen-induced cervical and vaginal squamous carcinogenesis in human papilloma virus type 16 transgenic mice. *Proc Natl Acad Sci USA* 1996; 93:2930–2933.

48. Arbeit JM, Riley RR, Huey B, Porter C, Kelloff G, Lubet RA, et al. Difluoromethylornithine chemoprevention of epidermal carcinogenesis in K14-HPV16 transgenic mice. *Cancer Res* 1999; 59:3610–3620.

49. Riley R, Lubet R, Pinkel D, Arbeit J. DFMO or 9-cis retinoic acid chemoprevention of cervical carcinogenesis in K14-HPV16 transgenic mice. *Proc Am Assoc Cancer Res* 2000; 41:A540.

50. Gonzalez FJ. Use of transgenic animals in carcinogenesis studies. *Mol Carcinog* 1996; 16:63–67.

51. McCormick DL, Johnson WD, Rao KV, Bowman-Green T, Steele V, Lubet RA, et al. Comparative activity of N-(4-hydroxyphenyl)-all trans-retinamide and alpha-difluoromethylornithine as inhibitors of lymphoma induction in PIM-transgenic mice. *Carcinogenesis* 1996; 17:2513–2517.

52. Clifford AJ, Ebeler SE, Ebeler JD, Bills ND, Hinrichs SH, Teissedre PP, et al. Delayed tumor onset in transgenic mice fed an amino-acid-based diet supplemented with red wine solids. *Am J Clin Nutr* 1996; 64:748–756.

53. Gingrich JR, Greenberg NM. A transgenic mouse prostate cancer model. *Toxicol Pathol* 1996; 24:502–504.

54. Shibata M, Ward JM, Devor DE, Liu M, Green JE. Progression of prostatic intraepithelial neoplasia to invasive carcinoma in C3(1)/SV40 large T antigen transgenic mice: histopathological and molecular biological alterations. *Cancer Res* 1996; 56:4894–4903.

55. Kasper S, Sheppard PC, Yan Y, Pettigrew N, Borowsky AD, Prins GS, et al. Development, progression and androgen dependence of prostate tumors in probasin large T antigen transgenic mice: a model for prostate cancer. *Lab Invest* 1998; 78:319–333.

56. DiGiovanni J, Kiguchi K, Frijhoff A, Wilker E, Bol DK, Beltrán L, et al. Deregulated expression of insulin-like growth factor 1 in prostate epithelium leads to neoplasia in transgenic mice. *Proc Natl Acad Sci USA* 2000; 97:3455–3460.

57. Wechter WJ, Leipold DD, Murray ED, Quiggle D, McCracken JD, Barrios RS, et al. E-7689 (R-Flurbiprofen) inhibits progression of prostate cancer in the TRAMP mouse. *Cancer Res* 2000; 60:2203–2208.

58. Chan JM, Stampfer MJ, Giovannucci E, Gann PH, Ma J, Wilkinson P, et al. Plasma insulin-like growth factor-1 and prostate cancer risk: a prospective study. *Science* 1998; 279:563–566.

59. Allemand I, Angulo JF. Transgenic and knockout models for studying DNA repair. *Biochimie* 1995; 77:826–832.

60. Reitmar AH, Cai J, Bjerknes M, Redston M, Cheng H, Pind M, MSH2 deficiency contributes to accelerated Apc-mediated intestinal tumorigenesis. *Cancer Res* 1996; 56:2922–2926.

VI   METASTASIS MODELS

16 Metastasis Models
Lungs, Spleen/Liver, Bone, and Brain

Krishna Menon, MS and Beverly A. Teicher, PhD

CONTENTS

1. INTRODUCTION

The metastatic spread of solid tumors is directly or indirectly responsible for most cancer-related deaths *(1)*. Approximately 30% of cancer patients have clinically detectable metastases at the time of initial diagnosis, and 30–40% harbor occult metastases *(2)*. There is an urgent clinical need to predict the metastatic potential of individual tumors, to identify occult metastatic foci, to prevent metastatic dissemination, and to prevent the transformation of tumors to more invasive phenotypes. Appropriate preclinical models can help to achieve these goals.

Metastasis is a multi-step process, in which the tumor cells from the primary tumor are detached and deposited into the development of a similar tumor lesion in a secondary organ *(1,3,4)*. Although the genetic basis of tumorigenesis can vary greatly, the steps required for metastasis are similar for all tumor cells. The detached cells from the primary site use lymphatic vessels and the bloodstream for transport. Metastasis at the cellular level is regulated by well-coordinated and highly orchestrated mechanisms of gene products *(5)*. Extracellular matrix (ECM) receptors, invasion of the basal-cell membrane by proteolytic enzymes, entry into the vasculature, and motility factors of organs are essential for tumor-cell migration. For organ-specific invasion, receptors are required. The development of micro-colonies in the secondary organ is facilitated by growth factors. Angiogenic factors are also essential to development metastasis.

From: *Tumor Models in Cancer Research*
Edited by: B. A. Teicher © Humana Press Inc., Totowa, NJ

In the metastatic cascade, tumor cells undergo a series of further alterations, resulting in the up- or down-regulation of cell-surface molecules, proteases, and their inhibitors, motility factors, growth-stimulating and organ-specificity determining factors from the microenvironment, and angiogenesis-promoting molecules. Many of the mechanisms applicable to the process of tumor progression have normal functions during embryonic development and tissue-regeneration (5). There are no qualitative differences between cancer cells and normal cells, such as macrophages, trophoblasts, and endothelial cells, with respect to the basic processes of cell detachment, migration, invasion, and formation of colonies at distant sites. However, cancer cells express the phenotypic traits characteristic for these processes at times and in locations incompatible with normal organism function (6). Cancer-directed tissue remodeling, such as angiogenesis and stimulation of fibroblast proliferation and deposition of extracellular matrix around tumor enclaves also reflects mis-activated normal processes. The urokinase-type plasminogen-activator, (uPA) pathway mis-activation appears to be central to metastasis (6). The uPA system does not support tumor metastasis by the unrestricted enzyme activity of u-PA and plasmin, but by pericellular molecular and functional interactions between u-PA, u-PAR, PAI-1, extracellular matrix proteins, integrins, endocytosis receptors, and growth factors regulated by paracrine mechanisms (6). The primary structures of cell-adhesion proteins in the extracellular matrix—such as fibronectin, vitronectin, and laminin—have been shown to have common core sequences that contribute to adhesion, spreading, and migration of cells (7). Peptides derived from fibronectin, such as RGDS, and peptides derived from laminin, such as YIGSR, have been shown to inhibit lung metastasis when co-administered with tumor cells (8). Among the extracellular matrix (ECM) components and cell-surface receptors, laminin, and the 67-kD laminin receptor appear to be involved in metastasis (9). The function of the 67-kD laminin receptor is to stabilize the binding of laminin to cell-surface integrins acting as an integrin-accessory molecule.

2. ORGAN TROPISM

The most frequent organ location of metastasis for many types of cancers is the first capillary bed encountered by circulating cells, leading to distribution patterns that follow the venous drainage (10). However, the distribution of metastases varies widely, depending upon the histologic type and anatomic location of the primary tumor. Although anatomy can explain lung metastases from sarcoma, brain metastases from lung carcinoma, and liver metastases from colorectal cancer, renal clear-cell carcinoma metastases to the thyroid, breast-cancer metastases to the ovary and bone, ocular melanoma metastases to the liver, and prostate carcinoma metastases to bone reflect organ tropism (11,12). Walther autopsied 3000 patients who died of cancer between 1927 and 1942, and reported that the organs most targeted for distant metastasis of cancer, in order, are lung, liver, and bone (13). Because Walther's study was conducted without the use of anticancer agents, it is a true reflection of the natural pattern of organ dissemination. Metastasis to distant organs is influenced by the inherent metastatic ability of the malignant cells and the environment of the host organs. The cancer cells may gradually acquire capabilities necessary to achieve metastasis, under the influence of the host environment, and the host environment may also change because of the metastatic cancer cells.

Clearly, metastases tend to grow preferentially in specific organs. Three major types of homing mechanisms are described for this phenomenon *(10)*. Selective growth involves tumor cells that extravasate ubiquitously but selectively, and grow in organs with growth factors and an ECM environment. The preferential growth may be facilitated by local growth factors or hormones present in the target organ. Selective adhesion allows the tumor cells to adhere to the endothelial luminal surface only at the site of organ homing, and to develop a metastatic lesion. The endothelial surface in certain organs may express adhesion molecules, to which circulating tumor cells adhere. Selective chemotaxis of circulating tumor cells directs them to the organ-producing soluble attraction factors. Target organs may secrete soluble factors that act as chemoattractants for circulating tumor cells *(11)*. More than 80% of cancers that spread to bone originate from the breast, prostate, lung, thyroid gland, and kidney *(14)*. Well-designed preclinical models can help to elucidate the mechanisms involved in these processes.

Metastasis has been found to be an inefficient process in both clinical and preclinical studies *(15,16)*. Large numbers of malignant cells come into circulation from a primary tumor, but few of these cells form metastases. When viable malignant cells are injected into the bloodstream of animals, a very small fraction of the cells succeed in forming metastases *(17–20)*.

The organ environment is an important determinant of tumor response to chemotherapy *(21)*. Lymph-node and skin metastases from breast cancer respond better to chemotherapy than lung or bone metastases *(22)*. Preclinical models have shown that the same tumor cells implanted in different organs express different levels of drug-resistance genes, and have a different response to the same chemotherapy *(23–28)*. Studies with a murine fibrosarcoma and with the CT-26 murine colon cancer showed that subcutaneous *(SC)* growing primary tumors were sensitive to system doxorubicin, but lung metastases from these tumors were not *(25,28)*. For the CT-26 colon cancer lung metastases, resistance to doxorubicin and the accompanying elevated expression of the mdr-1 protein found in cells growing in the lung were dependent upon interaction with the specific organ environment *(29)*. When removed from the lung, the cells reverted to a phenotype similar to that of the parental cells.

3. MODELS FOR CLINICAL GROWTH PATTERNS: ORTHOTOPIC IMPLANTATION

The NIH:OVCAR3 xenograft tumor model was developed by Hamilton et al. *(30)* from the ascites of a patient whose tumor progressed on chemotherapy. Upon intraperitoneal (ip) inoculation with NIH:OVCAR3 tumor cells, nude mice develop malignant ascites and tumor nodules involving the ovaries and bowel, and sometimes the liver and lungs. This pattern of tumor growth accurately models the growth of ovarian cancer in patients.

Surgical orthotopic implantation models provide a potential means of more accurately representing clinical cancer with regard to metastasis *(31–34)*. By this method, intact tumor fragments including tumors directly from patients are surgically attached to the corresponding organ. Surgical orthotopic implantation allows spontaneous bone metastasis from prostate cancer, breast cancer, and lung cancer, and spontaneous liver and lymph-node metastasis from colon cancer, as well as metastatic models of pancreatic, stomach, ovarian, bladder, and kidney cancer *(34, 35)*. When the human prostate PC-3 carcinoma tumor line was surgically implanted into the ventral lateral lobes of the prostate gland of nude mice, there was a high frequency of lymph-node and lung metastasis *(36)*. This finding contrasts with results obtained when human prostate PC-3 carcinoma cells were injected into the prostate, and few metastases were observed. The metastastic rate of the human renal-cell SN12C carcinoma has also been compared using orthotopic-cell implantation vs orthotopic tissue implantation *(37)*. The implantation of the tumor fragment allowed faster and more invasive primary-tumor growth, as well as a higher rate of lung, liver, and mediastinal lymph-node metastasis, thus providing a more accurate model of the clinical disease. Morioka et al. *(38)* used the orthotopic-tissue implantation method with the hamster HaP-T1 pancreatic-cancer cell line, and upon necropsy found spontaneous metastases in 100% of the animals, including invasion to adjacent organs and liver metastases.

Fidler et al. *(39)* demonstrated organ effect on response to chemotherapy in several experimental tumor-model systems. Tumor cells from a murine fibrosarcoma, a murine colon carcinoma, and a human colon carcinoma were implanted subcutaneously or into different visceral organs. The SC tumors were sensitive to doxorubicin, yet the lung metastases and liver metastases were not.

4. LUNG METASTASES MODELS

Fidler and Hart observed that intravenously injected murine B16-F10 melanoma cells colonized the lung *(40)*. Furthermore, these cells would selectively grow in SC lung-tissue grafts, indicating a clear organ selectivity for lung by the B16-F10 cells *(41)*. Yokoyama et al. *(42)* implanted B16-BL6 melanoma into the anterior chamber of the eye, subcutaneously in the foot-pad, intradermally in the flank, and subcutaneously at the base of the ear. Primary-tumor growth was much faster in the ear and the flank as compared to the other sites. The intra-ocular melanomas rapidly developed lung metastasis, whereas the SC melanomas primarily developed lymph-node metastasis. The effect of route of inoculation on tumor response was also examined using the B16-F10 murine melanoma and the murine Lewis Lung carcinoma (LLC) implanted intradermally, intravenously to form lung colonies, or intraperitoneally *(43)*. The treatment combination of genistein and cyclophosphamide was more effective against B16-F10 melanoma than against LLC, and was most effective when the B16-F10 was implanted intradermally or intravenously. The host effect on metastatic rate has also been examined. The growth and metastatic potential of three human tumor-cell lines—bladder T24B carcinoma, melanoma RPMI 7931, and lacZ gene-transduced breast MDA-MB-435 BAG cancer—were compared in nude and severe combined immunodeficiency (SCID) mice *(44)*. The growth of the primary tumors was similar in the nude and the SCID mice, and the incidence of spontaneous lung metastasis was much higher in the SCID mice (96%) than in the nude mice (27%). Inoue et al. *(45)* found that the presence of a subcutaneously growing murine colon 26 tumor in a host completely inhibited lung colony formation in mice injected with the same cells intravenously. The inhibition of lung metastases in tumor-bearing mice by colon 26 was closely associated with an increase in serum interleukin-6 levels. The effect of mammalian circadian time structure on SC tumor take-rate and the number of pulmonary nodules after intravenous (iv) tumor-cell injection were studied using the methylcholanthrene A-induced murine fibrosarcoma and the murine B16 melanoma cell lines *(46)*. For both tumors, the daily sleep/wake boundary was the time of day associated with the greatest resistance to metastatic spread. When 3T3 fibroblasts were transformed with c-jun or *ras*, the resulting cells were highly tumorigenic, and when implanted intravenously, numerous pulmonary metastases were observed *(47)*. In contrast, 3T3 cells transformed with SV40 or BPV1 resulted in very slow tumor growth and no pulmonary-nodule growth after iv injection of the cells.

The rat 13762 mammary carcinoma was originally induced with 7, 12-dimethylbenz(a)anthracene (DMBA) in female Fischer rats *(48)*. When implanted subcutaneously in the syngeneic host, the primary tumor grows progressively; however, if the primary tumor is removed, all of the animals will succumb to lung metastases with other organ metastases. In another study, when the parental 13762 mammary carcinoma cells were implanted subcutaneously into the mammary fat pads of female Fischer 344 rats, the tumor metastasized to the lymph nodes and lungs with a low frequency *(49)*. However, SC implantation of cells collected from the lung metastases were much more spontaneously metastatic than the parental cells. Generally, the growth of primary 13762 mammary carcinoma implanted subcutaneously is paralleled by the growth of the lung metastases *(50)*. Sublines of high and low metastatic potential have been developed from the parental 13762 mammary carcinoma and designated MTLn3 for high metastatic potential and MTC for low metastatic potential *(51)*. These sublines have been used to examine molecular characteristics associated with the metastatic phenotype. The 13762 mammary carcinoma will also grow if implanted intradermally in the syngeneic host, the female Fischer 344 rat *(52)*.

Lung metastasis models have been widely used in the search for potential antimetastatic treatment agents. Administration of granulocyte-macrophage colony-stimulating factor (GM-CSF) neutralizing antibodies diminished the ability of metastatic LLC cell injected intravenously to form lung nodules *(53)*. Treatment of artificially immunosuppressed mice bearing LLC, B16 melanoma, rat RWT-M nephroblastoma, or human colon HCR25 carcinoma with Avemar, a fermented wheat-germ extract along with vitamin C, resulted in a marked decrease in metastasis formation, both in the presence and absence of the primary tumor *(54)*. Exposure of the highly metastatic human renal-cell SN12Cpm6 carcinoma cells exposed to sodium5-amino-5-deoxy-D-glucosaccharic acid-delta-lactam (ND-2001) caused a 78% inhibition of lung-metastases formation *(55)*. Leupeptin and leupeptin analogs inhibited lung-colony formation after iv injection of hepatoma cells in rats *(56)*.

5. BONE METASTASIS MODELS

Bone metastasis is a catastrophic complication in many cancer patients *(12)*. Causing very serious pain, pathological bone fractures, spinal-cord compression, hypocalcemia, etc. It is significant that the process is incurable. Once the tumor cells have lodged in the bone, only palliative therapy is available. With this in mind, models have been developed to address this specific site of metastasis. Attempts have been made to develop appropriate animals models to mimic the disease and its progression *(57)*.

When solid tumors metastasize to the skeleton, they cause a variety of alterations, including osteolysis, diffuse osteopenia, osteoblastic lesions, and a combination of all these. All these changes are caused by the effect of tumor products on the normal bone-remodeling processes. There are two patterns of effects on the bone cells, reflected as osteoclast and osteoblast formation. Breast cancer tends to develop osteolytic metastasis, whereas prostate cancer tends to develop osteoblastic metastasis. In both cases, tumor cells interact with osteoclasts and osteoblasts inside the bone cavity. Since prostate-cancer produces osteoblastic metastasis, the metastatic malignant cells from this disease likely produce factors that stimulate bone formation. The primary prostate cancer grows relatively slowly, but in bone, the growth is often accelerated. There are many stimulating factors identified. On very careful histological examination of the lesions in bone, osteoclastic bone destruction can be found. Every primary metastatic lesion in the bone begins with osteolysis. Osteolysis can be inhibited experimentally in rats—PAIII rat prostate adenocarcinoma—by pretreating the animals with dichloramethylene biphosphonate, an inhibitor of osteoclasts. The osteolysis provides calcium, nutrients, and the space needed for future osteoblastic changes.

The usefulness of intracardiac injection of tumor cells to produce growth of tumor in the bone was recognized many years ago *(58, 59)*. Since that time, bone metastasis models have focused primarily, but not exclusively, on prostate and breast cancer. The Dunning R3327-Mat-LyLu rat prostate-carcinoma tumor line has been used as the basis for several approaches. Haq et al. *(60)* inoculated Dunning R3327-Mat-LyLu cells into the left ventricle of the heart of Copenhagen rats, leading to the development of spinal metastases in 100% of the inoculated animals. A subline of Mat-LyLu, Mat-LyLu-B5, was selected through the sequential inoculation of bone-marrow-derived carcinoma cells into the left ventricle, and was found to have increased metastastic potential compared to the parental line. The subline was found to have higher adhesion to a bone-marrow stromal cell culture highly enriched for endothelial cells than the parental Mat-LyLu line. Recently, the full-length cDNA-encoding rat Parathyroid-related protein (PTHRP) was stably transfected into the Dunning R3327Mat-LyLu prostate-cancer cell line *(61)*. Control (vector only transfected) and experimental cells were inoculated subcutaneously into the right flank or by the intracardiac route into the left ventricle of inbred male Copenhagen rats. No skeletal metastases occurred after SC injection with either the control or PTHRP-transfected cells. The intracardiac inoculation led to lumbar vertebra metastasis and consequent hind-limb paralysis. Histological examination showed a marked increase in osteoclastic activity that was increased in the PTHRP-transfected line. In an independent study, Blomme et al. *(62)* prepared a stably transfected subline of Mat-LyLu rat prostate-carcinoma cells expressing rat PTHRP. The transfected Mat-LyLu subline was injected into the left ventricle of Copenhagen rats to induce formation of bone metastases. All of the rats developed osteolytic metastases in long bones and vertebra by 2-wk post-tumor-cell injection. There was no observable difference between the control Mat-LyLu tumor cells and the PTHRP-transfected subline in this study.

The human LNCaP prostate carcinoma is an androgen-responsive cell line, and has been widely used as a model for the clinical disease, both in cell culture and grown as a xenograft in immunodeficient mice. Several androgen-independent human prostate-cancer-cell lines have been derived from the androgen-dependent LNCaP cells with androgen independence defined as the capability of the prostate-cancer cells to grow in castrated hosts *(63)*. One of the sublines, C4-2, was androgen-independent, highly tumorigenic, and metastastic, with a proclivity for metastasis to the bone. Thalmann et al. *(64)* established androgen-independent and bone metastatic-cell sublines B2, B3,

B4, and B5 from the C4-2 subline. This collection of cell lines has been described as a prostate-cancer progression model from the parental LNCaP androgen-responsive cell line to the LNCaP C4-2 androgen-independent cell line, and then to the further selected B2, B3, B4, and B5 sublines. When implanted subcutaneously in nude mice, the B sublines metastasize from the primary tumor to the lymph nodes, and to the axial skeleton with a predominant osteoblastic reaction phenotype. In 5–19 wk postimplantation of the SC B subline tumors, 25–37.5% of the animals developed paralegia. Molecular characteristics of the sublines compared with the parental LNCaP cell line indicate a progression toward a more malignant cell type.

Several models of breast-cancer metastasis to bone have been described focusing on osteoclastic metastasis. To produce bone metastasis from breast-cancer lines, introduction of the cancer cells directly into the arterial circulation through the left ventricle of the heart in young mice is used as described here for prostate cancer (65,66). The tumor line most frequently used as a breast-cancer model by this method is the human estrogen-independent MDA-MB-231 cell line. The MB-231 cell line develops radiologically distinctive osteolytic bone metastases that histologically demonstrate numerous osteoclasts and aggressive tumor colonization in bone 3–4-wk after cell inoculation (67). The MDA-MB-231 intracardiac injection model has been used to study the character of metastatic lesions of the mandible (68). The metastatic lesions in untreated mice were radiolographically observed at the body and angle of the mandible. Histology of the mandible of untreated mice revealed that most of the bone-marrow cavities had been occupied by the metastatic tumor, with active osteoclasts along the trabecular bone (68). An orthotopic metastasis model using the mouse 4T1 mammary tumor has also been established (69, 70). The 4T1 murine mammary carcinoma cells form tumors in 7–10 d after SC inoculation into the orthotopic mammary fat pad, and subsequently develop bone and visceral organ metastases 3–5 wk after inoculation into female Balb/c mice (67). The 4T1 model produces bone metastases in 100% of the animals, and allows the use of an immunocompetent host. A subline of 4T1 stably transfected with the reporter gene luciferase (4T1/Luc) has also been established.

Osteolytic bone destruction and its complications are a major source of morbidity and mortality in patients with multiple myeloma (71). The bone destruction in multiple myeloma is caused by increased osteoclast activity and decreased bone formation in areas of bone adjacent to myeloma cells. The human ARH-77 plasma-cell leukemia-cell line has disseminated growth in SCID mice. It expresses IgGk and has been used as a model for human multiple myeloma (71). The ARH-77 cells were injected intravenously into the tail vein of female SCID mice. Development of bone disease was assessed by blood-ionized calcium levels, X-rays, and histology. All of the ARH-77 implanted mice developed hind-limb paralysis 28–35 d after injection of 106 cells and developed hypercalcemia approx 5 d after becoming paraplegic. Lytic lesions were detectable on X-rays. Histologic examination of tissues showed infiltration of ARH-77 myeloma cells in the liver and spleen, and marked infiltration in vertebrae and long bones, with loss of bony trabeculae and increased osteoclast numbers.

6. SPLEEN/LIVER METASTASES MODELS

Liver tumors have been of interest to cancer researchers from several fields, including those who focus on carcinogens, biophysicists studying imaging techniques, and experimental therapists. In the 1980s, it was noted that treatment of rats with chemical carcinogens such as trans-4-acetylaminostilbene produced preneoplastic lesions in the liver that could become neoplastic upon healing from a partial hepatectomy *(72)*. Other chemical carcinogens, such as phenobarbital and barbital sodium administered in the drinking water to F344 rats, enhanced development of hepatocellular adenomas at 52 wk and hepatocellular adenomas and trabecular carcinomas at 78 wk in N-nitrosodiethylamine-treated rats *(73)*. The production of liver tumors by exposure of F344 rats to chemical carcinogens is a model that is sufficiently reliable to assess the potential of chemopreventative and chemoprotective agents *(74)*. Seglen et al. *(75)* transplanted cell suspensions or tissue fragments from primary hepatocellular carcinomas induced by treating rats with chemical carcinogens into syngeneic hosts by intraportal injection or subcapsular implantation. A high rate of tumor-take was observed, and tumor growth could be stimulated by further carcinogen administration or partial hepatectomy. In C3H mice, administration of N-nitroso compounds during pregnancy resulted in a high percentage of offspring with hepatocellular carcinomas, depending upon the gestational age at exposure *(76)*.

In the classic approach, a metastatic model for large-cell lymphoma/lymphosarcoma was developed by sequential selection in vivo of the murine RAW117 cell line for enhanced liver metastasis *(77)*. The high liver-colonizing line was designated RAW117-H10 and used to elucidate molecular differences with the RAW117-P parental line. A hepatic invasive human colorectal xenograft model was derived in nude mice by selection through the liver of the parental cell line, C170 *(78)*. Following (ip) injection, tumors selectively grew on the liver in >80% of the animals. The liver-invading xenograft line was named C170HM2, and produced more aggressive tumors than the parental line. The ability of the RPMI 4788 human colon-carcinoma cell line to produce experimental metastases in the lung ip cavity and liver was studied in nude mice. Lung tumors were produced by iv injection of 2 million cells, liver tumors were produced by intraportal injection of 5 million cells, and intra-abdominal tumors were produced by ip injection of 5 million cells *(78)*. Cohen et al. *(80)* found that inoculation of murine colon adenocarcinoma MCA-38 cells into the ileocolic vein resulted in the development of distinct hepatic foci within 21 ds in C57B1 mice. An iv injection of M5076 murine reticulosarcoma also produces a high level of liver metastasis *(81)*. The blood clearance, tissue uptake, and antitumor efficacy of liposomal doxorubicin was studied in liver metastasis of M5076 reticulosarcoma in mice *(82)*. The liposomal preparation of the drug was more effective than the free doxorubicin. The murine Neuro2a neuroblastoma line also produces 100% liver metastasis upon iv injection of the tumor cells *(83)*. Recently, murine L1210 leukemia was used to study liposomal topotecan, comparing the ascitic tumor response with an L1210 liver metastasis model *(84)*. With a tumor at either site, the liposomal preparation of topotecan was more effective than the free drug.

For radiological imaging research, solitary or multiple metastatic tumors produced in a controlled manner were achieved by trocar inoculation of tumor fragments into the liver or by fine-needle injection of single-cell suspensions directly into the liver to produce solitary lesions or injection of single-cell suspensions via the spleen or mesenteric vein to produce multiple liver metastases *(85)*. To decrease tumor dissemination from the liver, a piece of GelFoam was placed into a small incision in the liver of 583 ACI rats, and a Morris hepatoma 3924A fragment was implanted. By this method, the tumor grew locally before invading the surrounding tissues and lungs, allowing time for the study of therapies on the liver disease *(86)*. Qin et al. *(87)* used magnetic resonance imaging (MRI) to determine the volumes of hepatic metastatic tumors in the rat. Three different hepatic tumor models mimicking liver metastases were established in syngeneic BDIX rats by injection of DHD/K12 rat colon-cancer cells, either directly under the liver capsule or via the portal system. The liver-tumor volumes were estimated in vivo by using MR imaging of the liver, summing the individual tumor volumes in the sequential MR liver sections. In another study, tumor detection using a hepatocyte-specific contrast agent was evaluated in four experimental tumor models in rats, with a focus on tumor-liver contrast-to-noise ratios *(88)*. The potential of positron emission tomography (PET) for the detection and evaluation of hepatomas using murine and rat liver-tumor models was also assessed *(89)*. Brix et al. *(90)* compared ^{18}F PET and ^{19}F MRI for noninvasive monitoring of 5-fluorouracil (5-*FU*) in ACI and Buffalo rats with transplanted MH3924A and TC5123 Morris hepatomas, respectively. While the imaging techniques were fairly equivalent, the MR images yielded more information. In another study, the rat Novikoff hepatoma was used to study (5-*FU*) by ^{19}F-magnetic spectroscopy in vivo *(91)*.

Thorstensen et al. *(92)* introduced a method for tumor transplantation into the rabbit liver for experimental study. VX2 tumor cells were initially grown intraperitoneally in a New Zealand white rabbit. An automated biopsy instrument with an ultrathin-wall biopsy needle was used to take standardized tumor samples from the peritoneal tumor. Using the same technique, a tumor sample was transplanted into the left-liver lobe of the recipient animals. The resulting VX2 tumors were well delineated from the surrounding liver, and metastasized only late in the disease. In a study of the antiangiogenic agent TNP-470, Kuwata et al. *(93)* used 25 Japanese white rabbits with metastatic liver tumors produced by intraportal injection of VX2 carcinoma cells. The tumors responded best when treatment with TNP-470 was combined with a cytotoxic anticancer agent. In a gene-therapy study, VX-2 rabbit carcinoma cells were maintained by serial transplantation into the thigh muscles of New Zealand white rabbits, and disseminated liver metastases were established by direct injection of tumor cells into the portal vein of the animals. Different doses of a recombinant thymidine kinase-negative vaccinia-virus vector encoding the firefly luciferase reporter gene were injected into tumor-bearing rabbits *(94)*. Transgene expression was higher in the tumor than the normal tissue, but the period of expression was limited.

7. BRAIN METASTASES MODELS

Brain metastases occur in 20–40% of all patients with cancer, and are an important cause of cancer morbidity and mortality. Schabet et al. *(95)* developed an experimental model of leptomeningeal metastasis by intracisternal injection of 104 B16-F10 murine melanoma cells in nude rats. Although (ACNU (N′-[(4-amino-2-methyl-5-pyrimidinyl)methyl]-N-(2-chloroethyl)-N-nitrosourea) provided effective local treatment and increased survival, the drug-treated animals had increased spinal seeding and mass growth. To model brain metastasis, cells from six different human cancer-cell lines that were known to produce visceral metastasis, were injected into the internal carotid artery of nude mice *(96)*. Human colon carcinoma (KM12SM) and human lung adenocarcinoma (PC14PE6 and PC14Br) cells produced large, fast-growing parenchymal brain metastases. Human lung squamous-cell carcinoma *(SCC)* (H226), human renal-cell carcinoma (RCC) (SN12PM6) and human melanoma (TXM13) cells produced only a few slow-growing brain metastases. The rapidly progressing brain metastases contained many enlarged blood vessels, and expressed high levels of vascular endothelial growth factor (VEGF) *(97)*. PC12PE6 cells were isolated from pleural effusions developed in a nude mouse injected intravenously with parental PC14 lung adenocarcinoma cells *(96)*. PC14Br cells were isolated from brain metastases established in combined immunodeficient/beige mice subsequent to intracarotid artery injection of PC14 cells *(97)*. The human KM12SM colon carcinoma was established at the M.D. Anderson Cancer Center *(98)*.

To produce brain metastases, mice were anesthetized, restrained, and placed under a dissecting microscope *(99)*. The carotid artery was prepared for injection distal to the point of division into the internal and external carotid arteries. A ligature of 4-0 silk was placed in the distal part of the common carotid artery. A second ligature was placed and loosely tied proximal to the injection site to elevate the carotid artery. This procedure controlled bleeding from the carotid artery by regurgitation from distal vessels. The artery was nicked with a pair of microscissors and a <30-gauge glass cannula was inserted into the lumen. The cells ($2.5 \times 10^4/100$ µl Hank's Balanced Salt Solution HBSS) were injected slowly. The second ligature was tightened, and the skin was closed with sutures *(99)*.

8. MODELS FOR DETECTION OF OCCULT METASTASES

The detection of micrometastases is clinically important in preclinical models to assess tumor aggressiveness and to assess treatment efficacy. Interest in this issue can be traced to the 19th century, when it was first noted that tumor cells were detectable when circulating in the blood of cancer patients *(100)*. During the mid-20th century, a major effort was mounted to detect, count, and correlate with treatment outcome the number of circulating tumor cells in cancer patients. However, the limitations of the technology available at the time—primarily morphologic analysis—produced a high rate of false-positives, and the effort was terminated. Immunohistochemical methods have offered improved differentiation between tumor cells and normal cells in the blood and bone marrow, but are limited by the availability of antibodies specific for tumor cells or selective for tumor cells within a population of normal cells. More recently, polymerase chain reaction (PCR) amplification of tissue-specific messenger RNA present in tumor cells has been applied to the detection of circulating tumor cells and micrometastases in solid-tumor patients *(100)*. Use of *PCR* amplification for messenger RNA for prostate-specific antigen (PSA) and for tyrosinase in prostate-cancer patients and in melanoma patients, respectively, has increased the sensitivity for detection of small numbers of tumor cells. The prognostic value of these findings remains controversial.

Preclinically, tumors carrying marker genes are being developed. Rubio et al. *(101)* prepared a subline of PC-3 prostate carcinoma expressing the luciferase gene. When these cells were implanted intramuscularly in nude mice, metastatic cells in target organs were easily detected by their capacity to produce light. Tumor cells were detected in all of the target organs examined, including lymph nodes, brain, bone, lungs, liver, kidney, spleen, testicles, prostate, seminal vesicles, and scrotum. Distant organ colonization began about 14 ds after implant of the primary tumor when the primary tumor was still very small, containing 2×10^4 tumor-cell equivalents of light production *(101)*.

Although injection of murine B16 melanoma cells into the left cardiac ventricle can produce metastasis to bone tissue, this process is complicated. Thus, its use in large-scale studies is not convenient. Injection of murine B16 melanoma cells into the tail vein of mice produces large numbers of colonies in the lungs, but few other detectable metastases. Injection of the tumor cells orthotopically into bone produces lesions in the bone, but the cascade of metastasis is lacking in this model. Yang et al. *(102)* developed a stably transfected subline of murine B16 melanoma and a stably transfected subline of human (LOX) melanoma expressing green fluorescent protein *(GFP)*. These highly fluorescent malignant-melanoma-cell lines allowed visualization of skeletal and multi-organ metastases after iv injection of the transfected B16 cells into C57BL/6 mice and after intradermal implantation of the transfected LOX cells into nude mice.

Immunodeficient male mice were injected intradermally with 1×10^6 LOX-GFP cells (0.1 mL), on the dorsal skin with a 30-gauge 1/2 precision glide needle. Female C57BL/6 mice were injected with 5×10^6 (0.2 mL) B16F0-GFP C1 cells into the lateral tail vein. Tumor progression was observed with decreased performance. Light microscopy and fluorescence microscopy were conducted, using a GFP filter set. Single cells or colonies in the skeletal system could be visualized by GFP fluorescence. B16F0 tumors developed extensive skeletal and visceral metastases when the animals were sacrificed 3 wk. after the tail vein injection. The lesions were strongly fluorescent. Most striking were extensive bone and bone-marrow metastases of the transfected B16 cells visualized by the GFP when animals were sacrificed 3 wk after implantation. Metastases for both transfected lines were visualized in many organs, including the brain, lung, pleural membrane, liver, kidney, adrenal gland, lymph nodes, skeletal muscle, and skin *(102)*.

REFERENCES

1. Ahmad A, Hart IR. Mechanisms of metastasis. *Crit Rev Onocol/Hematol* 1997; 26:163–173.
2. Liotta LA, Kohn EC. Invasion and metastasis. In: Holland JF, Frei E III, Bast RC, Kufe DW, Morton DL, Weichselbaum RR, eds., *Cancer Medicine.* Lea & Fibiger: Philadelphia, *PA*, 1993, pp. 165–180.
3. Meyer T, Hart IR. Mechanisms of tumor metastasis. *Eur J Cancer* 1998; 34:214–221.
4. Morris VL, Schmidt EE, MacDonald IC, Groom AC, Chambers AF. Sequential steps in hematogenous metastasis of cancer cells studied by in vivo videomicroscopy. *Invasion Metastasis* 1997; 17:281–296.
5. Ruiz P, Gunthert U. The cellular basis of metastasis. *World J Urol* 1996; 14:141–150.
6. Andreasen PA, Kjoller L, Christensen L, Duffy MJ. The urokinase-type plasminogen activator system in cancer metastasis: a review. *Int J Cancer* 1997; 72:1–22.
7. Saiki I. Cell adhesion molecules and cancer metastasis. *Jpn J Pharmacol* 1997; 75:215–242.
8. Iwamoto Y, Robey FA, Graf J, Saski M, Kleinman HK, Yamada Y, et al. YIGSR, a synthetic laminin penta-peptide, inhibits experimental metastasis formation. *Science* 1987; 238:1132–1134.
9. Menard S, Castronovo V, Tagliabue E, Sobel ME. New insights into the metastasis-associated 67 kD laminin receptor. *J Cell Biochem* 1997; 67:155–165.
10. Woodhouse EC, Chuaqui RF, Liotta LA. General mechanisms of metastasis. *Cancer* 1997; 80:1529–1537.
11. Nicolson GL, Dulski K, Basson C, Welch DR. Preferential organ attachment and invasion in vitro by B16 melanoma cells selected for differing metastatic colonization and invasive properties. *Invasion Metastasis* 1985; 5:144–154.
12. Rubens RD. Bone metastases—the clinical problem. *Eur J Cancer* 1998; 34:210–213.
13. Yoneda T. Cellular and molecular mechanisms of breast and prostate cancer metastasis to bone. *Eur J Cancer* 1998; 34:240–245.

14. Resnick MI. Hemodynamics of prostate bone metastases. In: JP Karr, Yamanka H, eds., *Prostate Cancer and Bone Metastasis,* Plenum Press: New York, *NY,* 1992, pp. 77–83.

15. Chambers AF, Matrisian LM. Changing views of the role of matrix metalloproteinases in metastasis. *J Natl Cancer Inst* 1997; 89:1260–1270.

16. Weiss L. Metastatic inefficiency. *Adv Cancer Res* 1990; 54:159–211.

17. Liotta LA, Kleinerman J, Saidel GM. Quantitative relationships of intravascular tumor cells, tumor vessels and pulmonary metastases following tumor implantation. *Cancer Res* 1974; 34:997–1004.

18. Butler TP, Gullino PM. Quantitation of cell shedding into efferent blood of mammary adenocarcinoma. *Cancer Res* 1975; 35:512–516.

19. Tarin D, Vass AC, Kettlewell MG, Proce JE. Absence of metastatic sequalae during long-term treatment of malignant ascites by perineovenous shunting. A clinico-pathological report. *Invasion Metastasis* 1984; 4: 1–12.

20. Fidler IJ. Metastasis: quantitative analysis of distribution and fate of tumor emboli labeled with ^{125}I-5-iodo-2'-deoxyuridine. *J Natl Cancer Inst* 1970; 45:773–782.

21. Fidler IJ, Poste G. The cellular heterogeneity of malignant neoplasms: implications for adjuvant chemotherapy. *Semin Oncol* 1985; 12:207–221.

22. Slack NH, Bross JDJ. The influence of the site of metastasis on tumor growth and response to chemotherapy. *Br J Cancer* 1975; 78:32–41.

23. Pratesi G, Manzotti C, Tortoreto M, Audisio RA, Zunino F. Differential efficacy of flavone acetic acid against liver versus lung metastases in a human tumor xenograft. *Br J Cancer* 1991; 71:663–671.

24. Smith KA, Begg AC, Denekamp J. Differences in chemosensitivity between subcutaneous and pulmonary tumors. *Eur J Cancer Clin Oncol* 1985; 21:249–259.

25. Staroselsky A, Fan D, O'Brian CA, Bucana CD, Gupta KP, Fidler IJ. Site-dependent differences in response of the UV-2237 murine fibrosarcoma to systemic therapy with adriamycin. *Cancer Res* 1990; 40:7775–7782.

26. Donelli MG, Russo R, Garattini S. Selective chemotherapy in relation to the site of tumor transplantation. *Int J Cancer* 1975; 32:78–88.

27. Teicher BA, Herman TS, Holden SA, et al. Tumor resistance to alkylating agents conferred by mechanisms operative only in vivo. *Science* 1990; 247:1457–1461.

28. Wilmanns C, Fan D, O'Brian CA, Bucana CD, Fidler IJ. Orthotopic and ectopic organ environments differentially influence the sensitivity of murine colon carcinoma cells to doxorubicin and 5-fluorouracil. *Int J Cancer* 1992; 52:98–107.

29. Dong Z, Radinsky R, Fan D, et al. Organ-specific modulation of steady-state mdr-1 gene expression and drug resistance in murine colon cancer cells. *J Natl Cancer Inst* 1994; 86:913–920.

30. Hamilton TC, Young RC, Louie KG, Behrens BC, McKoy WM, Grotzinger KR, et al. Characterization of a xenograft model of human ovarian carcinoma which produces ascites and intra-abdominal carcinomatosis in mice. *Cancer Res* 1984; 44:5286–5295.

31. Manzotti C, Audisio RA, Pratesi G. Importance of orthoptopic implantation for human tumors as model systems: relevance to metastasis and invasion. *Clin Exp Metastasis* 1993; 11:5–14.

32. Hoffman RM. Orthotopic is orthodox: why are orthotopic-transplant metastatic models different from all other models? *J Cell Biochem* 1994; 56: 1–3.

33. Kubota T. Metastatic models of human cancer xenografted in the nude mouse: the importance of orthotopic transplantation. *J Cell Biochem* 1994; 56: 4–8.

34. Hoffman RM. Orthotopic metastatic mouse models for anticancer drug discovery and evaluation: a bridge to the clinic. *Investig New Drugs* 1999; 17:343–359.

35. Mitchell BS, Schumacher U. Use of immunodeficient mice in metastasis research. *Br J Biomed Sci* 1997; 54:278–286.

36. An Z, Wang X, Geller J, Moossa AR, Hoffman RM. Surgical orthotopic implantation allows high lung and lymph node metastatic expression of human prostate carcinoma cell line PC-3 in nude mice. *Prostate* 1998; 34:169–174.

37. An Z, Jiang P, Wang X, Moossa AR, Hoffman RM. Development of a high metastatic orthotopic model of human renal cell carcinoma in nude mice: benefits of fragment implantyation compared to cell-suspension injection. *Clin Exp Metastasis* 1999; 17:265–270.

38. Morioka CY, Saito S, Ohzawa K, Watanabe A. Homologous orthotopic implantation models of pancreatic ductal cancer in Syrian golden hamsters: which is better for metastasis research—cell implantation or tissue implantation? *Pancreas* 2000; 20:152–157.

39. Fidler IJ, Wilmanns C, Staroselsky A, Radinsky R, Dong Z, Fan D. Modulation of tumor cell response to chemotherapy by the organ environment. *Cancer Met Rev* 1994; 13:209–222.
40. Fidler IJ, Hart IP. Biologic diversity in metstatic neoplasms: origins and implications. *Science* 1982; 217:998–1002.
41. Fidler IJ, Poste G. The cellular heterogeneity of malignant neoplasms: implications for adjuvant chemotherapy. *Semin Oncol* 1985; 12:207–221.
42. Yokoyama T, Ohneseit P, Buchholz R, Santo-Holtje L, Schmidberger H. Intrathecal ACNU treatment of B16 melanoma leptomengeal metastasis in a new athymic rat model. *J Neuro-Oncol* 1992; 14:169–175.
43. Wietrzyk J, Opolski A, Madej J, Radzikowski C. Antitumor and antimetastatic effect of genistein alone or combined with cyclophosphamide in mice transplanted with various tumors depends on the route of tumor transplantation. *In Vivo* 2000; 14:357–362.
44. Xie X, Brunner N, Jensen G, Albrectsen J, Gotthardsen B, Rygaard J. Comparative studies between nude and scid mice on the growth and metastatic behavior of xenografted human tumors. *Clin Exp Metastasis* 1992; 10:201–210.
45. Inoue K, Okabe S, Sueoka E, Sueoka N, Tabei T, Suganuma M. The role of interleukin-6 in inhibition of lung metastasis in subcutaneous tumor-bearing mice. *Oncol Rep* 2000; 7:69–73.
46. Hrushesky WJ, Lester B, Lannin D. Circadian coordination of cancer growth and metastatic spread. *Int J Cancer* 1999; 83:365–373.
47. Kraemer M, Touraire R, Dejong V, Montreau N, Briane D, Derbin C, et al. Rat embryo fibroblasts transformed by c-jun display highly metastatic and angiogenic activities in vivo and deregulate gene expression of both angiogenic and antiangiogenic factors. *Cell Growth Differ* 1999; 10:193–200.
48. Bogden AE, Esber HJ, Taylor DJ, Gray JH. Comparative study on the effects of surgery, chemotherapy, and immunotherapy, alone and in combination, on metastases of the 13762 mammary adenocarcinoma. *Cancer Res* 1974; 34:1627–1631.
49. Neri A, Welch D, Kawaguchi T, Nicolson GL. Development and biologic properties of malignant cell sublines and clones of a spontaneously metastasizing rat mammary adenocarcinoma. *J Natl Cancer Inst* 1982; 68:507–517.
50. Stanko RT, Mullick P, Clarke MR, Contis LC, Janosky JE, Rmaasatry SS. Pyruvate inhibits growth of mammary adenocarcinoma 13762 in rats. *Cancer Res* 1994; 54:1004–1007.
51. Kaufmann AM, Khazaie K, Wiedemuth M, Rohde-Schultz B, Ullrich A, Schirrmacher V, et al. Expression of epidermal growth factor receptor correlates with metastatic potential of 13762NF rat mammary adenocarcinoma cells. *Int J Oncol* 1994; 4:1149–1155.
52. Ramasastry SS, Weinstein LW, Zerbe A, Narayanan K, LaPietra D, Futrell JW. Regression of local and distant tumor growth by tissue expansion: an experimental study of mammary carcinoma 13762 in rats. *Plast Recon Surg* 1991; 87:1–7.
53. Young MR, Lozano Y, Djordjevic A, Devata S, Matthews J, Young ME, et al. Granulocyte-macrophage colony-stimulating factor stimulates the metastatic properties of Lewis lung carcinoma through a protein kinase A signal-transduction pathway. *Int J Cancer* 1993; 53:667–671.
54. Hidvegi M, Raso E, Tomoskozi-Farkas R, Paku S, Lapis K, Szende B. Effect of Avemar and Avemar + vitamin C on tumor growth and metastasis in experimental animals. *Anticancer Res* 1998; 18:2353–2358.
55. Kuramitsu Y, Hamada J, Tsuruoka T, Morikawa K, Naito S, Kobayashi H, et al. ND-2001 suppresses lung metastasis of human renal cancer cells in athymic mice. *Anti-Cancer Drugs* 1998; 9:739–741.
56. Umezawa K. Inhibition of experimental metastasis by enzyme inhibitors from microorganisms and plants. *Adv Enzyme Reg* 1996; 36:267–281.
57. Mundy GR. Mechanisms of bone metastasis. *Cancer* 1997; 80:1546–1556.
58. Arguello F, Baggs RB, Frantz CN. A murine model of experimental metastasis to bone and bone marrow. *Cancer Res* 1988; 48:6876–6881.
59. Stakpole CW, Alterman AL, Fornabaio DM. Growth characteristics of clonal cell populations constituting a B16 melanoma metastasis model system. *Invasion Metastasis* 1985; 5:125–143.
60. Haq M, Goltzman D, Tremblay G, Brodt P. Rat prostate adenocarcinoma cells disseminate to bone and adhere preferentially to bone marrow-derived endothelial cells. *Cancer Res* 1992; 52:4613–4619.
61. Rabbani SA, Gladu J, Harakidas P, Jamison B, Goltzman D. Over-production of parathyroid hormone-related peptide results in increased osteolytic skeletal metastasis by prostate cancer cells in vivo. *Int J Cancer* 1999; 80:257–264.

62. Blomme EAG, Dougherty KM, Pienta KJ, Capen CC, Rosol TJ, McCauley LK. Skeletal metastasis of prostate adenocarcinoma in rats: morphometric analysis and role of parathyroid hormone-related protein. *The Prostate* 1999; 39:187–197.

63. Gleave ME, Hsieh JT, Gao C, von Eschenbach AC, Chung LWK. Acceleration of human prostate cancer growth in vivo by prostate and bone fibroblasts. *Cancer Res* 1991; 51:3753–3761.

64. Thalmann GN, Sikes RA, Wu TT, Degeorges A, Chang S-M, Ozen M, et al. LNCaP progression model of human prostate cancer: androgen-independence and osseous metastasis. *The Prostate* 2000; 44:91–103.

65. Yoneda T, Sasaki A, Mundy GR. Osteolytic bone disease in breast cancer. *Breast Cancer Res Treatment* 1994; 32:73–84.

66. Yoneda T. Arterial microvascularization and breast cancer colonization in bone. *Histol Histopathol* 1997; 12:1145–1149.

67. Yoneda T, Michigami T, Yi B, Williams PJ, Niewolna M, Hiraga T. Use of bisphosphonates for the treatment of bone metastasis in experimental animal models. *Cancer Treat Rev* 1999; 25:293–299.

68. Sasaki A, Boyce BF, Story B, Wright KR, Chapman M, Boyce R, et al. Bisphosphonate risedronate reduces metastatic human breast cancer burden in bone in nude mice. *Cancer Res* 1995; 55:3551–3557.

69. Aslakson CJ, Miller FR. Selective events in the metastatic process defined by analysis of the sequential dissemination of subpopulations of a mouse mammary tumor. *Cancer Res* 1992; 52:1399–1405.

70. Lelekakis M, Moseley JM, Martin JM, Hards D, Williams E, Ho P, et al. A novel orthotopic model of breast cancer metastasis to bone. *Clin Exp Metastasis* 1999; 17:163–170.

71. Alsina M, Boyce B, Devlin RD, Anderson JL, Craig F, Mundy GR, et al. Development of an in vivo model of human multiple myeloma bone disease. *Blood* 1996; 87:1495–1501.

72. Hilpert D, Romen W, Neumann HG. The role of partial hepatectomy and of promoters in the formation of tumors in non-target tissues of trans-4-acetylaminostilbene in rats. *Carcinogenesis* 1983; 4:1519–1525.

73. Diwan BA, Rice JM, Ohshima M, Ward JM, Dove LF. Comparative tumor-promoting activities of phenobarbital, amobarbital, barbital sodium and barbituric acid on livers and other organs of male F344/NCr rats following initiation with N-nitrosodiethylamine. *J Natl Cancer Inst* 1985; 74:509–516.

74. Fukushima S, Hagiwara A, Hirose M, Yamaguchi S, Tiwawech D, Ito N. Modifying effects of various chemicals on preneoplastic and neoplastic lesion development in a wide-spectrum organ carcinogenesis model using F344 rats. *Jpn J Cancer Res* 1991; 82:642–649.

75. Seglen PO, Saeter G, Schwartze PE. Liver tumor promoters stimulate growth of transplanted hepatocellular carcinomas. *Hepatology* 1990; 12:295–300.

76. Anderson LM, Hagiwara A, Kovatch RM, Rehm S, Rice JM. Transplacental initiation of liver, lung, neurogenic and connective tissue tumors by N-nitroso compounds in mice. *Fundam Appl Toxicol* 1989; 12:604–620.

77. Irimura T, Tressler RJ, Nicolson GL. Sialoglycoproteins of murine RAW117 large cell lymphoma/lymphosarcoma sublines of various metastastic colonization properties. *Cell Res* 1986; 165:403–416.

78. Watson SA, Morris TM, Crosbee DM, Hardcastle JD. A hepatic invasive human colorectal xenograft model. *Eur J Cancer* 1993; 29A:1740–1745.

79. Naomoto Y, Kondo H, Tanaka N, Orita K. Novel experimental models of human cancer metastasis in nude mice: lung metastasis, intraabdominal carcinomatosis with ascites and liver metastasis. *J Cancer Res Clin Oncol* 1987; 113:544–549.

80. Cohen SA, Goldrosen MH. Modulation of colon-derived experimental hepatic metastasis by murine nonparenchymal liver cells. *Immunol Investig* 1989; 18:351–363.

81. Sola F, Farao M, Ciomei M, Pastori A, Mongelli N, Grandi M. FCE27266, a sulfonic distamycin derivative, inhibits experimental and spontaneous lung and liver metastasis. *Invasion Metastasis* 1995; 15:222–231.

82. Shimizu K, Qi XR, Maitani Y, Yoshii M, Kawano K, Takayama K, et al. Targeting of soybean-derived sterylglucoside liposomes to liver tumors in rat and mouse models. *Biol Pharmaceut Bull* 1998; 21:741–746.

83. Amirkhosravi A, Warnes G, Biggerstaff J, Malik Z, May K, Francis JL. The effect of pentoxifylline on spontaneous and experimental metastases of the mouse Neuro2a neuroblastoma. *Clin Exp Metastasis* 1997; 15:453–461.

84. Tardi P, Choice E, Masin D, Redelmeier T, Bally M, Madden TD. Liposomal encapsulation of topotecan enhances anticancer efficacy in murine and human xenograft models. *Cancer Res* 2000; 60:3389–3393.

85. Chen MC, Tsang YM, Stark DD, Weissleder R, Saini S, Brandhorst J, et al. Hepatic metastases: rat models for imaging research. *Magnet Reson Imaging* 1989; 7:1–8.

86. Yang R, Rescorla FJ, Reilly CR, Faight PR, Sanghvi NT, Lumeng L, et al. A reproducible rat liver cancer model for experimental therapy: introducing a technique of intrahepatic tumor implantation. *J Surg Res* 1992; 52:193–198.

87. Qin Y, Van Cauteren M, Osteaux M, Willems G. Quantitative study of the growth of experimental hepatic tumors in rats by using magnetic resonance imaging. *Int J Cancer* 1992; 51:665–670.

88. Kreft BP, Tanimoto A, Stark DD, Baba Y, Zhao L, Chen JT, et al. Enhancement of tumor-liver contrast-to-noise ratio with gadobenate dimeglumine in MR imaging of rats. *J Magn Reson Imaging* 1993; 3:41–49.

89. Fukuda H, Takahashi J, Fujiwara T, Yamaguchi K, Abe Y, Kubota K, et al. High accumulation of 2-deoxy-2-fluorine-18-fluoro-D-galactose by well-differentiated hepatomas of mice and rats. *J Nucl Med* 1993; 34:780–786.

90. Brix G, Bellemann ME, Haberkorn U, Gerlach L, Lorenz WJ. Assessment of the biodistribution and metabolism of 5-fluorouracil as monitored by 18F PET and 19F MRI: a comparative animal study. *Nucl Med Biol* 1996; 23:897–906.

91. Katzir I, Shani J, Wolf W, Chatterjee-Parti S, Berman E. Enhancement of 5-fluorouracil anabolism by methotrexate and trimetrexate in two rat solid tumor models, Walker 256 carcinosarcoma and Novikoff hepatoma, as evaluated by 19F-magnetic resonance spectroscopy. *Cancer Investig* 2000; 18:20–27.

92. Thorstensen O, Isberg B, Svahn U, Jorulf H, Venizelos N, Jaremko G. Experimental tissue transplantation using a biopsy instrument and radiologic methods. *Investig Radiol* 1994; 29:469–471.

93. Kuwata Y, Hirota S, Sako M. Treatment of metastastic liver tumors by intermittent repetitive injection of an angiogenesis inhibitor using an implantable port system in a rabbit model. *Kobe J Med Sci* 1997; 43:83–98.

94. Gnant MF, Noll LA, Irvine KR, Puhlmann M, Terrill RE, Alexander HR Jr, et al. Tumor-specific gene delivery using recombinant vaccinia virus in a rabbit model of liver metastases. *J Natl Cancer Inst* 1999; 91:1744–1750.

95. Schabet M, Ohneseit P, Buchholz R, Santo-Holtje L, Schmidberger H. Intrathecal ACNU treatment of B16 melanoma leptomeningeal metastasis in a new athymic rat model. *Neurooncol* 1992; 14:207–211.

96. Yano S, Nokihara H, Hanibuchi M, Parajuli P, Shinohara T, Kawano T, et al. Model of malignant plueral effusion of human lung adenocarcinoma in SCID mice. *Oncol Res* 1997; 9:573–579.

97. Yano S, Shinohara H, Herbst RS, Kuniyasu H, Bucana CD, Ellis LM, et al. Expression of vascular endothelial growth factor is necessary but not sufficient for production and growth of brain metastasis. *Cancer Res* 2000; 60:4959–4967.

98. Morikawa K, Walker SM, Nakajima M, Pathak S, Jessup JM, Fidler IJ. Influence of organ environment on the growth, selection, and metastasis of human colon carcinoma cell in nude mice. *Cancer Res* 1988; 48:6863–6871.

99. Fujimaki T, Fan D, Staroselsky AH, Gohji K, Bucana CD, Fidler IJ. Critical factors regulating site-specific brain metastasis of murine melanomas. *Int J Oncol* 1993; 3:789–799.

100. Ghossein RA, Carusone L, Bhattacharya S. Review: polymerase chain reaction detection of micrometastases and circulating tumor cells: application to melanoma, prostate and thyroid carcinomas. *Diagn Mole Pathol* 1999; 8:165–175.

101. Rubio N, Villacampa MM, El Hilali, Blanco J. Metastatic burden in nude mice organs measured using prostate PC-3 cells expressing the luciferase gene as a quantifiable tumor cell marker. *The Prostate* 2000; 44:133–143.

102. Yang M, Jiang P, An Z, Baranov E, Li L, Hasegawa S, et al. Genetically fluorescent melanoma bone and organ metastasis models. *Clin Cancer Res* 1999; 5:3549–3559.

17

Models for Evaluation of Targeted Therapies of Metastatic Disease

Suzanne A. Eccles, PhD

1. INTRODUCTION

Metastasis is the most frequent cause of cancer death, and the majority of therapeutic agents are aimed against systemic disease. Therefore, it is surprising that only relatively recently have new therapies been tested with any degree of regularity in models that mimic metastatic human cancer, and even now, truly adjuvant preclinical studies are rare. Animal models have been criticized for failing to predict the response of patients to new agents *(1)*. However, with the growing realization of the importance of cellular context and microenvironment, in some cases the use of inappropriate models may be the cause of misleading results *(2,3)*.

For over 20 years, the mainstays of cancer research were a handful of transplanted rodent tumors. A few of these (most notably B16F10 and Lewis Lung Carcinoma (LLC) were used as metastasis models, generally by injecting the cells intravenously to produce lung colonies. In the 1980s, when it was decided that human tumors were a more appropriate model system than rodent tumors, and athymic mice were used as hosts for in vivo testing, it was found that these tumors rarely metastasized when grown subcutaneously. So, by gaining expression of human molecular targets (essential for the evaluation of clinically useful monoclonal antibodies (MAbs), for example) we lost one of the most critically important features of cancer, its disseminated growth pattern.

Fortunately, more recent studies have revealed that when human tumors are grown orthotopically (i.e., in the correct anatomical site), there is a much higher probability of metastasis. Athymic and severe combined immunodeficiency (SCID) mice, however,

From: *Tumor Models in Cancer Research*
Edited by: B. A. Teicher © Humana Press Inc., Totowa, NJ

have abnormal immune (and endocrine) systems, and therefore have limitations for some therapeutic applications. The introduction of transgenic strains is finally enabling the development of the most patient-like models of cancer. When a known genetic aberration is introduced into the germline, it is seen as self by the host, and in some cases leads to the development of metastatic disease. Yet, it remains to be proven in most cases that the strong overexpression of a single oncogene (or knockout of a suppressor gene) results in cancers whose biology accurately mimics that of the human diseases, in which multiple genetic and environmental factors contribute to tumor progression. Also, well-established and/or simpler models still have their place. A bolus intravenous (iv) injection of enzymatically prepared tumor cells may not be appropriate for studying the *process* of metastasis. However, the resulting tumor colonies of relatively uniform number, size, and organ location may be invaluable for comparing access and activity of drugs or biological agents; situations in which such variables need to be carefully controlled. The art of using models for targeted therapies involves choosing the most appropriate one for the particular problem being addressed.

Finally, the introduction of genetically tagged cells has enabled earlier detection and more accurate quantitation of micrometastases, and has greatly increased the sensitivity of metastasis assays. However, this and other new techniques have led to problems in determining whether the cells detected are truly clonogenic, and whether identification of cancer-associated genetic sequences are sufficient evidence of metastasis. Similar problems occur in the clinic. For example, polymerase chain reaction (PCR)-positive samples and single cancer cells identified in body fluids or tissues introduce dilemmas regarding the need (or otherwise) for therapeutic intervention.

This chapter explores molecular targets that may be appropriate for metastasis therapy, describes a variety of tumor models and their suitability for different therapeutic approaches, and briefly discusses various methods available for the identification and quantitation of metastases.

2. TARGETS FOR THERAPY OF METASTATIC DISEASE

2.1. General Tumor Markers

A wide range of tumor markers have been described over the last three decades or more. Depending on their specificity for cancer(s), stability of expression, and cellular location (membrane, intracellular, or secreted), many have been utilized as targets for therapy. These can broadly be categorized as tissue-specific differentiation antigens and tumor-selective antigens that are either shared between different cancers or unique to one histogenic type. Table 1 provides some examples of the most commonly used tumor targets. Several excellent recent reviews discuss the use of peptide libraries for target definition (4) the choice of antigen for development of vaccines and immunotherapeutic intervention (5,6) and the current problems and prospects of such approaches (7–9).

Few, if any, current targets for therapy are unique to metastases. Yet it is important to determine whether their expression is maintained at secondary sites. Some genetic changes that play a role early in oncogenesis may not be homogeneously expressed later in tumor progression. Both experimental and clinical observations suggest that gene expression varies with the site of tumor growth. This can be a result of natural selection of cells expressing certain molecules that give them a survival advantage in

Table 1
Examples of Tumor-Associated Molecules Used for Targeting

Antigen	Cancer type	Comment
PSA Shed molecule	Prostate	Also expressed on some normal secretory epithelia
PSMA Membrane/shed antigen	Prostate	Also expressed in normal tissues and TAN
EGFR **EGFRvIII** Membrane antigen	Squamous (and other) carcinomas	Expressed in basal cells of skin, liver. Deletion mutants in gliomas and some other cancers
c-*erb*B-2 p185 Membrane antigen	Adenocarcinomas (various)	Restricted expression in normal adult tissue
TAG-72 Membrane antigen	Adenocarcinomas	Glycoprotein antigen
CA125 Shed antigen	Adenocarcinomas	Secreted glycoprotein
NG2 Membrane antigen	Chondrosarcoma, melanoma	Also expressed on TAN
G(M3); GD3 Membrane ganglioside	Melanoma	Shed antigen, also expressed on lymphocytes
GD2 Membrane ganglioside	Neuroblastoma melanoma	Syngeneic mouse model mimics normal tissue expression and tumor heterogeneity
Somatostatin receptors Membrane antigen	Many adenocarcinomas	Somatostatin octapeptide analogs for targeting
CCK-B receptor Membrane antigen	MTC, SCLC, astrocytomas	Ligand = gastrin; suitable for targeting
Folate receptor	Adenocarcinomas, myeloid leukemias	Ligand = folic acid; suitable for targeting
CD44 variant exon 6 Membrane antigen	SCC	Other variants may also be differentially expressed in cancers
c-kit Membrane antigen	SCLC	Ligand = stem-cell factor
Ep-CAM Membrane antigen	Adenocarcinomas	MAb 17-1A epitope
MAGE family, MART **GAGE, RAGE**	Melanomas and other cancers	Defined by CTL reactivity
MUC family **mucins**	Breast, pancreatic, B cells	Antigenicity caused by altered glycosylation
CEA Shed antigen	Colon, breast, and other adenocarcinomas	Related molecules may also be expressed on TAN
Le^y Membrane antigen	Lung, breast, and bladder carcinomas	Rat displays Le^y on same normal tissues as human

SCLC = small-cell lung cancer

MTC = medullary thyroid cancer

TAN = tumour associated neovasculature

SCC = squamous-cell carcinoma

specific tissues, loss of expression of genes no longer required, and/or other epigenetic microenvironmental influences. However, encouragingly, a study in late-stage melanoma patients revealed a high homogeneity of expression of a variety of antigens in multiple metastases *(10)*.

One good reason for assaying novel therapies in metastatic models is the fact that many genes are downregulated in ectopic, or subcutaneous (sc), sites. Thus, in the correct physiological environment, the molecules of interest will be better displayed for the targeting drug or antibody to access. Table 2 illustrates examples in which different in vitro culture conditions, sites of tumor growth, or comparison of primary and secondary cancers in patients have demonstrated significant differences in target antigen expression. Thus, although metastatic models may be more technically challenging than simple sc models, they are likely to provide more accurate and sensitive readouts of novel therapeutic approaches.

2.2. Metastasis-Related Targets

It is generally accepted that further genetic changes (beyond those involved in cellular transformation) are required for a tumor cell to express a metastatic phenotype. Although themes can be discerned, tumor cells acquire the molecular machinery required for metastasis (such as angiogenesis, mis-regulated adhesion, motility, invasive capacity, and ectopic growth) through a variety of different pathways. Categories of molecules that are often upregulated in carcinoma metastases include angiogenic factors such as vascular endothelial growth factor (VEGF), basic fibroblast growth factor (bFGF), and angiopoeitins; enzymes such as matrix metalloproteinases (MMPs), serine and cysteine proteases and oncogenes, such as the tyrosine kinase growth-factor receptors EGFR/c-*erb*B family and IGF1-R and their downstream effectors (including ras, src, raf, MAP and P13 kinases). In tumors of mesenchymal and lymphoreticular origin, various growth-factor receptors (such as PDGF-R) drive proliferation and other cellular processes, but there is some commonality in downstream second messengers.

Many of these molecules provide excellent targets for therapeutic intervention, especially when their expression is causally linked to expression of the metastatic phenotype *(11,12)*. For example, it has been shown that overexpression of EGFR and one or more ligands results in upregulation of specific MMPs and angiogenic factors, which lead to enhanced tumor invasion, angiogenesis, and metastasis *(13–16)*. The related c-*erb*B-2 receptor has been shown to be involved in tumor-cell motility and angiogenesis. Interestingly, there are many parallels in the molecular mechanisms used by tumor cells and by endothelial cells to invade surrounding stroma, including similar MMP profiles, integrin expression and motility factors, suggesting that therapies directed against these activities may target both these aspects of metastasis. Recently, subtractive immunization has been used to generate MAbs that specifically inhibit metastasis. One of the targets was identified as the tetraspanin protein PETA-3/CD151, and MAbs were able to inhibit invasion in vitro and metastasis of Hep3 human epidermoid carcinoma cells grown in chick embryos *(17)*.

Angiogenesis itself is also an attractive target for intervention, and is an area of intense investigation. It is clear that metastasis is critically dependent on angiogenesis in the primary tumor, and—in at least some cases—dormancy of micrometastases has been linked to failure of angiogenesis. It is interesting that several tumor markers have

Table 2
Modulatory Effect of Microenvironment on Target Molecule Expression

Tumor	Metastasis	Target molecule	Expression	Ref
MDA MB 231 Breast cancer	Bone	Active MMP-2 and MMP-9	Induced specifically by culture on bone ECM, and in bone micrometastases	81
PC-3, LNCaP, DU145, PC3 prostate cancer	Bone	MT1-MMP, MMP-2, MMP-9	Increased when grown inside human bone fragments implanted in SCID mice	82
PC-3M prostate cancer	Nodes, Bone, Lung	EGFR, bFGF, type IV collagenase, mdr-1	Increased in orthotopic (prostate) vs ectopic (sc) site	83
SP6.5 uveal melanoma	Liver	gangliosides	GM3 increased; GD3 and GD2 decreased	84
LS174T colorectal cancer	Liver	CEA	Increased × 3 relative to sc and spleen; MAb localization doubled	85
KM12 colorectal cancer	Liver	EGFR	Increased 20–60%	86
		CEA	Increased	
		Collagenase iv	Increased 20–80%	
		PGY-1 mdr gene	Increased in liver metastases vs primary (spleen) site or tc cells	
KM12SM colorectal cancer	Liver	Activated EGFR	Increased relative to primary (cecal) or sc sites	87
B16 LS9 melanoma	Liver	c-Met	Increased levels relative to parental F1 or lung metastasis selected F10	88
Uveal melanoma	Liver	EGFR	Correlates with liver metastasis	89
CLINICAL				
Melanoma	Various sites	VEGF	VEGF expressed in 32% primary and 91% metastatic melanomas	90
Colon	Liver	MMP-9	Active (82-kDa) form only found in liver mets	91
Prostate	Bone, node	PSMA	Upregulated in metastases	92

recently been shown to be expressed on endothelial cells of tumor neovasculature. For example, PSMA *(18)*, NG2 *(19)*, and carcino-embryonic antigen (CEA)-related molecules *(20)*. The significance of this is not known, but potentially offers additional benefits of using these particular antigens as targets and expands the range of tumors for which they may be appropriate.

Metastatic cells have also been found by various experimental approaches (such as differential display, transfection, subtractive immunization, and microarrays) to have increased (in the case of P9Ka, osteopontin, MTA-1, and CD151) or decreased (in the case of nm23, KAI1, and KiSS-1) the expression of specific molecules. In general, these have not yet been developed as targets for therapeutic intervention. It is likely that exploitation of such molecules will lead to more selective therapies for disseminated disease.

2.3. Tissue Targeting

Because particular cancers have a predilection for metastasizing to specific organs (such as sarcoma to lung, colon to liver, and prostate to bone), it is important to mention tissue-specific targeting. The liver asialoglycoprotein has been used with galactose-linked moieties for targeting to the liver parenchyma, with the goal of increasing local concentrations of the drug in the vicinity of hepatic metastases. Similarly, hepatic arterial infusion combined with degradable starch microspheres has been used to target and hold the drug in the liver vasculature in the hope of enhancing the perfusion of metastases. Others have achieved different target-tissue (e.g., lung and kidney) specificity using immunoliposomes *(21)*. However, the most novel and exciting approach has been the use of peptide libraries to target and identify tissue addresses—specific epitopes on organ (and tumor) vasculature that can be exploited to deliver therapeutics to affected sites *(22)*.

3. ANIMAL METASTASIS MODELS FOR EVALUATING TARGETED THERAPY

A wide variety of animal models have been developed with the aim of better understanding the molecular mechanisms of metastasis, and to serve as test systems to evaluate novel therapies. Because of the multiplicity and complexity of human cancers, no single model can be expected to serve as an appropriate screen for all applications. The following section exemplifies some of the types of models available, their strengths and weaknesses, and their utilization in various experimental settings.

3.1. Syngeneic Rodent Models

Many of the early tumors were chemically induced, and others (such as the mammary tumors in CBA mice) were caused by oncogenic viruses [mouse mammary-tumor virus (MMTV)], and were not ideal models for human cancer. Often, the tumors were highly immunogenic, apparently failed to metastasize (although this was often a result of the practice of leaving the primary tumor *in situ* until the burden became excessive), and the latter did not usually show the same sensitivity to hormones as human cancers. Nevertheless, at least two tumors emerged to serve the scientific community for many years in drug evaluation and metastasis studies—B16 melanoma and LLC. Often, the tumor cells were injected intravenously to promote lung colonies, which were easily counted (particularly the melanotic B16) on the surface of fixed, inflated lungs.

Gradually, researchers began to recognize the importance of using strictly syngeneic, inbred strains and the fact that spontaneous tumors may be closer to their human counterparts than those induced with strongly oncogenic chemicals and viruses. It was also discovered that the immune responses directed against neoantigens induced by the carcinogenic agent could suppress metastases, since growth of the tumors in immunosuppressed hosts often led to an increased incidence of secondary disease (23–25). On the one hand, these observations encouraged the view that immunomodulatory approaches could be harnessed to inhibit the outgrowth of metastases, but they also cautioned that the results obtained with highly immunogenic rodent tumors were unlikely to be matched in weakly (or non-) immunogenic human cancers. Indeed, for many years, it was unclear whether human tumor antigens existed, because it was believed that the long latency of most cancers would have selected against such molecules. The discovery of the melanoma associated antigen genes (MAGE) series of peptides, and other examples of antigens capable of eliciting immune responses in humans has reawakened an interest in immunotherapy.

At the present time, it is recognized that in most cases it is not the lack of antigens that allows tumors to progress, but a failure in one or more components of the host response such as major histocompatibility complex (MHC), expression, antigen processing/presentation, costimulatory molecules, and helper cytokines. Several molecules first recognized in rodent tumors are now known to be important in the malignant process in human cancers, and in some cases are also capable of eliciting cell-mediated and/or humoral responses—c-erbB-2 p185; (11,12,26), (MUC-1) (27), and NG2 (28,29). These and similar targets are being explored in immunotherapeutic approaches utilizing MAbs and vaccines.

A wide variety of syngeneic tumor models are now available (Table 3). Although the trend recently has been toward the use of human tumor xenografts, there is no doubt that syngeneic tumor models are invaluable for certain applications. Strategies that depend upon an intact immune system will clearly require the use of immunocompetent hosts, but the fact that metastasis is more readily observed in syngeneic systems, (at least in tumors that do not express strongly immunogenic tumor antigens) suggests that there are certain failures of communication between a xenogeneic tumor and its immunodeprived host. It has been proven that some cytokines and growth factors are species-specific, and there is evidence that lack of specific molecular messages required for angiogenesis and metastasis—in addition to nonspecific host defenses such as natural killer (NK)-cells and macrophages—can limit expression of the metastatic phenotype in xenografted human tumors.

Difficulties in using syngeneic tumors arise because (for example) MAbs raised against a human antigen generally fail to cross-react with the rodent equivalent, and thus such studies generally use human tumors grown in immunodeprived hosts. In this case, the antigen is expressed on the xenograft tumor, but the normal tissue distribution is lacking, and does not allow discrimination of any potentially harmful cross-reactivities and toxicities. In some cases, a human gene has been transfected into a rodent tumor with the goal of providing a human target in a metastatic tumor. However, in many cases, this leads to unwanted immune responses to the xenogeneic

Table 3
Examples of Syngeneic Tumor Models Used for Targeted Therapy

Tumor	Primary site	Metastasis	Therapy	Ref
Melanoma				
B16: C57 bl mice	iv	Lung	Doxorubicin encapsulated in anti-Gm(3) immunoliposomes	93
	intraportal vein	Liver	Batimastat (MMPi)	69
	sc tail	Lung, nodes, bm	Tumor-cell vaccine	59
	iv	Lung	AG3340 MMPi	94
	iv	Lung	r-hTIMP-2	95
	footpad	Lung and nodes	MMPi (CGS27023A)	96
Lung				
Lewis lung: C57bl mice	sc or iv	Lung	Ab to uPA	34
	sc	Lung	Vaccination with cytokine-expressing tumor cells (adjuvant treatment)	60
	sc	Lung	Batimastat and captopril (MMPi)	97
	sc or iv	Lung	Vaccination with Flk-1 (anti angiogenic)	64
	Lung	Lymph nodes	TAC-101 anti-uPA/uPAR	98
Prostate				
Mat-Ly-Lu: rat	Prostate	Lung	Vaccination with plasmid DNA encoding neu p185	37
	sc	Lung	Plasma fibronectin PHSCN postop	99
Dunning model	sc	Lung, kidney,	B-428 uPA enzyme inhibitor	100
	sc	Spleen, nodes bone, lung	CMT-3 MMPi	101
Neuroblastoma				
NXS2	iv	Bone marrow	Anti-GD2 mab-IL-2 fusion protein	58
		Liver	Anti-GD2-calicheamycin conjugate	102
		Liver	Alpha V antagonist + MAb-IL-2 fusion protein	70

Urinogenital

Model	Site	Location	Therapy	Ref.
Renca: Balb/C mice	Iv	Lung	Cytokine-producing tumor vaccines + lung irradiation	103
Renca tranfected with human EGFR or vIII deletion mutant	Iv	Lung	ScFv anti-EGFR-ETA immunotoxin	50

Breast

Model	Site	Location	Therapy	Ref.
EMT6: mouse	Iv	Lung	Immunoliposomes: MAb 34A vs thrombomodulin liposomes carrying dpFUdR	104
66.3-neu: mouse	Iv or breast	Lung	Vaccination with neu gene	61
4T1: mouse	Breast	Lung, liver, brain	Vaccination with MHC class II and B7.1 transfected tumor cells and postop therapy	6
HOSP1: rat	Breast	Lung, nodes	MMPi	68
MAT B-III: rat	Breast	Nodes	Tamoxifen + uPA peptide	71

Colon

Model	Site	Location	Therapy	Ref.
CC-36: mouse	Spleen	Liver	Vaccinia oncolysate encoding IL-2	105
Colon 26: mouse	Spleen	Liver	MAbs to TF antigen	106
Colon 26: mouse	iv	Lung	KB-R7785 MMP	107
Colon 26: mouse	Spleen	Liver	TKI	108
Colon 26: mouse	Spleen	Liver	Retroviral producer cells encoding IL-4 and IL-2	109
Buffalo rat	Portal vein	Liver	G207 mutated Herpes simplex lytic virus	65
DHD/K12/PROb: rat	Mesenteric vein	Liver	PROb transfected with CD gene, then 5-FC	110

Sarcoma

Model	Site	Location	Therapy	Ref.
FS6: mouse	Sc	Lungs	Tumor/cytokines vaccination	111
HSN chondrosarcoma: rat	Mesenteric vein	Lung, nodes	MAbs to NG2; immunotoxins	112,46
	Intrahepatic	Liver	Focused ultrasound	35
Osteosarcoma: rat	Bone	Lung	HSV-TK + ganciclovir	113
Yoshida sarcoma: rat	Sc	Lymph nodes	AGM-1470	36

transgene product *(30)*. The same may in some cases apply to genetic tags (which are often of nonmammalian origin).

3.2. Xenograft Models

Table 4 illustrates some of the most commonly used xenograft "metastasis" models, and the therapeutic modalities that have been tested using them. Although *nu/nu* or SCID mice are the most commonly used host (replacing the thymectomized/irradiated animals that preceded them), some studies have employed *nu/nu* rats, and more recently, chick embryos and zebra fish embryos. Differences have been noted in the ease with which different types of human cancers form xenografts, and also in the ability of various types and strains of immunodeprived rodents to support metastasis. Although nude rats are useful for studies requiring surgical manipulations that would be difficult in mice, they appear to have more residual immune function, and thus can be less permissive of xenograft growth. Also, differences in the patterns of metastasis between athymic rats and mice injected with the same human tumor cells have been observed *(31)*. SCID mice, lacking both B- and T-cell immunity, and *bg* mice with lower NK activity, should theoretically be more susceptible than athymic mice. However, although they are the preferred host for lymphoreticular neoplasms—and some solid tumors more readily metastasize than in *nu/nu* hosts—they are not universally superior, and breast cancers, for example, generally do not grow and disseminate more readily than in other strains *(2)*.

It is now widely accepted that tumors grown subcutaneously are less likely to metastasize than those grown in the anatomically correct (orthotopic) site (*see* Subheading 3.5.). Several studies have shown that transfection of human angiogenic cytokines and sc implantation of xenogeneic tumor cells with Matrigel and/or helper host cells such as fibroblasts can increase tumor growth and/or malignant potential *(32)*. These devices presumably mimic to some extent the orthotopic microenvironment, or at least overcome some of the defects of the xenogeneic/ectopic environment. A note of caution is that SCIDs and *nu/nu* mice can develop spontaneous lymphoreticular neoplasms at a relatively early age. These frequently manifest as swellings in the groins and axillae, and could be mistaken for lymphatic metastases if they are not checked histologically.

3.3. Experimental Metastasis/Organ Colonization

The simplest "metastasis" assays are intended to mimic late stages of metastasis (dissemination, extravasation, and colonization), and depend upon the direct inoculation of a bolus of tumor cells directly into the peripheral circulation. The first method used was the injection of cells into the tail vein of mice. In most cases, resultant tumor colonies are confined to the lungs (the first capillary bed encountered) because of mechanical trapping. However, some sarcomas and carcinomas are able to traverse the lung and yield colonies downstream of this organ *(33)*. It should be noted that there is no direct correlation between lung colonization and spontaneous metastasis, and in some tumor models there are large discrepancies between these two functions *(2)*. Also, therapeutic interventions do not always yield the same results—e.g., antibodies against urokinase-type plasminogen activator (uPA) inhibited spontaneous metastases, but not lung colonies *(34)*. Results obtained in the "experimental metastasis" assay should therefore be treated with caution, and if possible, confirmed in spontaneous metastasis assays.

Table 4
Examples of Xenograft Models Used for Targeted Therapy

Human Tumor Xenografts	Primary site	Metastasis	Therapy	References
Colon:				
WiDr: nude mice	Spleen	Liver	MMP-7 antisense	67
GX-39: nude mice	Spleen	Liver	Radioimmunotherapy vs CEA	53
GW-39: nude mice	iv	Lung	Radioimmunotherapy vs CEA or AFP	51
LS174T: nude rat	Intraportal vein	Liver	Radioimmunotherapy vs CEA	114
LS174T: nude mice	Spleen	Liver	Radioimmunotherapy vs CEA	52
LS174T: nude mice	Spleen	Liver	CD44v6 antisense	66
HT-29	Spleen	Liver	Adenovirus delivery of uPA antagonist	64
TK-3, TK-4, TK-9	Cecal wall	Liver	TNP-470 antiangiogenic agent	115
HM7:SCID mice	Spleen	Liver	Anti-TAG72 MAb targeted LAK cells	116
LS180	Intraportal iv	Liver, LN	Daunomycin-dextran-MAb conjugate	117
C-1H	Spleen	Liver	BPHA MMPi	118
Melanoma:				
M24 met: SCID mice	iv/iportal	Lung/liver	Anti-EGFR- or anti-GD2-IL-2 fusion protein	119
Uveal melanoma	Eye	Liver	Anti GD2 MAb	120
Uveal melanoma	Eye	Liver	Adenoviral vector carrying PAI-1 gene	121
Uveal melanoma:nu/nu	Eye	Liver	TIL	89
A375: nu/nu mice	Left ventricle	Bone	Laminin-derived synthetic peptide	122
HX118	Skin	LN	211At labeled methylene blue targeted radiotherapy	123
Prostate:				
PC-3	Prostate	Lung, Bone marrow	Immunocytokine: MAb-cytokine fusion protein huKS1/4-IL-2	124
PC3ML	iv	Vertebrae	IL-10	125
Lung; NSCLC				
A431, A549: nude mice	iv	Lung	Mab 210B labeled with 213Bi to target lung vasculature	126
PC14: nu mice	Pleural cavity	Pleura, lung	HSVtk + gancyclovir	127
		Liver, kidneys, LN	Chimeric MAb vs GM-2 ganglioside	128
Lung; SCLC				
SBC-3	iv	Meninges	Effective via macrophage ADCC	129
Urinogenital				
NC 65 renal cell ca: nu mice	Intradermal	Lung, LN, liver	ND2001 (laminin haptotaxis inhibitor)	130
2537 B-V: nu mice	Bladder	Lung, LN	C225 anti EGFR MAb	131

(Table continues)

Table 4
(continued)

Human Tumor Xenografts	Primary site	Metastasis	Therapy	References
Bladder				
UCRU-BL-17 clone 2B8: Irradiated nude rats	Bladder wall	Lung	MAb BLCA-38 intravesical radioimmunotherapy	54
Breast:				
MDA MB 231: nude mice	Intracardiac	Bone	MMP inhibitor GM6001	132
JYG-A, JYG-B, KPL-1	Mammary fat	Lungs, nodes	TNP-470 angiogenesis inhibitor	86
MDA MB 435	Mammary fat	Lungs	CMDB7 angiogenesis inhibitor	133
GI 101	Mammary fat	Lung	Scfv of NovoMAb-G2	134
Pancreatic				
HPAC	Pancreas	Liver	BB-94 MMPi	135
Epidermoid ca				
HEp3: chick embryo	CAM	Chick embryo lung	Anti CD151 MAb inhibits migration and spontaneous mets	17
Squamous cell ca				
OSC-19: nude mice	Floor of mouth	Cervical LN	Human CTL or A-NK cells + IL-2	62

ETA = *Pseudomonaexotoxin A*
ScFv = single-chain antibody
IL-2 = interleukin 2
GD2 = ganglioside antigen
G(M3) = ganglioside antigen
MMP-7 = matrix metalloproteinase 7; matrilysin
EGFR = epidermal growth-factor receptor
Ad = adenovirus

DC = dendritic cells
CEA = carcinoembryonic antigen
AFP = alphafetoprotein
TF = Thomsen-Friedenreich antigen
LN = lymph node
CTL = cytotoxic T cells
NK = natural killer cells
PAI-1 = plasminogen activator inhibitor 1

(M)Ab = (monoclonal) antibody
uPA = urokinase plasminogen activator
PyMT = polyoma virus middle T
HSV-TK = *Herpes simplex* thymidine kinase
5-FC = 5-fluorocytosine
CD = cytosine deaminase gene
Tki = tyrosine kinase inhibitor

Not surprisingly, tumors derived from cells that are naturally migratory—such as leukemias, lymphomas, and plasmacytomas—or those that are severely de-differentiated more readily transmigrate and form colonies (or infiltrative deposits) in multiple sites, including bone marrow, spleen, and liver. Cells can also be introduced into the portal circulation (for liver colonies), or the left ventricle of the heart (for bone colonies and also other sites such as the adrenal glands). The spleen provides a simpler alternative site for the injection of tumor cells than the portal or mesenteric vein (especially in mice), because from this site the cells pass almost immediately into the portal circulation. The only disadvantages are that it is not known exactly how many of the injected cells reach the liver, and growth and intraperitoneal (ip) spread from the primary tumor can be a confounding factor if the spleen is not removed. For situations in which a small number of colonies are required in the liver (e.g., for focused ultrasound therapy *(35)* or photodynamic therapy), tumor cells can be injected directly into the liver parenchyma. Tumor cells have also been directly injected into the pleura, bone marrow, and brain, but there is a risk of morbidity/mortality, and quantitation of the metastatic burden is difficult.

3.4. Spontaneous Metastasis

"Spontaneous" metastasis generally refers to the seeding of cells from a primary site and their development into detectable lesions at distant sites. It is important to note that the primary tumor, while *in situ,* may inhibit the outgrowth of metastases. Studies have suggested that this is a result of the production of natural antiangiogenic factors, such as angiostatin and endostatin. However, tumor growth tends to follow an asymptotic curve, and when the primary tumor burden is high—if the animals are in poor condition—this will be also be reflected in slowed (primary and secondary) tumor-growth rates. Whatever the mechanism, two points are noteworthy: firstly, that for accurate determination of the full extent of metastasis, the primary tumor should ideally be surgically excised and the animals observed for a suitable period for the full development of metastases (this depends on the growth rate and malignant potential of individual tumors).

Secondly, all suspected deposits should be confirmed histologically. It is, I believe, unethical and unscientific to allow primary tumors, particularly those in vital organs, to reach such gross dimensions that metastasis into other sites cannot be distinguished from direct extension or transcoelomic seeding. Human patients (whenever possible) have their primary tumor removed (or irradiated) as soon as possible, and most antimetastatic therapy occurs in an adjuvant setting. There is no reason why animal experiments should not be similarly designed. Secondly, if therapy is instigated while the primary tumor is *in situ,* and results in a significant inhibition of tumor growth (and metastasis), it cannot be determined whether the latter is simply a consequence of the former.

Considering the prevalence of lymphatic metastases from human carcinomas, they are not particularly well-represented in nonlymphoid animal tumor models. Injection of cells into the footpad encourages seeding to the popliteal nodes, and although this process is probably artificially enhanced by pressure during movement, it has been used to study basic mechanisms of lymphatic metastasis, but less often for evaluation of targeted therapies. Several rat breast carcinomas give rise to spontaneous lymphatic metastases when grown in mammary fat pads, and lymphatic metastasis of PC3M grown orthotopically has also been observed. It is important to attempt to assay the effects of novel compounds against both hematogenous and lymphatic metastasis, because they may not be equally effective in both. Indeed, in one study an antiangiogenic agent—although it inhibited hematogenous metastasis—*increased* lymphatic metastasis *(36)*.

3.5. Orthotopic Models

The orthotopic implantation of breast-tumor cells into the mammary fat pad usually encourages the development of both lung and lymphatic metastases, and more recently, orthotopic implantation has yielded spontaneous metastases from the rat Mat-Ly-Lu prostate carcinoma *(37)*. Xenografted tumors also seem to yield a much higher frequency of metastases when implanted orthotopically (reviewed in refs. *38,39*) and models of human colorectal cancer metastatic to liver, melanoma metastatic to nodes, prostate cancer metastatic to nodes and bone, pancreatic cancer metastatic to liver, and many other syngeneic and xenogeneic models have now been described (*see* Tables 3 and 4). It is hoped that these will increasingly be used in the preclinical work-up of novel therapies.

3.6. Transgenic Models

Transgenic models are discussed in Chapters 11–18 but it is important to mention some models in which metastases have been generated that are useful for evaluation of targeted therapies. Several mouse strains have been produced in which a putative oncogene is targeted to a specific organ by the use of tissue-specific promoters. In many cases, this leads to a high incidence of tumors, but metastasis is not an inevitable consequence. Of particular interest are animals that express a human oncogene such as c-*erb*B-2, in which the gene not only provides the initiating stimulus for oncogenesis, but is also (by virtue of the fact that its product is a cell-surface protein) an ideal target for therapy. Early work used the rat *neu* gene (which is mutated) to induce metastatic tumors at high frequency, however, HER-2/*neu* was generally believed to be oncogenic by virtue of overexpression rather than mutation in humans. Recently, alternatively spliced forms of *erb*B-2 that closely resemble the spontaneous activated forms have been found in human cancers *(40)*.

There are now strains of wild-type c-*erb*B-2 transgenic mice that develop (with a long latency) mammary cancers that metastasize to the lung, although again a proportion carry somatic mutations in the transgene. Another transgenic mammary carcinoma model with a faster development kinetics is that induced by polyoma virus middle T-antigen. Both systems have been used to explore vaccination strategies and (in the case of *neu*) MAb therapy resulting in the development of Herceptin. In these examples, transgene expression was confined to the mammary gland by using the MMTV long terminal repeat (LTR) for tissue targeting. However, in humans, c-*erb*B-2 is also expressed at low levels in other cell types—such as gastrointestinal epithelia, bile and pancreatic ducts, and kidney—which is a possible drawback to these models (in common with xenografts), since normal tissue toxicities (e.g., cardiac with Herceptin) were not observed.

A second interesting system is a transgenic mouse model for prostate cancer—the TRAMP model—which targets Simian virus 40 (SV40) T-antigen to the prostate using regulatory elements of the rat probasin gene. Mice develop metastases primarily in the lung and lymph node, and the incidence can reach 100% by 28 wk *(41).* In this model, target antigens are murine. In a different approach, a genomic clone of prostate specific antigen (PSA) has been used to generate transgenic mice with a PSA tissue expression pattern very similar to that in humans *(42).* In these immunocompetent mice, PSA is a self-antigen, and if metastatic prostate tumors could be induced, this would represent an almost ideal model system for testing the feasibility of PSA-directed immunotherapies. Similar approaches have been taken with CEA: Clarke et al. *(43)* produced CEA-transgenic mice and transplanted into them a syngeneic tumor transfected with the human CEA gene, and Thompson et al. *(44)* crossed CEA-transgenic mice with Min mice which have a mutation in the *APC* gene and thus a predisposition to colorectal cancer. The incidence of metastases (if any) has not been reported in these mice, and have they not yet been used to assess therapies targeting CEA, although the combination of an immunocompetent host, expression of a human tumor antigen, and normal spatiotemporal tissue distribution of CEA would make this an interesting model.

The main drawbacks of the transgenic systems for testing targeted therapies are their relatively high variability relative to transplantable systems and the long latency and development of multiple tumors per animal. The frequency (and sites) of metastases are also unpredictable. In some cases, the tumors can be developed into cell lines and reintroduced into young mice of the transgenic strain (providing it is an inbred genetic background). The transgene is still be seen as self, but the tumors may grow more reliably. Such strategies have been used for tumors developing in both *neu* and CEA-transgenic strains *(45),* but the incidence of metastasis from these transplanted tumors is unclear.

4. THERAPEUTIC STRATEGIES FOR TARGETING METASTASES

4.1. Immunological Approaches

4.1.1. ANTIBODY-BASED THERAPIES

As mentioned in previous sections, MAbs have been one of the mainstays of targeted therapies. It has long been recognized that although immune effectors have exquisite specificity and should (in the absence of untoward cross-reactivity with normal tissues) be of low toxicity, they are most effective against low tumor burden—i.e., minimal residual disease or metastases. This makes them a useful adjunct to conventional therapies that are generally directed against recurrent tumors or overt metastases, but in which outgrowth of resistant cells ultimately produces life-threatening disseminated disease. Most of the common tumor antigens—including CEA, PSMA, EGFR, c-*erb*B-2, and gangliosides—have been used to generate MAbs for therapy.

Initially, antibodies were raised in rodents, and repeated treatments could readily be given to athymic hosts bearing human tumor xenografts. Yet it was recognized that in man these schedules would lead to the development of human antimouse (HAMA, or rat HARA) immune reactions, eliminating the therapeutic antibody. Later work resulted in the development of chimeric antibodies (rodent variable regions spliced onto human constant immunoglobulin (IgG) regions) and finally recombinant human antibodies and fragments, such as single-chain Fv. Throughout this phase of development, animal models were invaluable in studies of the effects of antibody specificity, size, isotype, valency, affinity, and various therapeutic strategies.

Studies in syngeneic systems have been highly instructive in illustrating the differences in antibody localization in tumors at various metastatic sites (lung, liver, and lymph node) and the influence of tumor mass on antibody penetration (46–48). Antibodies have been used alone, relying on their ability to block critical tumor cell (or endothelial-cell) functions such as proliferation signaled by growth-factor receptors (EGFR, c-erbB-2, VEGFR) and/or via recruitment of host effectors. Anti-EGFR and antiganglioside MAbs have been shown to inhibit liver metastases from intra-ocular melanoma (49). In addition, antibodies have been used to deliver cytotoxic agents to tumors, such as plant and bacterial toxins, radioisotopes, drugs, and more recently, enzymes to activate prodrugs at the tumor site. An interesting model consists of a syngeneic murine renal carcinoma engineered to express human EGFR or the EGFRvIII deletion mutant plus lacZ as a marker. The cells were iv-injected, and the mice were treated with anti-EGFR/or EGFRvIII single-chain variable fragment (scfv) fused to a truncated *Pseudomonas* exotoxin A (50). The therapy reduced the number of lung colonies, although the expression of both bacterial and human genes in a tumor grown in immunocompetent mice may complicate interpretation of the results.

Radioimmunotherapy has been explored in lung and liver metastasis models of colorectal cancer using MAbs directed against CEA (51–53), and also in a novel nude rat xenograft model of bladder cancer (54). In all cases, therapeutic effects against metastases were observed, although with these direct conjugates, normal tissue toxicity was a problem. Antibody-directed enzyme prodrug therapy (ADEPT) is one example of pretargeting (reviewed in ref. 55), in which an antibody conjugate is first allowed to localize to tumor deposits, then to clear from the circulation before a second moiety is administered (56). This strategy minimizes the problem of antibodies directly conjugated to a toxic warhead that could damage normal tissues as it circulates.

Recently, more sophisticated therapeutic strategies have been devised that require correspondingly elegant models. For example, chimeric antibodies designed to target both a human antigen and to recruit host effector cells have been assayed in a SCID/hu mouse model of neuroblastoma metastatic to liver (57), where the mouse bone marrow is reconstituted with human stem cells capable of maturing into effector cells. Other strategies have included the use of fusion proteins combining the targeting ability of antibodies with agents such as cytokines in pulmonary and hepatic metastasis models of syngeneic mouse melanomas, neuroblastomas, and colorectal carcinomas (58). These and other approaches are listed in Tables 3 and 4.

4.1.2. VACCINES, CYTOKINES AND CELL MEDIATED IMMUNOTHERAPY

B700 antigen on B16F10 mouse melanoma cells has been used to generate vaccines capable of inhibiting spontaneous lymph node and lung metastases from a primary tumor grown in the tail. Further studies showed that combination with cytokines such as IL-2, IL-12 or GM-CSF potentiated the effects. Although this model mimics the human disease in terms of primary growth, bone marrow invasion, regional node involvement, and distant dissemination, it suffers from the fact that effects on the primary tumor cannot be discounted, and quantitation of lung metastases (which developed over a 1–2-mo period) was difficult (59). In another mouse model, Eisenbach's group have also shown that autologous tumor cells modified to express IL-12 or other cytokines can protect against lung metastases developing after surgical excision of primary LLCs *(60)*. This model was used in an adjuvant mode, similar to regimes that could be applied clinically. However, in these models, the antigens are murine.

In other examples, however, antigens such as c-*erb*B-2/neu, which can be expressed in both rodent and human cancers, can be used to explore vaccination strategies that are of more immediate relevance. Price et al. *(61)* have shown that vaccination with plasmid *neu* DNA (albeit before tumor implantation) could protect against tumor growth and lung colonies of 66.3 mouse mammary carcinoma cells transfected with rodent *neu;* the effect on spontaneous metastases was not reported. In a similar study, vaccination with plasmid cDNA encoding a truncated version of human HER2/*neu* reduced the subsequent growth and metastasis of orthotopically implanted rat Mat-Ly-Lu Dunning prostate carcinoma *(37)*. Other strategies using c-*erb*B-2 as a target for immunotherapy have been recently reviewed *(12,26)*. Adoptive immunotherapy with IL-2 and human cytotoxic T-lymphocytes (CTLs) or A-NK cells injected into the tumor site (OSC-19 cells in the floor of the mouth) in athymic mice resulted in fewer lymph node metastases *(62)* and in another patient-like model, tumor-infiltrating lymphocytes (TIL) isolated from transgenic intra-ocular melanomas in immunocompetent mice were capable of preventing liver metastases from intra-ocular melanomas in athymic mice *(49)*. Both of these models are highly specialized, require a high degree of skill, and are impractical for routine screening. Cytokines, as briefly illustrated here, have been used alone, as a component of vaccines, and in fusion proteins in various strategies to enhance immune responses capable of inhibiting metastases. Their potential has been reviewed by Lode et al. *(63)*.

Although not strictly metastasis-targeting, angiogenic factors and their receptors are also a very active area of research, and anti-angiogenic strategies have been shown to inhibit metastasis in a variety of models. Relevant to this section is a recent report that active immunization of mice using dendritic cells pulsed with the VEGF receptor Flk-1 inhibited lung colonies of LLC *(64)*, with no overt effects on wound healing, but some effects on reproductive function.

The main considerations in the choice of model for immunotherapeutic trials are an understanding of the antigen(s) involved, and their relative immunogenicity in rodents vs humans. It is also important that the interventions are done (if possible) in animals which bear primary tumors (or have had them surgically removed), because the immunocompetence of naive animals does not compare with that of animals conditioned by the presence of a tumor. This can lead to either sensitization to tumor antigens (or possibly spurious responses to xenogeneic transfected genes) or in the later stages to either specific immune tolerance or anergy.

4.2. Anti-Gene and Anti-Sense Therapy

Several studies have shown that by transducing genes such as *Herpes simplex* thymidine kinase, followed by therapy with ganciclovir (which is activated by the enzyme), subsequent tumor growth and metastasis are inhibited. However, because of the current difficulties in generating vectors that are sufficiently stable to survive in the circulation and target metastases, most gene therapy experiments have thus far used local or regional delivery. Oncolytic viral therapy has been achieved in a rat model of hepatic metastasis, using hepatic portal infusion of a replication-competent adenovirus that targets proliferating cells and thus spares the hepatic parenchyma *(65)*.

There are some potentially interesting opportunities whereby viral (or nonviral) vectors could be targeted to organs using tumor-specific promoters such as AFP (hepatoma) c-*erb*B-2 (breast, ovarian and gastric cancer), and colorectal cancer. Alternatively, ligands or antibody fragments could redirect the vector to receptor-overexpressing tumor cells. Anti-sense approaches have mainly been directed against molecules associated with invasion and metastasis, such as CD44 v6 *(66)* and matrilysin (MMP-7) *(67)* in liver metastasis models of colorectal carcinoma. Anti-sense oligos against other targets (e.g., EGFR) have been tested in vitro, and will no doubt proceed to in vivo testing in similar models. Examples are given in Tables 3 and 4.

4.3. Targeting Metastasis-Related Tumor-Cell Activities

In this category anti-angiogenic strategies may be considered, as well as drugs or biologicals which target molecules associated with malignant progression—e.g., certain integrins, proteases, and motility factors. Many different approaches to inhibiting angiogenesis have been explored, and in some cases the agents have been tested against metastatic disease. These approaches are not covered in detail in this chapter—since the targets and strategies are not unique to metastatic disease—and the models have been used in other applications. Selected illustrations follow; other examples are given in Tables 3 and 4, and the references can be consulted for further information.

MMP inhibitors have been explored in detail. These include natural inhibitors (TIMPs), synthetic inhibitors, and anti-sense oligonucleotides. These enzymes are important both in tumor-cell invasion and angiogenesis, and particular models have been useful in determining their mode of action. For example, early studies in a rat mammary carcinoma showed that (as expected) lung colony numbers could be reduced with the broad-spectrum MMP inhibitor batimastat. In a spontaneous metastasis assay, a short peri-operative treatment in an adjuvant setting inhibited haematogenous metastases, but not lymphatic metastases. However, treatment continued postoperatively also prevented the outgrowth of lymph node metastases. This observation, combined with the fact that the lung colonies were reduced in size as well as number, suggested that mechanisms beyond inhibition of invasion were operative—putatively an anti-angiogenic effect *(68)*. Subsequent studies in a specialized videomicroscopy mouse liver olonization assay (and also direct angiogenesis assays) confirmed that such MMPs could inhibit tumor growth indirectly, via an anti-angiogenic effect. In some models, particularly in the liver where the fenestrated vasculature may offer less resistance, this mechanism (rather than inhibition of extravasation) may predominate *(69)*.

As with chemotherapy, where multiple drug regimes are now the norm, several studies are exploring combination therapy. For example, Reisfeld's group have shown that an angiogenic (αV) integrin antagonist plus an antibody-cytokine fusion protein gave synergistic activity against spontaneous liver metastases of a mouse neuroblastoma *(70)*. Guo et al. recently showed that an anti-angiogenic urokinase-derived peptide combined with tamoxifen inhibited the growth and lymphatic metastasis of a rat mammary carcinoma better than each agent alone *(71)*. Because of the requirement for a reproducibly high incidence of metastases, most of these complex studies have been performed in syngeneic systems.

5. DETECTION AND QUANTITATION OF METASTASES

Welch *(2)* has published a detailed description and critical comparison of available methodologies. Originally, metastases (or lung colonies) were directly observed, and the numbers (generally on the surface of organs) were counted. In some cases, organ weight was taken as an indicator of metastasis burden, but this could be highly inaccurate. If gross metastases were not evident, histological sections could be taken, and metastasis number (and in some cases, area) recorded. In order to improve quantitation and sensitivity, a variety of molecular techniques have recently been developed. For example, tumor cells can be detected by immunohistochemistry with antibodies directed against epithelial markers (for bone marrow or blood samples) or tumor antigens, and quantified by image analysis. Examination of a limited number of samples may miss small tumor deposits. More recently, PCR/RT-PCR probes for tumor markers have been used, but some primers may yield false positive results *(72,73)*. Examples of different techniques used experimentally are given in Table 5.

We have explored the use of human Alu sequences as a sensitive and quantitative indicator of the presence of human tumor cells in the lungs of nude mice following iv injection (based on methods described by Weisberg et al. *(74)*. There was a direct correlation between the numbers of cells injected and the signal detected, with a lower limit of detection of 100 cells per lung. However, we found that even when killed tumor cells were iv-injected, the lungs remained PCR-positive for a significant period (unpublished observations). Clearly this technique would have limitations for assessing the effects of therapy, at least in short-term assays. The results suggest that genetic material from dead cells can persist for longer than one would imagine, perhaps taken up by phagocytic cells, or otherwise protected from complete degradation. The implication is that a positive PCR signal cannot be assumed to indicate the presence of viable, clonogenic tumor cells.

In animal models, tumor cells have been genetically tagged with a variety of markers to assist their detection when subsequently inoculated into animals. Examples include the bacterial lac Z gene, whose product is a β-galactosidase enzyme—which produces a blue product in the presence of a chromogenic substrate—and green fluorescent protein (GFP) from the jellyfish *Aequorea victoria*. It is possible that expression of the tag may be downregulated, or the cells expressing it selectively destroyed (particularly in immunocompetent hosts) *(75)*, so that counting of positive lesions may underestimate the total number *(76)*. It is necessary to check that molecular detection and subsequent incidence of metastases correlate. This is not always the case *(77)*. These approaches seem to be most useful in tracking the early stages of tumor cell dissemination, and indeed mixed populations of differentially labeled cells have proven useful in comparative studies of cell fate *(78)*.

GFP-transduced cells offer an advantage—unlike the LacZ system, the cells can be visualized directly via fluorescence microscopy rather than requiring a staining procedure. They have been used to aid tumor cell detection in high resolution in vivo videomicroscopy *(79)*, and the latest generation of proteins have such high-intensity fluorescence that noninvasive whole-body optical imaging of metastases in nude mice

Table 5
Detection Systems for Metastases

Tumor	Site(s)	Method	Notes	Reference
MDA MB 231 (human breast ca)	Bone	CAT activity	May not correlate with clonogenic potential	81
DHD/K12 (rat colon ca)	Lung, liver, spleen, kidney	Genomic CAT tag	Presence of CAT tag did not correlate with overt metastases	77
MCF7 (human breast ca)	Multiple, including LN, brain, lung	Lac Z tag		136
Anip 973 (human lung ca)	Multiple including LN	GFP tag		137
PC-3 (human prostate ca)	Bone, lung, liver, adrenal, kidney	GFP		138
PC-3 (human prostate ca)	Lung, bone marrow	RT-PCR for human β-actin		124
B16F10 melanoma	Brain, liver, bone	GFP	Detected by whole-body optical imaging in live mice	138
AC3488	Liver, bone	GFP		139
C162 mouse melanoma and M109 lung carcinoma	Lung	Luciferase	Correlated with colony number and response to T-cell therapy	140
MH-PR1 (prostate)	Multiple sites; LN, BM, and L sublines generated	LacZ tag		141
COL-2-JCK (human colon ca) SCID mice	Liver	LDH-5 isozyme	Correlated with liver wt	74
HT29 (human colon ca) SCID mice	Liver and lung	Human *Alu-C* sequences Southern blotting	Persistence of DNA from dead cells?	142
B16 melanoma various	Liver, lung	Intravital videomicroscopy	Liver only?	79
NXS2 neuroblastoma	Liver, bone marrow	RT-PCR tyrosine hydroxylase	Combined with GFP	143
4T1.2 (breast)	Bone, lungs	Serum PTHrP radioimmunoassay	Quantitative?	144
3T3 mouse sarcoma, human neuroblastoma, human prostate ca	Various	Lac Z, placental alkaline phosphatase, Drosophila alcohol dehydrogenase	Allows tracking of multiple tumor-cell populations using PCR and LCM	78
CC531 rat colon carcinoma	Liver	LacZ	Immune response to transfected cells decreased tumorigenicity	75

PTHrP = parathyroid hormone-related protein

PCR = polymerase chain reaction

LCM = laser-capture microdissection

has recently been achieved *(80)*. This will potentially allow real-time quantitation of the growth of metastases and their inhibition by novel agents.

REFERENCES

1. Gura T. Systems for identifying new drugs are often faulty. *Science* 1997; 278:1041–1042.
2. Welch DR. Technical considerations for studying cancer metastasis *in vivo*. *Clin Exp Metastasis* 1997; 15:272–306.
3. Eccles SA. Basic principles for the study of metastasis. In: Brooks SA, Schumacher U, eds. *Methods in Molecular Medicine,* vol. 58, Metastasis Research Protocols volume 2, 2001. Schumacher, Humana Press Inc., Totowa NJ.
4. Monaci P, Bartoli F, Di Zenzo G, Nuzzo M, Urbanelli L. Random peptide libraries for target definition. *Tumor Targeting* 1999; 4:129–142.
5. Wang R-F, Rosenberg SA. Human tumor antigens for cancer vaccine development. *Immunol Rev* 1999; 170:85–100.
6. Ostrand-Rosenberg S, Pulaski BA, Clements VK, Ling Q, Pipeling MR, Hanyok LA. Cell based vaccines for the stimulation of immunity to metastatic cancers. *Immunol Rev* 1999; 170:101–114.
7. Dimitroff CJ, Sharma A, Bernacki R. Cancer metastasis: a search for therapeutic inhibition. *Cancer Investig* 1998; 16:279–290.
8. Panchal RG. Novel therapeutic strategies to selectively kill cancer cells. *Biochem Pharmacol* 1998; 55:247–252.
9. Boral AL, Dessain S, Chabner BA. Clinical evaluation of biologically targeted drugs: obstacles and opportunities. *Cancer Chemother Pharmacol* 1998; 42(Suppl.) S3–S21.
10. Dalerba P, Ricci A, Russo V, et al. High homogeneity of MAGE, BAGE, GAGE, tyrosinase and Melan-A/MART-1 gene expression in clusters of multiple metastases of human melanoma: implications for protocol design of therapeutic antigen-specific vaccination strategies. *Int J Cancer* 1998; 77:200–204.
11. Eccles SA, Modjtahedi H, Court W, Sandle J, Dean CJ. Significance of the c-*erb*B family of receptor tyrosine kinase in metastatic cancer and their potential as targets for immunotherapy. *Invasion Metastasis* 1995; 14:337–348.
12. Eccles S. c-*erb*B-2 as a target for immunotherapy. *Exp Opinion Invest Drugs* 1998; 7:1879–1896.
13. Petit A, Rak J, Hung M-C. Neutralizing antibodies against EGFR and erbB-2/neu receptor tyrosine kinases down-regulate vascular endothelial growth factor production by tumor cells in vitro and *in vivo. Am J Path* 1997; 151:1523–1530.
14. O-charoenrat P, Modjtahedi H, Rhys-Evans P, Court W, Box G, Eccles S. Epidermal growth factor-like ligands differentially upregulate matrix metalloproteinase-9 in head and neck squamous carcinoma cells. *Cancer Res* 2000; 60:1121–1128.
15. O-charoenrat P, Rhys-Evans P, Modjtahedi H, Court W, Box G, Eccles SA. Overexpression of epidermal growth factor receptor in human head and neck squamous carcinoma cell lines correlates with matrix metalloproteinase-9 expression and *in vitro* invasion. *Int J Cancer* 2000; 86:307–317.
16. O-charoenrat P, Rhys-Evans P, Modjtahedi H, Eccles SA. Vascular endothelial growth factor family members are differentially regulated by c-*erb*B signaling in head and neck squamous carcinoma cells. *Clin Exp Metastasis* 2000; 18:155–161.
17. Testa JE, Brooks PC, Lin JM, Quigley JP. Eukaryotic expression cloning with an antimetastatic monoclonal antibody identifies a tetraspanin (PETA-3/CD151) as an effector of human tumor cell migration and metastasis. *Cancer Res* 1999; 59:3812–3820.
18. Chang SS, Reuter VE, Heston WD, Bander NH, Grauer LS, Gaudin PB. Five different anti-prostate-specific membrane antigen (PSMA) antibodies confirm PSMA expression in tumor-associated neovasculature. *Cancer Res* 1999; 59:3192–3198.
19. Burg MA, Pasqualini R, Arap W, Ruoslahti E, Stallcup WB. NG2 proteoglycan binding peptides target tumor neovasculature. *Cancer Res* 1999; 59:2869–2874.
20. Ergun S, Kilic N, Ziegeler G, et al. CEA-related cell adhesion molecule 1: a potent angiogenic factor and a major effector of vascular endothelial growth factor. *Molec Cell* 2000; 5:311–320.
21. Maruyama K, Ishida O, Takizawa T, Moribe K. Possibility of active targeting to tumor tissues with liposomes. *Adv Drug Deliv Rev* 1999; 40:89–102.
22. Pasqualini R. Vascular targeting with phage peptide libraries. *J Nucl Med* 1999; 43:159–162.
23. Eccles SA, Alexander P. Immunologically-mediated restraint of latent tumour metastases. *Nature* 1975; 257:52–53.

24. Eccles SA, Styles JM, Hobbs SM, Dean CJ. Metastasis in the nude rat associated with lack of immune response. *Br J Cancer* 1979; 40:802–805.

25. Eccles SA, Heckford SE, Alexander P. Effect of cyclosporin A on the growth and spontaneous metastasis of syngeneic animal tumours. *Br J Cancer* 1980; 42:252–259.

26. Disis ML, Cheever MA, et al. HER-2/neu protein: a target for antigen-specific immunotherapy of human cancer. *Adv Cancer Res* 1997; 17:343–371.

27. Seigal-Eiras A, Croce MV. Breast cancer associated mucin: a review. *Allergol Immunopathol* 1997; 25:176–181.

28. Leger O, Johnson-Leger C, Jackson E, Coles B, Dean C. The chondroitin sulfate proteoglycan NG2 is a tumour-specific antigen on the chemically-induced rat chondrosarcoma HSN. *Int J Cancer* 1994; 58:700–705.

29. Burg MA, Grako K, Stallcup WB. Expression of the NG2 proteoglycan enhances the growth and metastatic properties of melanoma cells. *J Cell Physiol* 1998; 177:299–312.

30. Lalani E-N, Berdichevsky F, Boshell M, et al. Expression of the gene coding for a human mucin in mouse mammary tumor cells can affect their tumorigenicity. *J Biol Chem* 1991; 266:15,420–15,426.

31. Kjonniksen I, Hoifodt HK, Pihl A, Fodstad O. Different metastasis patterns of a human melanoma cell line in nude mice and rats: influence of microenvironment. *J Natl Cancer Inst* 1991; 83:1020–1024.

32. Noel A, De Pauw-Gillet MC, Purnell G, Nusgens B, Lapiere C-M, Foidart J-M. Enhancement of tumorigenicity of human breast adenocarcinoma cells in nude mice by matrigel and fibroblasts. *Br J Cancer* 1993; 68:909–915.

33. Barnett SC, Eccles SA. Studies of mammary carcinoma metastasis in a mouse model system II. Lectin binding properties of cells in relation to incidence and organ distribution of metastases. *Clin Exp Metastasis* 1984; 2:297–310.

34. Kobayashi H, Gotoh J, Shinohara H, Moniwa N, Terao T. Inhibition of the metastasis of Lewis lung carcinoma by antibody against urokinase-type plasminogen activator in the experimental and spontaneous metastasis model. *Thromb Haemost* 1994; 71:474–480.

35. Chen L, Ter Haar G, Hill CR, Eccles SA, Box G. Treatment of implanted liver tumors with focussed ultrasound. *Ultrasound Med Biol* 1998; 24:1475–1488.

36. Hori K, Li HC, Saito S, Sato Y. Increased growth and incidence of lymph node metastases due to the angiogenesis inhibitor AGM-1470. *Br J Cancer* 1997; 75:1730–1734.

37. Salup RR, Pirtskhalaishvili G, Deng DH, Batthacharya R, Tran S, Lotze MT. Vaccination with a plasmid DNA encoding for a truncated HER2/neu protein prevents the growth of prostate cancer in rats and induces a tumor antigen specific immune response in vivo. *Proc Am Assoc Cancer Res* 1999; 40:abs#1697.

38. Killion JJ, Radinsky R, Fidler IJ. Orthotopic models are necessary to predict therapy of transplantable tumors in mice. *Cancer Met Rev* 1998–9; 17:279–284.

39. Fidler IJ. Critical determinants of cancer metastasis: rationale for therapy. *Cancer Chemother Pharmacol* 1999; 43:S3–10.

40. Siegal PM, Ryan ED, Cardiff RD, Muller WJ. Elevated expression of activated forms of Neu/ErbB-2 and ErbB-3 are involved in the induction of mammary tumors in transgenic mice: implications for human breast cancer. *EMBO J* 1999; 18:2149–2164.

41. Gingrich JR, Barrios RJ, Morton RA, et al. Metastatic prostate cancer in a transgenic mouse. *Cancer Res* 1996; 56:4096–4102.

42. Willis RA, Wei C, Turner MJ, Callahan BP, Pugh AE, Barth RK, et al. A transgenic strategy for analyzing the regulatory regions of the human prostate-specific antigen gene: potential applications for the treatment of prostate cancer. *Int J Mol Med* 1998; 1:379–386.

43. Clarke P, Mann J, Simpson JF, Rickard-Dickson K, Primus FJ. Mice transgenic for human carcinoembryonic antigen as a model for immunotherapy. *Cancer Res* 1998; 58:1469–1477.

44. Thompson JA, Eades-Perner AM, Ditter M, Muller WJ, Zimmermann W. Expression of transgenic carcinoembryonic antigen in tumor-prone mice: an animal model for CEA-directed immunotherapy. *Int J Cancer* 1997; 72:197–202.

45. Kass E, Schlom J, Thompson J, Guadagni F, Graziano P, Greiner JW. Induction of protective immunity to carcinoembryonic antigen (CEA) a self antigen in CEA transgenic mice, by immunizing with a recombinant vaccinia-CEA virus. *Cancer Res* 1999; 59:676–683.

46. Eccles SA, Purvies HP, Styles JM, Hobbs SM, Dean CJ. Potential of monoclonal antibodies for localisation and treatment of disseminated disease: studies in syngeneic rat tumour systems. *Adv Exp Med Biol* 1988; 233:329–339.

47. Eccles SA, Purvies HP, Styles JM, Hobbs SM, Dean CJ. Pharmacokinetic studies of radiolabelled rat monoclonal antibodies recognising syngeneic sarcoma antigens. I. Comparison of IgG subclasses. *Cancer Immunol Immunother* 1989; 30:5–12.

48. Eccles SA, Purvies HP, Styles JM, Hobbs SM, Dean CJ. Pharmacokinetic studies of radiolabelled rat monoclonal antibodies recognising syngeneic sarcoma antigens. II. Effect of host age and immune status. *Cancer Immunol Immunother* 1989; 30:13–20.

49. Ma D, Niederkorn JY. Efficacy of tumor-infiltrating lymphocytes in the treatment of hepatic tumors arising from transgenic intraocular tumors in mice. *Investig Opthalmol* 1995; 36:1067–1075.

50. Schmidt M, Maurer-Gebhardt M, Groner B, Kohler G, Brochman-Santos G, Wels W. Suppression of metastasis formation by a recombinant single chain antibody-toxin targeted to full length and onco-genic variant EGF receptors. *Oncogene* 1999; 18:1711–1721.

51. Sharkey RM, Weadock KS, Natale A, et al. Successful radioimmunotherapy for lung metastasis of human colonic cancer in nude mice. *J Natl Cancer Inst* 1991; 83:627–632.

52. Saga T, Sakahara H, Nakamoto Y, et al. Radiotherapy for liver micrometastases in mice: pharmacoki-netics, dose estimation and long-term effects. *Jpn J Cancer Res* 1999; 90:342–348.

53. Behr TM, Salib AL, Liersch T, et al. Radioimmunotherapy of small volume disease of colorectal can-cer metastatic to the liver: preclinical evaluation in comparison to standard chemotherapy and initial results of a phase 1 clinical trial. *Clin Cancer Res* 1999; 5:(10 Suppl. 1) 3232s–3242s.

54. Russell PJ, Ho Shon I, Boniface GR, et al. Growth and metastasis of human bladder cancer xenografts in the bladder of nude rats. A model for intravesical radioimmunotherapy. *Urol Res* 1991; 19:201–213.

55. Goodwin DA, Meares CF. Pretargeting. *Cancer* (Suppl.)1997; 80:2675–2680.

56. Eccles SA, Court WJ, Box GA, Dean CJ, Melton RG, Springer CJ. Regression of established breast carcinoma xenografts with antibody-directed enzyme prodrug therapy against c-erbB2 p185. *Cancer Res* 1994; 54:5171–5177.

57. Sabzevari H, Gillies SD, Mueller BM, Pancock JD, Reisfeld RA. A recombinant antibody-interleukin 2 fusion protein suppresses growth of hepatic human neuroblastoma metastases in severe combined immune deficiency mice. *Proc Natl Acad Sci USA* 1994; 91:9626–9630.

58. Lode HN, Xiang R, Varki NM, Dolman CS, Gillies SD, Reisfeld RA. Targeted interleukin-2 ther-apy for spontaneous neuroblastoma metastases to bone marrow. *J Natl Cancer Inst* 1997; 89:1586–1594.

59. Shrayer DP, Cole B, Hearing VJ, Wolf SF, Wanebo HJ. Immunotherapy of mice with an irradiated melanoma vaccine coupled with interleukin 12. *Clin Exp Metastasis* 1999; 17:63–70.

60. El Shami KM, Tzehoval E, Vadai E, Feldman M, Eisenbach L. Induction of anti-tumor immunity with modified autologous cells expressing membrane-bound murine cytokines. *J Interferon Cytokine Res* 1999; 19:1391–1401.

61. Price JE, Kiriakova G, Rao X-M, Lachman LB. DNA vaccination protects against the growth and metastasis of neu-expressing mammary tumor cells. *Proc Am Assoc Cancer Res* 2000; 41:(Abs # 2988) 469.

62. Chikamatsu K, Reichert TE, Kashii Y, et al. Immunotherapy with effector cells and IL-2 of lymph node metastases of human squamous cell carcinoma of the head and neck established in nude mice. *Int J Cancer* 1999; 82:532–537.

63. Lode HN, Xiang R, Becker JC, Gillies SD, Reisfeld RA. Immunocytokines: a promising approach to cancer immunotherapy. *Pharmacol Ther* 1998; 80:277–292.

64. Li Y, Wang K, King A, et al. Active immunization against the angiogenic receptor Flk-1 inhibits tumor metastasis. *Proc Am Assoc Cancer Res* 2000; 698(Abs 4437).

65. Kooby DA, Carew JF, Halterman MW, et al. Oncolytic viral therapy for human colorectal cancer and liver metastases using a multi-mutated herpes simplex virus type 1 (G207). *FASEB J* 1999; 13:1325–1334.

66. Reeder JA, Gotley DC, Walsh MD, Fawcett J, Antalis TM. Expression of antisense CD44 variant 6 inhibits colorectal tumor metastasis and tumor growth in a wound environment. *Cancer Res* 1998; 58:3719–3726.

67. Miyazaki K, Koshikawa N, Hasegawa S, et al. Matrilysin as a target for chemotherapy for colon can-cer: use of antisense oligonucleotides as antimetastatic agents. *Cancer Chemother Pharmacol* 1999; (43 Suppl.)S52–S55.

68. Eccles SA, Box GM, Court WJ, Bone EA, Thomas W, Brown PD. Control of lymphatic and hematogenous metastasis of a rat mammary carcinoma by the matrix metalloproteinase inhibitor bati-mastat (BB-94). *Cancer Res* 1996; 56:2815–2822.

69. Wylie S, MacDonald IC, Varghese HJ. The matrix metalloproteinase inhibitor batimastat inhibits angiogenesis in liver metastases of B16F1 melanoma cells. *Clin Exp Metastasis* 1999; 17:111–117.

70. Lode HN, Moehler T, Xiang R, et al. Synergy between an antiangiogenic integrin alpha antagonist and an antibody-cytokine fusion protein eradicates spontaneous tumour metastasis. *Proc Natl Acad Sci USA* 1999; 96:1591–1596.

71. Guo YJ, Mazar AP, Rabbani SA, et al. An anti-angiogenic urokinase-derived peptide (A6) combined with tamoxifen (TAM) promotes tumor apoptosis resulting in decreased growth and metastasis in a syngeneic breast carcinoma model. *Proc Am Assoc Cancer Res* 2000; 41:(Abstract 2077:327.

72. Zippelius A, Kufer P, Honold G, et al. Limitations of reverse-transcriptase polymerase chain reaction analyses for detection of micrometastatic epithelial cancer cells in bone marrow. *J Clin Oncol* 1997; 15:806–807.

73. Bostick P, et al. Limitations of specific reverse-transcriptase polymerase chain reaction markers in the detection of metastases in the lymph nodes and blood of cancer patients. *J Clin Oncol* 1998; 16:2632–2640.

74. Weisberg T, Cahill BK, Vary CPH. Non-radioisotopic detection of human xenogeneic DNA in a mouse transplantation model. *Molec Cell Probes* 1996; 10:139–146.

75. Wittmer A, Khaziae K, Berger MR. Quantitative detection of laz-Z transfected CC531 colon carcinoma cells in an orthotopic rat colon carcinoma model. *Clin Exp Metastasis* 1999; 17:369–376.

76. Fujimaki T, Ellis LM, Bucana CD, Radinsky R, Price JE, Fidler IJ. Simultaneous radiolabel, genetic tagging and proliferation assays to study the organ distribution and fate of metastatic cells. *Int J Oncol* 1993; 2:895–901.

77. Garcia-Olmo D, Ontanon J, Garcia-Olmo DC, Atienzar M, Vallejo M. Detection of genomically-tagged cancer cells in different tissues at different stages of tumor development: lack of correlation with the formation of metastases. *Cancer Lett* 1999; 140:11–20.

78. Culp LA, Lin W, Kleinman NR, O'Connor KL, Lechner R. Earliest steps in primary tumor formation and micrometastasis resolved with histochemical markers of gene-tagged tumor cells. *J Histochem Cytochem* 1998; 46:557–568.

79. Naumov GN, Wilson SM, MacDonald IC, et al. Cellular expression of green fluorescent protein, coupled with high-resolution *in vivo* videomicroscopy to monitor steps in tumor metastasis. *J Cell Sci* 1999; 112:1835–1842.

80. Yang M, Baranov E, Jiang P, et al. Whole-body optical imaging of green fluorescent protein expressing tumors and metastases. *Proc Natl Acad Sci USA* 2000; 97:1206–1211.

81. Yoneda Y, Sasaki A, Mundy GR. Osteolytic bone metastasis in breast cancer. *Breast Cancer Res Treat* 1994; 32:73–84.

82. Cher ML, Upadhyay J, Shekarritz B, Nemeth JA, Dong Z, Fridman R. Membrane-type metalloproteinase, MMP-2, and MMP-9 are induced in prostate cancer cells by growth in human bone *in vivo*. *Proc Am Assoc Cancer Res* 1999; 40:(Abs 486).

83. Greene GF, Kitadai Y, Pettaway CA, et al. Correlation of metastasis-related gene expression with metastatic potential in human prostate carcinoam cells implanted in nude mice using an *in situ* messenger RNA hybridization technique. *Am J Pathol* 1997; 150:1571–1582.

84. Tardif M, Coulombe J, Soullieres D, Rousseau AP, Pelletier G. Gangliosides in human uveal melanoma metastatic process. *Int J Cancer* 1996; 68:97–101.

85. Vogel CA, Galmiche MC, Westerman P, et al. Carcinoembryonic antigen expression, antibody localisation and immunophotodetection of human colon cancer liver metastases in nude mice: a model for radioimmunotherapy. *Int J Cancer* 1996; 67:294–302.

86. Singh RK, Tsan R, Radinsky R. Influence of the host microenvironment on the clonal selection of human colon carcinoma cells during primary tumor growth and metastasis. *Clin Exp Metastasis* 1997; 15:140–150.

87. Parker C, Roseman BJ, Bucana CD, Tsan R, Radinsky R. Preferential activation of the epidermal growth factor receptor in human colon carcinoma liver metastases in nude mice. *J Histochem Cytochem* 1998; 46:595–602.

88. Rusciano D, Lorenzoni P, Burger M. Murine models of liver metastasis. *Invasion Metastasis* 1994–5; 14:349–361.

89. Ma D, Niederkorn JY. Role of epidermal growth factor receptor in the metastasis of intraocular melanomas. *Invest Ophthalmol Vis Sci* 1998; 39:1067–1075.

90. Salven P, Heikkila P, Joensuu H. Enhanced expression of vascular endothelial growth factor in metastatic melanoma. *Br J Cancer* 1997; 76:930–934.

91. Zeng ZS, Guilem JG. Unique activation of MMP-9 within human liver metastases from colorectal cancer. *Br J Cancer* 1998; 78:349–353.

92. Elgamel AA, Holmes EH, Su SL, et al. Prostate specific membrane antigen: current benefits and future value. *Semin Surg Oncol* 2000; 18:10–16.

93. Nam SM, Kim HS, Ahn WS, Park YS. Sterically stabilized anti-G(M3), anti-Le(x) immunoliposomes: targeting to B16BL6, HRT-18 cancer cells. *Oncol Res* 1999; 11:9–16.

94. Shalinsky DR, Brekken J, Zou H, et al. Broad anti-tumour and antiangiogenic activities of AG3340, a potent and selective MMP inhibitor undergoing advanced oncology clinical trials. *Ann NY Acad Sci USA* 1999; 878:236–270.

95. Oku T, Ata N, Yonezawa K, et al. Antimetastatic and antitumour effect of a recombinant human tissue inhibitor of metalloproteinase-2 in murine melanoma models. *Biol Pharm Bull* 1997; 20:843–849.

96. Kasaoka T, Nishiyama H, Okada M, Nakajima M. Matrix metalloproteinase inhibitor (MMPI) CGS27023A inhibited hematogenic metastasis of B16 melanoma cells in both experimental and spontaneous metastasis models. *Proc Am Assoc Cancer Res* 2000; 41:(Abs 852) 134.

97. Prontera C, Mariani B, Rossi C, Poggi A, Rotilio D. Inhibition of gelatinase A (MMP-2) by batimastat and captopril reduces tumor growth and lung metastases in mice bearing Lewis lung carcinoma. *Int J Cancer* 1999; 81:761–766.

98. Murakami K, Yamaura T, Suda K, et al. TAC-101 inhibits spontaneous mediastinal lymph node metastasis produced by orthotopic implantation of Lewis lung carcinoma. *Jpn J Cancer Res* 1999; 90:1254–1261.

99. Livant DL, Brabec RK, Pienta KJ. Anti-invasive, antitumorigenic and antimetastatic activities of the PHSCN sequence in prostate carcinoma. *Cancer Res* 2000; 60:309–320.

100. Rabbani SA, Harakidis P, Davidson DJ, Henkin J, Mazar AP. Prevention of prostate cancer metastasis in vivo by a novel synthetic inhibitor of urokinase-type plasminogen activator (uPA). *Int J Cancer* 1995; 63:840–845.

101. Lokeshwar BL. MMP inhibition in prostate cancer. *Ann NY Acad Sci USA* 1999; 878:271–289.

102. Lode HN, Reisfeld RA, Handgretiner R, et al. Targeted therapy with a novel enediyne antibiotic calicheamycin theta 1 effectively suppresses growth and dissemination of liver metastases in a syngeneic model of murine neuroblastoma. *Cancer Res* 1998; 58:2925–2928.

103. Nishisaka N, Maini A, Kinoshita Y, et al. Immunotherapy for lung metastases of murin renal cell carcinoma: synergy between radiation and cytokine-producing tumor vaccines. *J Immunother* 1999; 22:308–314.

104. Mori A, Kennel SJ, van Borssum Waalkes M, Scherphof GL, Huang L, Characterisation of organ-specific immunoliposomes for delivery of 3,5-O-dipalmitoyl-5-fluoro-2-deoxyuridines in a mouse lung metastasis model. *Cancer Chemother Pharmacol* 1995; 35:447–456.

105. Sivanandham M, Scoggin SD, Tanaka N, Wallack MK. Therapeutic effect of a Vaccinia colon oncolysate prepared with interleukin-2 gene encoded vaccinia virus studied in a syngeneic CC-36 murine colon hepatic metastasis model. *Cancer Immunol Immunother* 1994; 38:259–264.

106. Shigeoka H, Karsten U, Okuno K, Yasutomi M. Inhibition of liver metastases from neuraminidase-treated colon 26 cells by an anti-TF-specific monoclonal antibody. *Tumour Biol.* 1999; 20:139–146.

107. Lozonschi L, Sumamura M, Kobari M, et al. Controlling tumor angiogenesis and metastasis of C26 colon adenocarcinoma by a new matrix metalloproteinase inhibitor, KB-R7785, in two tumor models. *Cancer Res* 1999; 59:1252–1258.

108. Shaheen RM, Davis DW, Liu W, et al. Antiangiogenic therapy targeting the tyrosine kinase receptor for vascular endothelial growth factor receptor inhibits the growth of colon carcinoma liver metastasis and induces tumor and endothelial cell apoptosis. *Cancer Res* 1999; 59:5412–5416.

109. Hurford RK, Dranoff G, Mulligan RC, Tepper RI. Gene therapy of metastatic cancer by in vivo retroviral gene targeting. *Nat Genet* 1995; 10:430–435.

110. Pierrefite-Carle V, Gavelli A, Brossette N, et al. Cytosine-deaminase/5-fluorocytosine-based vaccination against liver tumors: evidence of distant bystander effect. *J Natl Cancer Inst* 2000; 92:494–495.

111. Patel PM, Flemming CL, Harris JD, Fisher C, Eccles SA, Gore ME, et al. Engineering autologous IL-2 secreting tumour cell vaccines for malignant melanoma. *Br J Cancer* 1994; 69 (Suppl. XX1) 55.

112. Eccles SA, McIntosh DP, Purvies HP, Cumber AJ, Parnell GD, Forrester JA, et al. An ineffective monoclonal antibody-ricin A chain conjugate is converted to a tumoricidal agent in vivo by subsequent systemic administration of ricin B chain. *Cancer Immunol Immunother* 1987; 24:37–41.

113. Charissoux JL, Grossin L, Leboutet MJ, Rigaud M. Treatment of experimental osteosarcoma tumors in rat by herpes simplex thymidine kinase gene transfer and ganciclovir. *Anticancer Res* 1999; 19:77–80.

114. Mahteme H, Lovqvist A, Graf W, Lundqvist H, Carlsson J, Sundin A. Adjuvant 131-I-anti-CEA-antibody radioimmunotherapy inhibits the development of experimental colonic carcinoma liver metastases. *Anticancer Res* 1998; 18:843–848.

115. Tanaka T, Konno H, Matsuda I, Nakamura S, Baba S. Prevention of hepatic metastasis of human colon cancer by angiogenesis inhibitor TNP-470. *Cancer Res* 1995; 55:836–839.

116. Qi Y, Moyana T, Bresalier R, Xiang J. Antibody-targeted lymphokine-activated killer cells inhibit liver micrometastases in severe combined immunodeficient mice. *Gastroenterology* 1995; 109:1950–1957.

117. Hurwitz E, Adler R, Shouval D, Takahashi H, Wands JR, Seal M. Immunotargeting of daunomycin to localized and metastatic human colon adenocarcinoma in athymic mice. *Cancer Immunol Immunother* 1992; 35:186–192.

118. Maekawa R, Maki H, Yoshida H, et al. Correlation of antiangiogenic and antitumour efficacy of N-biphenyl sulfonyl-phenylalanine hydroxamic acid (BPHA), an orally-active selective matrix metalloproteinase inhibitor. *Cancer Res* 1999; 59:1231–1235.

119. Becker JC, Pancook JD, Gillies SD, Mendelsohn J, Reisfeld RA. Eradication of human hepatic and pulmonary melanoma metastases in SCID mice by antibody-interleukin 2 fusion proteins. *Proc Natl Acad Sci USA* 1996; 93:2702–2707.

120. Niederkorn JY, Mellon J, Pidherney M, Mayhew E, Anand R. Effect of anti-ganglioside antibodies on the metastatic spread of intraocular melanomas in a nude mouse model of human uveal melanomas. *Curr Eye Res* 1993; 12:347–358.

121. Ma D, Gerard RD, Li XY, Alizadeh H, Niederkorn JY. Inhibition of metastasis of intraocular melanomas by adenovirus-mediated gene transfer of plasminogen activator type 1 (PAI-1) in an athymic mouse model. *Blood* 1997; 90:2738–2746.

122. Nakai M, Mundy GR, Williams PJ, Boyce B, Yoneda T. A synthetic antagonist to laminin inhibits the formation of osteolytic metastases by human melanoma cells in nude mice. *Cancer Res* 1992; 52:5395–5399.

123. Link EM. Targeting melanoma with 211At/131I-methylene blue: preclinical and clinical experience. *Hybridoma* 1999; 18:77–82.

124. Dolman CS, Mueller BM, Lode HN, Xiang R, Gillies SD, Reisfeld RA. Suppression of human prostate carcinoma metastases in severe combined immune deficiency mice by interleukin 2 immunocytokine therapy. *Clin Cancer Res* 1998; 4:2551–2557.

125. Stearns ME, Fudge K, Garcia F, Wang M. IL-10 inhibition of human prostate PC-3 ML cell metastases in SCID mice: IL-10 stimulation of TIMP-1 and inhibition of MMP-2/MMP-9 expression. *Invasion Metastasis* 1997; 17:62–74.

126. Kennel SJ, Boll R, Stabin M, Schuller HM, Mirzadeh S. Radioimmunotherapy of micrometastases in lung with vascular targeted 213Bi. *Br J Cancer* 1999; 71:474–480.

127. Nagamachi Y, Tani M, Shimizu K, Yoshida T, Yokota J. Suicidal gene therapy for pleural metastasis of lung cancer by liposome-mediated transfer of herpes simplex virus thymidine kinase gene. *Cancer Gene Ther* 1999; 6:546–553.

128. Hanibuchi M, Yano S, Nishioki Y, Yanagawa H, Kawano T, Sone S. Therapeutic efficacy of mouse-human chimeric anti-ganglioside GM2 monoclonal antibody against multiple organ micrometastases of human lung cancer in NK cell-depleted SCID mice. *Int J Cancer* 1998; 78:480–485.

129. Mycklebust AT, Godal A, Fodstad O. Targeted therapy with immunotoxins in a nude rat model for leptomeningeal growth of human small cell lung cancer. *Cancer Res* 1994; 54:2146–2150.

130. Nakatsugawa S, Okuda T, Muramoto H, et al. Inhibitory effect of ND2001 on spontaneous multiple metastasis of NC 65 tumors derived from human renal cancer cells intradermally transplanted into nude mice. *Anticancer Drugs* 1999; 10:229–233.

131. Perrotte P, Matsumoto T, Inoue K, et al. Anti-epidermal growth factor receptor antibody C225 inhibits angiogenesis in human transitional cell carcinoma growing orthotopically in nude mice. *Clin Cancer Res* 1999; 5:257–265.

132. Winding B, Therkildsen B, Jakobsen M, et al. Inhibition of matrix metalloproteinases prolong survival and decrease both bone metastasis and osteolytic lesion growth in human breast cancer-bearing mice. *Proc Am Assoc Cancer Res* 1999; 40: (Abs 0730).

133. Bagheri-Yarmand R, Kourbali Y, Rath AM, et al. Carboxymethyl dextran blocks angiogenesis of MDA MB435 breast carcinomas xenografted in fat pad and its lung metastases in nude mice. *Cancer Res* 1999; 59:507–510.

134. MacDonanld GC, Entwhistle J, Lewis K, et al. Effect of an unconjugated human scfv on growth and metastasis of a breast adenocarcinoma in athymic mice. *Proc Am Assoc Cancer Res* 2000; 41: (Abs 9), 2.

135. Zervos EE, Norman JG, Gower WR, Franz MG, Rosemurgy AS. Matrix metalloproteinase inhibition attenuates human pancreatic cancer growth in vitro and decreases mortality and tumorigenesis in vivo. *J Surg Res* 1997; 69:367–71.

136. Kurebayashi J, McLeskey SW, Johnson MD, et al. Quantitative demonstration of spontaneous metastasis by MCF-7 human breast cancer cells co-transfected with fibroblast growth factor 4 and *LacZ Cancer Res* 1993; 53:2178–2187.

137. Chishima T, Miyagi Y, Wang X, et al. Metastatic patterns of lung cancer visualized live and in process by green fluorescent protein expression. *Clin Exp Metastasis* 1997; 15: 547–552.

138. Yang M, Jiang P, Sun FX, et al. A fluorescent orthotopic bone metastasis model of human prostate cancer. *Cancer Res* 1999; 59:781–786.

139. Zhang L, Hellstrom KE, Chen L. Luciferase activity as a marker of tumor burden and as an indicator of tumor response to antineoplastic therapy in vivo. *Clin Exp Metastasis* 1994; 12:87–92.

140. Heller M, Ferrer K, Xue B-H, McCorquodale M, Nupponen N, et al. A new reporter-tagged prostate cell line and its use as a metastatic model. *Proc Am Assoc Cancer Res* 1999; 40: (Abs 487).

141. Kuo TH, Kubota T, Nishibori H, et al. Experimental cancer chemotherapy using a liver metastatic model of human colon cancer transplanted into the spleen of SCID mice. *J Surg Oncol* 1993; 52:92–96.

142. Chambers AF, MacDonald IC, Schmidt EE, Morris VL, Groom AC. Preclinical assessment of anti-cancer therapeutic strategies using *in vivo* videomicroscopy. *Cancer Metastasis Rev* 1998-9; 17:263–269.

143. Lode HN, Handgretiner R, Schuermann U, et al. Detection of neuroblastoma cells in CD34+ selected peripheral stem cells using a combination of tyrosine hydroxylase nested RT-PCR and anti-ganglioside GD2 immunocytochemistry *Eur J Cancer* 1997b, 33:2024–2030.

144. Lelekakis M, Mosely JM, Martin TJ, et al. A novel orthotopic model of breast cancer metastasis to bone. *Clin Exp Metastasis* 1999; 17:163–170.

VII | NORMAL TISSUE RESPONSE MODELS

18

Animal Models of Oral Mucositis Induced by Antineoplastic Drugs and Radiation

Stephen T. Sonis, DMD, DMSc

CONTENTS

1. OVERVIEW OF THE CLINICAL CONDITION

Oral mucositis is a common, troubling, and often dose-limiting toxicity of cancer chemotherapy *(1)*. In the case of patients receiving radiation to the head and neck, stomatotoxicity is a frequent cause of unplanned interruptions in treatment. In its most dramatic form, mucositis results in diffuse full-thickness ulceration of the oral mucosa, causing severe pain and loss of function. The lesions that develop are often a site of secondary infection. Importantly, in the myelosuppressed patient, the loss of mucosal integrity results in a systemic portal of entry for the mouth's indigenous bacterial flora *(2)*. Consequently, oral mucositis is a major risk factor for sepsis in this population. In addition to its physiologic cost, the results of a number of pharmacoeconomic studies have attached significant economic and outcome costs to the condition. The length of hospital stay, febrile days, days of total parenteral nutrition, antibiotic use, and analgesic use are all increased in-patients with mucositis *(3)*. Among bone-marrow transplant recipients, the difference in charges between patients with mucositis compared to those without the condition is over $25,000 *(4)*. The finding by Bellm et al. that mucositis was the most commonly cited negative outcome among bone-marrow transplant recipients is illustrative of its impact on patients' quality of life *(5)*.

From: *Tumor Models in Cancer Research*
Edited by: B. A. Teicher © Humana Press Inc., Totowa, NJ

2. THE BIOLOGY OF MUCOSITIS

The pathobiology of mucositis can be divided into four phases: an inflammatory/vascular phase, an epithelial phase, an ulcerative/infectious stage, and a healing phase *(6)*. The process is probably initiated by the generation of reactive oxygen species by exposure to stomatotoxic stimuli. Activation and expression of pro-inflammatory cytokines, particularly tumor necrosis factor-alpha (TNF-α) and interleukin-1 beta (IL-1β) and endothelial damage characterize the inflammatory/vascular phase *(7)*. Alternative mechanisms leading to cell death, such as the ceramide pathway, may also be involved *(8)*.

The epithelial phase results from the nonspecific effects of cytotoxic agents on the DNA of rapidly dividing cells of the oral basal epithelium. As a result, epithelial proliferation and renewal are retarded, resulting in atrophy. Functional trauma leads to epithelial breakdown and the formation of ulcers.

The ulcerative/bacteriologic phase is clinically the most dramatic. The integrity of the oral mucosa is breached, leading to marked discomfort. Lesions are often secondarily colonized by bacteria that shed cell products into the underlying ulcerated tissue. Macrophages and histiocytes are stimulated to produce TNF-α and IL-1β, which serves to amplify tissue injury.

In the uninfected patient, spontaneous healing occurs in about 3–4 wk after the administration of chemotherapy, two or more weeks after the cessation of radiation.

3. OBJECTIVES OF ANIMAL MODEL DESIGN FOR MUCOSITIS

Like many other diseases, mucositis represents a clinical continuum in its course and severity. In the case of chemotherapy-induced disease, mucositis is dependent on the drug used, its dose, and the schedule of administration. The age of the patient influences risk—young patients develop the condition at higher frequency than older patients, yet heal more quickly *(9)*. The extent of neutropenia influences the duration of mucositis, as well as the risk of sepsis. Typically, chemotherapy-induced mucositis begins with erythematous changes of the oral mucosa within 1 wk after drug administration. Lesions progress to ulceration, and usually peak 10–12 d after the start of treatment. These heal spontaneously, if there is no infection, by d 21. Clinically, mucositis peaks 2–3 d prior to the point at which maximum myelosuppression (nadir) is observed. The level of clinical mucositis is adversely affected by local irritation from minor biting trauma.

Mucositis induced by radiation is a function of dose and schedule *(10)*. Typically, patients receive a total dose in fractionated amounts spread over a 6–8-wk period. If patients do not receive concomitant chemotherapy, neutropenia is not an issue. Although the clinical presentation of radiation-induced mucositis does not differ appreciably from that induced by chemotherapy, the course of the condition is markedly prolonged in comparison. The lesions that develop are not based on time, but on the total dose of radiation to the tissue. Typically, early lesions are noted at about 20 Gy, and increase progressively in severity to become diffuse confluent lesions at 30–50 Gy. Once radiation is completed, the time to healing of the mucosa may vary, but is usually complete in about 3 wk.

The challenge in developing an animal model for mucositis has been based on three goals: (1) to provide clinically robust mucosal changes that mimic the course seen in humans, (2) to create a model that is sensitive to changes in bone-marrow status, and (3) to provide a model in which the local oral environment plays a role in the development, course, and resolution of the condition. Because we anticipated that the model would be used for translational and mechanistic studies, we wanted one in which outcomes could be observed clinically, and one in which the changes in the oral cavity corresponded to other measurable clinical end points.

Although a number of murine models have been used to study radiation-induced mucosal changes, they have relied heavily on histologic outcomes, since the levels of clinical changes have been subtle (11).

After considering a number of animals, we elected to focus on the Syrian hamster for five primary reasons:

1. The hamster cheek pouch consists of a renewing squamous epithelium, which in many ways is similar to humans and which had been studied extensively for other conditions, especially chemically induced carcinogenesis. (*see* Chapter 8)
2. The cheek pouch provides a large mucosal surface area that is easily accessible for examination, and an anatomical site to which potential topical therapeutics can be easily applied.
3. The oral bacterial flora of the hamster is, in many ways, similar to the human in that gram-positive bacteria are the predominant species. Additionally, other investigators had described the potential of the hamster cheek pouch as a model for oral fungal infections (12), something that is common in the oncology patient population.
4. The hamster is sensitive to chemotherapeutic agents that elicit toxicity in humans, in particular both antimetabolites and alkylating agents. The hamsters' marrow response to these agents is similar to humans, and thus the relationship of neutropenia to mucositis can be easily studied.
5. The similarity in blood-cell size between the hamster and human permits automated, instrument-based analysis of peripheral blood, which reduces the technician time in dealing with the model.

4. CHEMOTHERAPY-INDUCED MUCOSITIS

4.1. Background

Despite the major clinical significance of chemotherapy-induced mucositis, successful animal models for the condition were lacking until fairly recently. Initial studies to develop an animal model focused on methotrexate as the chemotherapeutic agent of choice. The reason for this drug selection involves the fact that most of the investigators had a specific interest in head and neck cancer for which methotrexate was the drug of choice and was associated with high levels of mucositis.

Shklar found that SC administration of 0.1 mg of methotrexate 3 times per wk for 4 wk to hamsters produced gross mucosal erythema (13). He also observed histologic changes of oral mucosa characterized by collagen degeneration and epithelial atrophy. However, ulcerative lesions failed to develop.

In a study designed to determine the effects of folic-acid deficiency on the oral mucosa of marmosets, Dreizen et al. (14) used methotrexate to supplement folic acid-free diets. They observed that low doses of methotrexate given three time per week plus folic-acid-free diets interfered with epithelial maturation, impaired keratinization, and increased susceptibility to ulceration and secondary infection.

Duperon *(15)* failed to produce significant mucositis in rats with methotrexate, but noted a significant reduction in the mitotic index of epithelial cells.

Although we found that methotrexate produced severe intestinal injury in rats, it did not produce oral lesions that were consistent or easy to evaluate. After confirming the lack of methotrexate-induced stomatotoxicity in the hamster, we elected to use 5-fluorouracil (5-FU) as the primary agent in the model. This choice was based on the hamsters' demonstrated sensitivity to fluorinated pyrimidines and the frequency of mucositis in patients treated with the drug.

4.2. Hamster Cheek-Pouch Model Development

In our study, we attempted to maximize stomatotoxicity, yet maintain an acceptable level of morbidity and mortality. Among the variables, that affected the frequency and severity of mucositis and systemic toxicities were 5-FU dose, frequency and interval between dosing, and animal age.

A number of preliminary studies were performed to identify the optimal dose and schedule for 5-FU administration. A single large bolus dose of the drug caused mortality without mucositis. Multiple dosing at intervals of 5 d with moderate dosages was stomatotoxic, with little mortality. Three 60 mg/kg, intraperitoneal (IP) doses of 5-FU administered on d 0, 5, and 10 were initially used. Since the cheek-pouch mucosa is anatomically protected from functional trauma, superficial irritation of the mucosa was performed using an 18-gauge needle on d 1 and 2. The combination of three doses of 5-FU and superficial irritation consistently produced ulcerative mucositis without significant mortality. Slight but insignificant weight loss was noted subsequent to the second injection of 5-FU on d 5. Evaluation of peripheral white blood cell (WBC) counts showed marked myelosuppression on d 10 and a second dip in white blood count on d 14. No changes in animal activity level were observed *(16)*.

Early mucositis was noted by d 7, after the initial injection of 5-FU. Control animals that had received only superficial mucosal irritation were completely healed within 24–48 h after injury. Marked progressive mucositis characterized by large areas of epithelial disruption and surface necrosis was present in 71% of animals by d 9, and 100% of animals had robust lesions by d 14.

Additional studies using this model demonstrated that the anecdotal data and clinical observations—suggesting a relationship between the oral changes noted in response to chemotherapy and the degree of myelosuppression—were not causal. Using this above scheme to induce mucositis, evaluation of femoral bone-marrow cellularity on d 8, 12, 16, and 20 demonstrated a temporal relationship between the development of ulcerative mucositis and the degree of myelosuppression. As in patients, mucosal breakdown preceded the maximum myelosuppression and healing of the oral mucosa occurred before the recovery of the marrow *(17,18)*.

4.3. Histologic Changes

Parakeratosis of the epithelium and areas of hydropic degeneration characterized early histologic changes (between d 2 and 5 after the first injection of 5-FU). Capillaries in the underlying connective tissue were dilated and engorged. An infiltrate consisting of lymphocytes and macrophages, often in a perivascular distribution, was present. Localized infiltrations of neutrophils were also present.

Parakeratosis and liquefaction necrosis (hydropic degeneration) of the stratum germinativum were seen 2 wk after the first 5-FU injection. Changes were also prominent in the connective tissue, in which collagen degeneration coupled with an cellularly diverse inflammatory infiltrate was present.

The most dramatic late change was epithelial destruction characterized by frank ulceration. Large ulcerated lesions with extensive fibrin deposition, underlying fibroblastic activity, extensive connective destruction and necrotic epithelium, and colonies of microorganisms were seen.

4.4. The Hamster Cheek-Pouch Model for 5-FU-Induced Mucositis

Although the regimen of three moderate doses of 5-FU administered 5 d apart consistently produced mucositis, its lack of significant systemic morbidity and mortality was a mixed blessing—it did not permit complete assessment of therapeutic interventions. Because we had noted that mucositis was present following fewer injections of chemotherapy, the model was modified to include two injections of 5-FU on d 0 and 2, followed by superficial irritation of the mucosa on day 4 *(19)*. Varying doses of 5-FU have been used in the model, but a first dose of 60 mg/kg to 75 mg/kg followed by a second dose of 60 mg/kg consistently produces robust mucositis. *Superficial* irritation is performed on d 4 by gently scoring the cheek pouch with a criss-cross (tic-tac-toe) pattern with care to avoid perforating the mucosa. With this regimen, ulcerative mucositis is achieved in virtually 100% of animals with peak lesions occurring on d 8 to 11, which corresponds well to results in humans.

Because of the increased intensity of 5-FU, changes in weight and survival are more pronounced than when more conservative dosing is used. Animals may lose 15–20% of starting body wt, with peak weight loss at approx d 9. Survival is also affected. Approximately 30% of animals succumb to this regimen.

Although mucositis can be achieved without the use of superficial irritation, the doses of chemotherapy that are required result in unacceptable mortality.

The objective assessment of mucositis is achieved through the use of a technique of blinded grading of clinical photographs. Following the induction of anesthesia, the cheek-pouch mucosa is everted and photographed using a standardized technique. This procedure is typically performed on alternate days of an experiment. At the conclusion of a study, the film is developed, and the resulting photographs are randomly numbered and then graded against a standardized scale by two or three blinded observers. The grading scale that is used is a six-point scale (Fig. 1):

0-Pouch completely healthy. No erythema or vasodilation.

1-Erythema and vasodilation, but mucosa intact.

2-Severe erythema with superficial mucosal erosion

3-Formation of mucosal ulceration with a cumulative size of about 25% of the pouch's surface area.

4-Ulceration with a cumulative size of about 50% of the pouch's surface area.

5-Contiguous ulceration involving almost the entire surface area of the pouch mucosa.

4.5. The Hamster Cheek-Pouch Model for Other Forms of Chemotherapy

The cheek-pouch model has been adapted for other antineoplastic drugs including cytarabine and cyclophosphamide (Fig. 2). As with 5-FU, dose and schedule are critical to achieving a balance between the successful induction of mucositis and acceptable levels of morbidity and mortality.

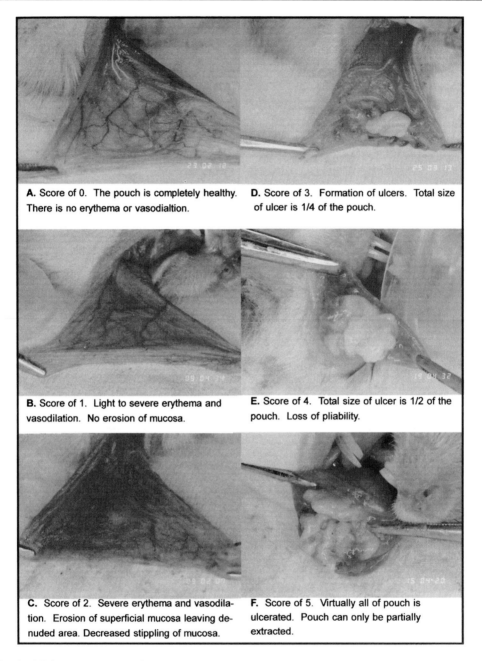

A. Score of 0. The pouch is completely healthy. There is no erythema or vasodialtion.

D. Score of 3. Formation of ulcers. Total size of ulcer is 1/4 of the pouch.

B. Score of 1. Light to severe erythema and vasodilation. No erosion of mucosa.

E. Score of 4. Total size of ulcer is 1/2 of the pouch. Loss of pliability.

C. Score of 2. Severe erythema and vasodilation. Erosion of superficial mucosa leaving denuded area. Decreased stippling of mucosa.

F. Score of 5. Virtually all of pouch is ulcerated. Pouch can only be partially extracted.

Fig. 1. Clinical Appearance of mucositis by severity. Lesions are graded on a six-point scale (0 to 5), in which 0 is normal and 5 is severe confluent mucositis. As in humans, ulcerative lesions are typically covered by a fibrinous pseudomembrane.

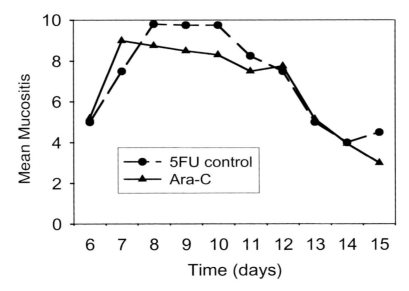

Fig. 2. The course of mucositis in hamsters treated with either 5-FU or cytosine arabinoside. Animals were injected with two doses of each drug. Two days later, with the hamsters anesthetized, the left buccal pouch was everted and superficially irritated with an 18-gauge needle to replicate functional trauma that occurs in humans. Beginning on d 6 (d 0 = the first day of chemotherapy), the animals were anesthetized and the left buccal pouch was exposed and scored using a 10-point scale, in which 10 is the most severe form of mucositis. A score of 10 corresponds to a 5 on the current scale described in the text. As seen in humans, peak mucositis occurred 7–10 d following the first drug exposure. The lesions resolve spontaneously, and are generally gone by 21 d.

4.6. The Hamster Cheek-Pouch Model for Radiation-Induced Mucositis

4.6.1. BACKGROUND

A number of studies focusing on the epithelial biology of oral radiation injury have been performed using murine lip or tongue models. Xu and his colleagues described the effects of single and fractionated radiation schedules on the lip mucosa of mice. They found that acute reactions of the lip mucosa, that is focal desquamation, could be reliably scored *(11)*. The mouse-tongue model described by Dorr et al. has been used to investigate the epithelial biology of radiation injury produced by acute, fractionated, and accelerated radiation regimens *(20)*. These models have been useful in defining responses to various radiation regimens, including cell repopulation studies, yet the limited anatomic area available for evaluation and the subtlety of clinical changes have limited their effectiveness in interventional studies. Given the efficacy of the hamster cheek-pouch model for translational studies of interventions for chemotherapy-induced mucositis, a model for radiation-induced disease was developed.

4.6.2. DEVELOPMENT OF A RADIATION MODEL FOR MUCOSITIS

In preliminary studies, we examined the morphology and histologic changes associated with large single-radiation fractions, and demonstrated that the criteria used to quantify the extent of mucositis following chemotherapy were valid and could be used to fully characterize the response under various radiation conditions. Using murine models as a basis, the initial model that we developed evaluated the effect of radiation exposure to the face and cheek of the Golden Syrian hamster and determined the practicality of using the hamster and identified the optimal conditions for radiation delivery. Animals were placed in a plastic stint (a modified 50-cc polyethylene centrifuge tube with the conical end removed) and shielded with lead so that only the facial region was exposed. Doses of 25 Gy or 30 Gy resulted in erythema, inflammation, and swelling of the mucosa, but within 1 wk following radiation, marked peri-oral inflammatory changes were seen, and the animals became moribund and demonstrated severe (>20%) weight loss. We concluded that this method was unsatisfactory. Consequently, we developed a technique in which only the cheek-pouch mucosa was exposed to radiation. A lead shield was fabricated with a slit at its base in the approximate length of the cheek-pouch base. Following anesthesia, the shield was positioned so that only the cheek-pouch mucosa protruded, and therefore was the only tissue exposed to radiation. The technique proved to be effective in producing consistent pseudomembranous ulcerative mucositis.

4.6.3. THE HAMSTER MODEL FOR ACUTE RADIATION-INDUCED MUCOSITIS

Golden Syrian hamsters, aged 5–6 wk and weighing between 80 g and 100 g, were obtained from Harlan Sprague Dawley or Charles River Laboratories. Animals were housed in small groups, fed standard hamster chow, and watered *ad libitum*.

Radiation was produced using an orthovoltage unit operating at 150 kVp at 14 mA, with 0.35 mm of Cu filtration and administered at a focal distance of 50 cm at a rate of 1.22 gy/min. Prior to irradiation, animals were anesthetized with pentobarbital (80–100 mg/kg given intraperitoneally). To preserve function, only one cheek pouch was radiated. The cheek-pouch mucosa was carefully exposed, and then pinned at the corners to a corkboard at the outer margin with two 27-gauge needles. Customized lead shields were then placed over the animal so that only the mucosa was exposed.

To establish a dosing curve, three doses of radiation (25 Gy, 30 Gy, and 35 Gy) were given at a rate of 121.5 gy/min. Direct irradiation of the buccal mucosa resulted in acute erythematous changes and mild mucositis from d 1 (d 0 = day of radiation) to d 10 in all groups. On d 11–32, dose-dependent changes were noted. Mucositis was most severe in all groups between d 13 and 18. Injury evaluation using the standardized mucositis six-point scale demonstrated mean scores between d 13 and 18 that were greater than four for the two higher-dosed groups, whereas the mean for animals irradiated with 25 Gy was 2.2. Mucositis induced by radiation persisted longer than that noted in the hamster chemotherapy model, and lasted beyond 2 wk. Radiation with lower doses failed to produce marked clinical changes, suggesting a dosing threshold of >20 Gy for spontaneous radiation-induced mucositis. Changes in weight varied and did not follow a typical dose-response. For the most part, animals continue to gain weight despite changes in their oral mucosa. Unlike chemotherapy models, mortality in this model is limited to that associated with anesthesia.

Mucositis produced by acute radiation follows a consistent course of about 35 d. Early mucosal changes, characterized by slight erythema and edema, are noted between d 8 and 10 (d 0 = d of radiation). A linear increase in mucositis severity

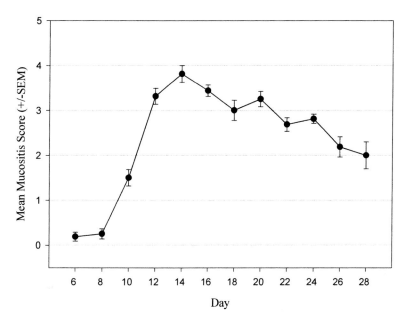

Fig. 3. The course of mucositis produced by a single mucosal exposure to 35 Gy of radiation. Following the induction of general anesthesia, the left buccal pouch was everted, and the mucosa was exposed. The remainder of the hamster's body was covered by a lead shield. The mucosa was then irradiated. Erythematous changes were first noted by d 10 (d 0 = day of radiation). As in this case, peak mucositis is typically noted on d 14–16. Lesions subsequently resolve. The error bars demonstrate the tightness of scores in groups of eight animals.

peaks between d 14 and 16. At an exposure dose of 35 Gy, typical peak mucositis scores range between 3 and 4. Higher levels of mucositis can be achieved by increasing the exposure dose. Ulcerative mucositis typically lasts for 1 wk, and then slowly resolves over the duration of a study (Fig. 3). Typically, mucositis does not influence survival, but weight gain may be blunted during the development and presence of ulcerative lesions.

4.6.4. THE HAMSTER MODEL FOR FRACTIONATED RADIATION-INDUCED MUCOSITIS

Radiation treatment in humans for cancers of the head and neck is typically given in small, daily fractionated doses over a period of weeks. A representative regimen may be 2 Gy/fraction administered five times per wk for 6–8 wk. Such a regimen results in a predictable pattern of mucositis that begins when the cumulative radiation dose reaches 20 Gy. At that level, the mucosa demonstrates inflammatory changes characterized by erythema and edema. Symptomatically, patients complain of discomfort similar to that experienced as a consequence of a mucosal burn caused by hot food such as pizza. As the cumulative dose increases, superficial erosion of the epithelium occurs, which progresses to full-thickness ulceration. A layer of necrotic tissue resulting in the formation of a pseudomembrane often covers ulcers. The pain that accompanies such lesions is profound. Patients are often unable to tolerate any solid food, and require aggressive pain management. Mucositis is of such severity in some patients that a temporary discontinuation of treatment is necessary.

Although the acute radiation model described here provides an excellent method to assess acute mucosal radiation injury, its clinical applicability can be questioned. Consequently, we modified the acute radiation model. Animals were prepared as previously described, and irradiated on four consecutive days, with daily doses ranging from 5 Gy to 15 Gy per animal. Consequently, total exposure ranged from 20 Gy to 60 Gy per animal.

The daily observation of animals between ds 7 and 35 (d 0 = the first day of radiation) is typically done for clinical evaluation. Photographs of the exposed cheek pouch provide documentation of studies, as well as a mechanism for blinded scoring at the conclusion of an experiment.

Mucositis severity is dose-dependent. Four daily doses of 5 Gy fail to produce any clinical changes in exposed mucosa, whereas nonulcerative mucositis characterized by erythema and edema is seen by d 9 in hamsters exposed to 7.5 Gy per day. Exposure to doses of 10 Gy per day results in a rapid increase in mucosal injury from d 9 to a peak at d 15. By d 15, consistent ulceration of less than 60% of the cheek-pouch mucosa is observed. Following peak injury on d 15, healing occurs slowly, with lesions lasting beyond 4 wk. Animals that receive a cumulative dose of 60 Gy (15 Gy per day) develop severe ulcerative mucositis more rapidly. Lesions are seen as early as d 7, and peak by d 15. Ulcerative lesions involving up to two-thirds of the cheek-pouch surface are present 5 wk after the initial radiation exposure. For the peak mucositis period (d 13–23) mean mucositis scores for animals receiving 10 Gy/d reflect severe nonulcerative mucositis. In contrast, higher radiation doses (15 Gy/d) result in marked ulcerative lesions. In general, the severity of mucositis in the high-dose group is statistically more pronounced than that noted in animals treated more conservatively. Because the duration of clinically significant mucositis is an important outcome for studies assessing potential interventional therapy, the number of animal days of ulcerative mucositis is often an important analysis. Animals radiated with 15 Gy/d have significantly more days of ulcerative mucositis than animals receiving lower doses (Fig. 4). Unlike the acute model described above, dose-dependent weight loss is seen and was dose-dependent. Hamsters that receive the two lower doses of radiation demonstrate equivalent linear weight gain from d 7 to d 35. In contrast, animals radiated with 10 Gy/d or 15 Gy/d lose weight between ds 11 and 15. Peak weight loss occurs on d 15, the same day as maximum mucositis. Subsequent to d 15, both high-dose groups demonstrate a linear weight gain of 1–2% per day until d 35, which is the same as is noted for low-dose animals. Survival is not a significant outcome in this model. No differences are observed between groups. Deaths, when they occur, are almost always attributable to anesthesia.

5. HISTOLOGIC OUTCOMES

Sequential histologic sampling from animals irradiated with 15 Gy/d provides a good representation of the longitudinal tissue changes associated with radiation-induced mucosal injury. Normal mucosal tissue from the cheek pouch is devoid of inflammatory elements. There are no inherent changes in the connective tissue or epithelium. In contrast, by d 4, focal areas of hyperkeratosis can be seen in irradiated tissue. Eight days after radiation, a slight inflammatory infiltrate is noted in the submucosa, as well as some edema and incipient breaks in the epithelium. Two days later, on d 10, localized areas of epithelial necrosis were accompanied by lifting of the epithelium from the underlying connective tissue. Epithelial atrophy and capillary engorge-

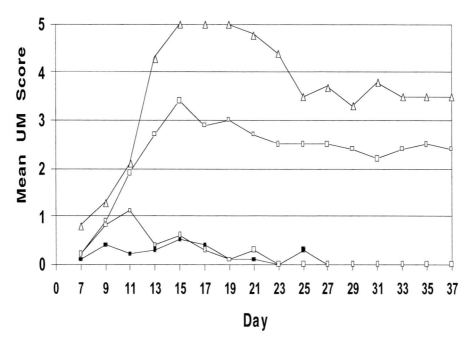

Fig. 4. Course of mucositis following fractionated radiation course. Following anesthesia, hamsters were irradiated with 5 Gy, 7.5 Gy, 10 Gy, or 15 Gy given to the left buccal pouch on four consecutive days. Beginning on d 7 and continuing until the end of the experiment, the animals were anesthetized, and the left buccal pouch was exposed and photographed. At the conclusion of the study, the film was developed, and the resulting photographs randomly numbered and then scored in blinded fashion by two observers. The results demonstrate a dose-response in both mucositis severity and duration. Mucositis produced by fractionated dosing is more dramatic in both severity and duration compared to the acute model.

ment are also present at this time. A moderately robust round-cell infiltrate with numerous mast cells is present. By d 12, more dramatic changes are seen. Pan-tissue necrosis involving connective tissue and epithelium can be seen. Other epithelial sites have hyperkeratosis and connective-tissue degeneration is present. Histiocytes and neutrophils characterize the inflammatory infiltrate. By d 15, when peak clinical mucositis is seen, severe inflammatory changes are noted. An intense neutrophil-rich infiltrate is present within the connective tissue. Rampant tissue destruction with necrosis and frank epithelial ulceration dominates. By d 28, histologic evidence of ulcer resolution can be seen, accompanied by healing of the connective tissue, although a chronic inflammatory infiltrate persists.

CONCLUSION

Mucositis is an increasingly important dose-limiting toxicity of cancer drug and radiation therapy. Because of its clinical significance—which impacts on patients' ability to tolerate treatment, and creates situations that result in less than optimal cancer therapy—there has been a great deal of interest in developing an effective intervention for the condition. Animal models have played an important role in leading to an understanding of the biologic complexities underlying the condition and in translational studies that have resulted in a number of potential therapies being in clinical trials. While murine models have been effective in helping to define the radiation biology of oral and lip mucosa, the hamster model has uniquely replicated the human condition.

The major limitations of the hamster are associated with its rather infrequent use in studying biologic end points. In particular, the absence of commercially available antibodies and other biologic reagents have limited the utility of the hamster for mechanistic studies to some degree. Fortunately, many homologies between mouse, hamster, and human have permitted some mechanistic studies to be performed in the hamster.

Although these hamster models offer the advantage of being reasonably predictable of the human experience, this strength is also their weakness, because they require a reasonably long period to run. As a result, for someone interested in quickly screening a large number of potential therapeutic compounds, the models are slow and somewhat expensive. Nevertheless, the hamster's large mucosal surface and robust mucosal response to antineoplastic drugs and radiation are so similar to the condition in humans that they remain a valuable tool for studying mucosal injury and repair and essential in the process of drug development for this condition.

ACKNOWLEDGMENTS

I am indebted to my colleagues, staff, and students who have contributed their ideas, technical skills, and hard work to the development of the models discussed: Jacqueline Mitus, Paul Busse, John Haley, Michael Ribera, Joseph Costa, Gerard Moses, Daphne Florine, James Jenson, Gerald Shklar, Andrew VanVugt, Lucas Edwards, Carolyn Lucey, Amy Muska, James O'Brien, Loryn Linquist, Susan Evitts, Elizabeth Dotoli, James McDonald, and Amy Koplowsky.

REFERENCES

1. Epstein JB, Schubert MM. Oral mucositis in myelosuppressive cancer therapy. *Oral Surg, Oral Med, Oral Pathol, Oral Radiol, Endod* 1999; 88:273–276.
2. Shenep JL. Viridans-group streptococcal infections in immunocompromised hosts. *Int J Antimicrob Agents* 2000; 14:129–135.
3. Horowitz M, Oster G, Fuchs H, Edelsberg J, McGarry L, Sonis S. Association between oral mucositis as measured by the Oral Mucositis Assessment Scale (OMAS) and clinical and economic outcomes of blood and marrow transplants. Presentation at the American Society of Hematology, December, 1999.
4. Ruescher TJ, Sodeifi A, Scrivani SJ, Kaban LB, Sonis ST. The impact of mucositis on alpha-hemolytic streptococcal infections in patients undergoing autologous bone marrow transplantation for hematologic malignancies. *Support Care Cancer* 1998; 82:2275–2281.
5. Bellm LA, Epstein JB, Rose-Ped A, Martin P, Fuchs HJ. Patient reports of complications of bone marrow transplantation. *Support Care Cancer* 2000; 8:33–39.
6. Sonis ST. Mucositis as a biological process: a new hypothesis for the development of chemotherapy-induced stomatotoxicity. *Oral Oncol* 1998; 34:39–43.
7. Sonis ST, Peterson RL, Edwards LJ, Lucey CA, Wang L, Mason L, et al. Defining mechanisms of action of Interleukin-11 on the progression of radiation-induced oral mucositis in hamsters. *Oral Oncol* 2000; 36:373–381.
8. Lin X, Fuks Z, Kolesnick R. Ceramide mediates radiation-induced death of endothelium. *Crit Care Med* 2000; 28:N87–N93.
9. Sonis ST, Sonis AL, Lieberman A. Oral complications in patients receiving treatment for malignancies other than of the head and neck. *J Am Dent Assoc* 1978; 97:468–472.
10. Trotti A. Toxicity in head and neck cancer: a review of trends and issues. *Int J Radiat Oncol Biol Phys* 2000; 47:1–12.

11. Xu FX, van der Schueren E, Ang KK. Acute reactions of the lip of mice to fractionated irradiations. *Radiother Oncol* 1984; 1:369–374.
12. McMillan CD, Lowell VM. Experimental candidiasis in the hamster cheek pouch. *Arch Oral Biol* 1985; 30:249–255.
13. Shklar G. The effect of 11-amino-N10-methyl-pterylglutamic acid on oral mucosa of experimental animals. *J Oral Ther* 1968; 4:374–377.
14. Dreizen S, Levy BM, Bernick S. Studies on the biology of the periodontium of marmosets VIII. The effect of folic acid deficiency on the marmoset oral mucosa. *J Dent Res* 1970; 49:616–620.
15. Duperon D. The effect of topical leukovorin on the gingiva of Long Evans rats undergoing methotrexate therapy. *J Oral Med* 1978; 33:12–16.
16. Sonis ST, Tracey C, Shklar G, Jenson J, Florine D. An animal model for mucositis induced by cancer chemotherapy. *Oral Surg, Oral Med, Oral Pathol* 1990; 69:437–443.
17. Sonis S, Koplowsky A, Mitus J, Rosenthal D, Brand M. Relationship of chemotherapy-induced mucositis and myelosuppression in hamsters. *Eur J Cancer B Oral Oncol* 1992; 28B:43.
18. Lockhart PB, Sonis ST. Relationship of oral complications to peripheral blood leukocyte and platelet counts in patients receiving cancer chemotherapy. *Oral Surg, Oral Med, Oral Pathol* 1979; 48:21–28.
19. Sonis ST, Van Vugt AG, McDonald J, Dotoli E, Schwertschlag V, Szklut P, et al. Mitigating effects of Interleukin-11 on consecutive courses of 5-fluorouracil-induced ulcerative mucositis in hamsters. *Cytokine* 1997; 9:605–612.
20. Dorr W, Emmendorf H, Weber-Frisch M. Tissue kinetics in mouse tongue mucosa during daily fractionated radiotherapy. *Cell Prolif* 1996; 495–504.

19 The Intestine as a Model for Studying Stem-Cell Behavior

Catherine Booth, PhD
and Christopher S. Potten, PhD, DSc

CONTENTS

1. NORMAL ADULT INTESTINAL EPITHELIAL ORGANIZATION

The intestine is lined by a simple columnar epithelium that folds into a number of cavities—the crypts of Lieberkühn—embedded in the connective tissue. In the small intestine, there are also finger-like protrusions known as villi, which are covered in this epithelium. The villi are approximately ten times larger than the crypts, but much less common (4–7× fewer, depending upon the intestinal region) *(1)*. The functional cells are located on the villus (or toward the top of the crypts of the large intestine), and are continuously sloughed off into the lumen. These cells are replaced by massive cell production within the bottom two-thirds of the crypt, where cells in the mouse are dividing approx twice daily. This crypt region is therefore frequently referred to as the proliferative zone.

In a healthy adult, the rate of cell production equates precisely to the rate of cell loss. Any change in this balance can result in a breach of mucosal integrity or creation of a hyperplastic epithelium, which may ultimately generate a tumor. Surprisingly, despite the enormous potential for error with such a high replication rate and large cell numbers, cancers of the small intestine are very rare.

The physical separation of the proliferative and functional regions creates a continuous upward linear migration of cells to the lumenal surface (except small-intestinal Paneth cells that migrate down to the crypt base). The migrational position can therefore be a useful

From: *Tumor Models in Cancer Research*
Edited by: B. A. Teicher © Humana Press Inc., Totowa, NJ

indicator of cellular age, with the youngest cells (and therefore the stem cells) at the origin of the migration—i.e., toward the crypt base. This linear map can also be used to monitor the various responses of cells of varying ages to different stimuli. Such a response is generally a measure of DNA synthesis, mitosis, or apoptosis, but can be the occurrence of cell types such as differentiation, or other labeled markers such as immunolabeled cells.

2. MEASURING PROLIFERATION IN THE NORMAL INTESTINE

Although individual crypts can be isolated using either chelating agents or enzymes and can ultimately yield single cells, fluorescence activated cell sorting (FACS) is not a very informative index of the proliferative or apoptotic status of the crypt. Such techniques lose any positional information (and therefore information regarding stem-cell vs daughter-cell responses), and are also limited by the presence of contaminating unrelated cell types. Positional information is crucial, because a small change in the cell-cycle parameters of only the stem cells at the origin of proliferative can, because of the exponential number of generations created, ultimately have a massive effect. Conversely, a similar change in a later generation will have little overall impact on the crypt.

Although it may be a much more laborious technique, examination of histological sections is a far more informative measurement of crypt-cell responses. Levels of mitosis can be measured in pathological specimens from human patients or from animal tissues. Such analysis requires a number of good transverse sections through the gut, a process that can be facilitated by "bundling" small pieces of gut together to provide—for example—10 cross sections of mouse ileum (Fig. 1).

Using a good longitudinal section through the entire length of the crypt (facilitated by good transverse sectioning of the gut) and designating the cell at the crypt base as position one, one can move up through the cell positions along one side of the crypt, counting whether the cell is mitotic. By counting about 50 half crypt sections per sample, the frequency of each event along the crypt axis, at each cell position can be plotted to provide a frequency distribution (Fig. 2).

Although measuring mitosis is a relatively simple indicator, it is not a particularly sensitive marker when used alone. The length of the mitotic phase of the cell cycle is relatively short (only about 30 min in the mouse ileum), and thus the probability of observing a mitotic cell is fairly low. A frequency distribution therefore analyzes very low numbers, and consequently provides poor material for statistical analysis.

The length of the S phase of the cell cycle is about 10× longer, and is therefore a more statistically valid marker of proliferation. However, endogenous markers of S phase in the intestine also have limitations. Proliferating-cell nuclear antigen (PCNA) and Ki67 are the two most frequently immunohistochemically labeled endogenous cell-cycle-related proteins. However, there are problems, associated with both proteins (2). The main problem is that neither simply measures the number of cells undergoing DNA synthesis. Because they are endogenous proteins, they are gradually accumulated in the cell during G1 and are not immediately degraded at the onset of G2—they can persist for a long period afterwards. Thus, in rapidly proliferating cells, such as in the crypt, the cells may be positive for most of the cycle time. PCNA is slightly worse than Ki67 in this regard, and has the added problem of extreme sensitivity to tissue fixation and processing (such endogenous proteins are also often expressed at low levels in cells undergoing DNA-repair synthesis). These markers may be a more useful marker of the crypt epithelial growth fraction rather than S phase. An additional problem in measuring the expres-

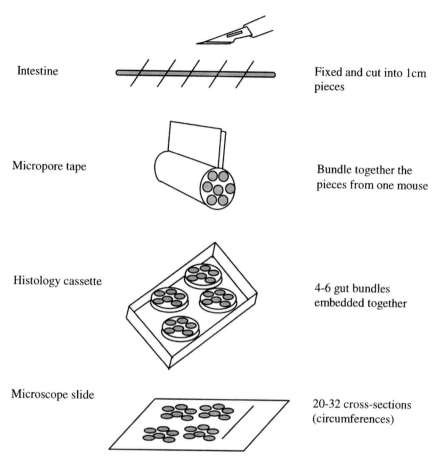

Intestine — Fixed and cut into 1cm pieces

Micropore tape — Bundle together the pieces from one mouse

Histology cassette — 4-6 gut bundles embedded together

Microscope slide — 20-32 cross-sections (circumferences)

Fig. 1. Cartoon of the "gut bundling" technique. Segments of intestine from the region of interest can be cut into small lengths (~1cm) and tightly held together by 3M Micropore tape as shown. Next, 4–6 bundles—i.e., samples from 4–6 mice—can be embedded together so that they are all in the same orientation, and good transverse sections of each segment can be observed in cut sections. Adapted from (ref. *36*).

sion patterns of such proteins is the need to be sure that the factor/drug under investigation does not directly modulate the turnover of the marker protein.

The most accurate indices of DNA synthesis measure the incorporation of an exogenous marker into the newly synthesized DNA strand during a short-term injected pulse. Clearly, this is not routinely possible in vivo in human tissue, and therefore the next best option—Ki67 expression—is often used. In other tissues short-term ex vivo incubation with the marker in physiological media is possible, but this is less ideal for intestinal tissue because of the rapid cell-cycle arrest and the onset of apoptosis and autolysis. Thus, the detection of bromodeoxyuridine or tritiated thymidine incorporation, via immunohistochemistry or autoradiography respectively, provide excellent cell positional information on the frequency of S-phase cells. Certain criteria must be used when scoring—only entire half crypts with a continuous lumen should be used (i.e., not crypts sectioned at an angle), and a positive cell must have a given threshold to be positive (3 autoradiographic silver grains or a given label intensity). Differences

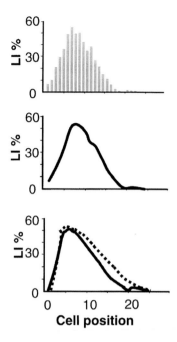

Fig. 2. Counting the frequency of a particular event along the full length of a number of half-crypt sections can generate a frequency distribution at each cell position. The results from individual animals within an experimental group can be pooled, and the distribution smoothed over a few (usually three) cell positions to generate a distribution curve—in this case a labeling index (LI) distribution. Comparisons of such curves after various treatments can reveal effects (e.g., changes in the number of labeled S-phase cells or apoptotic cells) at each cell position, which in turn can be related to the cellular hierarchy. In the lower diagram, the dotted line illustrates an increased labeling index between cell positions 10–20, equivalent to an effect on the transit amplifying cells.

between treatment samples can be easily detected, and small changes in the percentage of labeled cells (the labeling index or LI) at each crypt-cell position analyzed. A comparison of typical crypt-labeling profiles obtained with tritiated thymidine and Ki67, and the effect of a growth factor is shown in Fig. 3. These techniques, alone or in combination, can provide a huge amount of data on the proliferative characteristics of the crypt—e.g., the effects at specific cell positions can be analyzed (such as cell positions 4–7 for stem cells).

Application of a single pulse of tritiated thymidine provides a snapshot of the number of cells in S phase at that time (a single injection can be regarded as a pulse because the label is cleared within approx 20 min in a mouse). The cells can be heavily labeled with autoradiographic silver grains. However, by taking tissue at several subsequent time-points, the migration velocity of these labeled cells can be tracked and the lifetime of a cell estimated (a small intestinal-cell lifetime being about 5 d in total, or 2–3 d after its last cell division in the crypt). The origin of this migration can be extrapolated and assumed to be the site of the stem cells—cell position 4 in the small intestine, or cell position 1 in the large intestine (3).

The autoradiographic grain dilution as the cells continue to divide and migrate also provides information on the proliferative potential of cells within the crypt. For exam-

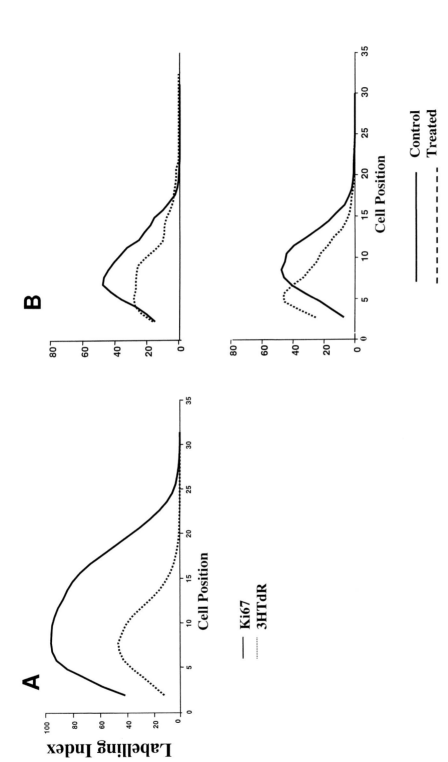

Fig. 3. The use of proliferation markers in the crypt. A single pulse of tritiated thymidine (dotted line, **A**), labels the cells in the S phase of the cell cycle, whereas Ki67 is expressed in a much larger population of cells, as denoted by the much larger area under the curve (solid line, **A**), an area approaching the size of the epithelial growth fraction. Ki67 is therefore a much less sensitive indicator of changes in the cell cycle. Using tritiated thymidine, any factor inducing inhibition of the cell cycle in the transit amplifying cells (dotted line, **B**, top panel) can be identified. Similarly, factors inducing stimulation in the stem-cell region, but inhibition in later generations can also be detected (**B**, bottom panel). Any such differences must be statistically verified, but this technique is a very powerful analytical tool.

ple, cells that are labeled in the upper region of the crypt only undergo one further mitotic division after the incorporating label during S phase, and the label is therefore only diluted by one-half. These cells then complete their differentiation program. They are cells with a very limited division potential, and retain this level of label as they move up the villus. Cells a little further down the crypt appear to dilute their thymidine-labeled DNA twice as they migrate; they undergo two rounds of division. Similarly, cells further down the crypt dilute their label through three rounds of division. Although such label-dilution studies cannot practically be taken any further, this experiment illustrates that cells in the upper region of the crypt have a very limited and defined number of divisions and shows the sensitivity of the technique.

Since the position of the stem cells within the crypts and the position of their daughter cells is known, any changes in their proliferative characteristics can be detected by these methods. Thus, the effect of a drug, growth factor, hormone, dietary constituent, or even a gene mutation can be measured directly, and its effects on stem cells and daughter cells can be quantitated.

Used in combination with S-phase analysis, measurements of the percentage of mitotic cells at each crypt position (the mitotic index [MI]) can provide supporting evidence for observed changes in crypt-cell proliferation. For example, although small changes in LI will not be reflected in the MI, larger changes should. Furthermore, an agent inducing G2 arrest may cause no reduction in LI, but will be detected by measuring the MI, where the reduced number of mitotic cells should become apparent.

The two types of measurements can also be used together in a technique for estimating the lengths of the cell-cycle phases (and the total length of the cell cycle) along the crypt axis—the percent labeled mitosis (PLM). In this procedure, a pulse of S-phase label, usually tritiated thymidine, is again applied to the tissue or animal. However, rather than counting labeled nuclei, only labeled *mitoses* are counted. Thus, with the passage of time the labeled S-phase cells will move into G2 and then into M, where their gradual appearance and eventual disappearance (as the cells leave M and move into Go/G1) will be counted at each position along the crypt axis. The length of time that the mitoses are labeled equates to the length of the S phase of the cell cycle. Eventually, labeled mitoses will reappear as these labeled daughter cells re-enter M (the period of time between the two M phases being equivalent the length of the cell cycle). This procedure is illustrated in Fig. 4. Using such procedures, the cells at positions 4–7 in the mouse small-intestinal crypt have been shown to have a cell-cycle time of about 24 h (although estimates vary from 12–32 h), whereas the daughter cells in mid-crypt have a cell-cycle time that is only about 12 h. *(4,5)*. In both cases the length of the S phase is fairly constant at 6–7 h. Thus, cells at position 4–7 are slowly cycling (slower than their daughters), and are the origin of cell migration—two typical characteristics of stem cells, although these alone are insufficient to define them.

The PLM technique has also been used to characterize cell-cycle changes along the crypt axis following exposure to various cytotoxic agents, thereby identifying the target cells and effects *(6–9)*. However, because these are damaged, repairing crypts over interpretation of these results should be avoided.

Further cell-cycle characteristics can be determined by double-labeling experiments—using, for example, application of tritiated thymidine and then bromodeoxyuridine (or vice versa, although there are arguments for the bromodeoxyuridine being the second pulse) at a later interval. Long time intervals can be used to determine

A

EVENT	PLM
● Pulse (label S phase cells)	
Remove pulse	0
● Cells move into G2	0
● Cells move into M	Increasing
● All labelled cells in M	Maximal
● Cells move out of M, into G1	Decreasing
● Cells move through S	0
● Cells move back into M	Increasing

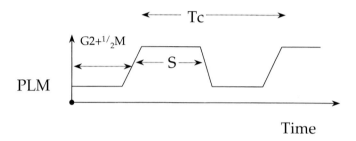

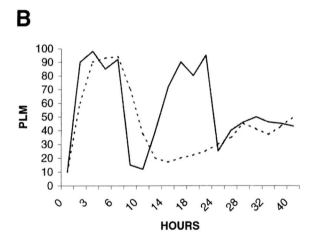

B

Fig. 4. Cell-cycle analysis by measuring the percent of labeled mitosis. A single pulse of tritiated thymidine initially labels S-phase cells. As these cells gradually move into the M phase of the cell cycle, the frequency of the labeled mitosis can be measured (at any cell position in the crypt). Cells will gradually exit M, and no labeled mitosis will be observed until these daughter cells re-enter M during the next cell cycle. This interval therefore corresponds to the cell-cycle time. The length of time one observes the maximum number of labeled mitosis corresponds to the length of the S phase. Typical PLM curves for the small intestine can be seen in the lower panel. These are generated by analyzing cells in the transit amplifying region (positions 12–16, solid line) or in the stem-cell region (positions 1–4, dotted line).

whether a cell is entering a second round of DNA synthesis, whereas shorter intervals can be used to monitor cell entry and exit from S. Repeated application of the same label can be equivalent to continuous labeling. For example, pulsing a mouse every 3–6 h for 48 h will tend to label almost all the cycling cells in the crypt, and again give an indication of the total proliferative region, similar to PCNA staining.

Such repeated injections of S-phase label can theoretically be used to label the slowly cycling stem-cell population. Over the next 4–6 d, all the labeled daughters will rapidly dilute their label as they migrate and be lost from the villus tip. Only labeled stem cells and the developing Paneth-cell lineage will remain labeled. Assuming that the stem cells are slowly cycling, it is likely that these cells will be exponentially losing label during this period (some Paneth cells will remain strongly labeled, but can easily be identified by the presence of their secretory granules and discounted from the analysis). However, by varying the autoradiography exposure times, it is possible to detect low levels of radioactivity and identify labeled non-Paneth cells (i.e., putative stem cells). This technique has been taken further to suggest that specific label-retaining stem cells exist.

Other techniques to measure cells in the S or M phase of the crypt cell cycle can involve cytotoxic agents, such as hydroxyurea or vincristine, respectively. Hydroxyurea kills S-phase cells somewhat specifically, and therefore can be a measure of the number of cells in or entering S over a given period. High specific-activity tritiated thymidine has also been used for this purpose. Vircristine and the related metaphase arrest agents cause the accumulation of cells in M (they cannot proceed through metaphase to cytokinesis). These agents can therefore be used to measure the crypt-cell production rate (CCPR), another frequently used index of crypt proliferative activity. In this procedure, the stathmokinetic approach, the number of mitotic figures can be counted in samples taken at various points after a dose of vincristine. The cell birth rate and the cell cycle can be estimated from the slope of the graph of mitotic figures vs time (at each cell position within the crypt, before and after a given treatment, if required).

3. CHARACTERIZING STEM CELLS

The observations that cell positions 4–7 (1–2 in the large intestine) are the origin of cell migration and are the location of the slower cycling cells suggests that this may be the position of the stem cells. However, further properties are needed to definitively prove this function. The first is that the cells at this position must be capable of regenerating the crypt. This has been tested by irradiating the crypt base with promethium 147—short-range β particle emitter *(10)*. Although the upper crypt cells survive, the crypt gradually dies away, since these cells cannot regenerate the crypt. Thus, the stem cells must reside in the few lower crypt positions penetrated by the β particles.

A stem cell must also be capable of regenerating all the differentiated phenotypes of the crypt epithelium (the enterocytes, Goblet cells, endocrine cells, Paneth cells, and M cells). To test this, a number of techniques have been employed. The simplest involves irradiation of the tissue to such a level that only one stem cell per crypt survives. The fact that the crypt regenerates and eventually contains all these cell types suggests that the original stem cell is pluripotent. Other techniques using chimeric mice with a labeled stem-cell output, and other naturally occurring human polymorphisms with a similar traceable output have also indicated that a stem cell produces all the differenti-ated phenotypes. Certain intestinal-cell lines also exhibit multipotency, although their relationship to true stem cells remains questionable.

For a stem-cell population to be maintained, each division must yield, on average, one daughter stem cell and one daughter cell committed to maturation and differentia-tion—an asymmetric division. Asymmetric division suggests that specific instructions are inherited by each daughter cell to direct its fate (direct maturation or remaining a stem cell). However, physical markers and definitive demonstration of such divisions have proven elusive and to date there are no reliable in vivo assays to monitor this phe-nomenon directly.

Alternatively, the asymmetry may be determined by the local environment. This leads to the elusive question: are stem cells intrinsically different, or merely instructed by the environment to behave differently?

3.1. Stem-Cell Marking

It is possible that an endogenous stem-cell marker has not been found because a stem cell has very restricted gene expression—a stem cell remains a stem cell because it cannot express certain genes (determined either intrinsically or by its environment). This may explain the number of failed subtractive hybridization attempts to identify such a marker. However, recent unpublished work in our laboratory investigating the expression of an RNA-binding protein, Msi-1, (involved in asymmetric divisions in neuroendocrine stem-cell development), has revealed that this protein is expressed in a few cells at the stem-cell region of steady-state crypts, but is expressed over the entire expanded clonogenic region following irradiation and during early crypt development. It is possible that Msi-1 is the first natural stem-cell marker to be identified.

Repeated application of an S-phase label has also been used in an attempt to identify stem cells as the label-retaining cells, based on their slower cell cycle or the fact that during asymmetric cell division the parental DNA strand may be retained within the daughter cell that is destined to remain a stem cell (11,12). Thus, any label in the tem-plate strand will be retained in this cell. Template strands could in principle be labeled when new stem cells are being made (during development or during tissue regenera-tion). Such experiments have, until recently, been largely unsuccessful in the small intestine, probably because of the extreme sensitivity of intestinal stem cells to dam-age—the act of label incorporation may itself compromise the stem cell. Indeed 25, µCi (0.925 MBq) is equivalent to 0.03 Gy, and can induce stem-cell apoptosis (5,13).

Recent work in our laboratory using crypts experiencing conditions specific for stem-cell expansion has suggested that this type of DNA-strand segregation may indeed occur in small-intestinal stem cells. During post-irradiation regeneration, stem cells divide symmetrically to repopulate the crypt—each stem cell divides to produces daughters that each retain stem-cell characteristics (stem-cell expansion). Application of tritiated thymidine during this time labels both of these stem cells, which at some point return to an asymmetric mode of division. Over time, all the maturing proliferat-ing cells labeled during the procedure will dilute their label and be shed into the lumen, and even any slowly cycling stem cells should have diluted labels below detection lim-its. However, persistent label-retaining cells can still be observed at positions 4–7, which are themselves cycling (as observed by double-labeling with bromodeoxyuri-dine). This suggests that selective DNA segregation has occurred in which the stem cells have preferentially retained the labeled template DNA during their subsequent divisions. Similar results are observed if young mice are labeled when undergoing stem-cell expansion (symmetrical division) in the growing intestine and then examined in later adult life. This may therefore represent one way in which stem cells can be marked, although the adult model is clearly perturbed in the initial stages, and therefore must be interpreted with some degree of caution.

3.2. Measuring Stem-Cell Number

Experiments using neonatal mice that are chimeras in which one strain expresses *Dolichos bifluros* lectin binding have indicated that at d 14 the crypts contain a single stem-cell (14,15), while at earlier times there may be more than one stem cell. At later times the single (d 14) stem cell expands the stem-cell population until the adult steady-state number is achieved. Similarly, experiments in which a crypt is exposed to irradiation such that only a single stem cell survives have indicated that the crypt can be completely regenerated from this single stem cell (16) (reviewed in refs. 17,18).

Neither of these experiments, however, reflect the normal adult situation. Indeed, the day-to-day maintenance of an adult crypt by a single stem cell is difficult to imagine, since it would tend to produce large oscillations in crypt size and asymmetry in crypt architecture. Cell-cycle and label-retaining experiments and mathematical modeling data suggest that the normal adult small-intestinal crypt contains 4–6 actual steady-state stem cells (equivalent to two–three symmetrical divisions during crypt development), (reviewed in ref. 19). Further experiments investigating the loss of expression of the *Dolichos bifluros* lectin binding site in F1 heterozygotes following mutations also suggest that crypts contain multiple stem cells. In this model mutation of the remaining lectin-binding allele in one stem cell produces a cell with daughters unable to bind *Dolichos bifluros*. A mixture of mutated and normal cells are produced in each crypt, which in turn produce a ribbon or stripe of unlabeled migrating cells up the villus. The width of this ribbon has been estimated to be equivalent to one-quarter of the output of a crypt. This model supports the proposal that a crypt contains four functioning stem cells (20). Over time, the crypts gradually become monophenotypic, but the long period needed to see such conversion (much longer than the cell-turnover time of the crypt) and the resultant change in the width of the villus ribbons, again confirm that there is more than one stem cell per crypt. The monophenotypic conversion indicates stem-cell competition within the crypt, so that the stem-cell population gradually changes as the daughters of one stem cell displace pre-existing stem cells. Again, it is important to consider that this behavior is the result of exposure to a mutagen, which may induce changes in stem cells (and indeed will kill some stem cells) and crypt behavior. However, these animals are a useful model for analyzing stem-cell number and the effects of various agents on stem-cell number and somatic-cell mutagenesis.

There are similar natural stem-cell markers that can be used as models for studying crypt and stem-cell kinetics. For example, there is a human polymorphism in which expression of G6PD can be seen in entire or only partial crypts, again with a distribution that indicates that adult crypts contain multiple stem cells (21–23). Unfortunately, in human situations the time-course of the crypt conversion cannot be followed. Ideally, this must be observed in real-time, possibly through the introduction of a reporter gene into a stem cell and the tracking of its behaviour either in vitro or in vivo using endoscopy. Such in vitro work may lead to information about the control of stem-cell division, with the number, clusters, lineages, radiosensitivity, and kinetics of labeled cells providing information on stem-cell generation and lifetime. To date, however, such studies are in their infancy and have not yet generated any reliable model systems.

These existing approaches indicate that a normal adult crypt contains 4–6 functioning or *actual* stem cells, sometimes referred to as lineage ancestor stem cells. Although these may be originally derived from a single stem cell in each crypt at approx d 14 postnatum, each crypt in the adult can be considered a distinct entity. Because a number of crypts feed their cellular output onto a single villus, these functional structures can be considered polyclonal.

3.3. Measuring Clonogenic Cell Number

Although a crypt normally contains 4–6 stem cells, various experimental approaches have been used to demonstrate that a number of cells in the subsequent generations can act as stem cells if necessary. These are *potential* stem cells—an additional range of clonogenic cells.

Clonogenic cells have been most extensively characterized by their responses to irradiation, although the clonogenic assays have also been used to measure clonogenic responses to other cytotoxic agents. A macrocolony assay, similar to the spleen-colony assay for hematopoietic cells, has now been superseded by a microcolony assay *(24–26)*. This latter assay measures crypt regeneration after a high dose of radiation or drugs. The number of regenerating crypts present after such an insult are counted per unit length of intestine (usually per intestinal cross-sectional circumference, ideally with 10 cross sections counted per mouse). A surviving, regenerating crypt can be identified (usually 3–5 ds post-insult, depending on the intestinal region) as a structure containing at least 10 viable non-Paneth cells. These post-irradiation periods are the earliest that allow one to distinguish between dying crypts (which tend to disappear over the first 2 d) and actively regenerating crypts. The structures are highly proliferative, and will ultimately repopulate the entire mucosa by a crypt fission and epithelial spreading process (providing bone-marrow toxicity does not kill the animal). By using varying doses of irradiation, one can measure the ability of crypts to survive, and by varying the time of assay, the speed with which it regenerates, or the clone-growth rate. With certain assumptions and correction factors related to counting regenerating foci of different sizes, this can be directly related to the surviving number of clonogenic cells. The bone-marrow toxicity problem can be overcome by bone-marrow transplants or by bone shielding.

This assay has been used for two related applications: to estimate the total number of clonogenic cells per crypt, and to determine the efficacy of various agents (such as growth factors and drugs) in modulating crypt survival and regeneration.

Using such assays, it has been estimated that there are as many as 36 clonogenic cells per mouse crypt (rather than just the 4–6 stem cells), with about 120 proliferative cells per crypt that possess no clonogenic potential. The clonogenic cells themselves differ in their radiosensitivity, and can therefore be subdivided into tiers of radiosensitivity *(27)*.

The first tier, the most radiosensitive cells, consists of 4–6 cells that are killed by very low doses of irradiation (<1 Gy γ irradiation). These can be identified by counting apoptotic cells within 6 h of exposure, rather than in a clonogenic assay, and are located at the putative stem-cell position in the crypt. These cells are apparently unable to initiate repair of any DNA damage. It is believed that these are the *actual,* day-to-day functioning stem cells, and that the inability to repair DNA is a property that has evolved to protect the integrity of DNA in this normally long-lived population. Cell death is the ultimate form of tumor prevention. This apoptotic cell death is *p53*-dependent; it is absent in *p53*-null mice (*see* ref. *28*).

The second tier, identified by clonogenic assays, consists of six additional cells per crypt, which are killed by doses of γ irradiation between 1 and 9 Gy *(18)*. These cells would therefore normally mature, divide, and differentiate, but because they are less radiosensitive than the *actual* stem cells, they may replace them if they are killed. They may be the immediate daughters of the actual stem cells, and therefore still possess stem-cell properties (i.e., they may not have differentiated). It is believed that these cells strongly express *p53* protein after irradiation and are using the *p53/p21* cell-cycle arrest pathway to achieve effective DNA repair.

The third tier of clonogenic cells are the most radioresistant, and are only called upon to act as clonogens in situations of high cytotoxic stress—such as radiation doses > 9 Gy. These are the least sensitive of the clonogenic cell population. This tier may therefore be a population of second- and third-tier daughter cells that are the final resource of cells retaining any clonogenic potential. After any particular insult, these tiers may re-establish over a period dependent upon the severity of the insult *(5)*.

It should be noted that these effects are only detectable under extreme experimental conditions, and are unlikely to be called into action in the natural state.

The potential for a crypt to use any number of these clonogenic cells depending upon its circumstances may explain the wide variety of estimates of stem-cell number in the literature. The stress experienced by each individual crypt will determine the number of stem cells functioning at that moment. Furthermore, it is still unclear how long it takes a crypt to re-establish a normal hierarchy after such a trauma.

3.4. Stem-Cell Location

In the small intestine, the actual stem cells are believed to reside at cell position 4. When interpreting results from the various model systems, it must be remembered that this is an average situation, and may represent a location between 2 and 7 cell positions from the crypt base. Unlike the large intestine, the stem cells do not reside around the first position because of the presence of the Paneth cells at the crypt base. It is therefore believed that the stem cells reside above the Paneth cells. Since these form an undulating circumference around the crypt, the stem cells may be discretely located at various points in this undulation annulus of approx 16 cells. Their daughter clonogenic cells may therefore also occupy some of this annulus. The remaining clonogenic cells will occupy the cell positions above this annulus (reviewed in ref. *29*).

In the large intestine, there is evidence that the clonogenic tiers are very similar *(30,31)*, although in this tissue they presumably occupy all the positions at the crypt base (probably from position 1 up to positions 3–4 because of the tapering of the crypt base).

By measuring crypt responses at these cellular positions, it is therefore possible to predict responses within the hierarchy.

4. SPONTANEOUS APOPTOSIS IN THE INTESTINAL EPITHELIUM

Cells undergoing apoptosis in the intestine can easily be measured because they exhibit a characteristic morphology. Although the organelles are intact, the cytoplasm and chromatin are condensed. In hematoxylin and eosin (H&E)-stained histological sections, these appear as cells with intensely pink cytoplasm and a smooth, crescent-shaped purple nuclear material. Over time, these cells gradually fragment and are engulfed by the neighboring epithelial cells. It is therefore fairly easy to count such cells or their fragments, using morphological criteria alone (although occasionally it can be difficult to distinguish them from mitotic cells). It has been estimated that, 60–80% of all apoptotic cells in a crypt can be identified by this method on sectioned material (32,33). Positional analysis can yield statistically valid results if enough (>200 half crypts or 50/mouse) are counted. Apoptotic cells can also be identified using end-labeling techniques such as TUNEL, although this labels internucleosomal DNA-strand breaks and thus can be prone to false-negatives and false-positives (and is particularly sensitive to tissue-fixation techniques).

Even in the apparent absence of any cytotoxic agents, at any one time a small number of cells in the small intestine can be seen to be apoptotic. This process is therefore called spontaneous apoptosis. When the positional frequency of this apoptosis is measured along the crypt axis, the apoptotic cells are concentrated around the stem-cell location at positions 4–7, as seen in radiation-induced apoptosis. Thus, it appears that the stem cells are particularly sensitive to apoptosis, with up to 5–10% of the cells in these positions constantly dying. It has been suggested that this process forms part of the homeostatic mechanism regulating stem-cell number within the small-intestinal crypt, a process that is vital because one extra stem cell could yield 60–120 extra cells per crypt. Similarly, if a damaged stem cell were allowed to survive, not only would the offspring express the mutation, but the mutation would persist in the long-lived stem cells. It is crucial that the crypt can somehow detect this and induce the appropriate apoptosis.

In contrast, spontaneouos apoptosis in the large intestine is less frequent and is not concentrated in the stem-cell zone at the crypt base, but occurs throughout the crypt. It is therefore possible that the stem-cell homeostatic controls in the colon are less effective, and their numbers may gradually drift upward as the animal ages. Since these cells are continuously providing a cellular output, the first visible sign would be a hyperplastic crypt. Furthermore, since these cells persist in the tissue, it is likely that they gradually accumulate mutations, and their failure to apoptose may ultimately lead to tumor formation.

Positional analysis of the frequency of spontaneous apoptosis in the crypts after exposure to—for example—different dietary constituents can provide an indication of altered increased cancer risk, especially if changes in proliferative behavior can be observed. Similarly, apoptotic and proliferative changes in animals of different ages (e.g., changed risk in geriatric animals) and in transgenic animals can yield information on cancer susceptibility. The effects of a number of apoptosis-controlling genes on the control of spontaneous apoptosis have been examined, using both homozygously null mice as model systems or examination of the expression of the proteins in wild-type animals. In the small intestine *p53*, bcl-2 and bax all seem to be unnecessary for this type of apoptosis. In the wild-type mouse, *p53* is not expressed at immunohistochemically detectable levels in the small intestinal crypt, and *p53*-null mice exhibit normal levels of spontaneous apoptosis *(28,34)*. In the colon, however, the *bcl-2* gene seems to play an important role. The protein is expressed at the stem-cell location at the crypt base and, importantly, *bcl-2*-null mice have elevated levels of spontaneous apoptosis at this position *(35)*. Thus, bcl-2 appears to suppress spontaneous apoptosis in the large intestine, but not in the small intestine. This may have evolved to protect the colonic crypts from a constant apoptosis-regeneration scenario in the fermenting cytotoxic environment of the colon. The repeated regeneration from the clonogenic cells is at extremely high risk of incurring a mutation. The bcl-2-induced suppression of apoptosis, however, may actually allow stem-cell numbers to drift upward over time, leading to a hyperplastic crypt and an increased cancer risk (caused by the presence of more stem cells) in the elderly. The use of such transgenic models, and analysis of the expression of the apoptosis patterns of regulatory proteins in the stem-cell regions, will obviously provide many future clues to the effects of growth factors, drugs, and environmental and dietary factors on stem-cell homeostasis (or more importantly, the disruption of this homeostasis).

5. DAMAGE-INDUCED APOPTOSIS

Interestingly, when the small intestine is exposed to a range of cytotoxic agents, the induced apoptosis does not occur on the villus, but just in the crypts (unless there is enough time for the crypt apoptotic fragments to migrate upwards). Thus, although these villus cells ultimately experience programmed cell death in terms of cellular senescence, they are not capable of executing damage-induced apoptosis. The cells in the crypt, are much more sensitive to apoptosis, with cells at various crypt positions (at different stages of maturation) sensitive to various agents *(36)*.

The effects of radiation on the intestinal crypts have already been addressed in some detail, and the extreme sensitivity of the actual stem cells to radiation-induced apoptosis (at 1–5 cGy) is a very useful stem-cell assay. A number of mutagens—isopropyl-methane sulphonate, bleomycin and adriamycin—also appear to have some apoptotic specificity for stem cells *(37–39)*. The target cells for other cytotoxic drugs appear to be higher up the crypt.

The response of the crypt to such damage appears to involve the induction of *p53* *(28)*. *p53*-null mice do not exhibit the rapid induction of apoptosis following irradiation, and *p53* levels are upregulated in wild-type mice, but curiously not in the apoptotic cells. Thus, it appears that the cell death is mediated via *p53,* although it also appears that the surviving clonogenic cells express *p53* in order to induce cell-cycle arrest and DNA repair.

In the colon, radiation-induced apoptosis is not clustered in the stem cells at the crypt base, but is dispersed along the crypt axis. Furthermore, the apoptotic yield does not begin to plateau until approx 6 Gy, rather than 1 Gy in the small intestine *(40,33)*. This is believed to be caused by the expression of bcl-2, since null animals have an increased apoptotic yield in the stem-cell location following damage.

These apoptotic induction properties can be used to assess crypt—and particularly stem-cell—characteristics, and can also be used as a marker characterizing these cells. Furthermore, increased understanding of the responses of normal tissue to cytotoxic agents will aid the selection and design of cancer-therapy drugs. Measurement of radiation-induced apoptosis may be used to directly monitor the effectiveness of putative radioprotective factors (and be complemented by use of the clonogenic assay). Anticancer drugs with minimal stem cell cytotoxicity will have lower levels of overall normal tissue damage and thereby improve the therapeutic index.

6. CIRCADIAN RHYTHM

The intestinal epithelium exhibits a strong circadian rhythm. Major changes in cell proliferation (LI, MI) and cell migration can be seen at various times of the day. In a nocturnal animal such as the mouse, the peak period of DNA synthesis in the small intestine is around 3 am, and in the large intestine it is a few hours later at approx 9 am *(29,41)*. The peak mitotic levels are slightly later than these times, reflecting the passage through G2 of the cell cycle. In each case, the nadir of proliferative activity occurs about 12h after the peak. Related to these daily changes in proliferative activity, the levels of spontaneous and radiation-induced apoptosis also appear to possess a circadian rhythm, and the two processes are intimately linked to crypt homeostasis *(42)*. Since the effects of many agents such as drugs and growth factors, affect particular stages of the cell cycle, the magnitude of any response may vary with the circadian rhythm. It is therefore crucial to optimize treatments for the time of day, and to always compare treated groups with those of a time-matched control.

7. NORMAL INTESTINAL TISSUE RESPONSES AND CANCER THERAPY

The majority of anticancer regimens currently in use are designed to kill rapidly dividing cells. Since one of the most rapidly dividing normal tissues in the body is the mucosa lining of the small intestine, it is inevitable that, in any systemic application, this tissue is the main casualty of such therapy. If the proliferating transit cells are the major target, the remaining stem cells will gradually repopulate the crypt and repair the tissue. However, if the stem cells are also the targets, the repair may be much slower or even non existent if the crypts are sterilized and all the clonogenic cells are killed. This is theoretically a problem with intermittent (fractionated) treatments, in which the normally slower cycling stem cells (those less susceptible to antiproliferative drugs than their daughters) will be stimulated to cycle much faster in order to repair the tissue—and are then hit by another lethal dose of the drug. This situation also incurs a high risk of inducing a mutation into such a stem cell, with the associated increased cancer risk.

The first macroscopic response of any crypt to a cytotoxic anticancer agent is cell-cycle arrest and cell death, as described previously. This inevitably leads to a reduced cellular output onto the villus, although cell migration is maintained. Therefore, both the crypt and villus shrink *(3,5)* (Fig. 5). In response to an as-yet undefined combination of endogenous growth factors, any surviving clonogenic cells will be stimulated to proliferate and will gradually cause mucosal regeneration until the tissue senses that enough cells have been produced and cell production is downregulated *(17)*. The kinetics of the first stages of this regeneration process are illustrated in Fig. 6. Curiously, this endogenous signaling results in upregulation of stem-cell proliferation within a few hours of cytotoxic exposure, before any major changes occur in tissue architecture. If all the clonogenic cells are killed, the crypt will gradually shrink and disappear until only the more radioresistant Paneth cells remain. The key to protecting normal tissue,

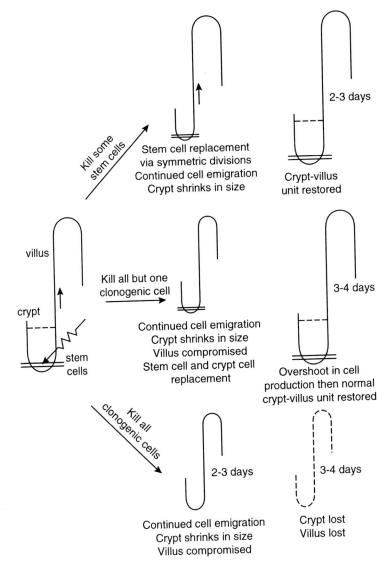

Fig. 5. Cartoon illustrating the response of the crypt to various doses of radiation. Low levels of irradiation kill only the most sensitive, actual stem cells. These can be replaced by symmetrical division of the remaining stem cells or their immediate daughters. Such symmetric division initially causes crypt shrinkage because of the reduced input into the transit population. However, this is a temporary effect and the crypt returns to its original size within 2–3 days.

If all but one of the clonogenic cells in a crypt are killed, a large number of symmetrical divisions are necessary before transit cells are produced. After the initial crypt shrinkage, a stem-cell population is re-established, and cellular input into the transit zone dramatically increases, resulting in a temporary increase in crypt-cell production and therefore in crypt size. If all the clonogenic cells are killed, the cells lost into the lumen cannot be replaced, and the crypt and villus eventually disappear, resulting in denudation and exposure of the lamina propria.

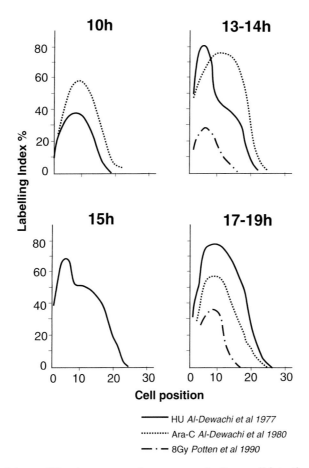

Fig. 6. Summary of the proliferative regenerative response in the small intestine of rodents. Representative time-points are presented from experiments in which the cell positional-proliferative index was measured over a range of times following cytotoxic insult. At approx 13–14 h postinsult, the regenerative response can be seen to begin at cell positions 4 to 5 for radiation and hydroxyurea (HU). The response following cytosine arabinocide (Ara-c) is less specific for an individual position, but even with this cytotoxic agent, a large relative change in proliferation occurs at approx cell position 4–5, and is associated with stem cells.

The data have been summarized from experiments by Al-Dewachi et al., 1977, in which 1,800 mg per kg of hydroxyurea was administered to rats (solid line), from experiments in which 400 mg per kg of cytosine arabinocide was administered to mice (dotted line) *(7)*, or a single dose of 8 Gy of caesium gamma rays was given to mice (interrupted line) *(17)*.

mimimizing damage, and maximizing repair, without compromising tumor-kill rates, is therefore to use all the information obtained in these assays that involve crypt-cell cycling, stem-cell apoptosis, and clonogen survival, to identify growth factors, drugs, or combinations of agents that will increase clonogen survival.

One example that we have been investigating is the potential use of TGFβ₃. This growth factor was initially shown to inhibit normal intestinal epithelial-cell growth in vitro, but have minimal effect on tumor cells (many of which have a disrupted TGFβ-signaling pathway). Application in vivo also demonstrated that the growth factor inhibited cell proliferation in the crypt, with the cells at stem-cell location also being

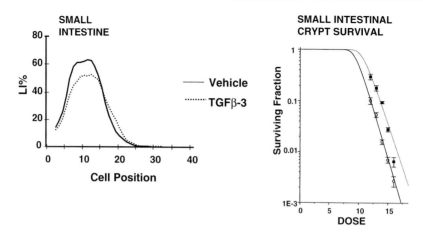

Fig. 7. Effect of TGFβ-3 on the small-intestinal crypt. Administration of TGFβ-3 (dotted line) clearly reduces the number of cycling cells in the mouse small-intestinal crypt, as seen by reduced tritiated thymidine labeling. Mice treated with the factor also exhibit increased crypt survival at high doses of irradiation, indicative of a greater number of surviving stem cells, presumably because of their exit from the radiosensitive cell cycle.

arrested (43,44). This could be a useful pretreatment, minimizing the response of these cells to antiproliferative cytotoxic agents. Using the clonogenic assay described here, mice pretreated with TGFβ₃ and then exposed to high-dose irradiation exhibited a greater number of surviving crypts and a greater number of surviving clonogenic cells than the controls not treated with TGFβ₃ (29,44) (Fig. 7). These animals also experienced less diarrhea, and survived for much longer than their controls. After 1 mo, the mucosa of these mice was histologically normal, whereas the severity of the mucositis in the controls was often lethal.

Other factors that might enhance proliferation (to be applied postcytotoxic treatment), or increase the number of clonogens or symmetrical divisions (to produce more stem cells per crypt and therefore increase the chances of both survival and regeneration) can similarly be investigated, and their therapeutic potential can be evaluated.

Clearly, any situation that enhances the survival of a cell after a cytotoxic insult increases the chances that that cell harbors a mutation. If this is a stem cell, then it is potentially an initiated cancer cell. The long-term effects of such treatments and an assessment of the risk and benefits for the patient must be carefully evaluated.

Any protection of normal tissue must not compromise tumor kill—it must enhance the therapeutic index. Analyses of normal tissue intestinal responses in mice carrying tumor xenografts is one option, but the use of a mutant or transgenic animals that develop intestinal tumors is also possible. The Min +/− mouse is one such animal, in which normal and naturally occurring tumor responses can theoretically be measured simultaneously in the same animal. With every change of mouse model, it is likely that the normal tissue responses will need to be recharacterized, since there are likely to be strain differences in their proliferative, apoptotic, and clonogenic characteristics.

8. NORMAL INTESTINE IN VITRO

Until recently, analysis of normal adult intestinal epithelium in vitro had been unsuccessful. The only ostensibly normal cell lines are from fetal/neonatal tissue, and many of these contain genetic mutations, such as mutated *p53*. They are also cultured away from their normal tissue context, and are removed from their neighbors, cloned, and selected for culture growth. To consider them normal is therefore highly controversial.

Primary culture models have advanced slowly over the last 10 years, with long-lived normal adult cultures reported in 1995 and 1999 (46–48). In addition to ex vivo maintenance, the former have now been grafted subcutaneously and shown to regenerate differentiated phenotypes and an intestinal topography similar to neonatal gut. Thus, these cultures also maintain stem cells ex vivo *(49)*. The development of in vitro colony-forming/clonogenic assays are now beginning to be reported *(48)* (Booth and Potten, unpublished observations). Such assays will have a tremendous impact on the study of the transformation of normal intestinal stem cells, providing an easily manipulated medium for characterizing the Fearon-Vogelstein transformation sequence.

These cultures should also allow detailed investigation and manipulation of the factors controlling asymmetric vs symmetric stem-cell division (and thus ultimately allow stem-cell expansion for transplantation), and factors controlling proliferation and apoptosis and stem-cell survival (providing new preclinical screens for anticancer drugs). In addition to transfecting genes into these cultures in order to mark stem cells and track their behavior, genes could be introduced or inactivated in order to determine their roles in stem-cell maintenance. This could also be the means to identify a true stem-cell marker—a gene that has to date proven so elusive.

REFERENCES

1. Wright NA, Alison M. The Biology of Epithelial Cell Populations. Clarendon Press, Oxford, UK, 1984.
2. Bromley M, Rew D, Becciolini A, Balzi M, Chadwick C, Hewitt D, et al. A comparison of proliferation markers (BrdUrd, Ki67, PCNA) determined at each cell position in the crypt of normal human colonic mucosa. *Eur J Histochem* 1996; 40:89–100.
3. Kaur P, Potten C.S. Cell migration velocities in the crypts of the small intestine after cytotoxic insult are not dependent on mitotic activity. *Cell Tissue Kinet* 1986; 19:601–610.
4. Potten CS. Cell cycles and hierarchies. *Int J Radiat Biol* 1986; 49:257–278.
5. Potten CS. A comprehensive study of the radiobiological response of the murine (BDF1) small intestine. *Int J Radiat Biol* 1990; 58:925–973.
6. Al-Dewachi HS, Wright NA, Appleton DR, Watson AJ. The effect of a single injection of hydroxyurea on cell population kinetics in the small bowel mucosa of the rat. *Cell and Tissue Kinetics* 1997; 10:203–213.
7. Al-Dewachi HS, Wright NA, Appleton DR, Watson AJ. The effect of a single injection of cytosine arabinoside on cell population kinetics in the mouse jejunal crypt. *Virchows Arch B Cell Pathol* 1980; 34:299–309.
8. Cairnie AB. Cell proliferation studies in the intestinal epithelium of the rat: response to continuous irradiation. *Radiat Res.* 1967; 32:240–264.
9. Cairnie AB. Further studies on the response of the small intestine to continuous irradiation. *Radiat Res.* 1969; 38:82–94.
10. Hendry JH, Potten CS, Ghaffor A, Moore JV, Roberts SA, Williams PC. The response of the murine intestinal crypts to short range prometheium-147 radiation. *Radiat Res* 1989; 118:364–374.
11. Cairns J. Mutation selection and the natural history of cancer. *Nature* 1975; 15:197–200.
12. Potten CS, Hume WJ, Reid P, Cairns J. The segregation of DNA in epithelial stem cells. *Cell* 1978; 15:899–906.
13. Potten CS. Extreme sensitivity of some intestinal crypt cells to X and γ irradiation. *Nature* 1977; 269:518–521.
14. Ponder BAJ, Schmidt GH, Wilkinson MM, Wood MJ, Monk M, Reid A. Derivation of mouse intestinal crypts from single progenitor cell. *Nature* 1985; 313:689–691.
15. Schmidt GH, Winton DJ, Ponder BAJ. Development of the pattern of cell renewal in the crypt villus unit of chimeric mouse small intestine. *Development* 1988; 103:785–790.

16. Inoue M, Imada M, Fukushima Y, Matsuura N, Shiozaki H, Mori T, et al. Macroscopic intestinal colonies of mice as a tool for studying differentiation of multipotential intestinal stem cells. *Am J Pathol* 1988; 132:49–58.

17. Potten CS, Owen G, Roberts S. The temporal and spatial changes in cell proliferation within the irradiated crypts of the murine small intestine. *Int J Radiat Biol* 1990; 57:185–199.

18. Roberts SA, Hendry JH, Potten CS. Deduction of the clonogen content of intestinal crypts: a direct comparison of two-dose and multiple dose methodologies. *Radiat Res* 1995; 141:303–308.

19. Potten CS, Loeffler M. Stem cells: attributes, cycles, spirals, pitfalls and uncertainties. Lessons for and from the crypt. *Development* 1990; 110:1001–1020.

20. Winton DJ. Intestinal stem cells and clonality. In: Halter F, Winton D, Wright N, eds. *The Gut as a Model in Cell and Molecular Biology.* Kluwer, Amsterdam, Netherland, 1997, pp. 3–13.

21. Williams ED, Lowes AP, Williams D, Williams GT. A stem cell niche theory of intestinal crypt maintenance based on a study of somatic mutation in colonic mucosa. *Am J Pathol* 1992; 141:773–776.

22. Park HS, Goodlad RA, Wright NA. Crypt fission in the small intestine and colon. A mechanism for the emergence of G6PD locus-mutated crypts after treatment with mutagens. *Am J Pathol* 1995; 147:1416–1427.

23. Wright NA. Stem cell repertoire in the intestine. In: Potten CS, ed. *Stem cells* Academic Press, London, 1996, pp. 315–330.

24. Withers HR, Elkind MM. Radiosensitivity and fractionation response of crypt cells of mouse jejunum. *Radiat Res* 1969; 38:598–613.

25. Withers HR, Elkind MM. Microcolony survival assay for cells of mouse intestinal mucosa exposed to radiation. *Int J Radiat Biol* 1970; 17:261–267.

26. Potten CS, Hendry JH. The microcolony assay in mouse small intestine. In: Potten CS, Hendry JH, eds. *Cell Clones: Manual of Mammalian Cell Techniques.* Churchill-Livingstone, Edinburgh, 1985, pp. 155–159.

27. Potten CS, Hendry JH. Clonal regeneration studies. In: Potten CS, Hendry JH. *Radiation and Gut.* Elsevier, Amsterdam, 1995, pp. 45–59.

28. Merritt AJ, Potten CS, Kemp CJ, Hickman JA, Ballmain A, Lane DP, et al. The role of p53 in spontaneous and radiation-induced apoptosis in the gastrointestinal tract of normal and p53-deficient mice. *Cancer Res* 1994; 54:614–617.

29. Potten CS, Booth D, Haley JD. Pretreatment with transforming growth factor beta-3 protects small intestinal stem cells against radiation damage in vivo. *Br J Cancer* 1997; 75:1454–1459.

30. Cai WB, Roberts SA, Bowley E, Hendry JH, Potten CS. Differential survival of murine small and large intestinal crypts following ionising radiation. *Int J Radiat Biol* 1997; 71:145–155.

31. Cai WB, Roberts SA, Potten CS. The number of clonogenic cells in crypts in three regions of murine large intestine. *Int J Radiat Biol* 1997; 71:573–579.

32. Merritt AJ, Jones LS, Potten CS. Apoptosis in murine intestinal crypts. In: Cotter TG, Martin SJ, eds. *Techniques in Apoptosis.* Portland Press Ltd., London, 1996, pp. 269–300.

33. Potten CS, Grant HK. The relationship between ionizing radiation induced apoptosis and stem cells in the small and large intestine. *Br J Cancer* 1998; 78:993–1003.

34. Clarke AR, Gledhill S, Hooper ML, Bird CC, Wyllie AH. p53 dependence of early apoptotic and proliferative responses within the mouse intestinal epithelium following γ irradiation. *Oncogene* 1994; 9: 1767–1773.

35. Merritt AJ, Potten CS, Watson AJM, Loh DY, Nakayama K, Nakayama K, et al. Differential expression of bcl-2 in intestinal epithelia—correlation with attenuation of apoptosis in colonic crypts and the incidence of colonic neoplasia. *J Cell Science* 1995; 108:2261–2271.

36. Ijiri K, Potten CS. Further studies on the response of intestinal crypt cells of different hierarchical status to eighteen different cytotoxic agents. *Br J Cancer* 1987; 55:113–123.

37. Ijiri K, Potten CS. Response of intestinal cells of differing topographical and hierarchical status to ten cytotoxic drugs and five sources of radiation. *Br J Cancer* 1983; 47:175–185.

38. Ijiri K, Potten CS. Stem cell death in cell hierarchies in adult mammalian tissue. In: Potten CS, ed. *Perspectives on Mammalian Cell Death.* Oxford University Press, New York, NY, 1987, pp. P325–P356.

39. Li YQ, Fan CY, O'Connor PJ, Winton DJ, Potten CS. Target cells for the cytotoxic effects of carcinogens in the murine small bowel. *Carcinogenesis* 1992; 13:361–368.

40. Potten CS. The significance of spontaneous and induced apoptosis in the gastrointestinal tract of mice. *Cancer Metastasis Reviews* 1992; 11:179–195.

41. Qiu JM, Roberts SA, Potten CS. Cell migration in the small and large bowel shows a strong circadian rhythm. *Epithelial Cell Biol* 1994; 3: 137–148.
42. Ijiri K, Potten CS. The circadian rhythm for the number and sensitivity of radiation-induced apoptosis in the crypts of mouse small intestine. *Int J Radiat Biol* 1990; 58:165–175.
43. Potten CS, Owen G, Hewitt D, Chadwick CA, Hendry J, Lord BI, et al. Stimulation and inhibition of proliferation in the small intestinal crypts of the mouse after in vivo administration of growth factors. *Gut* 1995; 36:864–873.
44. Booth D, Haley JD, Bruskin AM, Potten CS. Transforming growth factor β3 protects murine small intestinal crypt stem cells and animal survival after irradiation, possibly by reducing stem cell cycling. *Int J Cancer* 2000; 86:53–59.
45. Potten CS, Booth C, Pritchard DM. The intestinal epithelial stem cell: the mucosal governor. *Int J Exp Path* 1997; 78:219–243.
46. Booth C, Patel S, Bennion GR, Potten CS. The isolation and culture of adult mouse colonic epithelium. *Epithelial Cell Biol* 1995; 4: 76–86.
47. Whitehead RH, Brown A, Bhathal PS. A method for the isolation and culture of human colonic crypts in collagen gels. *In Vitro Cell Dev Biol* 1987; 23:436–442.
48. Whitehead RH, Demmler K, Rockman SP, Watson NK. Clonogenic growth of epithelial cells from normal colonic mucosa from both mice and humans. *Gastroenterology* 1999; 117:858–865.
49. Booth C, O'Shea JA, Potten CS. Maintenance of functional stem cells in isolated and cultured intestinal epithelium. *Exp Cell Res* 1999; 249:359–366.

20 SENCAR Mouse-Skin Tumorigenesis Model

Rana P. Singh, PhD and Rajesh Agarwal, PhD

CONTENTS

1. INTRODUCTION

Over the past few decades, the mouse has been established as the primary organism used to investigate the fundamental mechanisms of skin carcinogenesis and to model human neoplasia. Skin is the most important protective barrier against the harmful and lethal carcinogenic effects of physical (e.g., ultraviolet (UV) radiation), chemical (e.g., polycyclic aromatic hydrocarbons (PAHs)), and biological (e.g., oncogenic viruses) environmental factors. Carcinogenesis has been demonstrated by experimental and epidemiologic studies to be a multifactorial, multigenic, and multiphasic process composed of three major sequential stages: initiation, promotion, and progression *(1)*. A single exposure of a carcinogenic agent such as 7,12-dimethylbenz(a)anthracene (DMBA), benzo(a)pyrene B(a)P to epidermal cells may result in a small subset of initiating cells carrying irreversible mutations in critical gene(s) such as proto-oncogenes and tumor-suppressor genes, which control normal cellular growth and differentiation *(2)*. In the promotion stage, repeated applications of promoters such as phorbol esters that are generally nonmutagenic bring about many important epigenetic alterations in initiated cells, facilitating the clonal expansion of an initiated phenotype and leading to the formation of benign tumors or papillomas. The early stage of promotion is reversible, but promotion in late stage and progression represents the irreversible phases of carcinogenesis process *(3)*. In progression stage, papillomas acquire additional aberrant genetic and epigenetic changes, and develop into a rapidly growing

From: *Tumor Models in Cancer Research*
Edited by: B. A. Teicher © Humana Press Inc., Totowa, NJ

invasive lesion known as carcinoma. Because of an increasing trend in the incidence of human skin cancer, many laboratories have been involved in the process of developing a suitable skin carcinogenesis model to investigate and understand the tumorigenic factors and the cellular, biochemical, and molecular mechanisms involved in the process of human skin tumorigenesis. The ongoing search effort for genetically sensitive mice with a shorter latency period, in addition to increased tumor incidence and tumor multiplicity, has led to the development of the SENCAR mouse, which is the best currently available skin carcinogenesis model. Study of this skin carcinogenesis model has greatly advanced planning strategies to reduce or avoid the risk factors and search for chemopreventive and anticancer agents *(4)*.

2. DEVELOPMENT OF SENCAR MOUSE-SKIN TUMORIGENESIS MODEL

The most widely used skin-tumor-sensitive mouse is the outbred SENCAR (sensitive to skin carcinogen) mouse developed by Boutwell and Baird in early 1970s by the outbreeding method developed by Boutwell in the 1960s *(2,5)*. These mice respond more rapidly and uniformly to the chemical induction of skin tumors than other available inbred and outbred strains. SENCAR mice were selectively bred for sensitivity to skin-tumor induction by the two-stage tumorigenesis protocol. Coincidently, they were also found to be extremely sensitive to complete carcinogenesis, which is accomplished by application of either repetitive small doses or a single large dose of a chemical carcinogen *(6)*. The criteria employed for selection and breeding was the sensitivity of mice skin to DMBA-TPA (12-*O*-tetradecanoylphorbol-13-acetate) protocol. Skin-tumor-sensitive (STS) Rockland mice were obtained by selective breeding on the basis of tumor incidence and tumor multiplicity (100% tumor incidence and >12 papillomas per mouse at wk 12 of promotion in a classical DMBA-TPA skin carcinogenesis protocol) for eight generations. The resulted STS male mice were crossed with Charles CD-1 female mice and again selected for sensitivity to DMBA-TPA two-stage carcinogenesis for eight generations, leading to the development of the SENCAR mouse strain. In both cases, the mice developing the earliest and greatest number of papillomas after initiation-promotion treatment were selected for each breeding.

3. SENCAR MOUSE VS OTHER SKIN TUMORIGENESIS MODELS

A comparison of complete carcinogenesis and initiation-promotion protocols among the mouse, rat, and hamster has revealed that mice are more sensitive than rats and hamsters *(7,8)*. The high incidence of papillomas in mice and their subsequent conversion to squamous-cell carcinomas (SCCs), especially in two-stage protocol, has made this a suitable experimental model for skin carcinogenesis. Rats mainly produce basal-cell carcinomas in both protocols, whereas hamsters mainly give rise to SCCs in complete carcinogenesis and melanomas in initiation-promotion protocol *(8)*.

To date, several stocks and strains of mice have been used for skin tumorigenesis, but there is little data available for comparing the relative sensitivity of these stocks and strains of mice to various carcinogens. DiGiovanni and Colleagues have shown that for tumor initiation, SENCAR mice are 10–20 times more sensitive to DMBA and 3–5 times to B(a)P as compared to CD-1 mice *(5)*. On the basis of available studies, the susceptibility of various strains of mice to DMBA and B(a)P-induced skin carcinogenesis can be represented as: SENCAR > CD-1 > C57BL/6 ≥ Balb/c ≥ ICR/Ha Swiss > C3H for complete carcinogenesis, and SENCAR >> CD-1 > ICR/Ha Swiss > Balb/c ≥ C57BL/6 ≥ C3H ≥ DBA/2 for initiation-promotion carcinogenesis *(6,9)*. A number of carcinogens have been tested for their efficacy in SENCAR mouse skin. The relative potency of most commonly used carcinogens, such as DMBA, B(a)P, and 3-methyl-cholanthrene (MC) for complete and two-stage carcinogenesis, has been found in the order of DMBA >> MC > B(a)P, which is well correlated with their ability of covalent binding to epidermal DNA *(10)*.

Now, we know that different strains and stocks of mice differ in their overall response to both protocols of skin carcinogenesis, but at the same time they show similarity in some aspects of tumor initiation. This can be exemplified by the similar kinetics of DMBA binding to DNA (formation and removal of adducts) in C57BL/6, DBA/2 and Swiss mice *(11)*, and in SENCAR and CD-1 mice *(7)*. Therefore, It can be speculated that the difference in susceptibility to skin tumorigenesis among various stocks and strains of mice is mostly related to either promotion or progression or both stages of tumor development.

4. INBRED STRAINS OF SENCAR MICE AND SKIN TUMORIGENESIS

A SENCAR skin-sensitive inbred strain, SSIN, was developed by Fisher and colleagues in 1987 *(12)*. SSIN mice are reported to be at least three times more sensitive to two-stage tumorigenesis protocol as compared to their outbred parental SENCAR stock at the same doses of DMBA and TPA. Although the incidence of papillomagenesis was high in SSIN, the number of papillomas progressing to malignant carcinomas was very low compared to SENCAR mice *(13)*. The high sensitivity of SSIN to tumor promotion and resistance to progression suggest that during the processes of selection and inbreeding of these mice, a gene(s) involved in susceptibility to tumor promotion would have been dissociated from those involved in tumor progression. These observations and hypotheses have elucidated an important aspect of skin carcinogenesis—to study and identify the inheritance and expression patterns of various genes involved in tumor promotion and progression under various stress conditions. By using SENCAR, SSIN, and Balb/c strains, Conti and colleagues have demonstrated that susceptibility to TPA promotion is inherited as a dominant trait, and susceptibility to tumor progression is inherited as a dominant autosomal trait *(14)*.

Hennings and colleagues have derived three new inbred SENCAR strains by random inbreeding of outbred SENCAR mice for more than 20 generations. These strains are designated as SENCAR A/Pt, SENCAR B/Pt, and SENCAR C/Pt, evaluated for their susceptibility to a variety of initiators and promoters, including DMBA and TPA. These inbred strains are found to be at least twofold more sensitive to the development of both squamous papillomas and carcinomas by all protocols tested *(15)*. More recently, DiGiovanni and colleagues have developed and characterized five new inbred strains of SENCAR mice designated as SL2/sprd, SL5/sprd, SL7/sprd, SL8/sprd, and SL10/sprd. They have found the sensitivity of these inbred strains to DMBA-TPA carcinogenesis protocol in the order of SL2/sprd and SL8/sprd > SL7/sprd and SL10/sprd >> SL5/sprd in terms of number of papillomas per mouse. The tumor multiplicity of SL2/sprd and SL8/sprd were found to be very similar to SENCAR B/Pt, and the highest propensity of papillomas progression to SCCs in SL2/sprd was found to be similar to that observed in both outbred SENCAR and inbred SENCAR B/Pt *(16)*. Overall, these inbred strains are very important because they provide additional insight into the mechanistic studies of multistage skin carcinogenesis and the underlying genetic basis of susceptibility and resistance to tumor promotion and progression in the SENCAR mouse model system.

5. MECHANISMS OF SKIN CARCINOGENESIS IN SENCAR MICE

The mouse-skin carcinogenesis system has provided an important model for an understanding of the multistage nature and mechanisms involved in carcinogenesis. The mechanism is generally divided into three stages: initiation, promotion, and progression. In the two-stage SENCAR mouse-skin carcinogenesis model, skin tumors are induced by topical treatment of a single subcarcinogenic dose of genotoxic carcinogen followed by multiple applications of a nongenotoxic tumor promoter. Each of these stages has been discussed in detail under respective subheadings. Skin carcinogenesis is greatly influenced by several factors, such as differences in species and strains, the nature of carcinogens, route of carcinogen exposure, localization of target cells, and xenobiotic metabolism.

5.1. Factors Affecting Skin Carcinogenesis

It is important to note that the differences in the incidence of carcinogenesis between species—and even certain individuals of the same species or various regions in the same individual—are significantly influenced by immunosurveillance, repair mechanisms, and cell sensitivity, as well as their pharmacokinetic differences. Pharmacokinetic studies tell us about the distribution of xenobiotic compounds and their metabolic products in the body, which help to predict carcinogen/drug/chemical deposition with respect to dose, time, exposure regimen, organs, individuals, sexes, and species *(17)*. Female mouse skin is generally more sensitive to the carcinogenic effects of topically applied chemicals. The reason may be hormonal differences and variability in dermal penetration. It has been reported that the permeability constant for several chemicals was 2–3 times greater for female rats than for males, and that the female rat stratum corneum (primary rate-limiting barrier) was one-half the thickness of that of the male *(18)*. Pharmacokinetic and pharmacodynamic studies based on physiological parameters, permeability constant, tissue-partition coefficient, and metabolic and enzyme inhibition kinetics are employed to predict the effective absorbed tissue dose—i.e., the "target dose". The skin permeability for most of the xenobiotic compounds in laboratory animals and humans has been found in the order of rabbit > rat > mice > human. Thus, the close association between human and mouse skin made the latter the best relevant model to study various aspects of skin carcinogenesis *(19)*.

In experimental animals, cancer susceptibility depends largely on which animal and genetic strain of the animal is selected. Stratum corneum is the end point of epidermal differentiation, and consists of keratinized cells (corneoytes) surrounded by lipids containing cholesterol and free fatty acid and ceramide, but no phospholipid, which makes it exceptionally low in permeability *(20)*. In the murine epidermis, stem cells are considered to be located in the center of the basal layer in the so-called epidermal proliferative unit. Stem cells have great proliferative potential, and are usually located in the well-protected and well-vascularized areas. These cells have a large nucleus-to-cytoplasmic ratio, and contain a copious amount of ribosomes, melanosomes, and relatively few keratin filament bundles *(21)*. These cells are the main target for epithelial carcinogenesis, and they play a central role in tumor development. In the two-stage SENCAR mouse-skin carcinogenesis model, it has been demonstrated that the time lapse between the initiation and the start of promotion did not significantly affect tumor multiplicity until the interval become more than 1 yr *(22,23)*. This indicates that the carcinogen-initiated cells are long-lived and slow-cycled, which are the important features of stem cells, thus providing evidence that tumor initiation involves mainly stem cells. Miller and colleagues have shown that the hair cycle in SENCAR mouse significantly affects the yield of skin tumor. They found that anagen—i.e., growth phase of hair follicle is more susceptible to initiation as compared to telogen—i.e., resting phase of the hair follicle *(24)*.

5.2. Xenobiotic Metabolism and Formation of Ultimate Carcinogen

Most xenobiotics and endobiotics undergo an extensive biotransformation in mammals, in which lipophilic substances are converted into hydrophilic substances and then excreted from the body. Two classes of enzymes have been proposed by Williams in 1971 for the biotransformation of xenobiotics: phase I and phase II enzymes. Phase I enzymes introduce polar groups to the substrate compounds that make them more water-soluble. This reaction facilitates conjugation reaction by phase II enzymes *(25)*. The reactions for detoxifying foreign compounds are exceedingly important in preventing toxicity from a wide variety of xenobiotic compounds, including chemical carcinogens. With the vast variety of reactions catalyzed by phase I and phase II enzymes, it is anticipated that some adverse reactions may occur. These enzymes serve as biochemical indices for assessing the toxicity and carcinogenicity, as well as the chemopreventive ability, of a test compound.

Phase I metabolism generates reactive electrophilic species, which can interact with nucleophilic sites on target molecules (including DNA) of the cell. This task is accomplished by some of the monooxygenases of phase I machinery—cytochrome P450 system *(25–27)*. Any modulation in the levels/activities of these enzymes will affect the xenobiotic metabolism as well as the process of carcinogenesis. The xenobiotic compounds acted upon by the phase I enzymes become the substrates for phase II enzymes. This process of conjugation is biosynthetic, and produces the water-soluble nontoxic products that are easily excretable through bile or urine *(28)*. Under various stress conditions, the normal equilibrium between phase I and phase II enzymes induction becomes disturbed and shifts toward increased oxidative metabolism, and the outcome of which is mostly deleterious to the cell/organism.

Most of the carcinogens, especially those belonging to the PAH class, are chemically inert and need oxidative metabolic activation for their conversion from procarcinogen or proximate carcinogen to ultimate carcinogen in order to exert neoplastic effect (Fig. 1) *(29)*. The metabolic activation of PAHs occurs through several pathways. In a major pathway, it is catalyzed by nicotinamide-adenine dinucleotide phosphate (NADPH)-dependent cytochrome P450 monooxygenases and epoxide hydrolase, producing a non-K-region transdihydrodiol (proximate carcinogen) which is then converted to antidiol epoxides (ultimate carcinogen) with the potential to alkylate DNA. In this way, DMBA is predominantly metabolized by the CYP1A1 isozyme present in the endoplasmic reticulum of skin cells to its ultimate electrophilic carcinogenic form,

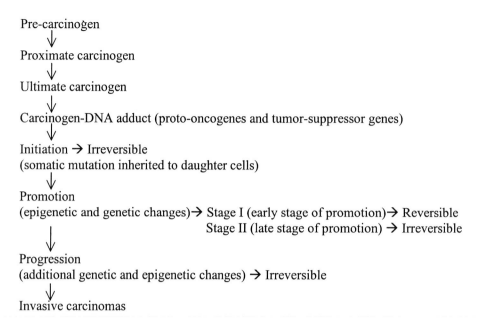

Fig. 1. Multistage chemical carcinogenesis in SENCAR mouse skin.

DMBA-3,4-diol 1,2-epoxide, which forms covalent DNA adducts by binding to the N^6 position of deoxyadenosine *(31,32)*. Carcinogen-DNA adducts represent an early, detectable, and critical step in the carcinogenic process, and thus may serve as an internal dosimeter of carcinogen exposure.

5.3. Oxidative Stress and Multistage Skin Carcinogenesis

The increase in highly reactive oxygen species (ROS), including free radicals such as superoxide anion radical, hydroxyl radical, peroxyl radical, alkoxyl radical, hydroperoxyl radical, and hydrogen peroxide, leads to oxidative stress—which can either directly or indirectly modify a number of biologically important molecules, and cause skin cancer and other diseases *(32,33)*. It has been shown that the epidermis is a major site for the ROS-mediated lipid peroxidation in mouse skin *(34)*. In addition to external sources, an array of enzymes (xanthine oxidase, NADPH oxidase, hemoprotein oxidases, and others) can inadvertently contribute to oxidative stress in a living system when the antioxidant defense fails to contain them. Thioredoxin reductase, glutathione peroxidase, glutathione reductase, superoxide dismutase, catalase, and thiols constitute major antioxidant defense mechanisms in skin, and the thioredoxin system is believed to form the first line of defense against ROS because of its localization at the outer membrane surface of keratinocytes *(35–37)*. It has been observed that tumor promoters shift the equilibrium toward the generation of ROS and organic peroxide, and that subsequent biochemical and biological effects are inhibited by the application of various antioxidants and free-radical scavengers *(38)*. Conversely, these effects are mimicked by some free-radical-generating system. Oxidative stress also helps to acquire multiple genetic mutations and alterations in epigenetic mechanisms during the progression stage of tumorigenesis *(39)*. Oxidative stress has a profound effect on car-

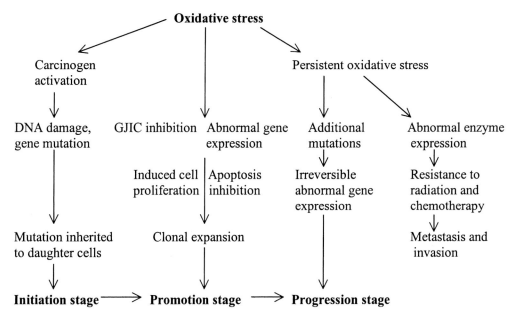

Fig. 2. Interaction of oxidative stress with all the three stages of carcinogenesis process. During the initiation stage, oxidative DNA damage may produce mutation and structural alterations in DNA resulting in a heritable mutation. During the promotion stage(s), in target gene(s), oxidative stress can contribute to abnormal gene expression, blocking of cell-to-cell communication, and alteration of mitogenic cell signaling, resulting in an increase in cell proliferation and/or decrease in apoptosis in the initiated cell population. This leads to clonal expansion of the initiated cells to preneoplastic focal lesions. Oxidative stress may also participate in the progression stage by importing further DNA alterations in the initiated cells resulting in changes in the enzyme activity and making the lesions resistant to normal growth control. (GJIC-gap junction intercellular communication).

cinogen activation, gene expression, and enzyme activity, which are closely linked to the process of carcinogenesis, as depicted in Fig. 2.

5.4 Genetic Changes Associated with Skin Tumor Initiation

Skin-tumor initiation essentially requires a mutation in the gene(s) controlling cell division, growth, and differentiation of the target-epithelial stem cell(s), and the resultant mutation should be heritable to daughter cells. SENCAR mice are specially developed to study the cellular, biochemical, and molecular mechanisms of chemical carcinogenesis. In a two-stage protocol, a single topical application of a subcarcinogenic dose of the pure PAH—DMBA—is used for initiation stage. DMBA is metabolized by cytochrome P450 monooxygenases and epoxide hydrolase to its ultimate carcinogenic form, DMBA-3,4-diol,1,2-epoxide, which forms carcinogen-DNA adduct in critical target gene(s) of stem cells *(40,41)*. The adduct formation results in an error during replication. If this aberration is not corrected by cellular machinery, it leads to an irreversible mutation, driving the cell into initiation stage. These initiated cells are long-lived—one of the characteristics of epithelial stem cells—and have been shown to yield a similar response to that of the standard initiation-promotion protocol, even after a period of 1 yr between the initiation event and the beginning of promoter application *(22,42)*.

Ras protooncogenes are the main target in epithelial-chemical carcinogenesis. There are three mammalian *ras* proto-oncogenes (Ha-, K-, and N-*ras*), which code for a 21-kDa protein that is involved in cell signaling, mediating the transfer of extracellular information to the nucleus for control of cellular growth and proliferation *(43)*. The *ras* genes are activated in tumors by the induction of specific point mutations clustered within specific codons in exons 1, 2, and 3. These point mutations usually occur at codons 12, 13, 59, 61, and 117, and have frequently been detected in human tumors as well as in spontaneous and chemically induced animal tumors. The frequency of the mutational spectrum varies with genotoxic carcinogens, as well as species and strains of mice *(44)*.

The initiation of tumorigenesis with DMBA induces a specific point mutation in codon 61 of the c-Ha-*ras* gene *(45,46)*. This mutation can be easily detected by the appearance of a XbaI RFLP (restriction enzyme fragment-length polymorphism), generated by the specific $A^{182} \rightarrow T$ transversion *(46,47)*. Mouse keratinocytes infected with v-Ha-*ras* oncogene in culture have also been shown to produce squamous papillomas in nude mice *(48)*. These early studies provided the basis for the development of transgenic K1.*ras* mice, which carry the v-Ha-*ras* oncogene fused to the regulatory element of the human keratin K1 gene, and TG.AC mice, which carry the v-Ha-*ras* oncogene fused to a ξ-globin promoter. These mice have the property of genetically initiated skin, and can develop benign tumors *(49,50)*.

This point mutation in the Ha-*ras* proto-oncogene has been observed in DMBA-initiated papillomas and carcinomas, regardless of the nature of promoters. Usually, the point mutation in c-Ha-*ras* carried out by different PAHs is not similar, showing the carcinogen specificity for point mutation during initiation stage. This can be exemplified by the methylnitrosourea (MNU) and B(a)P-caused skin carcinogenesis in SENCAR mice, which generate a point mutation only in codon 12 of c-Ha-*ras* *(51)*. In UV-skin carcinogenesis, a relatively low incidence of c-Ha-*ras* mutation has been observed *(52)*. UV ray-irradiation forms pyrimidine dimers and inactivates DNA photolyase, thereby impairing the photoreactivation pathway in initiated cells. Spontaneous initiation of epidermal cells, which leads to the development of tumorigenesis by multiple application of promoter, has been shown to contain mutated Ha-*ras* gene *(53)*. The initiation in complete skin carcinogenesis protocol is carried out by a topical application, either by a single large dose or by multiple smaller doses of carcinogen. This protocol results in a relatively higher incidence of papillomas in a short time (14±2 wk), but fewer carcinomas in long time (45±5 wk), as compared to two-stage carcinogenesis protocol *(42)*.

Cellular genes (proto-oncogenes and tumor-suppressor genes) controlling growth, differentiation, and mortality are the main targets of chemical carcinogens as well as oncogenic viruses. Phorbol esters are potent in expressing phenotypes of initiated cells. They function as activating ligands for protein kinase C, and significantly modify the signal transduction pathways toward preneoplastic development *(54)*.

5.5 Biochemical and Molecular Changes Associated with Tumor Promotion

Many compounds have been shown to have potential in skin-tumor promotion *(1)*. The unequal susceptibility to complete and two-stage carcinogenesis within a stock or strain of mice strongly suggests that promotional phases of two protocols are dissimilar. The use of phorbol esters as skin-tumor promoters in the study of SENCAR mouse-skin carcinogenesis has provided much of our current knowledge about mechanisms of tumor promotion. The tumor promotion stage has been studied most thoroughly by the use of TPA, which produces numerous cellular, biochemical, and molecular changes in initiated mouse skin, leading to the development of preneoplastic lesions. Now it has been shown that the promotion stage can be distinguished as an early stage of promotion in which the effects of promoter are mostly epigenetic and reversible, and the late stage of promotion, in which the additional genetic effects of promoter become responsible for its characteristic irreversible nature (55).

The short-term markers associated with the early stage of tumor promotion are the induction of skin edema, and epidermal hyperplasia, accompanied by increase in the proliferation index (especially an increase in the number of dark basal keratinocytes), neutrophil infiltration, expression of inflammatory cytokines, oxidative stress causing increases in hydrogen peroxide and lipid peroxidation, and lipoxygenase- and cyclooxygenase-dependent metabolism of arachidonic acid (27,38,56). The other characteristic responses of mouse skin to phorbol esters and other promoters in the later stage of promotion are: an increase in histone synthesis and phosphorylation, increase in ornithine decarboxylase (ODC) activity and polyamines, an increase in the activities of proteases, protein kinase C, and cyclic-AMP-independent protein kinase, and a decrease in the activities of superoxide dismutase and catalase (27,54). These diverse effects of tumor promoters directly or indirectly alter the gene expression, signal transduction, differentiation and intercellular communication, resulting in selection and growth of the initiated cell population.

5.5.1. ALTERED EXPRESSION OF CYTOKINES

Cytokines play an important role in immune and inflammatory reactions in skin. Tumor promoters are known to induce inflammation and hyperplasia in keratinocytes that are important to the promotion stage of skin carcinogenesis. The increased activity of interleukin-1α (IL-1α), which is also dependent on the other interleukin family members, has been observed in papillomas and SCC, and cancer-cell lines (57,58). Two IL-1 genes—IL-1α and IL-1β—have been identified. Human keratinocytes express both isoforms of IL-1, whereas only IL-1α mRNA is expressed in murine keratinocytes (58). An important component of the IL-1 system is the recently identified endogenous-receptor antagonist IL-1Ra (59), which competes with IL-1 for binding to its receptor IL-1R1. This endogenous inhibitor of IL-1 has been shown to induce with various kinetics with different tumor promoters, such as TPA, anthralin, and thapsigargin in SENCAR mouse epidermis and various keratinocyte tumor-cell lines (60). There are two distinct isoforms of IL-Ra—secretory and intracellular. Only the latter is produced by keratinocytes and other epidermal cells. The net pro-inflammatory effect of IL-1α in skin reflects the balance between the concentration of IL-1α and its receptor antagonist. It has been shown that subcutaneous (sc) injection of IL-1α into mouse skin increases vascular permeability and infiltration of inflammatory cells, and causes epidermal hyperplasia (58). Furthermore, IL-1Ra induction has been shown during keratinocyte differentiation, whereas IL-1 production remained unaltered (61). Increased IL-1Ra expression in papillomas suggests that IL-1Ra inhibits the IL-1 activity increased by repeated application of TPA during early tumor development. Therefore, an imbalance between IL-1α and IL-1Ra expression may significantly contribute to the development of tumorigenesis. Our laboratory has shown that cancer chemopreventive agents have the potential to significantly inhibit the TPA-generated induction of IL-1α protein and m-RNA in SENCAR mice *(62)*. Furthermore, our studies are directed toward evaluating the cancer chemopreventive potential of various phytochemicals which target the expression of both IL-1α and IL-1Ra, as well as other molecular events involved in epithelial carcinogenesis.

5.5.2. ALTERATION IN GROWTH FACTORS AND THEIR RECEPTORS

The treatment with promoters in tumor initiation-promotion protocol has been shown to alter the expression of multiple epidermal growth-factor receptor (EGFR) ligands, including transforming growth factor α (TGFα), heparin-binding epidermal growth factor (HB-EGF), amphiregulin (AR), and betacellulin (BTC) in SENCAR mouse epidermis, as well as primary skin tumors, both papillomas and SCCs *(63,64)*. TGFα, a member of the epidermal growth-factor (EGF) superfamily, like EGF, binds to and activates the EGFR and is expressed in skin as well as other normal tissues *(63,65,66)*. However, it has been found to be overexpressed in a variety of epithelial tumors and tumor-cell lines *(67)*. The elevated expression of TGFα has been detected in papillomas generated by transfection of normal keratinocytes with v-Ha-*ras*, followed by growth of these cells in chambers of nude mice and in primary skin tumors generated by initiation-promotion protocol in SENCAR mice *(68,69)*. Now, studies are focused on answering these questions: what are the similarities and dissimilarities in the mechanisms of induction of multiple EGFR ligands and their effects in mouse skin, papillomas, and SCCs against various types of tumor-promoting stimuli, and subsequently, are different EGFR ligands necessary to produce distinct effects during skin-tumor promotion in the SENCAR mouse model?

5.5.3. MODULATION IN EXPRESSION OF EARLY GROWTH RESPONSE GENES

The immediate early genes such as *fos, jun,* and early growth-response-1 *(Egr-1)* are believed to mediate processes of cell growth and differentiation. In particular, the modulation in *Egr-1* gene expression by TPA has been shown in both epidermis and dermis, as well as in papillomas and SCCs of female SENCAR mice in multistage skin carcinogenesis *(70)*. *Egr-1* is the member of the Egr family of zinc-finger transcription factors, and encodes a nuclear phosphoprotein that can modulate gene expression by binding a GC-rich DNA consensus sequence *(71)*. Riggs et al. has reported that the application of TPA dramatically elevated the level of *Egr-1* m-RNA by 28-fold in epidermis after just 2 h of treatment. A large proportion of papillomas and carcinomas generated in SENCAR mice by standard initiation promotion protocol also exhibited two- to threefold increase in the level of *Egr-1* m-RNA, as compared to that of skin *(70)*. Interestingly, *Egr-1* overexpression has been found to suppress growth and/or tumorigenicity in several human tumor-cell lines *(72,73)*. *Egr-1* participates in growth-regulation pathways through positive or negative regulation of gene expression, depending on cell type, and may significantly contribute to the process of skin-tumor promotion, although its precise function in growth regulation remains unclear.

5.5.4. ACTIVATION OF PROTEIN KINASE C

Protein kinase C (PKC) is a serine/threononine protein kinase and is present in all the tissues of the body, indicating their importance in cellular functions. In an important signal transduction pathway, PKC is activated by the naturally occurring endogenous ligand diacylglycerol (DAG), which is produced by phosphatidylinositol turnover by the action of phospholipase C when cells are stimulated. Phorbol esters, as well as other promoters, have also been shown to activate PKC directly, and to influence a wide range of biological processes such as tumor promotion *(54,74,75)*. This pathway regulates the expression of a number of growth factor receptors such as EGFR *(76)*, and certain oncogenes such as *fos* and *myc (77)*. The investigation of the mechanisms of pleiotropic effects on cellular functions by tumor promoters through the activation of PKC in the SENCAR mouse model has become an important field of research.

5.5.5. INDUCTION OF ORNITHINE DECARBOXYLASE

Ornithine decarboxylase (ODC) is a key regulator of the polyamine biosynthetic pathway, which plays an important role in cell growth, differentiation, and development of cancer *(78)*. ODC coverts ornithine to putrescine, the precursor of the other polyamines. Both the steady-state level of ODC gene transcripts and the constitutive level of ODC activity, as well as expression of c-*fos* and c-*myc,* are shown to be increased in the papillomas and carcinomas generated by the two-stage skin carcinogenesis protocol *(79,80)*. The ODC gene contains six potential Sp1 sites in the promoter region. It has been shown that transcription factor Sp1 is an important regulator of ODC expression, and that its function is antagonized by Sp3 in murine keratinocyte cell lines and epidermal tumors *(81)*. The increased expression of Sp1, and its binding to DNA and subsequent overexpression of Sp1-responsive genes such as ODC and keratin 18, have been implicated in epidermal carcinogenesis *(82,83)*. Overexpression of ODC in mouse epidermis helps in continued cell proliferation and/or inhibition of terminal-cell differentiation.

5.5.6. LOSS OF GLUCOCORTICOID RECEPTOR

Even a single treatment of phorbol esters to mouse skin has been shown to decrease the affinity and induce the loss of cytosolic glucocorticoid receptor (GR), which becomes permanent in tumors *(84)*. Generally, GRs are potent inhibitors of tumor promotion, as they inhibit cellular inflammation and proliferation. Upon ligand activation, GR forms a homodimer and migrates to the nucleus, where it binds to specific DNA sequences and glucocorticoid-response elements (GREs) and significantly influences the transcription-initiation complex *(85,86)*. The mechanism of loss of cytosolic GR in response to TPA is not yet clear. The increased level of AP-1 transcription factor in response to TPA results in the enhancement of GR/AP-1 complex formation, indicating possible biological interactions between glucocorticoids and tumor promoters *(87)*.

5.5.7. INCREASE IN OXIDATIVE STRESS AND DOWNREGULATION OF ANTIOXIDANT DEFENSE MECHANISMS

Tumor promoters also generate endogenous oxidative stress, causing downregulation of antioxidant enzyme systems (thioredoxin reductase, glutathione peroxidase, glutathione reductase, reduced glutathione, superoxide dismutase, and catalase) (reviewed in ref. *27*). The increased expression of hydrogen peroxide by TPA in mouse epidermis is well-documented *(88)*. Although 12-lipoxygenase is predominantly present in the normal mouse epidermis, the constitutive expression of 8-lipoxygenase has recently been shown in papillomas but not in carcinomas in two-stage mouse skin carcinogenesis, indicating the role of 8-lipoxygenase catalyzed-arachidonic-acid metabolic product 8-hydroxyeicosatatraenoic acid (HETE) in mouse skin-tumor promotion

(42,89). The oxidative metabolic products of arachidonic acid, including PGE$_2$, PGF$_2\alpha$, and PGD$_2$ catalyzed by cyclooxygenases (COX)—have also been shown to play an important role in skin-tumor promotion *(62,90)*. More recently, it has been found that the increase in COX activity during tumor promotion in mouse epidermis is only caused by constitutive overexpression of its inducible form known as COX-2, whereas COX-1 expression remains unchanged *(91)*. Our laboratory has shown that silymarin, a potential chemopreventive agent, significantly inhibits TPA-caused expression of COX-2 and formation of PGE$_2$ in the SENCAR mouse epidermis *(62)*. These results support a thorough exploration of COX-2 as molecular target for epithelial-cancer chemoprevention by this agent.

5.5.8. INHIBITION OF GAP-JUNCTIONAL INTERCELLULAR COMMUNICATIONS

Gap-junctional intercellular communications (GJIC) play a crucial role in the maintenance of cellular homeostasis and growth control. Gap junctions are intercellular channels formed by hexameric structural protein units called connexins (Cxs), and allow the passage of ions and small molecules such as Ca^{++}, inositol triphosphate and c-AMP between neighboring cells *(92)*. It has been shown that agents with tumor-promoting ability in multistage skin carcinogenesis inhibit GJIC. Yet the knowledge about the effect of tumor promoters on GJIC in target organs in vivo is very limited and primarily based upon a few experiments in the rat-liver carcinogenesis model *(93)*. Studies are underway to investigate the mechanisms and effects of tumor promoters on GJIC or connexin expression in SENCAR mouse skin. Budunova and colleagues *(94)* have shown that TPA, okadaic acid, chrysarobin, and benzoyl peroxide significantly change the expression of Cxs (Cx26, Cx31.1 and Cx43), as well as their localization in SENCAR mice epidermis, but possibly through different mechanisms. More detailed mechanistic studies are needed to explore the differential permeability and sensitivity of Cxs to various regulatory factors of different signal transduction pathways that control cell growth, differentiation, and death.

5.6. Biochemical and Molecular Events Associated with Tumor Progression

Premalignant progression is characterized by an increased proliferative compartment, loss of normal differentiative function, acquisition of migratory potential, and aberrant cell-cell interactions. Studies indicate that in humans suffering from or prone to cancer, the DNA repair mechanism(s) is defective. Now, we know that eukaryotic cellular DNA undergoes continuous damage, repair, and resynthesis. A homeostatic equilibrium exists to counterbalance the damage by multiple pathways for DNA repair. However, in neoplastic conversion, this equilibrium is lost, resulting in accumulation of multiple mutations—mainly through point mutation, gene amplification, microsatellite instability, and chromosomal aberrations (mostly translocation, deletion, and amplification) and aneuploidy *(95)*.

At the genetic level, progressing papillomas develop trisomies of chromosomes 6 and 7, and become aneuploid *(96)*. Tumor clones undergoing premalignant progression often display the duplication of the chromosome containing mutant Ha-*ras* allele, and carcinomas are frequently deleted from the chromosome containing the normal Ha-*ras* allele *(97)*. AP-1 transcription factor activity and its transcript level increases during premalignant progression of squamous papillomas, supporting the contributory role for this transcription factor in premalignant progression. It has been shown that experimentally produced genetic modifications can alter premalignant progression. Papillomas generated by introducing an oncogenic Ha-*ras* gene into normal keratinocytes become malignant when an oncogenic *fos* gene is added *(48)*. Conversely, genetic deletion of the normal *fos* allele prevents malignant progression of benign tumors induced by oncogenic Ha-*ras*, suggesting that AP-1 transcriptional activity is essential for progression *(98)*.

Specific tumor-induction protocols and defined phenotypic markers have been developed to explore the biological and molecular basis of low- and high-risk papillomas undergoing premalignant progression in the SENCAR mouse *(99)*. The alteration in the level and expression of gap-junctional proteins (connexins) is associated with both tumor promotion and progression *(94,100)*. Some of the phenotypic markers associated with premalignant progression have been identified, such as the appearance of α-glutamyl transpeptidase, loss of keratin 1 and 10, increased expression of keratin 13, an expansion of both the proliferative compartment and the number of cells expressing α6β4 integrin, and loss of TGF-β1 in the basal cells of tumor papillae *(100–102)*. It has been demonstrated that the molecular control of premalignant progression is similar in both the low- and high-risk papillomas, but the process is accelerated in the high-risk lesions *(101,102)*. Interestingly, in the SENCAR mouse, the angiogenesis switch is an early event, probably mechanistically related to the development of the exophytic lesions. Therefore, density of blood vessels cannot be used as a predictor of malignant progression *(103)*. Some important critical events providing the basis for tumor progression in the SENCAR mouse are discussed in the following section.

5.6.1. MULTIPLE MUTATIONS

The fact that cancer is heritable at cellular level and that cancer cells contain multiple mutations suggest that tumor progression is driven by mutagenesis. With each deeper-level exploration employing molecular techniques, more and more mutations are being documented in cancer cells which are involved in causing genetic instability manifested by extensive heterogeneity of cancer cells within each tumor. It has been hypothesized that there are thousands of mutations in cancer cells, and that there are many mechanisms for the generation of a mutator phenotype in the cells. Recent studies have suggested two pre-eminent mechanisms of generation of mutation in cancer cells—one involving deficits in DNA repair and other involving deficits in chromosomal partitioning during cell division *(104)*. There is an emerging theory that instability in the genome of cancer cells results in a cascade of mutations, including some that enable cancer cells to bypass the host-regulatory processes that controls cell location, division, expression, adaptation, and death.

During cell-cycle progression, several regulatory pathways function as checkpoints, and monitor the repair of the damage *(105)*. For example, mutations in *p53* result in decreasing the stringency of the DNA damage checkpoints, allowing cancer cells to replicate damaged DNA *(106)*. In presence of unrepairable damage, many cancers contain mutations that delay or prevent the apoptotic response and promote the survival of genetically unstable malignant cells.

5.6.2. INCREASED EXPRESSION OF MUTATED HA-*RAS*

The *ras*-proto-oncogene family products are membrane-associated, guanine nucleotide-binding proteins that serve a molecular switch for signal-transduction pathways. *Ras* proteins transduce mitogenic signals from tyrosine-kinase receptors. *Ras* protein containing activating mutations have been implicated in the transformation of cells both in vivo and in culture *(107,108)*. Important changes, including alterations in positive and negative regulators of the cell cycle in differentiated papillomas, occur at 20 wk of promotion when most of the papillomas become moderately dysplastic, and atypical cells appear in the basal and suprabasal layers *(109)*. Concomitant with the histologic changes, papilloma progression results in numerical chromosome alterations, including nonrandom trisomy of chromosome 6 and 7 *(96)*.

In SENCAR mouse epidermal lesions, quantitative increases in Ha-*ras* protein expression and m-RNA level, and in the expression of mutated Ha-*ras* allele, probably play an important role in papilloma progression. It has also been reported that this mutated allelic expression remained almost constant at 20, 30, and 40 wk of promotion *(110)*. More recently, it has been observed that *ras* activity, along with cyclin D1 overexpression, is an essential mechanism of mouse skin-tumor development *(111)*. It is widely accepted that during progression of premalignant lesions, several genetic changes that determine subsequent phenotypic alterations take place. Only some of these alterations have been studied in the mouse-skin two-stage carcinogenesis system; therefore, it provides an important field of study to search the target genes associated with conversion of benign cell type into malignant cell type acquiring metastatic potential.

5.6.3. Correlation of Positive and Negative Cell-Cycle Regulators

It is now evident that several regulatory genes controlling the mammalian cell cycle—particularly some that control the progression of quiescent cells through G1 and into S phase—are the targets for alteration during development of neoplasms. The events regulating the cell cycle are becoming clearer as more attention is given to this area of research. Cell-cycle progression is regulated by the combinations of cyclins and cyclin-dependent kinases (cdks) that form complexes at specific phases of the cell cycle *(112)*. G1 cyclin-cdk complexes phosphorylate the retinoblastoma (Rb) gene (tumor-suppressor gene) product, pRb, which has been implicated in the proliferation-regulation mechanism in keratinocytes and other cell types. The loss of growth control in various tumors has been attributed to the loss of Rb function *(113)*. It has been found that pRb and pRb-related proteins target E2F transcription factors with oncogenic potential. This interaction is correlated with the capacity of pRb to arrest cell growth in the G1 phase *(114)*. Wild-type *p53* is a growth-suppressor protein that inhibits the growth of both normal and transformed cells and leads to a G1 arrest when overexpressed. It is a sequence-specific DNA-binding protein, and modulates the replication and transcription of growth-regulatory genes *(115)*. Its multiple phosphorylation is brought about by protein kinases during mitosis. The majority of mice, as well as human tumors, lack the wild-type *p53* gene or its expression and possess its mutant form, which acts in a dominant negative fashion to suppress the wild-type *p53* activity by sequestering the wild-type protein in a multimeric complex *(116)*. The frequency and spectrum of *p53* mutation may provide evidence of carcinogen exposure and cancer risk, and may be useful as an early indicator of the success of cancer chemotherapeutic agents. In SENCAR mouse cyclin D1, D2, E2F family proteins, $p16^{INK4a}$, $p57^{Kip2}$ are overexpressed at 20 wk of promotion, whereas levels of cyclin D3, CDKs, $p21^{Cip1}$ and $p27^{Kip1}$ remain constant *(117,118)*. Cyclin D1, which is involved in cell-cycle progression, has been shown to be overexpressed in mouse-skin papillomas and carcinomas, but not in hyperplastic skin *(119)*. It has also been noted that cyclin D1-null mice have dramatically reduced susceptibility to develop skin tumors after DMBA-TPA treatment *(120)*. The multiplicity of known cyclin-cdk complexes implies that in addition to the defined G1-S and G2-M cell cycle transitions, there may be other important regulated cell-cycle transition(s) operative during cell-cycle progression. More detailed mechanistic studies are needed to establish the role and correlation of activation/inactivation among cyclins, cdks, cdkIs and associated proteins in premalignant progression.

5.6.4. OVEREXPRESSION OF TELOMERASE

The expression of telomerase has been postulated as a necessary event for malignant tumors to overcome cellular senescence and maintain their immortality. The SENCAR mouse-skin chemical carcinogenesis system is a well-characterized model for assaying the telomerase activity at various stages of premalignant progression of papilloma by employing recently developed PCR-mediated telomeric repeat amplification protocol (TRAP assay) *(121)*. However, the telomerase activity in normal mice skin is not detectable. It has been observed that papillomas at 10–30 wk of promotion and carcinomas possess increasing levels of telomerase activity *(122)*. The progressive increase in telomerase activity, is believed to be associated with the increased levels of genomic instability and the phenotypic progression of these premalignant tumors. This could be a reason for the absence of nonrandom chromosomal structural abnormalities that arise mostly from telomere-telomere fusion in mouse-skin papillomas or carcinomas *(96)*. Further studies are needed to develop a better understanding of mechanisms associated with increase in telomerase activity during papilloma progression in the SENCAR mouse model, which may be a very useful model to target telomerase for antitumor therapy in human beings.

6. UTILITY OF SENCAR MOUSE MODEL IN CANCER PREVENTION

Despite recent advances in cancer research, diagnosis, and therapy, the morbidity and mortality resulting from cancer remained almost the same. This has led to the urgency to find alternatives to control the spread of a deadly malignancy involving preventive measures. In chemoprevention, pharmacologic or natural agents are used that inhibit the development of invasive cancer, either by blocking the DNA damage that initiates carcinogenesis, or by arresting or reversing the progression of premalignant cells, in which the damage has occurred. Thus far the data provided by the SENCAR mouse model have proven quite beneficial in targeting and approaching the goals of chemoprevention: logical intervention for persons at genetic risk for cancer; inhibition of carcinogenesis; treatment of precancerous lesions; and confirmation and translation of leads from dietary epidemiology into intervention strategies *(123–125)*.

Most current cancer chemoprevention research is based on the concept of multistage carcinogenesis, which involves initiation, promotion, and progression. The enzymes can convert procarcinogen into ultimate carcinogen, which is mostly composed of reactive electrophiles. The inhibition of the rate-limiting multistep activation process of procarcinogens, and the activation of enzymes conjugating or facilitating the destruction of reactive electrophiles into innocuous excretable metabolites, have been employed as chemopreventive strategies *(124)*. Furthermore, studies are in progress to determine the critical events during promotion and progression, and the potential chemopreventive and anticancer agents that can inhibit these processes (125,126). Worldwide, there is a large consumption of chemopreventive agents, namely vitamins and minerals, but the scientific evidence of their effectiveness is limited. The dietary intake of nutrients and non-nutrients is specific to individuals, population, and countries. It is therefore necessary to identify dietary and other naturally occuring agents that may form a part of the lifestyle in prevention of cancer. In these respects, the majority of the available data has been contributed by the studies in SENCAR mice.

6.1. Prevention in the DMBA-TPA Model

The stepwise process of skin carcinogenesis in the SENCAR mouse model has made it suitable for chemopreventive studies. Our laboratory has screened and proven the effectiveness of various compounds with the potential of being a cancer chemopreventive agent by using DMBA-TPA SENCAR mouse-skin carcinogenesis model. The polyphenols such as ellagic acid, caffeic acid, tannic acid, quercetin, myricetin, epigallocatechin-3-gallate (EGCG), a green tea polyphenolic fraction (GTP), glycyrrhizin, 18α- and 18β-isomers of glycyrrhetinic acid, and nordihydroguaiaretic acid (NDGA) have shown to inhibit the covalent binding of PAH carcinogens and their metabolites to epidermal DNA (127 and references therein). These compounds, as well as silymarin and curcumin group, are also effective in inhibiting several biochemical events of TPA-caused promotion, such as epidermal hyperplasia, inflammation, cytokine activation, induction of cyclooxygenase, lipoxygenase, ornithine decorboxylase, activation of protein kinase C, and depletion of antioxidant defense (127 and references therein). Phytochemicals such as silymarin, silibinin, and phytic acid have been found to be most effective in inhibiting the process of mouse-skin carcinogenesis (38,62,128). Their chemopreventive action has also been proven in various mouse and human cancer cell lines (127,129–131). This model has also helped in studying the effect of retinoids on normal epidermal differentiation, as well as on skin cancer. Furthermore, the SENCAR mouse has provided valuable information regarding the mechanisms and efficacy of most of the chemopreventive agents which formed the basis of their clinical trials on human beings.

6.2. Prevention of Epithelial Cancers Other Than Skin

It has been observed that most of the agents with chemopreventive or antineoplastic activity in SENCAR mouse skin may also exert almost similar action in other cancers of epithelial origin, such as the lung, colon, breast, and prostate cancer. It can be best exemplified by the chemopreventive potential of silymarin, silibinin, green tea and its constituent ECGC, grape-seed extract, and phytic acid in skin cancer and other cancers.

CONCLUSION

This chapter summarizes various aspects of skin carcinogenesis in the SENCAR mouse model, and draws some useful conclusions and guidelines for future studies. The SENCAR mouse is one of the best models currently available for both complete and two-stage protocols, and provides the largest database for skin tumorigenesis. This system has also provided an important model for the study of cellular, biochemical, and molecular mechanisms involved in cancer induction and subsequent development, not only in skin but also in other epithelial cancers. This model has also provided a basis for identifying the antagonistic and synergistic effects of various agents that modify the process of carcinogenesis. The two-stage tumorigenesis protocol provides a reliable and relatively short-term bioassay for carcinogens, promoters, anti-carcinogens, and cancer chemopreventive agents. The main drawback of this mouse-skin model is that some carcinogens are tissue-specific, and this may not be a suitable system to study the effects of those carcinogens. However, this is also inherent in other carcinogenesis systems. Overall, this model has helped to form a remarkable picture of progress in understanding the mechanisms of carcinogenesis, in finding and applying chemopreventive as well as anticancer agents.

ACKNOWLEDGMENTS

Our original work was supported in part by USPHS Grants CA83741, CA64514, US Army Medical Research and Material Command DAMD17-98-1-8588, and AMC Cancer Research Center Institutional Funds.

REFERENCES

1. Mukhtar H, Mercurio MG, Agarwal R. Murine skin carcinogenesis: relevance to humans. In: Mukhtar H, ed. *Skin Cancer: Mechanisms and Human Relevance.* CRC Press, Boca Raton, FL, 1995, pp. 3–8.
2. Boutwell RK. Some biological effects of skin carcinogenesis. *Prog Exp Tumor Res* 1964; 4:207–250.
3. Agarwal R, Khan SG, Athar M, Zaidi SIA, Bickers DR, Mukhtar H. Ras protein p21 processing enzyme farnesyltransferase in chemical carcinogen-induced murine skin tumors. *Mol Carcinog* 1993; 8:290–298.
4. Agarwal R, Katiyar SK, Zaidi SIA, Mukhtar H. Inhibition of tumor promoter-caused induction of ornithine decarboxylase activity in SENCAR mice by polyphenolic fraction isolated from green tea and its individual epicatechin derivatives. *Cancer Res* 1992; 52:3582–3588.
5. DiGiovanni J, Slaga TJ, Boutwell RK. Comparision of the tumor initiating activity of 7,12-dimethylbenz(a)anthracene and benzo(a)pyrene in female SENCAR and CD-1 mice. *Carcinogenesis* 1980; 1:381–389.
6. Slaga TJ. SENCAR mouse skin tumorigenesis model versus other strains and stocks of mice. *Environ Health Persp* 1986; 68:27–32.
7. Slaga TJ, Fischer SM, Triplett LL, Nesnow S. Comparison of complete carcinogenesis and tumor initiation and promotion in mouse skin: the induction of papillomas by tumor initiation-promotion, a reliable short term assay. *J Environ Pathol Toxicol* 1981; 4:1025–1041.
8. Stenback F. Skin carcinogenesis as a model system, observations on species, strain and tissue sensitivity to 7,12-dimethylbenz(a)anthracene with and without promotion from croton oil. *Acta Pharmacol Toxicol* 1980; 46:89–97.
9. Reiners J, Davidson K, Nelson K, Mamrack M, Slaga TJ. Skin tumor promotion: a comparative study of several stocks and strains of mice. *Basic Life Sci* 1983; 24:173–178.
10. Slaga TJ, Fischer SM. Strain differences and solvent effects in mouse skin carcinogenesis experiments using carcinogens, tumor initiators and promoters. *Prog Exp Tumor Res* 1983; 26:85–109.
11. Phillips DH, Grover PL, Sims P. The covalent binding of polycyclic hydrocarbons to the DNA in the skin of mice of different strains. *Int J Cancer* 1987; 52:479–494.
12. Fischer SM, O'Connell JF, Conti CJ, Tacker KC, Fries JW, Patrick KE, et al. Characterization of an inbred strain of the SENCAR mouse that is highly sensitive to phorbol esters. *Carcinogenesis* 1987; 8:421–424.
13. Gimenez-Conti IB, Bianchi AB, Fischer SM, Reiners JJ Jr, Conti CJ, Slaga TJ. Dissociation of sensitivities to tumor promotion and progression in outbred and inbred SENCAR mice. *Cancer Res* 1992; 52:3432–3435.
14. Stern MC, Gimenez-Conti IB, Conti CJ. Genetic susceptibility to papilloma progression in SENCAR mice. *Carcinogenesis* 1995; 16:1947–1953.

15. Hennings H, Lowry DT, Yuspa SH, Bock B, Potter M. New strains of inbred SENCAR mice with increased susceptibility to induction of papillomas and squamous cell carcinomas in skin. *Mol Carcinog* 1997; 20:143–150.

16. Coghlan LG, Gimenez-Conti I, Kleiner HE, Fischer SM, Rundhaug JE, Conti CJ, et al. Development and initial characterization of several new inbred strains of SENCAR mice for studies of multistage skin carcinogenesis. *Carcinogenesis* 2000; 21:641–646.

17. Wester RC, Maibach HI. Animal models for percutaneous absorption. In: Wang RGM, Knaak JB, Maibach HI, eds. *Health Risk Assessment.* CRC Press, Boca Raton, FL, 1993, pp. 89–116.

18. Bronaugh RL, Steward RF, Congdon ER. Differences in the permeability of rat skin related to sex and body size. *J Soc Cosmet Chem* 1983; 34:1237–1240.

19. Clayson DB, Kitchin KT. Interspecies differences in response to chemical carcinogens. In: Kitchin KT, ed. *Carcinogenicity Testing, Predicting, and Interpreting Chemical Effects.* Marcel Dekker, Inc, New York, NY, 1999, pp. 837–880.

20. Potts RO, Francoeur ML. The influence of stratum corneum morphology on water permeability. *J Invest Dermatol* 1991; 96:495–499.

21. Lavker RM, Sun TT. Epidermal stem cells. *J Invest Dermatol* 1983; 81(1S):121–127.

22. Morris RJ, Fischer SM, Slaga TJ. Evidence that a slowly cycling subpopulation of adult murine epidermal cells retains carcinogens. *Cancer Res* 1986; 46:3061–3066.

23. Stenback F, Peto R, Shubik P. Initiation and promotion at different ages and doses in 2200 mice. I. Methods, and the apparent persistence of initiated cells. *Br J Cancer* 1981; 44:1–14.

24. Miller SJ, Wei ZG, Wilson C, Dzubow L, Sun TT, Lavker RM. Mouse skin is particularly susceptible to tumor initiation during early anagen of hair cycle: possible involvement of hair follicle stem cells. *J Invest Dermatol* 1993; 101:591–594.

25. Ahmed N, Agarwal R, Mukhtar H. Cytochrome P450 and drug development for skin diseases. *Skin Pharmacol* 1996; 9:231–241.

26. Anari MR, Khan S, Liu ZU, O'Brien PJ. Cytochrome P450 peroxidase/peroxygenase mediated xenobiotic metabolic activation and cytotoxicity in isolated hepatocytes. *Chem Res Toxicol* 1995; 8:997–1004.

27. Lahiri M, Mukhtar H, Agarwal R. Reactive intermediates and skin cancer. In: Kitchin KT, ed. *Carcinogenicity Testing, Predicting, and Interpreting Chemical Effects.* Marcel Dekker, Inc, New York, NY, 1999, pp. 679–714.

28. Nebert DW. Drug metabolizing enzymes in ligand-modulated transcription. *Biochem Pharmacol* 1994; 47:25–37.

29. Guengerich FP. Metabolic activation of carcinogens. *Pharmcol Ther* 1992; 54:17–61.

30. Chouroulinkov I, Gentil A, Tierney B, Grover PL, Sims P. The initiation of tumors on mouse skin by dihydrodiols derived from 7,12-dimethylbenz(a)anthracene and 3-methylcholanthrene. *Int J Cancer* 1979; 24:455–460.

31. Ramakrishna NV, Devanesan PD, Rogan EG, Cavalieri EL, Jeong H, Jankowiak R, et al. Mechanism of metabolic activation of the potent carcinogen 7,12-dimethylbenz(a)anthracene. *Chem Res Toxicol* 1992; 5:220–226.

32. Flagg EW, Coates RJ, Jones DP, Eley JW, Gunter EW, Jackson B, et al. Plasma total glutathione in humans and its association with demographic and health-related factors. *Br J Nutr* 1993; 70:797–808.

33. Witz G. Active oxygen species as factors in multistage carcinogenesis. *Proc Exp Biol Med* 1991; 198:675–682.

34. Dixit R, Mukhtar H, Bickers DR. Studies on the role of reactive oxygen species in mediating lipid peroxide formation in epidermal microsomes of rat skin. *J Invest Dermatol* 1983; 81:369–375.

35. Schallreuter KU, Wood JM. Role of thioredoxin reductase in the reduction of free radicals at the surface of the epidermis. *Biochem Biophys Res Commun* 1986; 136:630–637.

36. Carraro C, Pathak MA. Characterization of superoxide dismutase from mammalian skin epidermis. *J Invest Dermatol* 1988; 90:31–36.

37. Ketterer B. Protective role of glutathione and glutathione transferases in mutagenesis and carcinogenesis. *Mutat Res* 1988; 202:343–361.

38. Lahiri-Chatterjee, Katiyar SK, Mohan RR, Agarwal R. A flavonoid antioxidant, silymarin affords exceptionally high protection against tumor promotion in the SENCAR mouse skin tumorigenesis model. *Cancer Res* 1999; 59:622–632.

39. Hennings H, Shores R, Wenk ML, Spangler EF, Tarone R, Yuspa SH. Malignant conversion of mouse skin tumors is increased by tumor initiators and unaffected by tumor promoters. *Nature* 1983; 304:67–69.

40. Dipple A, Pigott M, Moschel RC, Constantino N. Evidence that binding of 7,12-dimethylbenz(a)anthracene to DNA in mouse cell cultures results in extensive substitution of both adenine and guaninine residues. *Cancer Res* 1983; 43:4132–4135.

41. Guengerich FP. Metabolism of chemical carcinogens. *Carcinogenesis* 2000; 21:345–351.

42. Agarwal R, Mukhtar H. Cutaneous chemical carcinogenesis. In: Mukhtar H, ed. *Pharmacology of the Skin.* CRC Press, Boca Raton, FL, 1992; pp. 371–387.

43. Balmain A, Brown K. Oncogene activation in chemical carcinogenesis. *Adv Cancer Res* 1988; 57:147–182.

44. Barrett JC, Anderson M. Molecular mechanisms of carcinogenesis in humans and rodents. *Mol Carcinog* 1993; 7:1–13.

45. Nelson MA, Futscher BW, Kinsella T, Wymer J, Bowden GT. Detection of mutant Ha-*ras* genes in chemically initiated mouse skin epidermis before the development of benign tumors. *Proc Natl Acad Sci USA* 1992; 89:6398–6402.

46. Roop DR, Lowy DR, Tambourin PE, Strickland J, Harper JR, Balaschak M, et al. An activated Harvey *ras* produces benign tumors on mouse epidermal tissue. *Nature* 1986; 323:822–824.

47. Quintanilla MI, Brown K, Ramsden M, Balmain A. Carcinogen specific mutation and amplification of Ha-*ras* during mouse skin carcinogenesis. *Nature* 1986; 322:78–80.

48. Greenhalgh DA, Welty DJ, Player A, Yuspa SH. Two oncogenes v-*fos* and v-*ras,* cooperate to convert normal keratinocyte to squamous cell carcinoma. *Proc Natl Acad Sci USA* 1990; 87:643–647.

49. Greenhalgh DA, Rothnagel JA, Quintanilla MI, Orengo CC, Gagne TA, Bundman DS, et al. Induction of epidermal hyperplasia, hyperkeratosis, and papillomas in transgenic mice by targeted v-Ha-*ras* oncogene. *Mol Carcinog* 1993; 7:99–110.

50. Spalding JW, Momma J, Elwell MR, Tennant RW. Chemically induced skin carcinogenesis in a transgenic mouse line (TG.AC) carrying a v-HA-*ras* gene. *Carcinogenesis* 1993; 14:1335–1341.

51. Brown K, Buchmann A, Balmain A. Carcinogen-induced mutations in the mouse c-Ha-*ras* gene provide evidence of multiple pathways for tumor progression. *Proc Natl Acad Sci USA* 1990; 87:538–542.

52. Husain Z, Yang Q, Biswas DK. C-Ha-*ras* proto-oncogene: amplification and overexpression in UV-B-induced mouse skin papillomas and carcinomas. *Arch Dermatol* 1990; 126:324–330.

53. Pelling JC, Neades R, Strawhecker J. Epidermal papillomas and carcinomas induced in uninitiated mouse skin by tumor promoters alone contain a point mutation in 61st codon of the Ha-*ras* oncogene. *Carcinogenesis* 1988; 9:665–667.

54. Nishizuka Y. The role of protein kinase C in cell surface signal transduction and tumor promotion. *Nature* 1984; 308:693–698.

55. Aldaz CM, Conti CJ, Jimenez IB, Slaga TJ, Klein-Szanto APJ. Cutaneous changes during prolonged application of 12-*O*-tetradecanoylphorbol-13-acetate on mouse skin and residual effects after cessation of treatment. *Cancer Res* 1985; 45:2753–2759.

56. Stanley PL, Steiner S, Havens M, Tramposch KM. Mouse skin inflammation induced by multiple topical application of 12-O-tetradecanoylphorbol-13-acetate. *Skin Pharmacol* 1991; 4:262–271.

57. Oberyszyn TM, Sabourin CLK, Bijur GN, Oberyszyn AS, Boros LG, Robertson FM. Interleukin-1α gene expression and localization of interleukin-1α protein during tumor promotion. *Mol Carcinog* 1993; 7:238–248.

58. Lee WY, Butler AP, Lockniskar MF, Fischer SM. Signal transduction pathway(s) involved in phorbol ester and autocrine induction of interleukin-1α mRNA in murine keratinocytes. *J Biol Chem* 1994; 269:17,971–17,980.

59. Eisenberg SP, Brewer MT, Verderber E, Heimdal P, Brandhuber BJ, Thomson RC. Interleukin-1 receptor antagonist is a member of the interleukin-1 gene family: evolution of a cytokine control mechanism. *Proc Natl Acad Sci USA* 1991; 88:5232–5236.

60. La E, Muga SJ, Locniskar MF, Fischer SM. Altered expression of interleukin-1 receptor antagonist in different stages of mouse skin carcinogenesis. *Mol Carcinog* 1999; 24:276–286.

61. Corradi A, Franzi AT, Rubartelli A. Synthesis and secretion of interleukin-1α and interleukin-1 receptor antagonist during differentiation of cultured keratinocytes. *Exp Cell Res* 1995; 217:255–362.

62. Zhao J, Sharma Y, Agarwal R. Significant inhibition by the flavonoid antioxidant silymarin against 12-*O*-tetradecanoyl-13-phorbol acetate-caused modulation of antioxidant and inflammatory enzymes, and cyclooxygenase 2 and interleukin-1α expression in SENCAR mouse epidermis: implications in the prevention of the stage I tumor promotion. *Mol Carcinog* 1999; 26:321–333.

63. Kiguchi K, Beltran LM, You J, Rho O, DiGiovanni J. Elevation of transforming growth factor-α mRNA and protein expression by diverse tumor promoters in SENCAR mouse epidermis. *Mol Carcinog* 1995; 12:225–235.

64. Kiguchi K, Beltran L, Rupp T, DiGiovanni J. Altered expression of epidermal growth factor receptor ligands in tumor promoter-treated mouse epidermis and in primary mouse skin tumors induced by an initiation-promotion protocol. *Mol Carcinog* 1998; 22:73–83.

65. Coffey RJ Jr, Derynck R, Wilcox JN, Bringman TS, Goustin AS, Moses HL, et al. Production and auto-induction of transforming growth factor-alpha in human keratinocytes. *Nature* 1987; 328:817–820.

66. Prigent SA, Lemoine MR. Type 1 (EGF-related) family of growth factor receptors and their ligands. *Prog Growth Factor Res* 1992; 4:1–24.

67. Derynck R, Goeddel DV, Ullrich A, Gutterman JU, Williams RD, Bringman TS, et al. Synthesis of mRNAs for transforming growth factors α and β, and the epidermal growth factor receptor by human tumors. *Cancer Res* 1987; 47:707–712.

68. Glick AB, Sporn MB, Yuspa SH. Altered expression of TGFβ1 and TGFα in primary keratinocytes and papillomas expressing v-Ha-*ras*. *Mol Carcinog* 1991; 4:210–219.

69. Rho O, Beltran LM, Gimenez-Conti IB, DiGiovanni J. Altered expression of the epidermal growth factor receptor and transforming growth factor during multistage skin carcinogenesis. *Mol Carcinog* 1994; 11:19–28.

70. Riggs PK, Rho O, DiGiovanni J. Alteration of *Egr-1* mRNA during multistage carcinogenesis in mouse skin. *Mol Carcinog* 2000; 27:247–251.

71. Gashler A, Sukhatme VP. Early growth response protein 1 *(Egr-1):* prototype of a zinc-finger family of transcription factors. *Prog Nucleic Acid Res Mol Biol* 1995; 50:191–224.

72. Huang RP, Liu C, Fan Y, Mercola D, Adamson ED. *Egr-1* negatively regulates human tumor cell growth via the DNA binding domain. *Cancer Res* 1995; 55:5054–5062.

73. Liu C, Fan Y, Adamson ED, Mercola D. Transcription factor *Egr-1* suppress the growth and transformation of human HT-1080 fibrosarcoma cells by induction of transforming growth factor β1. *Proc Natl Acad Sci USA* 1996; 93:11,831–11,836.

74. Castagna M, Takai Y, Kaibuchi K, Sano K, Kikkawa U, Nishizuka Y. Direct activation of calcium-activated, phospholipid-dependent protein kinase by tumor-promoting phorbol esters. *J Biol Chem* 1982; 257:7847–7851.

75. Miyake R, Tanaka Y, Tsuda T, Kaibuchi D, Kikkawa U, Nishizuka Y. Activation of protein kinase C by non-phorbol tumor promoter, mezerein. *Biochem Biophys Res Commun* 1984; 121:649–656.

76. Hunter T, Ling N, Cooper JA. Protein kinase C phosphorylation of the EGF receptor at a threonine residue close to the cytoplasmic face of the plasma membrane. *Nature* 1984; 311:480–483.

77. Grausz JD, Fradelizi D, Dautry F, Monier R, Lehn P. Modulation of c-*fos* and c-*myc* mRNA levels in normal human lymphocytes by calcium ionophore A23187 and phorbol ester. *Eur J Immunol* 1986; 16:1217–1221.

78. Auvinen M, Paasinen A, Anderson LC, Holtta E. Ornithine decarboxylase activity is critical for cell transformation. *Nature* 1992; 360:355–358.

79. Koza RA, Meghosh LC, Palmieri M, O'Brien T. Constitutively elevated levels of ornithine and polyamines in mouse epidermal papillomas. *Carcinogenesis* 1991; 12:1619–1625.

80. Rose-John S, Furstenberger G, Krieg P, Besemfelder E, Rincke C, Marks F. Differential effects of phorbol ester on c-*fos* and c-*myc,* and ornithine decarboxylase gene expression in mouse skin in vivo. *Carcinogenesis* 1988; 9:831–835.

81. Kumar AP, Butler AP. Enhanced DNA-binding activity in murine keratinocyte cell lines and epidermal tumors. *Cancer Lett* 1999; 137:159–165.

82. Hagen G, Mueller S, Beato M, Suske G. Spl-mediated transcriptional activation is repressed by Sp3. *EMBO J* 1994; 13:3843–3851.

83. Gunther M, Frebourg T, Laithier M, Fossar N, Bouziane-Quartini M, Lavialle C, et al. An Sp1 binding site and the minimal promoter contribute to overexpression of the cytokeratin 18 gene in tumorigenic clones relative to that in nontumorigenic clones of a human carcinoma cell line. *Mol Cell Biol* 1995; 15:2490–2499.

84. Warren BS, Naylor MF, Vo TKO, Sandoval A, Davis MM, Slaga TJ. Phorbol ester tumor promoter treated epidermis, papillomas, carcinomas, and tumor derived epidemial cell lines have decreased levels of the glucocorticoid receptor. *Proc Am Assoc Cancer Soc* 1991; 32:162–169.

85. Beato M, Herrlich P, Schultz G. Steroid hormone receptors: many actors in search of a pilot. *Cell* 1995; 83:851–857.

86. Diamond MI, Minor JN, Yoshinaga SK, Yamamoto KR. Transcriptional factor interactions: steroids of positive and negative regulation from a single DNA element. *Science* 1990; 249:1266–1272.
87. Jonat C, Rahmsdorf HJ, Park KK, Cato ACB, Gebel S, Ponta H, et al. Antitumor promotion and anti-inflammation: down-modulation of AP-1 *(fos/jun)* activity by glucocorticoid hormone. *Cell* 1990; 62:1189–1204.
88. Perchellet EM, Perchllet GP. Characterization of the hydrogen peroxide response observed in mouse skin treated with tumor promoters in vivo. *Cancer Res* 1989; 49:6193–6201.
89. Burger F, Krieg P, Kinzig A, Schurich B, Marks F, Furstenberger G. Constitutive expression of 8-lipoxigenase in papillomas and clastogenic effects of lipoxigenase-derived arachidonic acid metabolites in keratinocytes. *Mol Carcinog* 1999; 24:108–117.
90. Ruzicka T, Printz MP. Archidonic acid metabolism in skin: a review. *Rev Physiol Biochem Pharmacol* 1984; 100:121–132.
91. Muller-Decker K, Scholz K, Marks F, Furstenberger G. Differential expression of prostaglandin H synthase isoenzymes during multistage carcinogenesis in mouse epidermis. *Mol Carcinog* 1995; 12:31–41.
92. Beyer EC. Gap junctions. *Int Rev Cytol* 1993; 137C:1–37.
93. Yamasaki H, Krutovskikh V, Mesnil M, Columbano A, Tsuda H, Ito N. Gap junctional intercellular communication and cell proliferation during rat liver carcinogenesis. *Environ Health Perspect* 1993; 101S:191–198.
94. Budunova IV, Carbajal S, Slaga TJ. Effect of diverse tumor promoters on the expression of gap junctional proteins connexin (Cx)26, Cx31.1, and Cx43 in SENCAR mouse epidermis. *Mol Carcinog* 1996; 15:202–214.
95. Yokota J. Tumor progression and metastasis. *Carcinogenesis* 2000; 21:497–503.
96. Aldaz CM, Trono D, Larcher F, Slaga TJ, Conti CJ. Sequential trisomization of chromosomes 6 and 7 in mouse skin premalignant lesions. *Mol Carcinog* 1989; 2:22–26.
97. Bremner R, Balmain A. Genetic changes in skin tumor progression: correlation between the presence of a mutant *ras* and loss of heterozygosity on mouse chromosome 7. *Cell* 1990; 61:407–417.
98. Domann FE Jr, Levy JP, Finch JS, Bowden GT. Constitutive AP-1 DNA binding and transactivating ability of malignant but not benign mouse epidermal cells. *Mol Carcinog* 1994; 9:61–62.
99. DuBowski A, Jonston DA, Rupp T, Beltran L, Conti CJ, DiGiovanni J. Papillomas at high risk for malignant progression arising both early and late during two-stage carcinogenesis in SENCAR mice. *Carcinogenesis* 1998; 19:1141–1147.
100. Rundhaug JE, Gimenez-Conti I, Stern MC, Budunova IV, Kiguchi K, Bol DK, et al. Changes in protein expression during multistage mouse skin carcinogenesis. *Mol Carcinog* 1997; 20:125–136.
101. Tennenbaum T, Weiner AK, Belanger AJ, Glick AB, Hennings H, Yuspa SH. The suprabasal expression of $\alpha6\beta4$ integrin is associated with a high risk for malignant progression in mouse skin carcinogenesis. *Cancer Res* 1993; 53:4803–4810.
102. Glick AB, Kulkarni AB, Tennenbaum T, Hennings H, Flanders KC, O'Reilly M, et al. Loss of expression of transforming growth factor β in skin and skin tumors is associated with hyperproliferation and a high risk for malignant conversion. *Proc Natl Acad Sci USA* 1993; 90:6076–6080.
103. Bolontrade MF, Stern MC, Binder RL, Jenklusen JC, Gimenez-Conti IB, Conti CJ. Angiogenesis is an early event in the development of chemically induced skin tumors. *Carcinogenesis* 1998; 19:2107–2113.
104. Loeb KR, Loeb LA. Significance of multiple mutations in cancer. *Carcinogenesis* 2000; 21:379–385.
105. Hartwell LH, Kastan MB. Cell cycle control and cancer. *Science* 1994; 266:1821–1827.
106. Kuerbitz SJ, Plunkett BS, Walsh VW, Kastan MB. Wild type p53 is a cell cycle checkpoint determinant following irradiation. *Proc Natl Acad Sci USA* 1992; 89:7491–7495.
107. Balmain A, Pragnell I. Mouse skin carcinomas induced in vivo by chemical carcinogens have a transforming Harvey *ras* oncogene. *Nature* 1983; 303:72–74.
108. Nakazawa H, Aguelon A, Yamasaki H. Identification and quantification of a carcinogen-induced molecular initiation event in cell transformation. *Oncogene* 1992; 7:2295–2301.
109. Aldaz CM, Conti CJ, Klein-Szanto AJP, Slaga TJ. Progressive dysplasia and aneuploidy are hallmarks of mouse papillomas: relevance to malignancy. *Proc Natl Acad Sci USA* 1987; 84:2029–2034.
110. Rodriguez-Puebla ML, LaCava M, Bolontrade MF, Russell J. Increased expression of mutated Ha-*ras* during premalignant progression in SENCAR mouse skin. *Mol Carcinog* 1999; 26:150–156.
111. Rodriguez-Puebla ML, Robles AI, Conti CJ. Ras activity and cyclin D1 expression: an essential mechanism of mouse skin tumor development. *Mol Carcinog* 1999; 24:1–6.

112. Sherr CJ. Mammalian G1 cyclins. *Cell* 1993; 73:1059–1065.
113. Weinberg RA. Tumor suppressor genes. *Science* 1991; 254:1138–1146.
114. Hiebert S. Regions of the retinoblastoma gene product required for its interaction with the E2F transcription factor are necessary for E2 promoter repression and pRb-mediated growth suppression. *Mol Cell Biol* 1993; 13:3384–3391.
115. Lane DP. Cancer: *p53*, guardian of the genome. *Nature* 1992; 358;15–16.
116. Ruggeri B, Caamano J, Goodrow T, DiRado M, Bianchi A, Trono D, et al. Alterations of the *p53* tumor suppressor gene during mouse skin tumor progression. *Cancer Res* 1991; 51:6615–6621.
117. Rodriguez-Puebla ML, LaCava M, Gimenez-Conti IB, Johnson DG, Conti CJ. Deregulated expression of cell cycle proteins during premalignant progression in SENCAR mouse skin. *Oncogene* 1998; 17:2251–2258.
118. Sherr CJ. The pezcoller lecture: cancer cell cycle revisited. *Cancer Res* 2000; 60:3689–3695.
119. Robles AI, Conti CJ. Early overexpression of cyclin D1 protein in mouse skin carcinogenesis. *Carcinogenesis* 1995; 16:781–786.
120. Robles AI, Rodriguez-Puebla ML, Glick AB, Trempus C, Hansen L, Sicinski P, et al. Reduced tumor development in cyclin D1-deficient mice highlights the oncogenic ras pathway in vivo. *Genes Dev* 1998; 12:2469–2474.
121. Kim NY, Piatyszek MA, Prowse KR, Harley CB, West MD, Ho PLC, et al. Specific association of human telomerase activity with immortal cells and cancer. *Science* 1994; 266:2011–2115.
122. Bednarek A, Budunova I, Slaga TJ, Aldaz CM. Increased telomerase activity in mouse skin premalignant progression. *Cancer Res* 1995; 55:4566–4569.
123. Wattenberg LW. An overview of chemoprevention: current status and future prospects. *Proc Soc Exp Biol Med* 1997; 216:133–141.
124. Kelloff GJ, Hawk ET, Karp JE, Crowell JA, Boone CW, Steele VE, et al. Progress in chemical chemoprevention. *Semin Oncol* 1997; 24:241–252.
125. Sporn MB, Suh N. Chemoprevention of cancer. *Carcinogenesis* 2000; 21:525–530.
126. Kelloff GJ. Perspectives on cancer chemoprevention research and drug development. *Adv Cancer Res* 1999; 78:199–334.
127. Agarwal R, Katiyar SK, Mukhtar H. Skin cancer chemoprevention by naturally occurring polyphenols. In: Mukhtar H, ed. *Skin Cancer: Mechanisms and Human relevance.* CRC Press, Boca Raton, FL, 1995, pp. 391–399.
128. Ishikawa T, Nakatsuru Y, Zarkovic M, Shamsuddin AM. Inhibition of skin cancer by IP6 in vivo: initiation-promotion model. *Anticancer Res* 1999; 19:3749–3752.
129. Zi X, Agarwal R. Modulation of mitogen-activated protein kinase activation and cell cycle regulators by the potent skin cancer preventive agent silymarin. *Biochem Biophys Res Commun* 1999; 263:528–536.
130. Shamsuddin AM, Vusenic I, Cole KE. IP6: a novel anti-cancer agent. *Life Sci* 1997; 61:343–354.
131. Bhatia N, Zhao J, Wolf DM, Agarwal R. Inhibition of human carcinoma cell growth and DNA synthesis by silibinin, an active constituent of milk thistle: comparison with silymarin. *Cancer Lett* 1999; 147:77–84.

21

Murine Models of Bone-Marrow Transplant Conditioning

Ronald van Os, PhD and Julian D. Down, PhD

1. INTRODUCTION

Hematopoietic stem-cell transplantation (SCT) is a rapidly evolving clinical strategy for treating a variety of malignancies or disorders of the lymphohematopoietic system. Bone-marrow cells or, more recently, mobilized peripheral blood (MPB) stem cells, are used as a vital source of hematopoietic cells that can reconstitute the host and rescue the patient from an otherwise fatal bone-marrow aplasia induced by intensive cancer therapy. SCT is also envisaged as an essential prerequisite toward the induction of immunological tolerance in organ transplantation, and as a vehicle for gene therapy in the correction of a number of genetic diseases.

The conditioning of leukemia patients prior to stem-cell transplantation often includes total body irradiation (TBI), which serves to deplete host bone-marrow cells, to suppress immunity, and to eradicate leukemic cells. The addition of cyclophosphamide to TBI is commonly used to provide the immune suppression required for accepting allogeneic stem cells. The remaining problems may vary according to the type of disease and the type of HSCT used for hematopoietic reconstitution. For exam-

From: *Tumor Models in Cancer Research*
Edited by: B. A. Teicher © Humana Press Inc., Totowa, NJ

ple, autologous HSCT has fewer treatment-related complications, but carries the risk of re-introducing malignant cells and does not benefit from a graft-vs-leukemia (GVL) effect. In the case of allogeneic HSCT from healthy donors, the immunological disparities bring the risk of graft-vs-host-disease (GVHD) or graft rejection. In human leukocyte antigen (HLA)-matched transplants, depletion of T-lymphocytes from the donor-marrow inoculum has been successful in reducing the incidence of GVHD, but is complicated by an accompanying increase in graft rejection and leukemic relapse. The limited eligibility of patients for SCT therapy according to HLA typing represents another problem. Most successful allogeneic transplants are confined to matched patients, while the stronger immunological reactions posed by HLA-mismatched transplants offer a worse prognosis. Many of these problems may theoretically be overcome by intensifying the pretransplant conditioning regimen, but this would then be frustrated by the onset of unacceptable toxicities.

The different variables encountered in the clinical treatment and outcome of HSCT are certainly complex, and very difficult to resolve. These concerns emphasize the need for continuing experimental research using animal models of bone-marrow transplantation (BMT). Much of our theoretical understanding in this area has been built on the basic principles of experimental hematology, immunology, and radiation biology as applied to inbred strains of mice. This chapter is therefore devoted to the topic of establishing donor-type chimerism in various murine BMT combinations, with a particular focus on the use of radiation in pretransplant conditioning.

2. HETEROGENEITY AND RADIATION SENSITIVITY OF HEMATOPOIETIC STEM CELLS

The hematopoietic system is organized in a hierarchy of stem- and progenitor-cell populations with differing proliferative potential, and is well-known for its high sensitivity toward ionizing radiation. After whole-body exposure, death can occur between 10 and 30 d after exposure as a result of infection, hemorrhage, and anemia caused by depression of circulating leukocytes, platelets, and erythrocytes. Radiation sterilizes progenitors that usually maintain normal blood cellularity. The probability of an animal dying from hematopoietic failure increases upon increasing the radiation dose. The dose estimated at 50% incidence of mortality within 30 d ($LD_{50/30}$) was one of the first recognized quantified effects of radiation on the hematopoietic system (1,2). The $LD_{50/30}$ was found to vary for different species, with a value of approx 4 gy for humans and approx 7 gy for mice (3).

The colony-forming unit (spleen) (CFU-S) assay introduced by Till and McCulloch (4) was the first in vivo clonogenic assay to determine cell survival for normal tissue. In this assay, mouse bone-marrow cells are injected into lethally irradiated syngeneic recipients, and a fraction of the cells home to the spleen and develop into visible colonies after a period of 8–14 d. The radiation survival curve of colony-forming unit (spleen) (CFU-S) typically shows an almost linear relationship between log survival and dose, and the slope (D_0) is between 0.7 and 0.9 gy, indicative of a relatively radiosensitive cell population (5). The position of this curve is not significantly altered by fractionated or protracted irradiation, implying little or no cellular recovery or repair during extended treatments (6,7). Increasing the interval time to more than 3 d in split-dose experiments allows repopulation of CFU-S consistent with rapid proliferation (6,8,9). Fractionation effects on the $LD_{50/30}$ end point are also minimal within overall treatment times of 1 wk, but rapid recovery from repopulation of proliferating cells can occur thereafter *(10–12)*. More direct evidence for the rapid proliferation of the CFU-S population comes from their high sensitivity to 5-fluorouracil (5-FU), an agent known for its selective cytotoxic effect on rapidly dividing cells *(13)*.

The recognition of any earlier pre-CFU-S population of distinctly different radiobiological characteristics came from the special ability of stem cells to provide for continuous and long-term repopulation of all lineages—myeloid and lymphoid—in an irradiated recipient after BMT—long-term repopulating ability (LTRA). This stem-cell function can only be adequately shown in chimera models that are able to distinguish descendents from two competing stem-cell pools, either between two donor-cell populations in the competitive repopulation assay as first described by Harrison *(14)*, or between donor cells and endogenous stem cells in the treated recipient. Short-term repopulating ability, (STRA), as opposed to LTRA, can only produce new peripheral blood cells in the first few weeks after BMT, and are probably CFU-S-like cells *(15–19)*. These cells are necessary for rescuing lethally irradiated animals from radiation-induced bone-marrow aplasia, which that without a marrow-cell transplant would lead to mortality, and are therefore said to have a radioprotective ability. The frequency of LTRA stem cells is extremely low (estimated to be about 1 or 2 per 100,000 marrow cells) *(20,21)*, presenting a great challenge for studies aimed at their true definitive isolation. These cells are also proliferatively quiescent under normal steady-state conditions, rendering them resistant to the effects of 5-FU *(22,23)*. The essential stages of hematopoietic cells within a hierarchical organization is schematically shown in 1 to indicate how depletion of primitive LTRA stem cells in the recipient allows for a permanent state of chimerism from engrafted donor stem cells, and eradication of transit populations—including CFU-S and their progeny—provides for only temporary growth of donor-type cells.

Also shown in Fig. 1 are the different stages of hematopoietic cell development according to the time of appearance of mouse cobblestone-area-forming cells (CAFC) using a miniaturized long-term bone-marrow culture system devised by Ploemacher and colleagues *(24,25)*. This requires growth of stem cells on pre-established stroma, where the correlation between late-developing CAFC and LTRA has been demonstrated from cell-separation experiments using rhodamine or wheat-germ agglutinin *(23,25)* and on variations in chemosensitivity *(23,26)*. The time-dependent formation of cobblestone areas was found to reflect the renewal and primitive nature of hematopoietic cells, and can be related to other standard stem cell assays. CAFC developing early on d5 is found to correlate with CFU-GM frequencies, whereas CAFC-10 shows a good correlation with CFU-S-12. Late-developing CAFC (≥28 d) represent the most primitive stem cell, which agrees with MRA as well as LTRA measurements *(16,18,25,27)*.

The importance of depleting the primitive LTRA stem-cell population by pretransplant conditioning and of establishing a relationship between the chimerism and CAFC assays have been demonstrated under conditions of radiation-dose fractionation using single doses, split doses, and multiple 2- and 1.2-gy fractions (Fig. 2). The CAFC d 12 subset in this case shows little change in survival, and the later-appearing CAFC d 35 exhibits a high recovery in survival with increasing dose fractionation. Such recovery is clearly reflected by a parallel shift in the dose-responses for syngeneic engraftment, for which the fractionated treatments allow greater ability of the host stem cells to out-compete the transplanted donor stem cells and necessitated

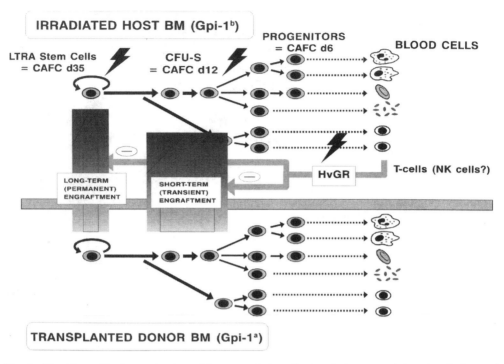

Fig. 1. The hierarchical organization of hematopoietic cells in relation to recipient irradiation and short- and long-term engraftment of donor stem cells. In this scheme the CFU-S as well as progenitors (e.g., CFU-GM) are regarded as transit populations whose ablation in the host by radiation allows rapid but transient growth of composite populations from the donor bone marrow. The CFU-S population arises from an earlier and more primitive population that is characterized by extensive self-renewal and long-term repopulation ability (LTRA). Thus, ablation of this stem-cell subset in the host is often required before achieving permanent engraftment on behalf of primitive donor stem cells. In allogeneic BMT radiation-induced depletion of certain lymphocyte progenitors is also required to reduce host-vs-graft reactivity (HvGR).

higher total radiation doses to establish equivalent engraftment. Thus, primitive stem cells can be identified as a population separate from their CFU-S-like descendants that are involved in acute marrow failure by their much higher capacity for repairing radiation damage. Indeed, application of the linear-quadratic (LQ) model of cell survival *(28,29)* gives an α/β value (a parameter that is an inverse measure of repair during fractionation) that is more in keeping with a late radiation-responding tissue system of slow turnover (Table 1).

3. ASSAYS TO DETERMINE CHIMERISM IN EXPERIMENTAL BMT

Several approaches developed for the detection of donor or host cells in the treated recipient utilize cytogenetic, immunological, or biochemical markers. Cytological examination of metaphases for the presence of the T6 marker was the first method for the identification of donor cells in a transplanted host *(45)*. T6 is an unequal translocation between chromosome 14 and 15. However, this is a laborious technique, and it remains uncertain whether the chromosomal abnormality confers a competitive disadvantage over normal cells. Another method investigates chimerism in sex-mismatched

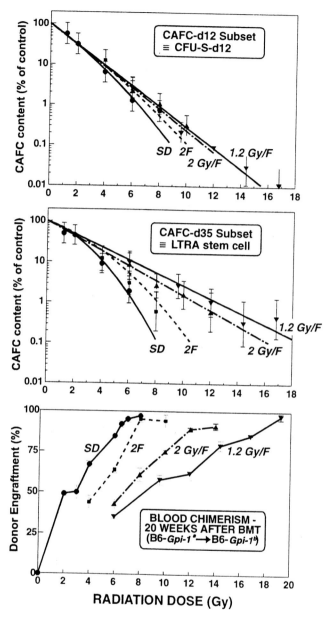

Fig. 2. Changing survival of bone-marrow CAFC d-12 and d-35 subsets with radiation-dose fractionation and their comparison with long-term donor engraftment after BMT. TBI was delivered as single doses (●), split-doses (■) and multiple 2 gy (▲) and 1.2 gy (▼) fractions. In the CAFC assay the marrow cells were harvested at 1 d after TBI treatment, and survival curves were obtained for (A) CAFC-d 12 (equivalent to CFU-S) and (B) CAFC d 35 (equivalent to LTRA stem cells) (after Down et al. *(38)*. In the chimerism assay (C) 10 million marrow cells from untreated congenically marked donors (B6-*Gpi-1ᵃ*) were transplanted into B6-*Gpi-1ᵇ* recipients at 1 d after TBI treatment, and the extent of donor-type chimerism in the blood was determined at 5 mo (after van Os et al. *(37))*.

Table 1
α/β Ratios for Various Normal Tissue Responses in Rodents

Tissue	α/β	Reference
Early-responding		
Mucosa	8–16 Gy	Stuben et al. *(30)*
		Chougule and Supe *(31)*
Skin epidermis	10 Gy	Douglas and Fowler *(32)*
Gut	8–9 Gy	Withers et al. *(33)*
		Peck and Gibbs *(34)*
Bone marrow (LD$_{50/30}$)	8 Gy	Brown et al. *(35)*
		Travis et al. *(36)*
Late-responding		
Long-term hematopoietic	2 Gy	Van Os et al. *(37)*
chimerism (LTRA stem cells)		Down et al. *(38)*
Lung	3–4 Gy	Down et al. *(39)*
		Travis et al. *(40)*
		Vegesna et al. *(41)*
Kidney	2–3 Gy	Stewart et al. *(42)*
		Thames et al. *(43)*
Spinal cord	3 Gy	Thames et al. *(43)*
Skin dermis	2 Gy	Bentzen et al. *(44)*

BMT by detecting the male Y-chromosome after *in situ* hybridization *(46)* or after Southern blotting for Y-chromosome-specific DNA sequences on Southern blots *(47)*.

Immunological markers use differences in membrane antigens between donor and host that are tagged with specific monoclonal antibodies (MAbs). The difference in MHC (H-2) is one of the most widely used markers in transplantation research. Lysis of labeled cells with complement in a microcytotoxicity assay and flow-cytometric analysis of antibody binding are alternately used to measure donor chimerism *(48–50)*. However, H-2 antibody typing is restricted to MHC-mismatched allogeneic BMT, and host-vs-graft and graft-vs-host reactions can influence bone-marrow engraftment. Flow-cytometric analysis of other surface markers (Ly-1, Ly-5, and Thy-1) was developed as a method for determination of long-term chimerism in congenic recipients *(51,52)*. The Ly-1 and Thy-1 markers can only be used for measurement of lymphoid chimerism, whereas the Ly-5 antigen (CD45) is expressed on all bone-marrow-derived cells, except erythrocytes and erythroblasts *(53)*. More recent research, has indicated a certain level of immune-mediated rejection of transplanted Ly5 congenic bone marrow at low doses of TBI *(54)*.

Biochemical markers have exploited electrophoretic differences in erythrocyte proteins such as hemoglobin *(14,55)* or carbonic anhydrase *(56)* to distinguish donor from host-derived mature red blood cells (RBCs). Hemoglobin and carbonic anhydrase are erythrocyte-specific enzymes, and thus cannot be used for measuring engraftment along other lineages. Other biochemical markers that can be used to measure engraftment in all living cells are the glycolytic enzymes phosphoglycerate kinase (PGK) or glucose-phosphate isomerase (Gpi) *(20,57–59)*, and these can be used in congenically marked syngeneic as well as allogeneic (MHC-matched and mismatched) BMT.

Developments in molecular biology have increased the number of genetic markers used in mouse models of stem-cell transplantation. The use of transgenic mice to monitor donor engraftment in transplanted recipients has been reported *(60)*. DNA sequences introduced into the genome of these mice serve as genetic markers to detect the presence of donor-derived repopulation in nucleated cells. Also, reporter genes, such as the gene for nerve growth-factor receptor (NGFR) or green fluorescent protein (GFP), are increasingly used to follow transplanted cells following gene transduction *(61–63)*. In theory, mice transgenic for these or other marker genes would be valuable as donors for future studies on hematopoietic repopulation of a transplanted recipient.

4. MULTILINEAGE ENGRAFTMENT AND THE PHENOMENON OF SPLIT CHIMERISM

Marrow cells that give rise to CFU-S are already known to be multipotent through production of erythrocytes, granulocytes, and megakaryocytes *(4,64)*. Morphologically, splenic colonies appearing on d 8 are mostly erythroid, and the majority of colonies appearing on d 12 are megakaryocytic and/or granulocytic, with a minority of erythroid colonies *(65,66)*. From these investigations, it has been proposed that CFU-S-8 and CFU-S-12 were lineage-restricted—i.e. committed to form only a few hematopoietic lineages. The more primitive pre-CFU-S cells are believed to be truly pluripotent. Thus, they should be able to repopulate erythroid, myeloid, and lymphoid lineages *(20,67)*. The ability of a chimerism assay to measure the donor-type cells in hematopoietic tissues other than blood offers the opportunity to investigate repopulation in various lineages within one assay system. To study chimerism, it should be considered that engraftment is dependent on the rate of cell renewal of the different lineages. In the mouse, monocytes, granulocytes, and B-lymphocytes are replaced in about 2 wk *(68,69)* and erythrocytes are completely replaced every 4 wk *(70)*. Most T-lymphocytes have a short lifetime of a few weeks, but a subpopulation of T cells can persist for up to 6 mo *(68)*.

Lemischka recently suggested that small numbers of stem cells can give rise to lineage-restricted hematopoiesis or fluctuations in the contribution of stem-cell clones, because of a demand for commitment rather than self-renewal shortly after BMT. This was followed by stabilization through the activation of stem cells that had undergone self-renewal rather than commitment *(71–73)*. It was stated that fluctuations in stem-cell activation generally lasted 4–6 mo, but in a small fraction of animals, this fluctuation persisted until 9 mo post-BMT *(72)*. In allogeneic BMT, only small numbers of stem cells of donor or recipient type could have remained, since both are heavily depleted by immune rejection or high radiation doses. This combined with the long lifetime of a subpopulation of T-lymphocytes may therefore require very late measurements of donor chimerism before evaluating stable engraftment among cells of the lymphoid lineage in allogeneic BMT.

In cases of genetic hematological disorders that affect a particular stem-cell-derived lineage, a selective growth advantage for donor cells may help to preferentially correct the defect. This phenomenon results in discordant levels of chimerism among the progeny of engrafted cells, a condition appropriately termed as split chimerism. This

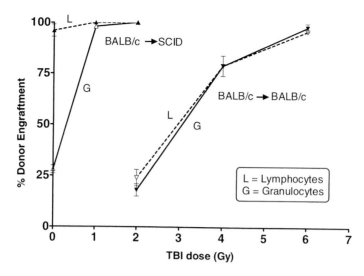

Fig. 3. Syngeneic donor engraftment in Balb/c or SCID mice. Female Balb/c bone marrow (10×10^6 cells) was transplanted into male syngeneic Balb/c (▼,▽) or male congenic C.B-17 *scid/scid* (SCID)-mice (▲,△) after various doses of TBI. Engraftment was determined from FISH-chimerism in blood granulocytes (closed symbols) and blood lymphocytes (open symbols) (van Os and Down).

has been well-documented to occur in allogeneic transplant patients with severe combined immunodeficiency (SCID) disease *(74–76)* and patients with DiGeorge syndrome *(77)*. Similarly, the immunodeficiency of SCID mice can be easily corrected with syngeneic BMT, as shown from restoration of lymphoid-organ cellularity in unirradiated recipients, as well as in recipients prepared with 1 or 2 gy TBI. Transplantation of only a moderate dose of bone-marrow cells (10×10^6 cells) into unirradiated SCID mice led to a donor engraftment of approx 25% in granulocytes, but more than 90% engraftment in lymphocytes (Fig. 3). Thus split chimerism is clearly evident to indicate preferential growth and differentiation of donor stem cells along the lymphoid lineage. The bone-marrow cavities of SCID mice therefore seem to have enough space to allow for engraftment, even without prior TBI. After radiation doses of only 1 or 2 gy, more than 95% donor engaftment was also observed in nonlymphoid cells in the SCID recipients, and much higher doses were required for engaftment in normal mice. This additional factor is consistent with the higher sensitivity of SCID stem cells toward ionizing radiation *(78,79)* that is now known to be specifically attributed to deregulation of DNA-dependent protein kinase (DNA-PK) involved in DNA double-strand break repair *(80,81)*. A selective advantage for the correction of defective progenitor populations from a few engrafted stem cells has also been documented for the erythroid lineage in mouse models for genetic anemia exemplified in W/Wv-mice *(58,82,83)* and thalassemic mice *(84–86)*. Mouse models have been developed for correction of chronic granulomatous disease with genetically modified syngeneic stem cells *(87,88)*. These studies have shown that reconstitution with as few as 5% genetically corrected donor neutrophils can ameliorate the disease *(87)*, but long-term expression of the healthy gene after retroviral gene transduction in primitive stem cells may depend on the retroviral vector used and the conditioning of the recipient *(88,89)*. With the advent of more effective gene-transduction protocols, these observations offer a basis for current attempts to correct a variety of hematological defects using milder BMT-conditioning regimes.

5. BMT ACROSS VARIOUS GENETIC BARRIERS: THE ROLE OF TRANSPLANTATION IMMUNITY

Suppression of immune-mediated graft rejection, as well as ablation of malignant and nonmalignant lymphohematopoietic stem cells, is required in allogeneic BMT. In this case, ineffective radiation conditioning can lead to graft rejection, followed by death from bone-marrow aplasia or regrowth of host stem cells and malignancies. The immune response responsible for rejection of allogeneic stem cells is directed against so-called transplantation antigens encoded for by histocompatibility genes *(90)*. As many as 40 loci have now been identified in mice designated as H-1, H-2, and H-3. The locus encoding for H-2 is called the major histocompatibility complex (MHC) because the gene products of H-2 generally elicit a stronger allogeneic reaction than the products of the other genes, and are analogous to the human leukocyte antigen (HLA) system in humans. The other minor histocompatibility loci also play a role in the immune reaction against allogeneic cells, and their cumulative reactivity can sometimes exceed reactivity against H-2 antigens *(91)*. The level of host-vs-graft reactivity remaining after radiation determines whether donor cells are accepted or rejected by BMT recipients. Rejection of allogeneic bone marrow is a relatively radioresistant process and often requires radiation doses greater than 8 gy for donor engraftment *(92–95)*. The actual phenotype of cells responsible for rejecting allogeneic marrow grafts in mice has not been fully resolved. It has been suggested that T-lymphocytes and possibly natural killer (NK) cells are involved in rejecting H-2 disparate cells or parental bone-marrow grafts *(93,96–98)*. Rejection in clinical BMT is often associated with the presence of primarily CD8$^+$ effector cells of host origin *(99–102)*.

The use of various donor-host-strain combinations with increasing genetic disparity can discriminate the effects of TBI on hematopoietic stem cells responsible for host repopulation (syngeneic BMT) from the effects on immunocytes capable of allograft rejection (allogeneic BMT). It is especially informative to compare various donor-host combinations in terms of how the level of long-term chimerism varies according to radiation dose, as shown in Fig. 4 *(103)*. In syngeneic transplantation, partial engraftment can be easily achieved at low radiation doses, and progressively increased to attain 100% donor engraftment at 8 gy. H-2-compatible BMT (Balb.b → B6) required at least 5.5 gy for partial (mixed) donor hematopoietic chimerism, and showed a steeper radiation dose-response relationship. In H-2-incompatible transplantation (Balb/c → B6), no mixed chimeras were observed: either complete donor engraftment or complete host repopulation was found. The dose-response curve of engraftment for this combination was also very steep, but positioned at higher radiation doses. When the BMT combinations were reversed (B6 → Balb/c and B6 → Balb.b), lower doses were sufficient to produce engraftment, and were consistent with both lower reactivity in mixed lymphocyte cultures (MLC) and lower T-cell precursor (pPTL) numbers in the spleens of Balb/c mice. Fig. 4B shows radiation dose-response curves for sex-mismatched donor engraftment where Y-chromosome fluorescent *in situ* hybridization (FISH) on blood leukocytes allowed for an estimation of resistance conferred exclusively by an H-2 disparity in the Balb/c (H-2^d) → Balb.b (H-2^b) combination. Also

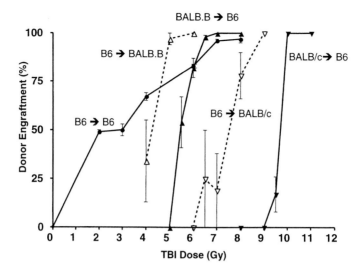

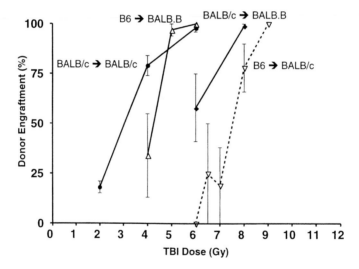

Fig. 4. TBI dose-responses at 20 wk for erythroid engraftment of bone marrow (10×10^6 cells) transplanted over different genetic barriers. (A) Syngeneic engraftment was performed in the combination B6 (Gpi-1^a) → B6 (Gpi-1^b) (●). H-2 compatible engraftment is shown for Balb.B marrow in B6 recipients (▲) and the reverse combination B6 → Balb.b (△) and H-2 incompatible transplantation was performed in the combinations Balb/c → B6 (▼) and B6 → BALB/c (▽). (B) TBI dose-responses for leukocyte (Y-chromosome FISH) and erythroid (Gpi-1 electrophoresis) donor chimerism in male Balb/c or Balb.B recipients. Female donors and male recipients were used for detection of Y-chromosome (host) leukocytes at 18 wk after the syngeneic combination Balb/c → Balb/c (●) and the H-2 incompatible, non-H-2-compatible combination Balb/c (H-2^d) → Balb.b (H-2^b) (◆). For comparison, results from Gpi-1 phenotyping of erythrocytes performed at 20 wk after the H-2 compatible, non-H-2-incompatible combination B6 → Balb.b (△), and the full H-2- and non-H-2-incompatible combination B6 (H-2^b) → Balb/c (H-2^d) (▽) are also shown in this panel.

shown for comparison are the data obtained from the corresponding sex-mismatched syngeneic combination (Balb/c ♀ → Balb/c ♂), and from erythrocyte chimerism in allogeneic BMT involving Balb.b and Balb/c hosts. The relative position of these curves indicates a higher resistance across the major H-2 difference (Balb/c → Balb.b) than across minor non-H-2 differences (B6 → Balb.b). The greater resistance of H-2 over non-H-2 mismatching can be equated to a radiation dose of approx 2 gy. The TBI dose needed to be increased further (by approx 1 to 2 gy) in the fully allogeneic combination B6 → Balb/c to compensate for the cumulative resistance conferred by both H-2 and non-H-2 disparities.

There is evidence from experimental studies that pre-immunization (presensitization) from prior blood transfusions may render the recipient even more susceptible to bone-marrow graft rejection *(104,105)*. The enhanced rejection is associated with increased alloreactivity in vitro, as determined from both MLC and pPTL assays, in which once again the radiation dose is very critical for allogeneic engraftment and survival in animals presensitized with irradiated donor splenocytes *(106)*. In this case, H-2 matched bone marrow was promptly rejected in presensitized animals, but the low TBI dose allowed survival through recovery of host hematopoiesis. Raising the TBI dose to 9.5 gy was shown to be inadequate to prevent rejection of allogeneic bone marrow in presensitized mice, and this led to death from acute bone-marrow aplasia *(106)*.

In a separate study, the syngeneic and allogeneic murine BMT combinations were used to determine the dose-sparing effect of low-dose-rate TBI (at 2 cgy/min) treatments and to provide insights regarding the radiation repair characteristics of the critical target-cell population(s) *(107)*. The radiation dose-dependent depletion of alloreactive T-lymphocyte precursors (pPTL) in the host after both high- and low-dose-rate TBI was also measured in vitro for comparison with the appearance of donor chimerism in vivo. It was found that pPTL reactive against H-2-compatible Balb.b donor cells showed similar radiation dose-sparing as long-term chimerism to suggest involvement of these cells in bone-marrow rejection (Fig. 5).

Comparison of this low-dose-rate (LDR) effect with syngeneic BMT suggests that the radiation-repair parameters in the immune cells capable of allograft rejection are different from those found in bone-marrow stem cells. A dose-rate of 2 cgy/min appears to spare immunocytes more than HSC, and this difference is enhanced as the genetic barrier between donor and host is increased *(107)*. An earlier investigation into fractionated TBI has demonstrated more dose-sparing in H-2 compatible allogeneic than in syngeneic BMT *(108)*. Other studies in mice *(50)* and dogs *(109,110)* have similarly shown that the probability of rejection increases when TBI is fractionated. Although further studies are still needed to more precisely define the limiting host-cell type(s) involved in bone-marrow transplant immunity, the present results highlight potential problems in attempting to improve on BMT conditioning in the clinic through dose-modification with protracted or fractionated TBI. An intracellular repair process—either occurring during LDR exposures or between dose fractions—therefore appears to reside in the target-cell population responsible for host-vs-graft reactivity. Indeed, comparison of several clinical reports have also indicated a higher incidence of rejection after altered TBI schedules *(111–113)* and emphasizes that graft rejection is critically dependent on total radiation dose and dose fractionation, as used in the conditioning regimen.

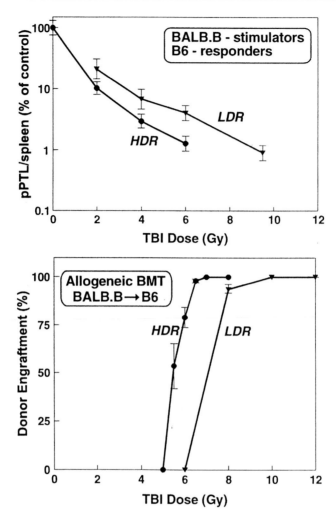

Fig. 5. Similar low dose-rate-sparing for proliferating precursors of T-lymphocytes (pPTL) and allo-geneic-marrow engraftment (Balb.B → B6). (A) pPTL frequencies were determined from limiting dilution analysis of splenocytes from irradiated host (B6) mice that proliferate in response to allo-geneic splenocytes from donor (Balb.b) mice. (B) Donor-type engraftment was determined from Gpi-1 chimerism in the blood at 5 mo after TBI and BMT (10^7 bone-marrow cells). TBI was delivered either at a high dose-rate (HDR, 40 cgy/min) or a low dose-rate (LDR, 2 cgy/min). (Adapted from van Os et al., *(107)*).

6. THE ACTIVE ROLE OF DONOR LYMPHOCYTES IN ALLOGENEIC BMT

Alloreactivity on behalf of cells that have been cotransplanted with the donor stem cells is also important in allogeneic BMT. A major concern in the clinical scenario is the manifestation of graft-vs-host disease (GVHD), a particularly disturbing and life-threat-ening complication. Considerable research on the pathophysiology of GVHD has accu-mulated in mice. Skin, gut, liver, and lung represent the critical target tissues, wherein a complex interplay can occur between various donor- and host-cell types and inflammatory cytokines (114). Many of these GVH-related reactions are difficult to discern from the effects of radiation conditioning. Indeed, an interdependency of donor T-cell dose and radiation dose for the induction of lethal GVHD, principally in the lung, has been shown in an H-2 matched allogeneic BMT combination (115). Subsequent studies have confirmed the enhanced susceptibility of the lung toward alloreactive donor T-cells after both radiation (116,117) and cyclophosphamide (118,119). Another important variable in the incidence and severity of GVHD in mice is the microbiological flora of the gut. Injury to the intestinal lining by radiation and/or cyclophosphamide can result in increased absorption of bacterial lipopolysaccharide (LPS) that in turn can stimulate lymphocytes and macrophages to produce inflammatory cytokines (120,121).

The primary role of donor T cells in eliciting GVHD was first recognized in a murine BMT model by Korngold and Sprent (122), which consequently encouraged clinical studies in which removal of T cells from the donor-marrow inoculum greatly reduced the incidence of GVHD. However, this procedure was accompanied by an increase in both graft rejection and leukemic relapse (123–125) prompting further experimental studies in an attempt to nurture the beneficial effects of donor T cells in promoting engraftment and eliminating leukemia (termed the graft-vs-leukemia, GVL, effect), while avoiding GVHD. Various strategies for separating GVL from GVHD have been proposed form rodent models, including the separation of various T-cell subsets, delayed donor lympho-cyte infusions (DLI), and administration of certain cytokines such as IL-2, IL-11, and IL-12 (126–133), although results may differ depending on the particular host-donor strain combination and the type of leukemia used.

The facilitating role of donor T cells, in particular the CD8 subset, in improving the engraftment of donor stem cells but without causing GVHD, have now been demon-strated in the context of murine allogeneic BMT (134–137). At a moderate radiation dose of 6 Gy, suppression of recipient hematopoiesis by donor CD4 T-cells in an MHC class II-specific manner has been shown (138, 139) and this may at least partially explain how donor-type chimerism can be facilitated after stem cell transplantation. Interferon (IFN)-γ is required for CD4$^+$ T-cell mediated GVH reactions against both marrow and intestinal tissues after 6 GY TBI whereas this cytokine appears to be protective against GVHD after the radiation dose was raised to 8 Gy (139). However, there are reports of no effect on engraftment after adding back T cells to T-cell-depleted marrow grafts (106,115,138), but in these cases the reactivity of the donor lymphocytes may have been compromised by immunological resistance of the host at relatively low TBI doses. It is therefore apparent that the type and magnitude of the conditioning regimen should not be overlooked in the continuing efforts to harness the alloreactivity of donor lymphocytes toward improving stem-cell engraftment and eradicating malignant disease.

7. CONDITIONING WITH DIFFERENT CYTOTOXIC AGENTS: EFFECTS ON BONE-MARROW STEM CELLS AND TRANSPLANT IMMUNITY

Studies using radiation alone clearly indicate that successful engraftment of allogeneic stem cells is dependent on the provision of both depletion of primitive stem cells and sup-pression of immunity. The application of other pretransplant conditioning agents has enabled a number of investigators to further dissect the relative requirements of these two processes, and allows the evaluation of therapies with possible merits for clinical applica-tion. Indeed, the dual-function of combining the alkylating drug cyclophosphamide—a

Table 2
Relative Effects of Different BMT Conditioning Agents in Mice

	Immune suppression	Myelodepression	Stem-cell depletion
Single dose irradiation	++	+++	+++
Multiple dose irradiation	+	+++	++
Busulfan	−	++	+++
Cyclophosphamide	+++	++	−
Thiotepa	+++	+++	−
Melphalan	−	++	−

potent immune suppressant—with TBI has had a long history in the treatment of allogeneic BMT patients. Thus, the addition of cyclophosphamide in mice can reduce the radiation dose required for allogeneic engraftment *(139,140)*, although large variations in the effectiveness of this drug have been documented, depending on its sequence and timing with TBI *(140)*. While cyclophosphamide is also well-known for its acute myelotoxicity *(141)*, it has little effect against the primitive cells of the host, and is incapable of inducing significant levels of donor engraftment in syngeneic models *(26,140)*. These properties are shared among a large number of other chemotherapeutic drugs, including 5-FU, melphalan, and thiotepa—probably related to the refractory nature of quiescent stem cells *(23,26,142)*. Busulfan and related compounds stand out as being particularly toxic to long-term repopulating (LTR) stem cells and can consequently allow for long-term donor engraftment *(23,26,143)*. Busulfan and dimethylbusulfan are poorly immune-suppressive *(144–147)*. Such agents therefore require addition of cyclophosphamide or anti-T-cell antibodies to achieve allo-engraftment in rodents *(143,146,148)*, and have now become an established alternative conditioning protocol in patients *(149,150)*. The relative contributions of the three principal effects on the lymphohematopoietic system are summarized in Table 2 for various agents commonly included in pretransplant conditioning protocols. 1) immune suppression leading to allograft acceptance, 2) acute myelodepression commonly associated with early but transient donor-cell engraftment, and 3) depletion of stem cells required for long-term chimerism.

An appreciation of which target cells in the host determine the outcome of hematopoietic engraftment has led to the exploration of potential therapies with greater specificity. Selectivity may be achieved with radiotherapy by localizing the radiation field to principal target tissues—such as lymphoid tissues and sanctuary sites—while shielding the organs that are commonly at risk, such as lung, gut, liver, and kidneys. The application of immune-suppressive courses of total lymphoid irradiation (TLI) constitutes such a strategy, which has already shown some clinical potential in combination with TLI for HLA-mismatched as well as matched allogeneic bone marrow *(151–153)*. Although the application of TLI in mice has also indicated its usefulness in allowing for allogeneic engraftment *(154)*, it is difficult to extrapolate such experimental studies to humans because of the small anatomical dimensions of the mouse and the effects of incident radiation exposure on a large component of the bone marrow. An alternative and perhaps more attractive approach to further abrogate antidonor reactivity may be the use of monoclonal antibodies (MAbs) against host immune-effector cells *(155–157)* or against adhesion molecules *(158–160)*. Antibodies can also be directed against host stem cells, and allow for engraftment without the necessity for high-dose

TBI. Voralia and colleagues *(161)* found that administration of an anti-class I antibody alone was able to facilitate the engraftment of syngeneic stem cells. A more recent study has shown that anti-CD45 antibody radioactively labeled with ^{131}I was effective in targeting lymphohematopoietic-specific antigens and in enabling engraftment of Ly5 congenic marrow *(162)*. ^{131}I-labeled anti-CD45 was also able to partially replace TBI when transplanting H-2 disparate marrow, forming the basis for on a clinical study that applies the human equivalent of radiolabeled antibody as a supplement to standard cyclophosphamide and TBI *(163)*.

8. NON-MYELOABLATIVE CONDITIONING

There is an obvious desire to reduce the intensity of pretransplant conditioning away from the treatment-related toxicities commonly encountered in conventional SCT. Preparative regimes that become mild enough to allow for recipient survival from endogenous hematopoietic repopulation alone—i.e., without SCT—are termed non-myeloablative. Other terms include "minimal ablative," "reduced-intensity," "sub-lethal" or "Nonlethal Conditioning" and, perhaps with more ambiguity, "mini-transplant" and "transplant-lite." One approach to achieving this lower level of conditioning while maintaining donor-type chimerism which has come to the forefront of both clinical and animal research has been to increase the number of infused stem cells. A competitive relationship between the donor and host stem cells has been studied in a syngeneic BMT model by varying the donor marrow as well as the radiation dose (van Os and Down, unpublished observations). In this case, increasing the bone-marrow-cell dose shifted the TBI dose-response curve for engraftment to lower doses because less stem-cell killing was presumably necessary given the higher competitive advantage of the transplanted stem cells (Fig. 6). Thus, at the radiation dose needed for equivalent engraftment, the number of surviving stem cells in the host is related to the competing number of transplanted cells. With marrow doses ranging from 10^5 to 10^7 cells, a 10-fold increase in cell number was able to reduce the radiation dose by approx 2 gy. This relationship produced a slope of relative stem-cell survival with radiation dose, from which a D_0 value of approx 1.3 Gy was obtained—a value in agreement with other assays of stem-cell radiosensitivity *(27,164)*. When very high bone-marrow cell doses (4×10^7 cells) are transplanted, donor-type chimerism can be detected even without the need for irradiation. Numerous other reports have similarly shown syngeneic stem-cell engraftment in unirradiated recipients when the donor cells are given at high doses *(161,165,166)*, to denote that donor stem cells can still occupy niches in the marrow without the need for stem-cell depletion. However, these conditions are extreme, requiring high doses of infused marrow that are unrealistic to attain in current clinical transplantation. A compromise may be reached by delivering radiation doses as low as 1 gy and obtaining reasonably high levels of donor-type chimerism (40%) at a more moderate marrow-cell dose (10×10^6 cells) *(167)*. Further improvement of long-term engraftment has been observed after combinations of G-CSF and/or SCF with low-dose TBI *(168,169)*. This phenomenon was not associated with an increase in stem-cell depletion, signifying that some other process, possibly an alteration in the supporting microenvironment and an enhancement in seeding efficiency of the transplanted donor stem cells, may play a role that could be exploited for clinical use.

In allogeneic BMT, non-myeloablative regimes offer the prospect of inducing stable mixed hematopoietic chimerism and creating a state of specific immune tolerance. In

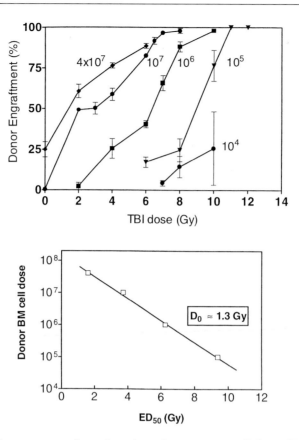

Fig. 6. Radiation dose-responses for various donor bone-marrow-cell doses (B6-*Gpi-1^a* → B6-*Gpi-1^b*). (A) Donor engraftment as a function of TBI dose is plotted for each bone-marrow-cell dose transplanted. It is assumed that the extra dose required for equivalent engraftment on lowering the donor-cell number corresponds to a proportional decrease in host LTRA survival. (B) The ED_{50} estimate (at 80% engraftment level) for each bone-marrow-cell dose was used to obtain a relative cell-survival curve and to calculate a D_0 for LTRA *in situ.* (van Os and Down, Unpublished data).

this case, extra immune suppression is often necessary to overcome the initial barrier imposed by host-vs-graft reactivity. This was first achieved by Cobbold and colleagues at a sublethal dose of 6 gy TBI by pretreating the recipients with depleting doses of anti-CD4 and anti-CD8 MAbs *(155).* Subsequently, Sharabi and Sachs *(170)* also used these antibodies, but were able to induce stable chimerism at a lower TBI dose of 3 gy if an additional dose of 7 gy was given locally to the thymus. Chimeric mice prepared with these regimens require a moderate dose of H-2-mismatched marrow cells (15×10^6), demonstrate donor-specific tolerance by their acceptance of donor-skin grafts and retain immunocompetence by their rejection of third-party grafts. The approach of pretreating recipients with a basic protocol of T-cell-depletion, 7 gy thymic irradiation, and 3 gy TBI has now been successfully extended to miniature swines *(171)* and cynomolgus monkeys *(172).* As in mice, these two large animal models demonstrated hematopoietic chimerism and donor-specific tolerance after infusion of allogeneic stem-cell grafts. In the murine allogeneic BMT model, TBI can be avoided altogether by raising the donor marrow-cell dose to the very high levels previously reported for syngeneic transplants. Sykes et al.

(173) were able to create tolerance-inducing levels of donor-type chimerism across an MHC-mismatched barrier by administering an extended course of the T-cell-depleting antibodies, local thymic irradiation, and 200×10^6 marrow cells delivered in five daily infusions. The addition of costimulatory blocking agents such as CTLA4lg or anti-CD154 (anti-CD40 ligand) to 3 gy TBI has recently proved to be valuable in overcoming the requirement for thymic irradiation or repeated injections of T-cell-depleting antibodies *(174)*. Another study showed that anti-CD154 antibody treatment could promote allogeneic chimerism (up to 40%) in presensitized recipients receiving only 1 gy TBI and a moderate high dose (40×10^6) of marrow cells *(177)*. Administration of anti-CD154 antibody and repeated marrow transplants (8 doses of 20×10^6 cells) can achieve lower levels of chimerism (6–12%) without TBI *(178)*. Finally, TBI has been replaced with cyclophosphamide in the T-cell depletion and thymic irradiation protocol, and this still permitted low levels of stem-cell engraftment that could then be converted to full chimeras after donor leukocyte infusion (DLI). All these studies dealing with non-myeloablative BMT preparation in mice have a direct bearing on the very current clinical efforts to reduce or even exclude the radiation conditioning in cancer patients receiving allogeneic SCT (177–180). Mixed donor-type chimerism is a notable feature in many of these patients, and the concurrent induction of immune tolerance with the less intensive preparative regimens opens up new opportunities to broaden the application of stem-cell transplants to include organ transplantation, autoimmune disease, and gene therapy.

REFERENCES

1. Ellinger F. Lethal dose studies with X-rays. *Radiology* 1945; 44:125–144.
2. Quastler H. Studies on roentgen death in mice. I. Survival time and dosage. *Am J Roentgenol* 1945; 54:449–456.
3. Hall E. Radiobiology for the Radiobiologist. JB Lippincott, Philadelphia, PA, 1988.
4. Till JE, McCulloch EA. A direct measurement of the radiation sensitivity of normal mouse bone marrow cells. *Radiat Res* 1961; 14:213–222.
5. Hendry J, Lord B. The analysis of the early and late response to cytotoxic insults in the haematopoietic cell hierarchy. In: Potten C, Hendry J. *Cytotoxic Insult to Tissues: Effects on Cell Lineages,* vol. 2. Churchill Livingstone, New York, NY, 1983, 1–66.
6. Hendry JH, Howard A. The response of haemopoietic colony-forming units to single and split-doses of gamma-rays or D-T neutrons. *Int J Radiat Biol* 1971; 19:51–64.
7. Tarbell NJ, Amato DA, Down JD, Mauch P, Hellman S. Fractionation and dose-rate effects in mice: a model for bone marrow transplantation in man. *Int J Radiat Oncol Biol Phys* 1987; 13:1065–1069.
8. Till JE, McCulloch EA. Early repair processes in marrow cells irradiated and proliferating *in vivo*. *Radiat Res* 1963; 18:96–105.
9. Imai Y, Nakao I. *In vivo* radiosensitivity and recovery pattern of the hematopoietic precursor cells and stem cells in mouse bone marrow. *Exp Hematol* 1987; 15:890–895.
10. Kaplan HS, Brown MB. Mortality of mice after total body irradiation as influenced by alterations in total dose, fractionation and periodicity of treatment. *J Natl Cancer Inst* 1952; 12:765–775.
11. Paterson E, Gilbert CW, Matthews J. Time intensity factors and whole body irradiation. *Br J Radiol* 1952; 25:427–433.
12. Krebs JS, Brauer RW. Accumulation of lethal irradiation doses by fractionated exposure to X-rays. *Radiat Res* 1965; 25:480–488.
13. Hodgson GS, Bradley TR. Properties of haematopoietic stem cells surviving 5-fluorouracil treatment: evidence for a pre-CFU-S cell? *Nature* 1979; 281:381–382.
14. Harrison DE. Competitive repopulation: a new assay for long-term stem cell functional capacity. *Blood* 1980; 55:77–81.
15. Ploemacher RE, Brons NHC. Isolation of hemopoietic stem cell subsets from murine bone marrow: II. evidence for an early precursor of day-12 CFU-S and cells associated with radioprotective ability. *Exp Hematol* 1988; 16:27–32.

16. Ploemacher RE, Brons NHC. Separation of CFU-S from primitive cells responsible for reconstitution of the bone marrow hemopoietic stem cell compartment following irradiation: evidence for a pre-CFU-S cell. *Exp Hematol* 1989; 17:263–266.

17. Jones R, Wagner J, Celano P, Zicha M, Sharkis S. Separation of pluripotent hematopoietic stem cells from spleen colony-forming cells. *Nature* 1990; 347:188–189.

18. Ploemacher RE, van der Loo JCM, Van Beurden CAJ, Baert MRM. Wheat germ agglutinin affinity of murine hemopoietic stem cell subpopulations is an inverse function of their long-term repopulating ability in vitro and in vivo. *Leukemia* 1993; 7:120–130.

19. Pallavicini MG, Redfearn W, Necas E, Brecher G. Rescue from lethal irradiation correlates with transplantation of 10–20 CFU-S-day 12. *Blood Cells Mol Dis* 1997; 23:157–168.

20. Harrison D, Astle C, Lerner C. Number and continuous proliferative pattern of transplanted primitive immunohematopoietic stem cells. *Proc Natl Acad Sci USA* 1988; 85:822–826.

21. Harrison D, Jordan C, Zhong R-K, Astle C. Primitive hemopoietic stem cells: direct assay of most productive populations by competitive repopulation with simple binomial, correlation and covariance calculations. *Exp Hematol* 1993; 21:206–219.

22. Harrison D, Lerner C. Most primitive hematopoietic stem cells are stimulated to cycle rapidly after treatment with 5-fluorouracil. *Blood* 1991; 78:1237–1240.

23. Down JD, Ploemacher RE. Transient and permanent engraftment potential of murine hematopoietic stem cell subsets: differential effects of host conditioning with gamma radiation and cytotoxic drugs. *Exp Hematol* 1993; 21:913–921.

24. Ploemacher RE, van der Sluijs JP, Voerman JSA, Brons NHC. An in vitro limiting-dilution assay of long-term repopulating hematopoietic stem cells in the mouse. *Blood* 1989; 74:2755–2763.

25. Ploemacher RE, van der Sluijs JP, Van Beurden CAJ, Baert MRM, Chan PL. Use of limiting-dilution type long-term marrow cultures in frequency analysis of marrow-repopulating and spleen colony-forming hematopoietic stem cells in the mouse. *Blood* 1991; 10:2527–2533.

26. Down J, Boudewijn A, Dillingh J, Fox B, Ploemacher R. Relationship between ablation of distinct haematopoietic cell subsets and the development of donor bone marrow engraftment following recipient pretreatment with different alkylating drugs. *Br J Cancer* 1994; 70:611–616.

27. Ploemacher RE, van Os RP, Van Beurden CAJ, Down JD. Murine hematopoietic stem cells with long-term engraftment and marrow repopulating ability are less radiosensitive to gamma radiation than are spleen colony forming cells. *Int J Radiat Biol* 1992; 61:489–499.

28. Barendsen GW. Dose fractionation, dose rate and iso-effect relationships for normal tissue responses. *Int. J Radiat Oncol Biol Phys* 1982; 8:1981–1987.

29. Thames HD, Jr, Rozell ME, Tucker SL, Ang KK, Fisher DR, Travis EL. Direct analysis of quantal radiation response data. *Int J Radiat Biol Relat Stud Phys Chem Med* 1986; 49:999–1009.

30. Stuben G, Landuyt W, van der SE, van der Kogel AJ, Reijnders A. Estimation of repair parameters in mouse lip mucosa during continuous and fractionated low dose-rate irradiation. *Radiother Oncol* 1991; 20:38–45.

31. Chougule A, Supe SJ. Linear quadratic model—estimation of alpha/beta ratio for mucosal reaction. *Strahlenther Onkol* 1993; 169:427–430.

32. Douglas BG, Fowler JF. The effect of multiple small doses of x rays on skin reactions in the mouse and a basic interpretation. *Radiat Res* 1976; 66:401–426.

33. Withers HR, Reid BO, Hussey DH. Response of mouse jejunum to multifraction radiation. *Int J Radiat Oncol Biol Phys* 1975; 1:41–52.

34. Peck JW, Gibbs FA. Mechanical assay of consequential and primary late radiation effects in murine small intestine: alpha/beta analysis. *Radiat Res* 1994; 138:272–281.

35. Brown JAH, Corp MJ, Mole RH. The effect of dose-rate and fractionation on acute mortality in X-irradiated mice. Part II. *Int J Radiat Biol* 1962; 5:369–377.

36. Travis EL, Fang MZ, Basic I. Protection of mouse bone marrow by WR-2721 after fractionated irradiation. *Int Radiat Oncol Biol Phys* 1988; 15:377–382.

37. van Os R, Thames HD, Konings AW, Down JD. Radiation dose-fractionation and dose-rate relationships for long-term repopulating hemopoietic stem cells in a murine bone marrow transplant model. *Radiat Res* 1993; 136:118–125.

38. Down JD, Boudewijn A, van Os R, Thames HD, Ploemacher RE. Variations in radiation sensitivity and repair among different hematopoietic stem cell subsets following fractionated irradiation. *Blood* 1995; 86:122–127.

39. Down JD, Easton DF, Steel GG. Repair in the mouse lung during low dose-rate irradiation. *Radiother Oncol* 1986; 6:29–42.

40. Travis EL, Thames HD, Watkins TL, Kiss I. The kinetics of repair in mouse lung after fractionated irradiation. *Int J Radiat Biol Relat Stud Phys Chem Med* 1987; 52:903–919.

41. Vegesna V, Withers HR, Taylor JM. Repair kinetics of mouse lung. *Radiother Oncol* 1989; 15:115–123.

42. Stewart FA, Soranson JA, Alpen EL, Williams MV, Denekamp J. Radiation-induced renal damage: the effects of hyperfractionation. *Radiat Res* 1984; 98:407–420.

43. Thames HD, Ang KK, Stewart FA, van der Schueren E. Does incomplete repair explain the apparent failure of the basic LQ model to predict spinal cord and kidney responses to low doses per fraction? *Int J Radiat Biol* 1988; 54:13–19.

44. Bentzen SM, Thames HD, Overgaard M. Latent-time estimation for late cutaneous and subcutaneous radiation reactions in a single-follow-up clinical study. *Radiother Oncol* 1989; 15:267–274.

45. Ford CE, Hamerton JL, Barnes DWH, Loutit JF. Cytological identification of radiation chimaeras. *Nature* 1956; 177:452–454.

46. van der Sluijs J, van den Bos C, Baert M, Van Beurden C, Ploemacher R. Loss of long-term repopulating ability in long-term bone marrow culture. *Leukemia* 1993; 7:725–732.

47. Hampson IN, Spooncer E, Dexter TM. Evaluation of a mouse Y chromosome probe for assessing marrow transplantation. *Exp Hematol* 1989; 17:313–315.

48. Soderling CC, Song CW, Blazar BR, Vallera DA. A correlation between conditioning and engraftment in recipients of MHC-mismatched T cell-depleted murine bone marrow transplants. *J Immunol* 1985; 135:941–946.

49. Lapidot T, Singer T, Reisner Y. Transient engraftment of T cell depleted allogeneic bone marrow in mice improves survival rate following lethal irradiation. *Bone Marrow Transplant* 1988; 3:157–164.

50. Salomon O, Lapidot T, Terenzi A, Lubin I, Rabi I, Reisner Y. Induction of donor-type chimerism in murine recipients of bone marrow allografts by different radiation regimens currently used in treatment of leukemia patients. *Blood* 1990; 76:1872–1888.

51. Sprangrude GJ, Heimfeld S, Weissman IL. Purification and characterization of mouse hematopoietic stem cells [published erratum appears in *Science* 1989 Jun 2;244(4908):1030]. *Science* 1988; 241:58–62.

52. Li CL, Johnson GR. Long-term hemopoietic repopulation by Thy-1lo, Lin-, Ly6A/E+ cells. *Exp Hematol* 1992; 20:1309–1319.

53. Sprangrude GJ, Johnson GR. Resting and activated subsets of mouse multipotent hematopoietic stem cells. *Proc Natl Acad Sci USA* 1990; 87:7433–7437.

54. van Os R, Sheridan TM, Robinson S, Drukteinis D, Ferrara JL, Mauch PM. Immunogenicity of Ly5 (CD45)-antigens hampers long-term engraftment following minimal conditioning in a murine bone marrow transplantation model. *Stem cells* 2001; 19:80–87.

55. Ferrara JLM, Lipton J, Hellman S, Burakoff S, Mauch P. Engraftment following T-cell-depleted bone marrow transplantation. I. The role of major and minor histocompatibility barriers. *Transplantation* 1987; 43:461–467.

56. Ferrara JLM, Mauch P, Mclntyre J, Michaelson J, Burakoff S. Engraftment following T-cell-depleted bone marrow transplantation. II. Stability of mixed chimerism in semiallogeneic recipients after total-body irradiation. *Transplantation* 1987; 44:495–499.

57. Francescutti LH, Gambel P, Wegmann TG. Characterization of hemopoietic stem cell chimerism in antibody-facilitated bone marrow chimeras. *Transplantation* 1985; 40:7–11.

58. Barker JE, Braun J, McFarland-Starr E. Erythrocyte replacement precedes leukocyte replacement during repopulation of W/W^v mice with limiting dilutions of +/+ donor marrow cells. *Proc Natl Acad Sci USA* 1988; 85:7332–7335.

59. Ansell J, Micklem H. Genetic markers for following cell populations. In: Weir DM, Herzenberg LA, Blackwell CC. *Handbook of Experimental Immunology,* vol. 2, 4th ed. Blackwell, Edinburgh, 1986, pp. 56.1–56.18.

60. Sigounas G, MacVittie TJ. Transgenic marrow transplantation: A new *in vivo* and *in vitro* system for experimental hemopoiesis and radiobiology which employs sequential molecular monitoring of multiple genetic markers. *Radiat Res* 1993; 135:206–211.

61. Phillips K, Gentry T, McCowage G, Gilboa E, Smith C. Cell-surface markers for assessing gene transfer into human hematopoietic cells. *Nat Med* 1996; 2:1154–1156.

62. Persons DA, Allay JA, Riberdy JM, Wersto RP, Donahue RE, Sorrentino BP et al. Use of the green fluorescent protein as a marker to identify and track genetically modified hematopoietic cells. *Nat Med* 1998; 4:1201–1205.

63. Van Hennik PB, Verstegen MM, Bierhuizen MF, Limon A, Wognum AW, Cancelas JA, et al. Highly efficient transduction of the green fluorescent protein gene in human umbilical cord blood stem cells

capable of cobblestone formation in long-term cultures and multilineage engraftment of immunodeficient mice. *Blood* 1998; 92:4013–4022.

64. Wu AM, Till JE, Siminovich L, McCulloch EA. A cytological study of the capacity for differentiation of normal hemopoietic colony-forming cells. *J Cell Physiol* 1967; 69:177–184.

65. Magli MC, Iscove NN, Odartchenko N. Transient nature of early haematopoietic spleen colonies. *Nature* 1982; 295:527–529.

66. Ploemacher RE, Brons NHC. In vivo proliferative and differential properties of murine bone marrow cells separated on the basis of rhodamine-123 retention. *Exp Hematol* 1988; 16:903–907.

67. Harrison D, Zhong R-K. The same exhaustible multilineage precursor produces both myeloid and lymphoid cells as early as 3–4 weeks after marrow transplantation. *Proc Natl Acad Sci USA* 1992; 89:10,134–10,138.

68. Stutman O. Intrathymic and extrathymic T cell maturation. *Immunol Rev* 1978; 42:138–184.

69. Van Furth R. Origin and turnover of monocytes and macrophages. *Curr Top Pathol* 1989; 79P:125–150.

70. Down J, Berman A, Warhol M, Yeap B, Mauch P. Late complications following total-body irradiation and bone marrow rescue in mice: predominance of glomerular nephropathy and hemolytic anemia. *Int J Radiat Biol* 1990; 57:551–565.

71. Lemischka I, Raulet D, Mulligan R. Developmental potential and dynamic behavior of hematopoietic stem cells. *Cell* 1986; 45:917–927.

72. Jordan CT, Lemischka IR. Clonal and systemic analysis of long-term hematopoiesis in the mouse. *Genes Dev* 1990; 4:220–232.

73. Lemischka I. The haematopoietic stem cell and its clonal progeny: mechanisms regulating the hierarchy of primitive haematopoietic cells. *Cancer Surv* 1992; 15:3–18.

74. Parkman R, Gelfand EW, Rosen FS, Sanderson A, Hirschhorn, R. Severe combined immunodeficiency and adenosine deaminase deficiency. *N Engl J Med* 1975; 292:714–719.

75. van Leeuwen JE, van Tol MJ, Joosten AM, Schellekens PT, van den Bergh RL, Waaijer JL, et al. Relationship between patterns of engraftment in peripheral blood and immune reconstitution after allogeneic bone marrow transplantation for (severe) combined immunodeficiency. *Blood* 1994; 84:3936–3947.

76. Minegishi Y, Ishii N, Tsuchida M, Okawa H, Sugamura K, Yata J. T cell reconstitution by haploidentical BMT does not restore the diversification of the Ig heavy chain gene in patients with X-linked SCID. *Bone Marrow Transplant* 1995; 16:801–806.

77. Borzy MS, Ridgway D, Noya FJ, Shearer WT. Successful bone marrow transplantation with split lymphoid chimerism in DiGeorge syndrome. *J Clin Immunol* 1989; 9,386–392.

78. Fulop G, Phillips R. The scid mutation in mice causes a general defect in DNA repair. *Nature* 1990; 347:479–482.

79. Biederman K, Sun J, Giaccia A, Tosto L, Brown J. SCID-mutation in mice confers hypersensitivity to ionizing radiation and a deficiency in DNA double-strand break repair. *Proc Natl Acad Sci USA* 1991; 88:1394–1397.

80. Blunt T, Finnie NJ, Taccioli GE, Smith GC, Demengeot J, Gottlieb TM, et al. Defective DNA-dependent protein kinase activity is linked to V(D)J recombination and DNA repair defects associated with the murine scid mutation. *Cell* 1995; 80:813–823.

81. Kirchgessner CU, Patil CK, Evans JW, Cuomo CA, Fried LM, Carter T, et al. DNA-dependent kinase (p350) as a candidate gene for the murine SCID defect. *Science* 1995; 267:1178–1183.

82. Nakano T, Waki N, Asai H, Kitamura Y. Different repopulation profile between erythroid and nonerythroid progenitor cells in genetically anemic W/Wv mice after bone marrow transplantation. *Blood* 1989; 74:1552–1556.

83. Nakano T, Waki N, Asai H, Kitamura Y. Lymphoid differentiation of the hematopoietic stem cell that reconstitutes total erythropoiesis of a genetically anemic W/Wv mouse. *Blood* 1989; 73:1175–1179.

84. Barker JE, Compton ST. Hematopoietic repopulation of adult mice with beta-thalassemia. *Blood* 1994; 83:828–832.

85. van den BC, Kieboom D, van der Sluijs JP, Baert MR, Ploemacher RE, Wagemaker G. Selective advantage of normal erythrocyte production after bone marrow transplantation of alpha-thalassemic mice. *Exp Hematol* 1994; 22:441–446.

86. van der Loo JC, van den BC, Baert MR, Wagemaker G, Ploemacher RE. Stable multilineage hematopoietic chimerism in alpha-thalassemic mice induced by a bone marrow subpopulation that excludes the majority of day-12 spleen colony-forming units. *Blood* 1994; 83:1769–1777.

87. Bjorgvinsdottir H, Ding C, Pech N, Gifford MA, Li LL, Dinauer MC. Retroviral-mediated gene transfer of gp91phox into bone marrow cells rescues defect in host defense against Aspergillus fumigatus in murine X-linked chronic granulomatous disease. *Blood* 1997; 89:41–48.

88. Mardiney M III, Jackson SH, Spratt SK, Li F, Holland SM, Malech HL. Enhanced host defense after gene transfer in the murine p47phox-deficient model of chronic granulomatous disease. *Blood* 1997; 89:2268–2275.

89. Dinauer MC, Li LL, Bjorgvinsdottir H, Ding C, Pech N. Long-term correction of phagocyte NADPH oxidase activity by retroviral-mediated gene transfer in murine X-linked chronic granulomatous disease. *Blood* 1999; 94:914–922.

90. Snell G, Stimpling J. Genetics of tissue transplantation. In: Green E. *Biology of the Laboratory Mouse,* 2nd ed. McGraw Hill, New York, NY, 1966; 457–491.

91. Michaelson J, Lawrence M, Dorf M. Genetics of bone marrow engraftment in mice. *J Cell Biochem* 1988 (Suppl. 12C) abstract #K126.

92. Gengozian N, Carlson D, Allen E. Transplantation of allogeneic and xenogeneic (rat) marrow in irradiated mice as affected by radiation exposure rates. *Transplantation* 1969; 7:259–273.

93. Cudkowicz G, Bennett M. Peculiar immunobiology of bone marrow allografts. I. Graft rejection by irradiated responder mice. *J Exp Med* 1971; 134:83–102.

94. Sado T, Kamisuka H, Kubo E. Strain difference in the radiosensitivity of immunocompetent cells and its influence on the residual host-vs-graft reaction in lethally irradiated mice grafted with semiallogeneic bone marrow. *J Immunol* 1985; 134:704–710.

95. Schwartz E, Lapidot T, Gozes D, Singer T, Reisner Y. Abrogation of bone marrow allograft resistance in mice by increased total body irradiation correlates with eradication of host clonable T cells and alloreactive cytotoxic precursors. *J Immunol* 1987; 138:460–465.

96. Dennert G, Anderson C, Warner J. T killer cells play a role in allogeneic bone marrow graft rejection but not in hybrid resistance. *J Immunol* 1985; 135:3729–3734.

97. Sentman C, Kumar V, Koo G, Bennett M. Effector cell expression of NK1.1, a murine natural killer cell-specific molecule, and ability of mice to reject bone marrow allografts. *J Immunol* 1989; 142:1847–1853.

98. Nakamura H, Gress R. Graft rejection by cytolytic T cells. Specificity of the effector mechanism in the rejection of allogeneic marrow. *Transplantation* 1990; 49:453–458.

99. Bunjes D, Heit W, Arnold R, Schmeiser T, Wiesneth M, Carbonell F, et al. Evidence for the involvement of host-derived OKT8-positive T, cells in the rejection of T-depleted, HLA-identical bone marrow grafts. *Transplantation* 1987; 43:501–505.

100. Marijt WA, Kernan NA, Diaz-Barrientos T, Veenhof WF, O'Reilly RJ, Willemze R, et al. Multiple minor histocompatibility antigen-specific cytotoxic T lymphocyte clones can be generated during graft rejection after HLA-identical bone marrow transplantation. *Bone Marrow Transplant* 1995; 16:125–132.

101. Lamb LS, Jr., Szafer F, Henslee-Downey PJ, Walker M, King S, Godder K, et al. Characterization of acute bone marrow graft rejection in T cell-depleted, partially mismatched related donor bone marrow transplantation. *Exp Hematol* 1995; 23:1595–1600.

102. Lamb LS, Jr., Gee AP, Parrish RS, Lee C, Walker M, Geier S, et al. Acute rejection of marrow grafts in patients transplanted from a partially mismatched related donor: clinical and immunologic characteristics. *Bone Marrow Transplant* 1996; 17:1021–1027.

103. van Os R, Konings AW, Down JD. Radiation dose as a factor in host preparation for bone marrow transplantation across different genetic barriers. *Int J Radiat Biol* 1992; 61:501–510.

104. Van Putten LM, Van Bekkum DW, Vries Md, Balner H. The effect of preceding blood transfusions on the fate of homologous bone marrow grafts in lethally irradiated monkeys. *Blood* 1967; 30:749–757.

105. Weiden PL, Storb R, Thomas ED, Graham TC, Lerner KG, Buckner CD, et al. Preceding transfusions and marrow graft rejection in dogs and man. *Transplant Proc* 1976; 8:551–554.

106. van Os R, de Witte T, Dillingh JH, Mauch PM, Down JD. Increased rejection of murine allogeneic bone marrow in presensitized recipients. *Leukemia* 1997; 11:1045–1048.

107. van Os R, Konings AW, Down JD. Compromising effect of low dose-rate total body irradiation on allogeneic bone marrow engraftment. *Int J Radiat Biol* 1993; 64:761–770.

108. Down J, Tarbell N, Thames H, Mauch P. Syngeneic and allogeneic bone marrow engraftment after total body irradiation: Dependence on dose, dose-rate, and fractionation. *Blood* 1991; 77:661–669.

109. Lösslein L, Kolb HJ, Porzsolt S. Hyperfractionation of total-body irradiation and engraftment of marrow from DLA-haploidentical littermates. *Transplant Proc* 1987; XIX:2707–2708.

110. Storb R, Raff RF, Appelbaum FR, Graham TC, Schuening FG, Sale G, et al. Comparison of fraction-ated to single-dose total body irradiation in conditioning canine littermates for DLA-identical marrow grafts. *Blood* 1989; 74:1139–1143.

111. Patterson J, Prentice HG, Brenner MK, Gilmore M, Janossy G, Ivory K, et al. Graft rejection follow-ing HLA matched T-lymphocyte depleted bone marrow transplantation. *Br J Haematol* 1986; 63:221–230.

112. Guyotat D, Dutou L, Ehrsam A, Campos L, Archimbaud E, Fiere D. Graft rejection after T-cell depleted marrow transplantation: role of fractionated irradiation [letter]. *Br J Haematol* 1987; 65:499.

113. Iriondo A, Hermosa V, Richard C, Conde E, Bello C, Garijo J, et al. Graft rejection following T lym-phocyte depleted bone marrow transplantation with two different TBI regimens [letter]. *Br J Haema-tol* 1987; 65:246–248.

114. Ferrara JL, Levy R, Chao NJ. Pathophysiologic mechanisms of acute graft-vs.-host disease. *Biol Blood Marrow Transplant* 1999; 5:347–356.

115. Down J, Mauch P, Warhol M, Neben S, Ferrara J. The effect of donor T lymphocytes and total-body irradiation on hemopoietic engraftment and pulmonary toxicity following experimental allogeneic bone marrow transplantation. *Transplantation* 1992; 54:802–808.

116. Cooke KR, Krenger W, Hill G, Martin TR, Kobzik L, Brewer J, et al. Host reactive donor T cells are associated with lung injury after experimental allogeneic bone marrow transplantation. *Blood* 1998; 92:2571–80.

117. Shankar G, Scott BJ, Darrell JC, Kaplan AM, Cohen DA. Idiopathic pneumonia syndrome after allo-geneic bone marrow transplantation in mice. Role of pretransplant radiation conditioning. *Am J Respir Cell Mol Biol* 1999; 20:1116–1124.

118. Panoskaltsis-Mortari A, Taylor PA, Yaeger TM, Wangensteen OD, Bitterman PB, Ingbar DH, et al. The critical early proinflammatory events associated with idiopathic pneumonia syndrome in irradi-ated murine allogeneic recipients are due to donor T cell infusion and potentiated by cyclophos-phamide. *J Clin Invest* 1997; 100:1015–1027.

119. Haddad IY, Panoskaltsis-Mortari A, Ingbar DH, Yang S, Milla CE, Blazar BR. High levels of perox-ynitrite are generated in the lungs of irradiated mice given cyclophosphamide and allogeneic T cells. A potential mechanism of injury after marrow transplantation. *Am J Respir Cell Mol Biol* 1999; 20:1125–1135.

120. Hill GR, Crawford JM, Cooke KR, Brinson YS, Pan L, Ferrara JL. Total body irradiation and acute graft-versus-host disease: the role of gastrointestinal damage and inflammatory cytokines. *Blood* 1997; 90:3204–3213.

121. Hill GR, Cooke KR, Brinson YS, Bungard D, Ferrara JL. Pretransplant chemotherapy reduces inflam-matory cytokine production and acute graft-versus-host disease after allogeneic bone marrow trans-plantation. *Transplantation* 1999; 67:1478–1480.

122. Korngold B, Sprent J. Lethal graft-versus-host disease after bone marrow transplantation across minor histocompatibility barriers in mice. Prevention by removing mature T cells from marrow. *J Exp Med* 1978; 148:1687–1698.

123. Trigg ME, Billing R, Sondel PM, Exten R, Hong R, Bozdech MJ, et al. Clinical trial depleting T lym-phocytes from donor marrow for matched and mismatched allogeneic bone marrow transplants. *Can-cer Treat Rep* 1985; 69:377–386.

124. Mitsuyasu RT, Champlin RE, Gale RP, Ho WG, Lenarsky C, Winston D, et al. Treatment of donor bone marrow with monoclonal anti-T-cell antibody and complement for the prevention of graft-ver-sus-host disease. A prospective, randomized, double-blind trial. *Ann Intern Med* 1986; 105:20–26.

125. Champlin R. T-cell depletion to prevent graft-versus-host disease after bone marrow transplantation. *Hematol Oncol Clin N Am* 1990; 4:687–698.

126. Kloosterman TC, Tielemans MJ, Martens AC, Van Bekkum DW, Hagenbeek A. Quantitative studies on graft-versus-leukemia after allogeneic bone marrow transplantation in rat models for acute myelo-cytic and lymphocytic leukemia. *Bone Marrow Transplant* 1994; 14:15–22.

127. Blazar BR, Taylor PA, Boyer MW, Panoskaltsis-Mortari A, Allison JP, Vallera DA. CD28/B7 interac-tions are required for sustaining the graft-versus-leukemia effect of delayed post-bone marrow trans-plantation splenocyte infusion in murine recipients of myeloid or lymphoid leukemia cells. *J Immunol* 1997; 159:3460–3473.

128. Johnson BD, Drobyski WR, Truitt RL. Delayed infusion of normal donor cells after MHC-matched bone marrow transplantation provides an antileukemia reaction without graft-versus-host disease. *Bone Marrow Transplant* 1993; 11:329–336.

129. Sykes M, Romick ML, Sachs DH. Interleukin 2 prevents graft-versus-host disease while preserving the graft-versus-leukemia effect of allogeneic T cells. *Proc Natl Acad Sci USA* 1990; 87:5633–5637.

130. Yang YG, Sergio JJ, Pearson DA, Szot GL, Shimizu A, Sykes M. Interleukin-12 preserves the graft-versus-leukemia effect of allogeneic CD8 T cells while inhibiting CD4-dependent graft-versus-host disease in mice. *Blood* 1997; 90:4651–4660.

131. Johnson BD, Becker EE, LaBelle JL, Truitt RL. Role of immunoregulatory donor T cells in suppression of graft-versus-host disease following donor leukocyte infusion therapy. *J Immunol* 1999; 163:6479–6487.

132. Johnson BD, Becker EE, Truitt RL. Graft-vs.-host and graft-vs.-leukemia reactions after delayed infusions of donor T-subsets. *Biol Blood Marrow Transplant* 1999; 5:123–132.

133. Ito M, Shizuru JA. Graft-vs-lymphoma effect in an allogeneic hematopoietic stem cell transplantation model. *Biol Blood Marrow Transplant* 1999; 5:357–368.

134. Bacchetta R, Vandekerckhove BA, Touraine JL, Bigler M, Martino S, Gebuhrer L, et al. Chimerism and tolerance to host and donor in severe combined immunodeficiencies transplanted with fetal liver stem cells. *J Clin Invest* 1993; 91:1067–1078.

135. Kaufman CL, Colson YL, Wren SM, Watkins S, Simmons RL, Ildstad ST. Phenotypic characterization of a novel bone marrow-derived cell that facilitates engraftment of allogeneic bone marrow stem cells. *Blood* 1994; 84:2436–2446.

136. Gandy KL, Domen J, Aguila H, Weissman IL. CD8+TCR+ and CD8+TCR-cells in whole bone marrow facilitate the engraftment of hematopoietic stem cells across allogeneic barriers. *Immunity* 1999; 11:579–590.

137. Martin PJ. Winning the battle of graft versus host [news]. *Nat Med* 2000; 6:18–19.

138. Sprent J, Surh CD, Agus D, Hurd M, Sutton S, Heath WR. Profound atrophy of the bone marrow reflecting major histocompatibility complex class II-restricted destruction of stem cells by CD4+ cells. *J Exp Med* 1994; 180:307–317.

139. Welniak LA, Blazar BR, Anver MR, Wiltrout RH, Murphy WJ. Opposing roles of interferon-gamma on CD4+ T cell-mediated graft-versus-host disease: effects of conditioning. *Biol Blood Marrow Transplant* 2000; 6:604–612.

140. Uharek L, Glass B, Gassmann W, Eckstein V, Steinmann J, Loeffler H, et al. Engraftment of allogeneic bone marrow cells: experimental investigations on the role of cell dose, graft-versus-host reactive T cells and pretransplant immunosuppression. *Transplant Proc* 1992; 24:3023–3025.

141. Colson YL, Wren SM, Schuchert MJ, Patrene KD, Johnson PC, Boggs SS, et al. A nonlethal conditioning approach to achieve durable multilineage mixed chimerism and tolerance across major, minor, and hematopoietic histocompatibility barriers. *J Immunol* 1995; 155:4179–4188.

142. Down J, Mauch P. The effect of combining cyclophosphamide with total body irradiation on donor bone marrow engraftment. *Transplantation* 1991; 51:1309–1311.

143. Botnick L, Hannon E, Viognuelle R, Hellman S. Differential effects of cytotoxic agents on hematopoietic progenitors. *Cancer Res* 1981; 41:2338–2342.

144. Down JD, Westerhof GR, Boudewijn A, Setroikromo R, Ploemacher RE. Thiotepa improves allogeneic bone marrow engraftment without enhancing stem cell depletion in irradiated mice. *Bone Marrow Transplant* 1998; 21:327–330.

145. Westerhof GR, Ploemacher RE, Boudewijn A, Blokland I, Dillingh JH, McGown AT, et al. Comparison of different busulfan analogues for depletion of hematopoietic stem cells and promotion of donor-type chimerism in murine bone marrow transplant recipients. *Cancer Res* 2000; 60:5470–5478.

146. Floersheim GL, Ruszkiewicz M. Bone-marrow transplantation after antilymphocytic serum and lethal chemotherapy. *Nature* 1969; 222:854–857.

147. Kolb HJ, Storb R, Weiden PL, Ochs HD, Kolb H, Graham TC, et al. Immunologic, toxicologic and marrow transplantation studies in dogs given dimethyl myleran. *Biomedicine* 1974; 20:341–351.

148. Santos GW. Immunosuppression for clinical marrow transplantation. *Semin Hematol* 1974; 11:341–351.

149. Samlowski WE, Araneo BA, Butler MO, Fung MC, Johnson HM. Peripheral lymph node helper T-cell recovery after syngeneic bone marrow transplantation in mice prepared with either gamma-irradiation or busulfan. *Blood* 1989; 74:1436–1445.

150. Leong LY, Qin S, Cobbold SP, Waldmann H. Classical transplantation tolerance in the adult: the interaction between myeloablation and immunosuppression. *Eur J Immunol* 1992; 22:2825–2830.

151. Bortin MM, Horowitz MM, Gale RP, Barrett AJ, Champlin RE, Dicke KA, et al., Changing trends in allogeneic bone marrow transplantation for leukemia in the 1980s. *JAMA* 1992; 268:607–612.

152. Copelan EA, Deeg HJ. Conditioning for allogeneic marrow transplantation in patients with lympho-hematopoietic malignancies without the use of total body irradiation. *Blood* 1992; 80:1648–1658.

153. Champlin RE, Ho WG, Mitsuyasu R, Burnison M, Greenberg P, Holly G, et al. Graft failure and leukemia relapse following T lymphocyte-depleted bone marrow transplants: effect of intensification of immunosuppressive conditioning. *Transplant Proc* 1987; 19:2616–2619.

154. Ganem G, Kuentz M, Beaujean F, Lebourgeois JP, Vinci G, Cordonnier C, et al. Additional total-lymphoid irradiation in preventing graft failure of T-cell-depleted bone marrow transplantation from HLA-identical siblings. Results of a prospective randomized study. *Transplantation* 1988; 45:244–248.

155. Soiffer RJ, Mauch P, Tarbell NJ, Anderson KC, Freedman AS, Rabinowe SN, et al. Total lymphoid irradiation to prevent graft rejection in recipients of HLA non-identical T cell-depleted allogeneic marrow. *Bone Marrow Transplant* 1991; 7:23–33.

156. Slavin S, Fuks Z, Kaplan HS, Strober S. Transplantation of allogeneic bone marrow without graft-versus-host disease using total lymphoid irradiation. *J Exp Med* 1978; 147:963–972.

157. Cobbold SP, Martin G, Qin S, Waldmann H. Monoclonal antibodies to promote marrow engraftment and tissue graft tolerance. *Nature* 1986; 323:164–166.

158. Ferrara JLM, Mauch P, van Dijken PJ. Evidence that anti-asialo GM1 in vivo improves engraftment of T cell depleted bone marrow in hybrid recipients. *Transplantation* 1990; 49:134–138.

159. Hiruma K, Hirsch R, Patchen M, Bluestone JA, Gress RE. Effects of anti-CD3 monoclonal antibody on engraftment of T-cell-depleted bone marrow allografts in mice: host T-cell suppression, growth factors, and space. *Blood* 1992; 79:3050–3058.

160. Fischer A, Griscelli C, Blanche S, Le Deist F, Veber F, Lopez M, et al. Prevention of graft failure by an anti-HLFA-1 monoclonal antibody in HLA-mismatched bone-marrow transplantation. *Lancet* 1986; 2:1058–1061.

161. van Dijken PJ, Ghayur T, Mauch P, Down J, Burakoff SJ, Ferrara JL. Evidence that anti-LFA-1 in vivo improves engraftment and survival after allogeneic bone marrow transplantation. *Transplantation* 1990; 49:882–886.

162. Blazar BR, Carroll SF, Vallera DA. Prevention of murine graft-versus-host disease and bone marrow alloengraftment across the major histocompatibility barrier after donor graft preincubation with anti-LFA1 immunotoxin. *Blood* 1991; 78:3093–3102.

163. Voralia M, Semeluk A, Wegmann T. Facilitation of syngeneic stem cell engraftment by anti-class monoclonal antibody pre-treatment of unirradiated recipients. *Transplantation* 1987; 44:487–494.

164. Matthews DC, Martin PJ, Nourigat C, Appelbaum FR, Fisher DR, Bernstein ID. Marrow ablative and immunosuppressive effects of (231) I-anti-CD45 antibody in congenic and H2-mismatched murine transplant models. *Blood* 1999; 93:737–745.

165. Matthews DC, Appelbaum FR, Eary JF, Fisher DR, Durack LD, Hui TE, et al. Phase I study of (131)I-anti-CD45 antibody plus cyclophosphamide and total body irradiation for advanced acute leukemia and myelodysplastic syndrome. *Blood* 1999; 94:1237–1247.

166. Meijne EI, Winden-van Groenewegen RJ, Ploemacher RE, Vos O, David JA, Huiskamp R. The effects of x-irradiation on hematopoietic stem cell compartments in the mouse. *Exp Hematol* 1991; 19:617–623.

167. Brecher G, Ansell J, Micklem H, Tjio J, Cronkite E. Special proliferative sites are not needed for seeding and proliferation of transfused bone marrow cells in normal syngeneic mice. *Proc Natl Acad Sci USA* 1982; 79: 5085–5087.

168. Stewart FM, Crittenden RB, Lowry P, Pearson-White S, Quesenberry PJ. Long-term engraftment of normal and post-5-Fluorouracil murine marrow into normal nonmyeloablated mice. *Blood* 1993; 81:2566–2571.

169. Stewart FM, Zhong S, Wuu J, Hsieh C, Nilsson SK, Quesenberry PJ. Lymphohematopoietic engraftment in minimally myeloablated hosts. *Blood* 1998; 91:3681–3687.

170. Mardiney M, Malech HL. Enhanced engraftment of hematopoietic progenitor cells in mice treated with granulocyte colony-stimulating factor before low-dose irradiation—Implications for gene therapy. *Blood* 1996; 87:4049–4056.

171. Down JD, de Haan G, Dillingh JH, Dontje B, Nijhof W. Stem cell factor has contrasting effects in combination with 5-fluorouracil or total-body irradiation on frequencies of different hemopoietic cell subsets and engraftment of transplanted bone marrow. *Radiat Res* 1997; 147:680–685.

172. Sharabi Y, Sachs DH. Mixed chimerism and permanent specific transplantation tolerance induced by a nonlethal preparative regimen. *J Exp Med* 1989; 169:493–502.

173. Huang CA, Fuchimoto Y, Scheier-Dolberg R, Murphy MC, Neville DM, Jr., Sachs DH. Stable mixed chimerism and tolerance using a nonmyeloablative preparative regimen in a large-animal model. *J Clin Invest* 2000; 105:173–181.

174. Kimikawa M, Sachs DH, Colvin RB, Bartholomew A, Kawai T, Cosimi AB. Modifications of the conditioning regimen for achieving mixed chimerism and donor-specific tolerance in cynomolgus monkeys. *Transplantation* 1997; 64:709–716.

175. Sykes M, Szot GL, Swenson KA, Pearson DA. Induction of high levels of allogeneic hematopoietic reconstitution and donor-specific tolerance without myelosuppressive conditioning. *Nat Med* 1997; 3:783–787.

176. Wekerle T, Sachs DH, Sykes M. Mixed chimerism for the induction of tolerance: potential applicability in clinical composite tissue grafting. *Transplant Proc* 1998; 30:2708–2710.

177. Quesenberry PJ, Zhong S, Wang H, Stewart M. Allogeneic chimerism with low-dose irradiation, antigen presensitization, and costimulator blockade in H-2 mismatched mice. *Blood,* 2001; 97:557–564.

178. Durham MM, Bingaman AW, Adams AB, Ha J, Waitze SY, Pearson TC, Larsen CP. Cutting edge: administration of anti-CD40 ligand and donor bone marrow leads to hemopoietic chimerism and donor-specific tolerance without cytoreductive conditioning. *J Immunol,* 2000; 165:1–4.

179. Pelot MR, Pearson DA, Swenson K, Zhao G, Sachs J, Yang YG, et al. Lymphohematopoietic graft-vs.-host reactions can be induced without graft-vs.-host disease in murine mixed chimeras established with a cyclophosphamide-based nonmyeloablative conditioning regimen. *Biol Blood Marrow Transplant* 1999; 5:133–143.

180. Slavin S, Nagler A, Naparstek E, Kapelushnik Y, Aker M, Cividalli G, et al. Nonmyeloablative stem cell transplantation and cell therapy as an alternative to conventional bone marrow transplantation with lethal cytoreduction for the treatment of malignant and nonmalignant hematologic diseases. *Blood* 1998; 91:756–763.

181. Khouri IF, Keating M, Korbling M, Przepiorka D, Anderlini P, O'Brien S, et al. Transplant-lite: induction of graft-versus-malignancy using fludarabine- based nonablative chemotherapy and allogeneic blood progenitor-cell-transplantation as treatment for lymphoid malignancies. *J Clin Oncol* 1998; 16:2817–2824.

182. Spitzer TR, McAfee S, Sackstein R, Colby C, Toh HC, Multani P et al. Intentional induction of mixed chimerism and achievement of antitumor responses after nonmyeloablative conditioning therapy and HLA-matched donor marrow transplantation for refractory hematologic malignancies. *Bio Blood Marrow Transplant* 2000; 6:309–320.

183. Bornhauser M, Thiede C, Schuler U, Platzbecker U, Freiberg-Richter J, Helwig A, et al. Dose-reduced conditioning for allogeneic blood stem cell transplantation: durable engraftment without antithymocyte globulin *Bone marrow Transplant* 2000; 26:119–125.

184. Sandmaier BM, McSweeney P, Yu C, Storb R. Nonmyeloablative transplants; preclinical and clinical results. *Semin Oncol* 2000; 27 (2 Suppl 5):78–81.

185. Childs R, Chernoff A, Contentin N, Bahceci E, Schrump D, Leitman S et al. Regression of metastatic renal-cell carcinoma after nonmyeloablative allogeneic peripheral-blood stem-cell transplantation. *N Engl J Med* 2000; 343:750–758.

22 Anesthetic Considerations for the Study of Murine Tumor Models

Robert E. Meyer, DVM, Rod D. Braun, PhD, and Mark W. Dewhirst, DVM, PhD

CONTENTS

1. INTRODUCTION

"There are no safe anesthetic agents; there are no safe anesthetic procedures; there are only safe anesthetists." – Robert Smith

The choice and validation of anesthesia are important considerations in the study of whole-animal tumor models. Anesthesia is often necessary for humane restraint, and is absolutely required for invasive or noxious procedures. Ideally, anesthesia itself should exert little or no effect on normal tissue or tumor homeostasis. However, just as there are no "safe" anesthetic agents or procedures, there is no "ideal" or "best" anesthetic choice for the study of tumors in rats and mice. Anesthetic suitability for any given study is largely determined by the knowledge and skill of the user.

Determining the appropriateness of a specific anesthetic agent for a particular experiment or tumor model is a difficult task (Table 1). The researcher must determine which physiological parameters are most important for the validity of the proposed study, and then determine the optimal anesthetic approach to preserve these parameters. This information can be gained only through a careful search of the literature. Merely adopting an anesthetic method described in previous publications will not necessarily ensure that an appropriate anesthetic method is used, and the effects of anesthetics on the model should be critically reviewed as part of the experimental design.

From: *Tumor Models in Cancer Research*
Edited by: B. A. Teicher © Humana Press Inc., Totowa, NJ

Table 1
Issues to Consider When Choosing An Anesthetic

- Anesthesia for restraint vs anesthesia for invasive surgery
- Acute experiment vs recovery from anesthesia
- Species, sex, and strain differences in anesthetic effect
- Duration of procedure
- Dose of anesthetic required and appropriate monitoring signs
- Effect of anesthetic redosing (if necessary)
- Anesthetic effect on target-tissue blood flow
- Anesthetic side effects on physiologic and metabolic homeostasis
- Maintenance of body temperature

For example, maintenance of blood pressure at wakeful levels is often a goal during murine tumor studies. Compared to conscious Fischer 344 rats, pentobarbital anesthesia increases systemic arterial blood pressure 14% (1). Skeletal-muscle blood flow is reduced 83%, yet cardiac output is unchanged. In contrast, systemic blood pressure with Hypnorm™ (a combination of fentanyl and the butyrophenone tranquilizer fluanisone) is 25% lower than with pentobarbital (2). Skeletal-muscle blood flow, increases fivefold in Hypnorm™ anesthetized rats, and cardiac output is nearly doubled. Although pentobarbital and Hypnorm™ can be reasonable anesthetic choices, any conclusions about the uptake and distribution of anticancer drugs or the antitumor effect of radiation are likely to differ considerably.

Similarly, regardless of blood pressure and perfusion effects, pentobarbital is the preferred anesthetic, and fentanyl-containing agents such as Hypnorm™ should be avoided if one is interested in primary leukocyte-endothelial-cell interactions. Leukocyte rolling in postcapillary venules is adversely affected by fentanyl but not pentobarbital (3).

The decision whether to use anesthesia should be made in the context of the animal's overall physiologic response to experimental conditions. Physical restraint without anesthesia can induce severe stress (4) and produce deleterious effects on experimental outcome. Blood-vessel cannulation in rats elevates plasma corticosteroid levels for several days (5). Hand restraint of awake mice is associated with a 30% decrease in heart rate (6); since heart rate is a major component of cardiac output, tissue blood flow can be compromised. Indeed, awake mouse restraint, even without immobilizing the tumor-bearing leg, increased squamous-cell carcinoma (SCC) VII tumor hypoxic fraction from 5.4–13% (7).

It is pointless to carefully design an experiment, and then allow the animal to become physiologically or metabolically deranged because of poor perioperative management (8). Peripheral sympathetic nervous system activity is altered by anesthetic agents, surgical procedures, hemorrhage, metabolic or respiratory acidosis, hypothermia, and hypoxia (9). Hypothermia reduces cellular metabolic rate and leads to an apparent increase in oxygen levels. Severe hypercarbia caused by anesthetic-induced respiratory inadequacy will lead to acute decreases in arterial, interstitial, and tumor pH. Similarly, stress and certain anesthetic agents such as the alpha-2 agonists and ketamine have well-described effects on mobilization of glucose reserves and blood glucose levels (10). Ketamine, diethyl ether (rarely used today due to explosion hazard)

Table 2
Partial List of Murine Anesthetics[a]

- Alpha-chlorolose (hypnosis only, no analgesia)
- Althesin™, Saffan™ (alphaxolone-alphadolone; not available in the United States)
- Chloral hydrate (hypnosis only, no analgesia)
- EMTU (Inactin™, ethyl (1-methylpropyl) malonylthiourea salt)
- Etomidate (Amidate™; hypnosis only, no analgesia)
- Hypnorm™ (fentanyl and fluanisone; not available in the United States)
- Inhaled anesthetics:
  - Halothane
  - Isoflurane
  - Enflurane
  - Methoxyflurane (currently not available in the United States)
  - Sevoflurane
  - Desflurane
- Immobilon™ (etorphine and methotrimeprazine; not available in the United States)
- Innovar-Vet™ (fentanyl and droperidol; no longer available in the United States)
- Ketamine (Vetalar™, Ketalar™, Ketaset™)
  - Combined with an alpha-2 adrenergic agonist (e.g., xylazine, medetomidine)
  - Combined with a benzodiazepine (e.g., diazepam, midazolam; suitable for restraint only)
- Pentobarbital (Nembutal™)
- Propofol (Diprivan™, Rapidovet™; hypnosis only, no analgesia)
- Telazol™ (zolazepam and tiletamine)
- Tribromoethanol (Avertin™; mice; short procedures only)
- Urethane (ethyl carbamate)

[a]After Wixson and Smiler (35)

and urethane all increase plasma catecholamine levels through central mediated sympathetic nervous system stimulation (9).

It is easy to be overwhelmed by the sheer number of murine tumor studies reported and the wide range of anesthetic agents and doses used (Table 2). The purpose of this chapter is to review the physiological effects of anesthetics commonly used in the study of murine tumors, and to provide a starting context for rational anesthetic choices. The general effects of anesthesia are discussed, and the inhalant anesthetics and the three injectable anesthetics pentobarbital, urethane, and ketamine are examined in detail. Comprehensive information on laboratory animal anesthesia—including pharmacology, administration technique, and recommended anesthetic and postsurgical analgesic drug dosages—is provided (8,11–13).

2. DEFINING AND QUANTIFYING THE ANESTHETIC STATE

Anesthesia, by definition, changes the integrated responses of an intact animal to external stimuli. The components of the anesthetic state include unconsciousness, amnesia, analgesia, immobility, and attenuation of autonomic responses to noxious stimulation. A wide variety of structurally unrelated compounds ranging from steroids to the elemental gas xenon are capable of producing anesthesia, and the molecular mechanisms responsible for producing the anesthetic state are diverse and not yet fully known.

Anesthetic uptake, distribution, and effect are governed by the pharmacokinetic and pharmacodynamic properties of the anesthetic agent in that strain or species. Anesthetic drugs that produce adequate anesthesia and analgesia in one strain or species may be insufficient or may provide different clinical signs of anesthesia at similar doses in other strains or species. For example, the benzodiazepine tranquilizers diazepam and midazolam are effective sedative and anxiolytic agents in humans, but in most animal species, they have a variable tranquilizing effect, and are ineffective anesthetics when used alone. Higher doses of hypnotic agents, such as propofol or the barbiturates, do not induce additional analgesia commensurate with increased central nervous system (CNS) and cardiopulmonary depression.

It has proven to be very difficult to definitively link in vitro anesthetic effects to the anesthetic state observed in vivo. Individual anesthetic agents do not produce equivalent depression of all sensory modalities. Likewise, anesthetics do not produce equivalent cardiovascular and respiratory effects. Although all anesthetics reversibly depress membrane and neuronal excitability, there are no common structure-activity relationships among anesthetics. In comparison to drugs, neurotransmitters, and hormones that act at specific receptors, anesthetics exert their effect at very high concentrations, which implies that if anesthetics act by specific receptor-site binding, this binding must be low-affinity and short-lived.

Nearly everyone is familiar with Guedel's four classic stages of anesthesia, which range from sedated (stage 1) through medullary overdose (stage 4). Guedel's original observations were based on observations made during diethyl ether anesthesia in humans. Although conceptually useful, these signs do not necessarily hold true and consistent for all anesthetics in all species. Level, or depth, of anesthesia is characterized by a continuum of progressive increases in CNS and cardiopulmonary depression. This continuum can differ substantially between anesthetic drugs or drug combinations, and can therefore influence observer interpretation. The withdrawal response to a toe pinch is one commonly used indicator of anesthetic depth. Although withdrawal indicates insufficient anesthesia, absence of response could be interpreted either as adequate anesthesia or as excessively deep anesthesia. Anesthetics that increase sympathetic activity cause dose-dependent pupillary dilation, yet this sign is absent with the inhalant anesthetics halothane and isoflurane. Dissociative agents, such as ketamine, do not induce the characteristic reduction of ocular signs and reflexes associated with increasing CNS depression. The assumption that equipotent levels of anesthetic drugs have been administered based solely on the observation of similar clinical signs, although traditional, can be a risky business.

In order to make meaningful comparisons of anesthetic effect on tumor physiology, it is essential that equally potent doses of anesthesia are administered under well-defined conditions. Determining an equivalent dose for different anesthetic agents, however, can be difficult for several reasons. For inhalant anesthetics, the ability to quantitatively determine potency was resolved by Eger and colleagues with the definition of the concept of MAC, or minimum alveolar concentration (14). MAC is defined as the alveolar partial pressure of a gas at which 50% of humans will not purposefully respond to a surgical incision. In animals, MAC is defined as the alveolar partial pressure of a gas at which 50% of animals will not purposefully respond to a noxious stimulus, such as a tail clamp with defined pressure and duration. Purposeful response is defined as movement of the head, torso, or legs, and does not include stiffening, cough-

Table 3
Physical Properties for Inhaled Anesthetics in Rats

Agent	Chemical Class	MAC (as percent in carrier gas)[b]	Blood: Gas Solubility	Biometabolism (% recovered as metabolites)[b]
Nitrous Oxide	inorganic gas	136–235	0.47	0.004% N2O inhibits methionine synthase; oxidizes vitamin B12
Diethyl ether	ethyl ether	3.2	15.2	20% Up to 24 h for complete elimination
Methoxyflurane	halogenated methyl ethyl ether	0.27	15.0	40–50% High levels of fluoride ion can cause acute renal toxicity
Halothane	halogenated alkane	0.81–1.23	2.54	15–20% trifluoroacetyl chloride
Enflurane	halogenated methyl ethyl ether	2.17	2.00	2.4% fluoride ion
Isoflurane	halogenated methyl ethyl ether	1.17–1.52	1.46	0.17% fluoride ion
Sevoflurane	fluorinated methyl ethyl ether	2.4–2.5	0.68	3.0% fluoride ion
Desflurane	fluorinated methyl ethyl ether	5.72–7.10	0.42	0.02% fluoride ion

[b]MAC and biometabolism data from Steffey (104).

ing, or hyperventilation. For surgical anesthesia, 1.3 MAC prevents movement in at least 95% of subjects. Thus, MAC provides a quantitative measure of anesthetic potency for all inhalant anesthetics.

A major advantage of MAC is that it is an extremely reproducible measurement that is remarkably constant over a wide range of species (Table 3). Another advantage is that MAC can be readily determined from the end-tidal gas concentration. Under steady-state conditions, the end-tidal anesthetic gas concentration, the blood and plasma gas concentration, and the partial pressure of the anesthetic at the brain and spinal cord, are in equilibrium. MAC is potentially influenced by a number of factors, including body temperature, catecholamines, electrolytes, oxygen and carbon dioxide levels, concurrently administered parenteral anesthetic drugs, pregnancy, and increasing age.

The ability to deliver a quantifiable, equipotent anesthesia dose has obvious advantages for all experimental systems. However, there are important limitations to the MAC concept. MAC is quantal in that an individual either responds or does not respond to a noxious stimulus at a given end-anesthetic tidal concentration. MAC, however, is reported as the average value for a population of subjects rather than the response of a specific individual. MAC represents only one point on the anesthetic dose-response curve. The quantal nature of MAC makes it difficult to compare in vivo MAC measurements to in vitro anesthetic concentration-response curves, for which the graded response of a single preparation is measured as a function of concentration. Although similar MACs produce equivalent *CNS* depression for all inhalant anesthetics, cardiopulmonary effects can differ substantially between individual agents. Furthermore, the concept of MAC cannot be applied to injectable anesthetics. A MAC equivalent for injectable anesthetics would be the free concentration of the drug in plasma required to prevent response to noxious stimulus in 50% of subjects, which is a difficult measurement to make. Comparisons between injectable anesthetics, or injectable and inhalant anesthetics, are therefore difficult for these reasons.

3. CARDIOVASCULAR EFFECTS OF ANESTHESIA

As a general rule, anesthetics tend to produce drug-specific and dose-dependent circulatory, respiratory, and CNS effects. These effects can vary substantially between different anesthetics, even at what appears to be equivalent doses, and will greatly affect uptake and distribution of concurrently administered pharmaceuticals. For example, Sancho and colleagues examined the effect of three commonly used anesthetics on biodistribution of carboplatin in female Wistar rats *(15)*. They observed that percentage values of the injected dose of platinum per mL in plasma at the final time-point were 0.557%, 0.156%, 0.115%, and 0.086%, respectively, in pentobarbital-, ketamine/xylazine-, and thiopental-anesthetized rats, and awake animals. The percentage values of injected platinum per mL in the cumulative urine were 0.001%, 0.619%, 0.184%, and 0.118%, respectively. Rats that received pentobarbital showed a nearly 100-fold increase in platinum uptake in the kidneys, cerebrum, and cerebellum over the awake control group, which led Sancho and colleagues to conclude that anesthetic selection can significantly influence biodistribution and the pharmacokinetic profile of drugs.

In an ideal world, cardiac output, arterial blood pressure, and tissue temperature and blood flows would be reported in experiments in which anesthesia or treatment may alter perfusion *(16)*. Unfortunately, methods to measure cardiac output or blood flow (surgically implanted vascular flow probes, microspheres, indicator washout methods, laser Doppler flowmetry, nuclear magnetic resonance, etc.) are invasive, expensive, and can be technically difficult to apply to small rodent models. Blood-pressure monitoring is often substituted for these more difficult methods of assessing perfusion. Blood-pressure monitoring permits an indirect assessment of circulatory function, and provides insight into the depth of anesthesia. Monitoring for laboratory animal anesthesia has been reviewed by Flecknell *(8)* and Mason and Brown *(17)*.

Delivery of blood-borne substances (D) is the product of perfusion or flow (Q) and blood content (C) where $D = Q * C$. With no convenient method to directly determine aortic flow or cardiac output (CO), blood pressure (BP) is often substituted as an indicator of cardiovascular homeostasis, where $BP = CO * PVR$ (peripheral vascular resistance). It is important to remember that blood pressure is the product of two independent variables. If flow and/or resistance increases, so will BP. For example, flow and pressure are both increased when relatively large volumes of intravenous (iv) fluid (10–20% of the circulating blood volume) are given rapidly; cardiac output is augmented under these conditions by increased venous return to the heart and the Starling effect. Blood pressure is increased when vasoconstriction occurs and resistance is increased; yet in this case, cardiac output and tissue perfusion may decrease. This is the case with the alpha-2 adrenergic agonists xylazine and medetomidine.

Blood pressure is reduced by vasodilation and decreased vascular resistance. Perfusion may decrease, remain unchanged, or selectively increase to specific organs and tissues in the face of vasodilation. The potent nitrovasodilator sodium nitroprusside reduces blood pressure, yet cardiac output and normal organ perfusion remain unchanged or increase because of reduced afterload (18–20). Likewise, the inhalant anesthetic isoflurane is a potent vasodilator, but cardiac output is maintained better than with halothane and skeletal-muscle perfusion is increased *(21)*. On the other hand, if cardiac output decreases as a result of either direct anesthetic depression of the myocardium or decreased ventricular filling pressure, without compensatory increases in arteriolar tone, perfusion and blood pressure will also fall. Thus, changes in blood pressure, although useful in monitoring anesthetic effect, must be interpreted cautiously because of specific myocardial and vascular effects.

It is exceedingly difficult to make sweeping generalizations regarding the cardiovascular and pulmonary effects of anesthetics. Anesthetic dose-response curves tend to be quite steep, and are not necessarily parallel. The mechanisms by which anesthetics exert their systemic effects in the intact animal are modified by their direct and indirect effects on myocardial contractility, peripheral smooth-muscle tone, and autonomic nervous-system activity. For example, ketamine, like many anesthetics, is a myocardial depressant. Yet this is offset in the intact animal through increased sympathetic nervous-system activity *(9)*. Halothane and isoflurane both decrease blood pressure in a dose-dependent manner—halothane through myocardial depression and isoflurane through vasodilation *(21)*. Anesthetic agents generally decrease the response of the respiratory centers to carbon dioxide, resulting in hypoventilation and—by definition—increased arterial CO_2. There are several excellent sources available for readers who wish to obtain further information on the pharmacology and physiology of specific anesthetic agents (11,12,22–24).

4. ANESTHESIA AND HYPOTHERMIA

4.1. Rodents and Hypothermia

Small rodents are normally endothermic, but can lose body heat rapidly because of their high ratio of surface area to body wt. Heat can be lost through infrared radiation to cooler surroundings, by conduction to colder objects, through convection to surrounding air, and by surface evaporation of liquids. Tumor temperature in awake, restrained C3H/HeDub mice decreased 1–1.5°C *(25)*, and rectal and tumor temperatures of awake C3Hf/Sed mice restrained on brass plates inserted into stainless steel or brass hyperbaric pressure chambers fell to 31°C and 27°C, respectively *(26)*. Hypothermia develops quickly in anesthetized mice, and body temperature can fall 10°C within 15–20 min *(8)*. Long lasting anesthetics, such as pentobarbital and urethane, will tend to produce greater hypothermia than shorter-acting anesthetics which allow quicker return of thermoregulation and movement. Male Wistar rats anesthetized with 1.5 g/kg urethane intraperitoneal (ip) were unable to maintain body temperature in a 32°C or 9°C laboratory environment *(27)*. Likewise, recovery from anesthesia will be prolonged in hypothermic individuals. In Balb/c mice anesthetized with 60 mg/kg ip pentobarbital, sleep time varied from 100 min at an ambient temperature of 26°C to 195 min at 18°C *(28)*. Methods to supply exogenous heat to maintain normothermia are therefore critical for optimal physiological function during awake restraint as well as during anesthesia.

4.2. Hypothermia and Metabolism

Nearly all anesthetics cause hypothermia by inhibiting central and peripheral thermoregulatory mechanisms. Hypothermia reduces metabolic rate and anesthetic metabolism and clearance, and decreases tissue oxygen use. Inhalant anesthetic MAC requirement is reduced 5.3% for each degree Celsus over the range 37–27°C (29) and oxygen utilization by Chinese hamster V79 cells decreases with temperature 7% per degree Celsius over the range 37–25°C °C *(30)*. Further, reduction in body temperature alone can improve apparent tissue pO2 provided that DO2 is not affected; a 10°C reduction in body temperature increases the amount of oxygen dissolved in plasma by about 20% in air-breathing animals at atmospheric pressure *(31)*.

4.3. Hypothermia and Immune Response

Hypothermia has been linked to decreased immune response. In normothermic Fischer 344 rats, anesthesia with the barbiturate thiopental (70 mg/kg ip) reduced natural killer (NK) cell activity to 40% of the control value *(32)*. Hypothermia at 30–32°C further reduced killer-cell activity to 15% of control, increased MADB106 tumor retention to 250% of control levels, and increased the number of distant metastases *(32)*. These changes were not accompanied by alterations in the numbers of circulating NK cells. In humans, hypothermia increases the risk of perioperative infectious complications *(33)*. A reduction in body temperature of 1°C has been shown to suppress mitogen-induced activation of lymphocytes and to reduce the production of IL-1beta and IL-2 in humans undergoing abdominal surgery *(34)*.

5. INHALANT ANESTHETICS

Inhalant anesthetics can be safely administered to rats and mice, and have the advantage over injectable anesthetics in greater control of anesthetic depth, as well as the previously discussed ability to consistently deliver a defined level of anesthesia for the duration of an experiment. Unlike injectable anesthetics and the potential for accumulation and prolonged effect with redosing, there is very little difference between administering an inhalant anesthetic for 30 min or for 10 h. Uptake, distribution, and recovery from inhalant anesthesia depends on agent solubility in blood and tissues (Table 3), cardiac output, and ventilation *(14)*. As previously stated, MAC for inhalant anesthetics is influenced by several factors, including body temperature, catecholamines, electrolytes, oxygen and carbon dioxide levels, concurrently administered parenteral anesthetic drugs, pregnancy, and increasing age. Methods for administering inhalant anesthetics to rodents have been reviewed by Flecknell *(8)* and Wixson and Smiler *(35)*.

5.1. Cardiopulmonary Effects

Like all anesthetics, inhalant anesthetics can exert influence on tumor models through depression of circulation and ventilation. These effects vary between inhalant anesthetics based on dose (MAC) and chemical structure. As a general rule, the halogenated ethers, such as isoflurane or sevoflurane, support cardiac output better but tend to cause greater vasodilation for a given MAC than the alkane halothane. Spontaneous ventilation is depressed by all inhalant anesthetics in a dose-dependent manner; however, it is important to remember that adequacy of ventilation is determined by arterial carbon dioxide levels and not by respiratory frequency.

5.2. Status of Inhalant Anesthetic Carcinogenicity

Currently used volatile anesthetics, which include the halogenated anesthetics halothane, isoflurane, methoxyflurane (not presently available in the United States), enflurane, and sevoflurane, are themselves not mutagenic or carcinogenic. Nitrous oxide, a gaseous anesthetic that is not halogenated or considered a volatile anesthetic, is teratogenic to experimental animals at subanesthetic concentrations, but relatively prolonged exposure is required. Both the chronic toxicity of nitrous oxide and its teratogenic effects are likely a result of reduced methionine synthase, which controls interrelations between vitamin B12 and folic acid metabolism. Findings from tests for genetic and related effects and from studies of DNA damage, chromosomal effects, and mutation in humans and for carcinogenicity in humans and experimental animals were summarized and updated by the 1986–1987 IARC Working Group *(36)*. Individual volatile anesthetics have insufficient or no data for classification as carcinogens in experimental animals. As a class, the inhalation anesthetics have inadequate evidence for carcinogenicity and are classified in class 3. The only mutagenic volatile anesthetics are those which contain a vinyl moiety or acquire a vinyl group during metabolism (divinyl ether, fluroxene, and trichloroethylene, none of which are currently used clinically). The volatile anesthetics currently in clinical use are not mutagenic, based on existing data *(37)*.

5.3. Inhalant Anesthetic Biometabolism

Halogenated inhalant anesthetic agents have widely differing chemical properties, which can influence their potential for retention within the body and their subsequent metabolism (Table 3). This is important, because it is the intermediate or end-metabolites of halogenated inhaled anesthetics that are implicated in chronic effects on the kidneys, liver, and reproductive organs. Generally speaking, highly lipid-soluble volatile anesthetics, such as methoxyflurane and halothane, are taken up and eliminated from the body more slowly than less soluble agents, such as isoflurane and sevoflurane. Thus, a highly lipid-soluble inhaled anesthetic will tend to undergo more biotransformation, simply because it is presented to metabolically active tissues within the body for a longer period of time. There are differences in the ability of various rat strains to respond to the nephrotoxic effects of inorganic fluoride, a metabolic end product of methoxyflurane and enflurane, and to a lesser extent, sevoflurane. Fischer 344 rats are particularly susceptible to fluoride, and Long-Evans and Sprague Dawley strains are not *(38)*.

5.4. Inhalant Anesthesia and Immune Function

Many normal functions of the immune system are depressed after exposure to the combination of anesthesia and surgery *(39)*. Many of these changes appear to be primarily the result of surgical trauma, hypothermia, and increased catecholamines and corticosteroids resulting from pain and endocrine responses, rather than the result of anesthetic exposure itself. Inhaled anesthetics—particularly—nitrous oxide—produce dose-dependent inhibition of polymorphonuclear leukocytes and their subsequent migration for phagocytosis. Reduced resistance to bacterial infection is unlikely, however, because of the short duration and dose of inhaled anesthetics. Furthermore, when leukocytes reach the site of infection, their ability to phagocytize bacteria appears unaffected following inhaled anesthesia exposure *(22)*. Exposure to halothane or isoflurane anesthesia increases the number of B16 melanoma pulmonary metastases in C57B1 mice compared with an oxygen breathing control group; there was no difference in number of metastases among animals treated with halothane or isoflurane *(40)*. Inhaled anesthetics, in doses as low as 0.2 MAC, produce dose-dependent inhibition of measles virus replication and reduce mortality of mice receiving intranasal influenza virus *(41)*. This inhibition may reflect anesthetic-induced decreases in DNA synthesis, and may have particular relevance to models where adenoviruses are used as vectors for gene therapy.

5.5. Halothane Effect on O_2 Electrodes

Quantification of blood or tissue oxygen is commonly performed using polarographic oxygen electrodes. The halogenated ether anesthetics—which include methoxyflurane, isoflurane, enflurane, and sevoflurane (Table 3)—do not affect the oxygen electrode current *(42)*. The halogenated alkane anesthetic halothane, however, has been shown to increase the oxygen current of microelectrodes, with the increase in electrode signal proportional to the halothane concentration *(43)*. Although this effect is caused by reduction of halothane at the cathode, it cannot be inhibited by coating the electrode with a membrane *(44)*. Thus, use of oxygen microelectrodes under halothane anesthesia would indicate a higher oxygen tension than is actually present in the tissue.

5.6. Protecting Laboratory Workers from Inhalant Anesthetics

Laboratories wishing to use inhalant anesthetics must take steps to limit worker exposure to these agents. In 1977, the National Institute of Occupational Safety and Health (NIOSH) estimated that over 200,000 workers were at risk for exposure to waste-inhalation anesthetics *(45)*. Based on then-current knowledge, NIOSH published a criteria statement recommending standards for reducing occupational waste anesthetic gas exposure to halogenated anesthetic agents *(45)*. These standards remain in effect today, although their relevance has been questioned in light of more recent knowledge *(46)*. Exposure to halogenated anesthetics was set to not exceed 2 ppm (1 hour ceiling) for halogenated anesthetic agents when used alone, or 0.5 ppm for a halogenated agent and 25 ppm nitrous oxide (time-weighted average during use) *(45)*. Anesthetic risk to animal workers has been reviewed by Meyer *(47)*, and detailed methods to reduce veterinary workplace exposure to anesthetic gases have been published by the American College of Veterinary Anesthesiologists *(48)*.

6. INJECTABLE ANESTHETIC AGENTS

6.1. Pentobarbital

6.1.1. MECHANISM OF ACTION

Pentobarbital is an oxybarbiturate that continues to be extensively used to produce rodent anesthesia. The barbiturates are generally good hypnotic agents, but relatively poor analgesics. The wide use of pentobarbital stems from its generalized availability, modest cost, widely available database encompassing decades of use, rapid anesthetic onset, nonirritant nature, and ease of ip injection to rodents of varying ages and body wt *(35)*. Commercial preparations of pentobarbital are racemic mixtures. The (+) isomer causes a transient period of hyperexcitability before depressing the CNS, while the (–) isomer produces relatively smooth and progressively deeper hypnosis *(49)*. The (–) isomer potentiates g-aminobutyric acid (GABA)-induced increases in chloride conductance and depresses voltage-activated Ca2+ currents. Barbiturates increase GABA-induced chloride currents by prolonging periods in which bursts of channel opening occur, rather than by increasing the frequency of these bursts, as benzodiazepines do. At anesthetic doses, pentobarbital suppresses high-frequency neuronal firing by inhibiting voltage-dependent Na+ channels; higher doses reduce voltage-dependent K+ conductances *(24)*. The mechanism of action of barbiturates has been reviewed (50–52). Pentobarbital is metabolized primarily by hepatic microsomal enzymes and hydroxylation of the 3-carbon methylbutyl side chain *(53)*.

6.1.2. ROUTE OF ADMINISTRATION AND CARDIOVASCULAR EFFECTS

Pentobarbital can be administered either intravenously or intraperitoneally. Kawaue and Iriuchijima *(54)* examined the effect iv of 30 mg/kg pentobarbital in rats chronically implanted with electromagnetic flow probes. Intravenous administration was associated initially with an acute decrease in blood pressure, from 105 mmHg to 75 mmHg, with recovery to 90 mmHg during the next 30 min. Cardiac output gradually decreased 30% by 30 min; hindquarter blood flow decreased 25%, and splanchnic blood flow initially increased 40%, then recovered to baseline by 30 min.

Cardiovascular effects of pentobarbital are less pronounced following ip administration. Peak blood concentration is reached more slowly than with iv injection, and the portion of drug absorbed into the portal system is subject to early destruction in the liver. Tuma et al. *(1)* examined the cardiovascular and tissue-perfusion effects of 35 mg/kg ip pentobarbital in 12-mo-old female Fischer 344 rats. Compared with awake controls, ip injection increased mean arterial blood pressure to 130 mmHg (awake control 114 mmHg) and cardiac output decreased insignificantly (to 22 mL/min/100 g, awake control 26 mL/min/100 g). Renal perfusion was maintained at awake levels; however, blood flow to most organs decreased from awake levels, with the exception of the liver. Skeletal-muscle blood flow showed the greatest decrease, with a four- to six-fold reduction from the awake state (to 3 mL/min/100 g, awake control 18 mL/min/100 g). Similar results were described by Skolleborg et al. *(2)* for cardiac output and organ blood flow following 50 mg/kg pentobarbital in male (WIST) rats.

Stable mean arterial pressures centered around 100 mmHg were reported during a 90-min observation period in male Sprague Dawley rats anesthetized with 40 mg/kg ip pentobarbital; 80 mg/kg reduced mean arterial pressure to around 90 mmHg, which was also stable during a 180-min observation period *(55)*. In contrast, Wixson et al. *(56)* found that ip injections of 30- and 40-mg/kg pentobarbital in male Sprague Dawley rats resulted in sustained MAP decreases of approx 20% (30 mmHg). The lower dose of pentobarbital showed minimal effect on heart rate, and the 40 mg/kg dose initially decreased heart rate by 9.2%, with mild tachycardia at later times.

In SvEv/Tac mice, 50 mg/kg ip pentobarbital reduced heart rate, from 658 beats/min (awake) to 377 beats/min, and reduced cardiac output, from 13 mL/min/g to 8.6

mL/min/g *(6)*. In comparison, ip 15/150 mg/kg xylazine/ketamine produced greater reduction in heart rate and cardiac output in SvEv/Tac mice than 50 mg/kg pentobarbital, to 293 beats/min and 7.2 mL/min/g *(6)*. At a dose of 50 mg/kg, which was insufficient to induce surgical-level anesthesia, pentobarbital decreased MAP in male adult Balb/c mice from 129 to 107 mmHg, and heart rate from 509 to 228 beats/min *(57)*. Respiratory rate was also depressed, decreasing from 195 breaths/min to 71 breaths/min.

6.1.3. EFFECT ON VENTILATION AND BLOOD GASES

Although pentobarbital can be a potent dose-dependent ventilatory depressant, Skolleborg et al. reported arterial blood-gas values for pH, pCO2, and pO2 within the normal awake range following 50 mg/kg ip administration in male WIST rats *(2)*. Similar findings of minimal respiratory depression have been reported for female Fischer 344 rats anesthetized with 50 mg/kg ip pentobarbital *(58)* and for male Sprague Dawley rats anesthetized with 40 mg/kg ip pentobarbital *(55)*. These reports are in contrast to findings by Wixson et al. in male Sprague-Dawley rats, where ip 40 mg/kg pentobarbital decreased pH by 1.2% or 0.09–0.10 pH units and increased $paCO_2$ by 46% (11 mmHg), and 30- and 40 mg/kg pentobarbital decreased paO_2 by 19–20% (34 mmHg) *(56)*.

Similar ventilatory effects were found in mice, even at dosages insufficient to produce analgesia. Intraperitoneal pentobarbital in male adult Balb/c mice at 50 mg/kg decreased arterial pH almost 0.15 units, from 7.285 to 7.137 *(57)*. Arterial pCO_2 increased from 26.5 to 38.8 mm Hg, and paO_2 dropped from 111.7 to 93.0 mmHg *(57)*.

6.1.4. TOLERANCE AND STRAIN DIFFERENCES

Tolerance of rats to pentobarbital is sex and strain-dependent *(59)*. At doses of 30–55 mg/kg, female rats take three times longer to recover than males, and mortality is higher in the females *(60)*. The use of pentobarbital in mice is slightly riskier than in rats. A dose of 50 mg/kg provides adequate sedation, but insufficient analgesia in male adult Balb/c mice *(57)*. These authors noted some mortality at doses of 60 mg/kg, indicating a narrow safety margin for pentobarbital in mice.

There are substantial differences in pentobarbital dose response between strains of mice, so that underdosage or overdosage frequently occurs. Lovell studied the effects of 60 mg/kg pentobarbital administered ip to 23 strains of inbred mice *(61,62,28)*. The variation in sleep time between different strains of mice is considerable, ranging from 50 min for female NZW mice to 250 min for male (DBA) mice. Male mice generally sleep longer than female mice, and C57B1/6 mice sleep longer than (CBA) mice, which sleep longer than Balb/c mice. Strain differences are also present for age, sex, litter size, and fasting prior to anesthesia. Environmental variables that affect sleep time include diet, environmental temperature, and bedding material, and inbred strains are more variable to the environment than F1 hybrids. At an environmental temperature of 18°C, sleep time in Balb/c mice administered 60 mg/kg ip pentobarbital is 195 min, and raising environmental temperature to 26°C decreases sleep time to 100 min. However, at an environmental temperature of 18°C, C57BL/10ScSn mice sleep over 400 min. It is likely that strain and environmental factors have contributed to the confusion surrounding anesthetic effect on tumor physiology and radiotherapy outcome.

6.1.5. EFFECT ON TUMOR PHYSIOLOGY AND RADIOSENSITIVITY

Pentobarbital anesthesia is reported to have variable effects on normal or tumor tissue response to radiation, producing radioprotection of tumors and some normal tissue during air breathing, but enhancing radiation effect during hyperbaric oxygen breathing at 3 atmospheres pressure. Differences in the hypoxic fractions for assays without anesthesia (15%) and with barbiturate anesthesia (20%) have been noted by several authors, and suggest that barbiturate anesthesia may result in a small, statistically insignificant increase in the hypoxic fraction *(16,63,64)*. These responses have been attributed to a direct effect of pentobarbital on cellular respiration, hypothermia, and increased tumor oxygen supply secondary to anesthesia, and cardiovascular depression with subsequent reduction of tumor blood flow. At this time, it appears that the in vivo radioprotective effect of pentobarbital anesthesia is largely because of anesthetic-mediated reduction and redistribution of tumor blood flow, rather than a direct anesthetic effect at the cellular level.

Gullino, Grantham, and Courtney reported oxygen utilization of the Walker carcinoma 256, Hepatoma 5123, and Fibrosarcoma 4956 in pentobarbital-anesthetized Sprague-Dawley rats *(65)*. They found that a reduced ratio of oxygen consumed to oxygen supplied (O2RR) for tumors only when pentobarbital dose was greater than 30 mg/kg, and concluded the effect of anesthesia was minor if the right conditions were met. Sheldon et al. attributed radioprotection for the MT1 tumor in (WHT)/Ht mice given 60 mg/kg ip pentobarbital to reduced tumor blood flow and a 4–9°C reduction in body temperature during radiation *(66)*. Unlike pentobarbital, there was no change in radiosensitivity of the MT1 tumor in WHT/Ht mice anesthetized with 200 mg/kg ip tribromoethanol or with 6 mL/kg subcutaneous (sc) injection of a 1:1 mixture of diazepam and Hypnorm *(67)*. Denekamp et al. examined the response of the squamous carcinoma D and slow carcinoma Rh in WHT/Ht mice and the carcinoma Neurotensin (NT) and slow sarcoma S in CBA/Ht mice *(68)*. Intraperitoneal pentobarbital at 60 mg/kg was found to have no influence on radiation response of the squamous carcinoma D and the sarcoma S, but there was evidence of radioprotection in the carcinoma NT and carcinoma Rh.

One proposed mechanism for the radioprotection observed with pentobarbital is suppression of oxygen utilization. The barbiturates are reported to uncouple oxidative phosphorylation in cellular respiration *(69)*. Using preparations of mitochondria from the liver and brain, Aldridge and Parker reported that when pyruvate is the substrate, the oxybarbiturates amytal, phenobarbital, and hexobarbital inhibit, but do not uncouple, in vitro oxidative phosphorylation *(69)*. It must be noted that Aldridge and Parker did not specifically examine pentobarbital effects in their report.

Pentobarbital at anesthetically relevant concentrations is not an important contributor to direct suppression of in vivo or in vitro tumor cellular oxygen utilization. The LD50 for C3Hf/Sed mice for pentobarbital is 90–100 mg/kg or 0.35 mM; a dose of 50 mg/kg corresponds to approx 0.2 mM *(26)*. Cellular oxygen utilization by V79 and Ehrlich ascites cells *(70)* and FsaII and McaIV cells *(30)* is inhibited less than 10% by 0.2 mM pentobarbital. The concentration of pentobarbital necessary to reduce cellular oxygen utilization by 50% in FSaII and MCaIV cells is greater than 1.3 mM *(26)*, a lethal dose for mice or rats. Rockwell and Loomis showed that pentobarbital in concentrations of 0.050 mg/mL and 0.25 mg/mL has no direct effect on the radiation response of EMT6 tumor cells, and does not alter the radiation dose-response curves of aerated or hypoxic EMT6 tumor cells in vitro *(71)*. Anesthesia of air-breathing Balb/c KaRw mice with 50 mg/kg ip pentobarbital did not alter the survival curve for EMT6 tumor cells. Rockwell and Loomis concluded that pentobarbital has no direct effect on the radiation response of EMT6 cells in culture or in tumors. They attributed the physiologic effects of pentobarbital on environmental alterations in the host, including changes in temperature and oxygenation of the tumor, which subsequently altered tumor-cell response to radiation.

Radioprotection with pentobarbital is likely caused by a reduction in blood flow. Pallavicini and Hill examined the effect of ip pentobarbital 70 mg/kg on ^{133}xenon washout in C3H/HeDub mice implanted with the (KHT) sarcoma *(25)*. Tumor blood flow decreased 59% with pentobarbital. Pentobarbital reduced body and tumor temperature 8–10°C. The hypoxic tumor-cell fraction increased threefold with anesthesia, but the magnitude of increase was not correlated with decrease in blood flow, supporting the concept of an upper limit to the proportion of hypoxic cells. Shibamoto, Sasai, and Abe compared radiation response of SCCVII tumor cells in C3H/He mice *(7)*. When mice were irradiated without anesthesia or physical restraint, tumors had a hypoxic fraction of 5.4%. Anesthesia with 50 mg/kg ip pentobarbital increased the hypoxic fraction to 23%, and taping the leg of anesthetized mice further increased the hypoxic fraction to 28%. However, simply restraining the awake mouse without immobilizing the tumor-bearing leg increased the hypoxic fraction to 13%.

6.2. Urethane

6.2.1. MECHANISM OF ACTION

Urethane, or ethyl carbamate, was initially introduced as an anesthetic in 1885. Urethane is widely used for rodent anesthesia because of its long duration of action (6–10 h), skeletal-muscle relaxant properties, and minimal cardiovascular and ventilatory depression *(72)*. Analgesia from urethane is sufficient to permit surgical procedures. Unlike barbiturates, urethane produces little or no enhancement of GABAergic neurotransmission in the central and peripheral nervous systems. Urethane has slight depressant effects on autonomic reflexes and the activity of subcortical structures of the CNS. Cardiovascular stability with urethane is partly caused by sustained sympathetic nervous system activity, and is associated with high circulating catecholamine levels *(9)*. Urethane is still a valuable anesthetic for providing long-lasting, stable surgical anesthesia in rodents; however, in light of its carcinogenic activity, it is inadvisable to allow animals to recover from urethane anesthesia *(8,11)*.

6.2.2. ROUTE OF ADMINISTRATION AND CARDIOVASCULAR EFFECTS

Blood-pressure effects of urethane are dependent on the route of administration. To achieve a surgical stage of anesthesia, it was necessary to inject female Cpb:Wu(WI) rats with the following doses: 1.0 g/kg ip, 1.8 g/kg subcutaneous (SQ), 1.8 g/kg per os, and 1.2 g/kg intra-arterially (IA) *(73)*. When urethane was iv-injected to male Wistar rats at a dose of 1.3 g/kg, blood pressure transiently dropped, but it recovered to near baseline by 5 min after the infusion *(74)*. This was accompanied by a transient rise in heart rate, which also recovered *(74)*. Intravenous injection of 0.2–0.8 g/kg urethane also resulted in a 5–10-min drop in arterial pressure, followed by a progressive increase in pressure *(75)*. Intraperitoneal injection of 1.2 g/kg in female Wistar rats resulted in a drop in mean blood pressure, which persisted for at least 1 h after injection (Hillebrand et al., 1971). Pressure in the urethane-treated group was 95 mmHg compared to 125 mmHg in unanesthetized animals. In some animals, pressure dropped below 80 mmHg and had to be excluded from the study (76). In contrast, ip injection of 1.2 g/kg urethane to male Wistar and Sprague Dawley rats caused no change in mean arterial blood pressure and heart rate (9). The fall in blood pressure after ip injection of 25% urethane at 1 g/kg can be reduced by slow injection and is absent if the dose is given rapidly IA (73).

6.2.3. EFFECT ON VENTILATION

Urethane is not a physiologically inactive drug, and its use is accompanied by decreases in respiratory, cardiovascular, and renal function. In Sprague Dawley rats, 1.2- and 1.5 g/kg ip urethane provided sleep time in excess of 24 h, anesthesia was characterized by progressive acidosis, hypocapnea, hyperoxia, hypotension, and brady-cardia (77). In decerebrate male Wistar rats, 750 mg/kg iv urethane had no effect on respiratory frequency or tidal volume, although blood pressure and heart rate decreased (78). In male Sprague-Dawley and Wistar rats, 1.2 g/kg ip urethane had minimal effects on blood-gas parameters until 4 h after anesthesia (9). There was a tendency for pH to decrease and arterial pO_2 and pCO_2 to rise during the anesthesia. Within 3–4 h under anesthesia, pCO_2 had significantly risen from a baseline value of 40 mmHg to 49 mmHg, and pO_2 had increased from 80 to 105 mmHg.

In another study, male Sprague-Dawley rats were injected with 1.5 g/kg ip urethane, and blood-gas parameters were measured under normothermic and hypothermic conditions (79). If the rats were maintained at normal body temperature, changes in blood parameters were minimal. Arterial pO_2 and pCO_2 remained unchanged, and arterial pH dropped from 7.48 to 7.42. Bicarbonate levels decreased from 21.8 to 18.9 mmol/L, and arterial lactate increased from 0.89 to 2.78 mmol/L. If the rats were not warmed, body temperature dropped from 37°C to 30°C within 2 h. The hypothermic rats showed a progressive increase in P_aO_2 over time, with an increase of 20–30 mmHg after 2 h. The changes in arterial bicarbonate, lactate, and pH were similar in the hypothermic group to those seen in the normothermic animals. The hypothermia-induced increase in arterial PO_2 suggests that the increase in arterial PO_2 seen in an earlier study (9) may have been caused by hypothermia.

6.2.4. EFFECT ON HEMATOCRIT AND BLOOD-GLUCOSE LEVELS

Urethane is known to affect hematocrit in rats. Rats injected with 1.5 g/kg urethane using a 50 wt% urethane solution showed "marked hemoconcentration" after 8 h (80). In a study investigating the effect of administration route on urethane-induced hemo-concentration, urethane was administered at doses sufficient to induce surgical anesthe-sia via four different routes: ip, sc, per os and ia (73). After 60 min, the hematocrit in the rats had changed by the following amounts: +21.7%, +8.0%, –2.8%, and +1.5%, respectively. The large increase in hematocrit following ip injection was attributed to plasma loss to the peritoneal cavity. An approximately linear relationship between dose of ip-injected urethane and relative increase in hematocrit was also found, with a slope 2.1 percent increase in hematocrit for every 0.1 g/kg increase in urethane dose. Severs et al. showed that ip urethane causes peritoneal fluid accumulation, hyperosmolality of body fluids, osmotic toxicity to the mesenteric vasculature, and increased plasma renin activity and aldosterone levels (81).

Urethane has also been found to have an effect on blood glucose levels. One of the earliest notations of urethane-induced hyperglycemia in rats was made by Reinert in 1964, who noted that blood-glucose level of fasting rats increased from 58 mg/dL to 168 mg/dL 1 h after ip injection of urethane at a dose of 1.25 g/kg *(75)*. Later, a more detailed study of this effect was performed by van der Meer and colleagues *(73)*. In that study, 25 wt% urethane (2.8 *M*) was injected either ip or ia at a dose of 1 g/kg, and the effects on blood glucose levels were examined. Before ip urethane injection, the mean blood glucose was 117 + 5 mg/dL. At 30, 60, and 120 minutes after ip injection, the blood-glucose values 150 + 12, 195 + 17, and 243 + 15 mg/dL, respectively. Before ia urethane injection, the mean blood glucose was 124 + 7 mg/dL. At 30, 60, and 120 min after ia injection, the blood-glucose values were 106 + 8, 108 + 8, and 142 + 8 mg/dL, respectively. In a later study, a 24 wt% urethane solution was administered sc to male rats at a dose of 1.6 g/kg, and blood glucose rose from 85 + 8 mg/dL (mean + SD, n=6) to 194 + 73 mg/dL at 60–120 min after injection *(82)*. Van der Meer speculated that urethane induced hyperglycemia through "stimuli arising in the damaged tissues" at the injection site *(73)*, although increased peripheral sympathetic activity and increased circulating catecholamine levels would be a more plausible explanation *(9)*.

6.2.5. TOLERANCE AND STRAIN DIFFERENCES

As with other anesthetics, there are strain and sex differences in the dose of urethane needed to induce surgical levels of anesthesia in rats. As noted previously, there are differences in urethane dosage based on the route of administration. The threshold blood urethane concentration for narcosis in rats was determined by injecting rats sc with 1.0 g/kg urethane and measuring blood levels of urethane at various times *(83)*. It was found that the anesthetic blood urethane concentration was between 60 and 80 mg/100 mL blood. Rats with blood concentrations below 60 mg/100 mL were not anesthetized, while those with concentrations of at least 80 mg/100 mL (10 m*M*) were anesthetized. A sc dose of 1 g/kg urethane was sufficient to induce anesthesia for 8–12 h in an unspecified fraction of rats *(83)*.

A sc dose of 1.6 g/kg urethane was required to surgically anesthetize male Sprague-Dawley rats *(82)*. Female WU (WI) rats required a sc urethane dose of 1.8 g/kg to reach a surgical level of anesthesia *(73)*. In male Wistar Morini rats, 1.0 g/kg sc urethane produced surgical levels of anesthesia in only 30% of the rats after 3 h, and 90% after 6 h *(84)*. In contrast, a sc dose of 1.2 g/kg resulted in surgical anesthesia in 100% of the same rats after 3 h; the anesthetic effect lasted at least 6 h.

The necessary ip urethane dose ranges from 0.8–1.2 g/kg. In one study, only 0.8 g/kg ip urethane was required to achieve surgical levels of anesthesia in male Wistar rats *(85)*. In another case, a surgical level of anesthesia in female CD (Sprague-Dawley) rats was achieved with 0.8–1.0 g/kg ip, urethane although 1.2 g/kg was required to ensure anesthesia of all animals *(86)*. Lincoln et al. reported that 1.1 g/kg intraperitoneally provided anesthesia levels suitable for sterotaxic manipulation and neurosurgery for at least 8 h in female Wistar rats *(87)*. Female WU (WI) rats required an ip dose of 1.0 g/kg to reach a surgical level of anesthesia *(73)*.

6.2.6. EFFECT ON TUMOR PHYSIOLOGY AND RADIOSENSITIVITY

Urethane decreases tumor blood flow and increases tumor-cell survival following radiation, but the tumor blood-flow reduction is not as pronounced as with pentobarbital. An ip dose of urethane 0.9 g/kg reduced DS-carcinosarcoma ^{85}Kr clearance in Sprague Dawley rats by 36%, increased tumor vascular resistance 35% and decreased mean arterial blood pressure 12.5% compared with conscious controls *(16)*. In C3H/HeDub mice, ip urethane 1.2 mg/kg reduced (KHT) sarcoma ^{133}Xe clearance 24% compared to the pretreatment value *(25)*; in comparison, ip pentobarbital 70 mg/kg reduced tumor blood flow 59% in the same study *(25)*. Tumor and core temperature were reduced by 1–2°C by urethane, compared to the 10°C decrease observed with pentobarbital. Anesthesia with urethane resulted in a threefold increase in tumor-cell survival following radiation; tumor hypoxic fraction was not directly correlated with the magnitude of urethane-induced decrease in blood flow *(25)*. It must be noted that 1.2 mg/kg urethane cited by Palavincini and Hill is likely an error, because 1.2 mg/kg would not be expected to induce anesthesia *(25)*. Johnson and colleagues reported similar findings during ip urethane 1.2–1.6 g/kg and ip pentobarbital 72 mg/kg anesthesia for tumor blood flow in sarcoma-implanted CBA and WHT mice *(88)*.

An interesting observation of increased duration of urethane anesthesia in tumor-bearing rats was made by Boyland and Rhoden *(83)*. A sc dose of 1 g/kg urethane resulted in 24 h of anesthesia in Walker carcinoma-bearing rats, compared to 8–12 h in normal rats. Traces of urethane were still present in the blood of tumor-bearing rats 48 h after injection, and urethane was absent from the blood of normal rats by 24 h.

6.2.7. PROTECTING LABORATORY WORKERS FROM URETHANE

Urethane is both mutagenic and carcinogenic *(89)*, and is regarded as a potential hazard to technical staff. Before using urethane, alternative anesthetics should be considered whenever possible. Precautions suitable for handling a moderate carcinogen should be utilized, including the use of appropriate breathing masks, gloves, and fume hoods for preparing solutions from the powdered drug. With the adoption of adequate precautions, urethane can be used in a reasonably safe manner.

6.3. Ketamine

6.3.1. MECHANISM OF ACTION

Ketamine is a cyclohexamine anesthetic that has been widely used for murine anesthesia since its introduction over 30 years ago. Ketamine anesthetic effects are best described as dose-dependent CNS depression that leads to a "dissociative" state characterized by profound analgesia and amnesia, but not necessarily loss of consciousness. The subject seems completely unaware of the environment, and suggested mechanisms include electrophysiologic inhibition of the thalamocortical pathways and stimulation of the limbic system. With ketamine, ocular and pharyngeal reflexes are retained, or attenuated less, than with other anesthetic agents, which can make monitoring of anesthetic depth through observation of physical signs misleading.

The wide use of ketamine can be attributed to its initial introduction as a Drug Enforcement Administration noncontrolled anesthetic (now reclassified DEA Class III), and its low cost, wide margin of safety, and ease of administration. Commercial ketamine is a racemic mixture of two optical enantiomers, R(–) and S(+), which differ in anesthetic potency and effect. The neuropharmacology of ketamine is complex with interactions at N-methyl D-aspartate (NMDA) and non-NMDA glutamate/nitric oxide/cyclic GMP (cGMP)-receptors, as well as nicotinic and muscarinic cholinergic receptors and monoaminergic and opioid receptors *(90)*. In addition, interactions with voltage-dependent Na^+ and L-type Ca^{++} channels have been described. Pharmacokinetically, ketamine has relatively short distribution and elimination half-lives. It is metabolized extensively by the hepatic cytochrome p450 system, and ketamine pretreatment can cause hepatic microsomal enzyme induction and tolerance. Norketamine, the primary metabolite, is one-third to one-fifth as potent as ketamine, and is excreted by the kidneys. Reduced renal output can result in prolonged ketamine action.

Muscle relaxation with ketamine is quite poor, and ketamine given alone does not produce satisfactory surgical anesthesia in rats or mice. To overcome this, ketamine is often combined with either alpha-2 adrenergic agonists, such as xylazine or medetomidine, or benzodiazepines, such as diazepam or midazolam, which further modifies cardiovascular and ventilatory effects.

The alpha-2 adrenergic agonists act by decreasing central noradrenergic neurotransmission through inhibition of presynaptic calcium influx and neurotransmitter release. Peripheral effects of alpha-2 agonists include vasoconstriction, hyperglycemia caused by decreased insulin release, diuresis, and decreased gastrointestinal motility. Bradycardia and hypertension commonly occur following alpha-2 adrenergic agonist administration, and severe respiratory and cardiovascular depression can occur when alpha-2 agonists are administered in combination with most anesthetic drugs.

Benzodiazepines act in the CNS at the $GABA_A$ receptor to modulate release of the excitatory neurotransmitters norepinephrine, dopamine, and serotonin. Although benzodiazepines can produce marked sedation in rodents, they are not analgesic. In general, benzodiazepines have minimal cardiovascular and respiratory effects. The phenothiazine tranquilizer acetylpromazine is sometimes combined with ketamine; yet acetylpromazine provides no additional analgesia, and can cause alpha-1 adrenergic-receptor blockade and hypotension. The combination of ketamine with an alpha-2 adrenergic agonist is preferred for surgical anesthesia, and combinations of ketamine with benzodiazepines or phenothiazines can only be recommended for procedures that are not painful (35).

6.3.2. Route of Administration and Cardiovascular Effects

Ketamine can be administered through intramuscular (im), iv, or ip methods. However, there is concern that im injection of ketamine can cause discomfort and tissue reactions in small rodents, and therefore this route should be avoided (8,35). Ketamine potentiates restraint-induced stress ulcers in the stomachs of rats, presumably because of splanchnic vasoconstriction (91).

The cardiovascular effects of ketamine are determined by dose and modified by concurrent administration with other anesthetic agents. Ketamine in vitro causes direct myocardial depression (92). Because of its receptor profile, however, ketamine increases myocardial contractility through increased sympathetic nervous system activity. The sympathetically mediated positive inotropic and chronotropic effects of ketamine can be blocked by inhaled anesthetics, ganglionic blockade, cervical epidural anesthesia, and spinal-cord transection (93,94). Ketamine has been reported to open arteriovenous shunts, so that microsphere-based methods of determining cardiac output and organ perfusion may be unreliable. Miller et al. reported that trapped microspheres were released from muscle and skin in Wistar rats given ip doses of ketamine 125 mg/kg, resulting in an apparent decrease in the distribution of cardiac output to muscle and an apparent increase in flow to the lung (95).

In a detailed study on the anesthetic effects of ketamine/xylazine mixtures in rats, Wixson and colleagues investigated three different dose combinations: 40/5 mg/kg, 60/7.5 mg/kg, and 80/10 mg/kg ketamine/xylazine *(56)*. All three doses produced deep levels of anesthesia, which persisted for 80–115 min. No mortality resulted from use of the mixture, and the authors recommended it for "procedures involving excessive manipulation of the animal." The major disadvantage of this anesthetic regimen was the presence of significant salivation, defecation, and urination with all doses. General recommended doses for ketamine/xylazine in rats range from 75–100 mg/kg ip ketamine + 10 mg/kg xylazine *(8)*, to 40–60 mg/kg ketamine + 3–5 mg/kg xylazine *(35)*. These doses provide surgical levels of anesthesia for 20–30 min.

In mice, an im dose of 100/5 mg/kg ketamine/xylazine was found to produce "excellent relaxation, sedation, and analgesia" in adult male Balb/c mice *(57)*. The mice remained at a surgical level of anesthesia for about 80 min. Although im injections have been used in mice, ip injections are now favored as a route of administration for this drug mixture *(8,35)*.

Ketamine alone results in a short vasodepression followed by a longer-lasting potent pressor response *(96)*. Ketamine-xylazine mixtures have variable effects on blood pressure and cardiac output in rats and mice. In male Sprague Dawley rats, an ip injection of 40/5 mg/kg ketamine/xylazine resulted in a 32.3% decrease in mean arterial pressure (MAP) *(56)*. A dose of 60/7.5 mg/kg ketamine/xylazine decreased MAP by 26.7% or 30–35 mmHg. MAP remained decreased until recovery, which was more than 2 h at the high dose. An ip injection of 40/5 and 60/7.5 mg/kg ketamine/xylazine decreased heart rate by 6% and 27%, respectively. Thus, both doses of ketamine/xylazine lowered MAP and heart rate *(56)*. Compared to awake rats, MAP decreased 11% and DS carcinosarcoma blood flow decreased 15.5% in Sprague Dawley rats given sc xylazine 1 mg/kg with ip ketamine 50 mg/kg, *(16)*. In contrast, an im dose of 50/5 mg/kg ketamine/xylazine maintained mean arterial pressure at approx 110 mmHg for 90 min in male Sprague Dawley rats, and an im dose of 100/10 mg/kg ketamine/xylazine maintained mean arterial pressure between 85 and 100 mmHg for 150 min *(55)*.

An im injection of 100/5 mg/kg ketamine/xylazine in Balb/c mice resulted in a decrease in MAP from 129 to 100 mmHg—a decrease of 22.5% *(57)*. Heart rate decreased from 509 to 159 beats/min, and the respiratory rate dropped from 195 to 109 breaths/min. In comparison, an ip dose of 150/15 mg/kg ketamine/xylazine reduced heart rate and cardiac output in SvEv/Tac mice from 658 to 293 beats/min, and cardiac output from 13.0 to 7.2 mL/min/g *(6)*.

Intraperitoneal injections of mixtures of ketamine/diazepam result in modest decreases in MAP in rats. A dose of 40/5 mg/kg ketamine/diazepam decreased MAP by 12%. A higher dose of 60/7.5 mg/kg resulted in a transient decrease of 31%, but the MAP was back to baseline value within 30–45 min after the injection *(56)*. Neither mixture had significant effects on heart rate, with heart-rate decreases of 9% and 12% at the two doses.

6.3.3. EFFECT ON VENTILATION AND BLOOD GASES

In male Sprague Dawley rats, ip ketamine/xylazine doses of 40/5 and 60/7.5 mg/kg decreased arterial pH by about 0.1 pH units, with slow recovery back to pre-anesthetic levels *(56)*. These same doses of ketamine/xylazine increased P_aCO_2 by 35%, and P_aO_2 decreased by 23–24%, or approx 18 mmHg. Both P_aCO_2 and P_aO_2 recovered within 60 min after the injection. In contrast, ketamine/xylazine im doses of 50/5 mg/kg in male Sprague Dawley rats maintained arterial blood-gas values within the physiologically normal range *(55)*.

Ketamine/xylazine mixtures also affect blood-gas values in mice. An im injection of a 100/5 mg/kg mixture of ketamine/xylazine into Balb/c mice decreased arterial blood pH from 7.285 to 7.122, or 0.16 pH units *(57)*. Arterial pCO_2 increased from 26.5 to 41.0 mmHg (55%), and p_aO_2 decreased from 111.7 to 97.3 mmHg, or approx 13% *(57)*.

Ketamine/diazepam mixtures have also been shown to affect blood-gas values in rats *(56)*. Intraperitoneal doses of 40/5 and 60/7.5 mg/kg decreased arterial pH in male Sprague Dawley rats by about 0.05 and 0.08 pH units, respectively. The lower dose of ketamine/diazepam (40/5 mg/kg) resulted in a P_aCO_2 increase of 20–30%. The higher dose (60/7.5 mg/kg) transiently increased P_aCO_2 by 4.9% (about 3–4 mmHg), respectively. The 40/5 and 60/7.5 mg/kg doses of ketamine/diazepam resulted in P_aO_2 decreases of 23% and 11.5% (8–9 mmHg), respectively.

6.3.4. TOLERANCE AND STRAIN DIFFERENCES

There are age and sex differences in the response of rats to ketamine *(97)*. Ketamine sleeping time decreases as young rats mature from 1–3 wk. This decrease in sleeping time seems to be associated with the increased production of norketamine, the cyclohexanone oxidation metabolite of ketamine. After 3 wk, females sleep longer in response to ketamine than males. Again, this seems to be associated with a greater ability of the male to produce the cyclohexanone oxidation metabolite.

6.3.5. EFFECTS ON BLOOD-GLUCOSE LEVELS AND HEMATOCRIT

Ketamine, alone or combined with xylazine, can increase blood-glucose levels. Blood-glucose levels following an iv glucose challenge are increased by ketamine *(98–100)*. Blood-glucose levels in male Sprague-Dawley rats injected with an ip 50/10 mg//kg ketamine/xylazine mixture rose to 256 mg/dL, compared to 131 mg/dL in pentobarbital-injected rats *(101)*. In the 9L glioma, xylazine alone or in combination with ketamine resulted in hyperglycemia and intratumor pH acidification *(10)*. The hyperglycemic response to xylazine is caused by reduced insulin secretion from pancreatic islets *(102)*.

Erhardt reported no effect of ketamine/xylazine (100/5 mg/kg) on hematocrit when injected intramuscularly into mice *(57)*. However, administration of alpha-2 agonists causes inhibition of antidiuretic hormone, antagonism of renal tubular action, and an increase in glomerular filtration, resulting in increased urine output *(103)*. In light of this, dehydration and increased hematocrit are certainly possible because of alpha-2 adrenergic agonist-induced diuresis.

6.3.6. EFFECT ON TUMOR PHYSIOLOGY AND RADIOSENSITIVITY

Compared to ip pentobarbital 60 mg/kg, ketamine 45 mg/kg combined with diazepam 20 mg/kg ip anesthesia increased radiosensitivity of the C3H mouse mammary adenocarcinoma in hyperbaric oxygen *(31)*. Body temperature of anesthetized mice in this study fell to 27°C, which may have contributed to radiosensitization. Interestingly, there was no difference in tumor radiosensitivity between ketamine/diazepam and pentobarbital anesthesia when mice were allowed to breathe air, implying that ketamine/diazepam anesthesia likely did not improve radiosensitivity over pentobarbital through improvement in tumor perfusion and oxygen delivery.

SUMMARY

It can be readily seen that both anesthesia and anesthetic management play major roles in defining a useful murine tumor model. It is the investigator's responsibility to assure that an anesthetic is appropriate, to determine sex and strain differences, to understand the effect of the anesthetic on the physiologic systems under study, and to control for known or predictable side effects in the particular tumor model.

The inhaled anesthetics, although rarely used in the study of murine tumors, are readily available in the United States, and have the unique advantage of providing a consistent, well-defined anesthetic dose during prolonged experiments. Administration of inhaled anesthetics to rats and mice, however, is not as easy or convenient as administration of injectable anesthetics. Therefore, pentobarbital, urethane, and ketamine will continue to be useful anesthetics in the study of murine tumors for many years to come.

As Smith reminds us, the suitability of any particular anesthetic agent is primarily a function of the user. Although no anesthetic agent can be considered truly ideal, careful choice and skillful application can define and minimize adverse physiological and pharmacological effects on tumor and normal tissue homeostasis.

REFERENCES

1. Tuma RF, Irion GL, Vasthare US, Heinel LA. Age-related changes in regional blood flow in the rat. *Am J Physiol* 1985; 249(3 Pt 2):H485–H491.
2. Skolleborg KC, Gronbech JE, Grong K, Abyholm FE, Lekven J. Distribution of cardiac output during pentobarbital versus midazolam/fentanyl/fluanisone anaesthesia in the rat. *Lab Anim* 1990; 24:221–227.
3. Janssen GH, Tangelder GJ, oude Egbrink MG, Reneman RS. Different effects of anesthetics on spontaneous leukocyte rolling in rat skin. *Int J Microcirc Clin Exp* 1997; 17:305–313.
4. Zanelli GD, Lucas PB. The effect of stress on blood perfusion and blood volume in transplanted mouse tumours. *Br J Radiol* 1976; 49:382–384.
5. Fagin KD, Shinsako J, Dallman MF. Effects of housing and chronic cannulation on plasma ACTH and corticosterone in the rat. *Am J Physiol* 1983; 245:E515–E520.
6. Yang XP, Liu YH, Rhaleb NE, Kurihara N, Kim HE, Carretero OA. Echocardiographic assessment of cardiac function in conscious and anesthetized mice. *Am J Physiol* 1999; 277(5 Pt 2):H1967–H974.
7. Shibamoto Y, Sasai K, Abe M. The radiation response of SCCVII tumor cells in C3H/He mice varies with the irradiation conditions. *Radiat Res* 1987; 109:352–354.
8. Flecknell PA. *Laboratory Animal Anaesthesia: A practical introduction for research workers and technicians,* 2nd ed., Academic Press, London, 1996.
9. Carruba MO, Bondiolotti G, Picotti GB, Catteruccia N, Da Prada M. Effects of diethyl ether, halothane, ketamine and urethane on sympathetic activity in the rat. *Eur J Pharmacol* 1987; 134:15–24.
10. Pavlovic M, Wroblewski K, Manevich Y, Kim S, Biaglow JE. The importance of choice of anaesthetics in studying radiation effects in the 9L rat glioma. *Br J Cancer Suppl* 1996; 27:S222–S225.
11. Kohn DF, Wixson SK, White WJ, Benson GJ, eds. *Anesthesia and Analgesia in Laboratory Animals.* Academic Press, San Diego, CA, 1997.
12. Thurmon JC, Tranquilli WJ, Benson GJ, eds. *Lumb and Jones' Veterinary Anesthesia,* 3rd ed., Williams and Wilkins, Philadelphia, PA, 1996.
13. Muir WW III, Hubbell JAE, Skarda RT, Bednarski RM, eds. *Handbook of Veterinary Anesthesia,* 3rd ed., Mosby, St. Louis, MO, 1000, pp. 394–401.
14. Eger EI. II *Anesthetic Uptake and Action.* Williams and Wilkins, Baltimore, MD, 1974.
15. Sancho AR, Dowell JA, Wolf W. The effects of anesthesia on the biodistribution of drugs in rats: a study. *Cancer Chemother Pharmacol* 1997; 40:521–525.
16. Menke H, Vaupel P. Effect of injectable or inhalational anesthetics and of neuroleptic, neuroleptanalgesic, and sedative agents on tumor blood flow. *Radiat Res* 1988; 114:64–76.

17. Mason DE, Brown MJ. Monitoring of Anesthesia. In: *Anesthesia and Analgesia in Laboratory Animals* (Kohn DF, Wixson SK, White WJ, Benson GJ, eds., Academic Press, San Diego, CA, 1997; pp. 73–82.

18. Styles M, Coleman AJ, Leary WP. Some hemodynamic effects of sodium nitroprusside. *Anesthesiology* 1973; 38:173–176.

19. Banic A, Krejci V, Erni D, Wheatley AM, Sigurdsson GH. Effects of sodium nitroprusside and phenylephrine on blood flow in free musculocutaneous flaps during general anesthesia. *Anesthesiology* 1999; 90:147–155.

20. Bendo AA, Kass IS, Hartung J, Cotrell JE. Anesthesia for neurosurgery. In: Barash PG, Cullen BF, Stoelting RK, eds., *Clinical Anesthesia,* 3rd ed. Lippincott-Raven, Philadelphia, PA, 1997; pp. 730.

21. Eger EI II. Isoflurane: a review. *Anesthesiology* 1981; 55:559–576.

22. Stoelting RK. *Pharmacology and Physiology in Anesthetic Practice,* 2nd ed., JB. Lippincott, Philadelphia, PA, 1991.

23. Barash PG, Cullen BF, Stoelting RK, eds. *Clinical Anesthesia,* 3rd ed., Lippincott-Raven, Philadelphia, PA, 1997.

24. Hardman JG, Limbird LE, Molinoff PB, Ruddon RW, Gilman AG, eds. *Goodman and Gilmans' The Pharmacological Basis of Therapeutics,* 9th ed., McGraw-Hill, New York, NY, 1996.

25. Pallavicini MG, Hill RP. Effect of tumor blood flow manipulations on radiation response. *Int J Radiat Oncol Biol Phys* 1983; 9:1321–1325.

26. Suit HD, Sedlacek RS, Silver G, Dosoretz D. Pentobarbital anesthesia and the response of tumor and normal tissue in the C3Hf/sed mouse to radiation. *Radiat Res* 1985; 104:47–65.

27. Malkinson TJ, Cooper KE, Veale WL. Physiological changes during thermoregulation and fever in urethan-anesthetized rats. *Am J Physiol* 1988; 255(1 Pt 2):R73–R81.

28. Lovell DP. Variation in barbiturate sleeping time in mice. 3. Strain X environment interactions. *Lab Anim* 1986c; 20:307–312.

29. Vitez TS, White PF, Eger EI II. Effects of hypothermia on halothane MAC and isoflurane MAC in the rat. *Anesthesiology* 1974; 41:80–81.

30. Biaglow JE, Suit HD, Durand RE, Dosoretz DE. On the mechanism for enhancement of tumor radiation to hyperbaric oxygen in sodium pentobarbital anesthetized rodents. *Adv Exp Med Biol* 1984; 180:301–310.

31. Tozer GM, Penhaligon M, Nias AH. The use of ketamine plus diazepam anaesthesia to increase the radiosensitivity of a C3H mouse mammary adenocarcinoma in hyperbaric oxygen. *Br J Radiol* 1984; 57:75–80.

32. Ben-Eliyahu S, Shakhar G, Rosenne E, Levinson Y, Beilin B. Hypothermia in barbiturate-anesthetized rats suppresses natural killer cell activity and compromises resistance to tumor metastasis: a role for adrenergic mechanisms. *Anesthesiology* 1999; 91:732–740.

33. Kurz A, Sessler DI, Lenhardt R. Perioperative normothermia to reduce the incidence of surgical-wound infection and shorten hospitalization. Study of Wound Infection and Temperature Group. *N Engl J Med* 1996; 334:1209–1215.

34. Beilin B, Shavit Y, Razumovsky J, Wolloch Y, Zeidel A, Bessler H. Effects of mild perioperative hypothermia on cellular immune responses. *Anesthesiology* 1998; 89:1133–1140.

35. Wixson SK, Smiler KL. Anesthesia and analgesia in rodents: In: Kohn DF, Wixson SK, White WJ, Benson GJ, eds. *Anesthesia and Analgesia in Laboratory Animals* Academic Press, San Diego, CA, 1997; pp. 165–203.

36. IARC (1987). IARC monographs on the evaluation of carcinogenic risks to humans, overall evaluations of carcinogenicity; an updating of IARC monographs. Suppl 7, vol. 1–42, Lyon, IARC Press, France pp. 38–57.

37. Rice SA. Reproductive and developmental toxicity of anesthetics in animals: In: Rice SA, Fish KJ, eds., *Anesthetic Toxicity* Raven Press, New York, NY, 1994; pp. 157–174.

38. Cousins MJ, Mazze RI, Barr GA, Kosek JC. A comparison of the renal effects of isoflurane and methoxyflurane in Fischer 344 rats. *Anesthesiology* 1973; 38:557–563.

39. Stevenson GW, Hall SC, Rudnick S, Seleny FL, Stevenson HC. The effect of anesthetic agents on the human immune response. *Anesthesiology* 1990; 72:542–552.

40. Moudgil GC, Singal DP. Halothane and isoflurane enhance melanoma tumour metastasis in mice. *Can J Anaesth* 1997; 44:90–94.

41. Knight PR, Bedows E, Nahrwold ML, Maassab HF, Smitka CW, Busch MT. Alterations in influenza virus pulmonary pathology induced by diethyl ether, halothane, enflurane, and pentobarbital anesthesia in mice. *Anesthesiology* 1983; 58:209–215.

42. Bates ML, Feingold A, Gold MI. The effects of anesthetics on an in-vivo oxygen electrode. *Am J Clin Pathol* 1975; 64:448–451.

43. Dent JG, Netter KJ. Errors in oxygen tension measurements caused by halothane. *Br J Anaesth* 1976; 48:195–197.

44. McHugh RD, Epstein RM, Longnecker DE. Halothane mimics oxygen in oxygen microelectrodes. *Anesthesiology* 1979; 50:47–49.

45. National Institute for Occupational Safety and Health (NIOSH). A Recommended Standard for Occupational Exposure to … Waste Anesthetic Gases and Vapors. Cincinnati, DHHS (NIOSH), 1977; Publication No. 77–140.

46. Berry AJ, Katz JD. Hazards of working in the operating room. In: Barash PG, Cullen BF, Stoelting RK, eds., *Clinical Anesthesia,* 3rd ed. Lippincott-Raven, Philadelphia, PA, 1997; pp. 69–91.

47. Meyer RE. Anesthesia hazards to animal workers. *Occup Med* 1999; 14:225–234.

48. Special report from the American College of Veterinary Anesthesiologists Commentary and recommendations on control of waste anesthetic gases in the workplace. *J Am Vet Med Assoc* 1996; 209:75–77.

49. Huang LY, Barker JL. Pentobarbital: stereospecific actions of (+) and (–) isomers revealed on cultured mammalian neurons. *Science* 1980; 207:195–197.

50. Macdonald RL, McLean MJ. Anticonvulsant drugs: mechanisms of action. *Adv Neurol* 1986; 44:713–736.

51. Olsen RW. GABA-drug interactions. *Prog Drug Res* 1987; 31:223–241.

52. Saunders PA, Ho IK. Barbiturates and the GABAA receptor complex. *Prog Drug Res* 1990; 34:261–286.

53. Freudenthal RI, Carroll FI. Metabolism of certain commonly used barbiturates. *Drug Metab Rev* 1973; 2:265–278.

54. Kawaue Y, Iriuchijima J. Changes in cardiac output and peripheral flows on pentobarbital anesthesia in the rat. *Jpn J Physiol* 1984; 34:283–294.

55. Taie S, Leichtweis SB, Liu KJ, Miyake M, Grinberg O, Demidenko E, et al. Effects of ketamine/xylazine and pentobarbital anesthesia on cerebral tissue oxygen tension, blood pressure, and arterial blood gas in rats. *Adv Exp Med Biol* 1999; 471:189–198.

56. Wixson SK, White WJ, Hughes HC Jr, Lang CM, Marshall WK. The effects of pentobarbital, fentanyl-droperidol, ketamine-xylazine and ketamine-diazepam on arterial blood pH, blood gases, mean arterial blood pressure and heart rate in adult male rats. *Lab Anim Sci* 1987; 37:736–742.

57. Erhardt W, Hebestedt A, Aschenbrenner G, Pichotka B, Blumel G. A comparative study with various anesthetics in mice (pentobarbitone, ketamine-xylazine, carfentanyl-etomidate). *Res Exp Med (Berl)* 1984; 184:159–169.

58. Dewhirst MW, Ong E, Rosner G, Rehmus S, Shan S, Braun R, et al. Arteriolar oxygenation in tumor and subcutaneous arterioles: Effects of inspired air oxygen content, *Br J Cancer* 1996; 74:S247–S251.

59. Collins TB Jr, Lott DF. Stock and sex specificity in the response of rats to pentobarbital sodium. *Lab Anim Care* 1968; 18:192–194.

60. Holck HGO, Kanân MA, Mills LM, Smith EL. Studies upon the sex-difference in rats in tolerance to certain barbiturates and to nicotine. *J Pharmacol Exp Ther* 1937; 60:323–346.

61. Lovell DP. Variation in pentobarbitone sleeping time in mice. 1. Strain and sex differences. *Lab Anim* 1986a; 20:85–90.

62. Lovell DP. Variation in pentobarbitone sleeping time in mice. 2. Variables affecting test results. *Lab Anim* 1986b; 20:91–96.

63. Rockwell S, Moulder JE, Martin DF. Tumor-to-tumor variability in the hypoxic fraction of experimental rodent tumors. *Radiother Oncol* 1984; 2:57–64.

64. Moulder JE, Rockwell S. Hypoxic fractions of solid tumors: experimental techniques, methods of analysis, and a survey of existing data. *Int J Radiat Oncol Biol Phys* 1984; 10:695–712.

65. Gullino PM, Grantham FH, Courtney AH. Utilization of oxygen by transplanted tumor in vivo. *Cancer Res* 1967; 27:1020–1030.

66. Sheldon PW, Hill SA, Moulder JE. Radioprotection by pentobarbitone sodium of a murine tumour in vivo. *Int J Radiat Biol* 1977; 32:571–575.

67. Sheldon PW, Chu AM. The effect of anesthetics on the radiosensitivity of a murine tumor. *Radiat Res* 1979; 79:568–578.

68. Denekamp J, Terry NHA, Sheldon PW, Chu AM. The effect of pentobarbital anaesthesia on the radiosensitivity of four mouse tumours. *Int J Radiat Biol* 1979; 35:277–280.

69. Aldridge WN, Parker VH. Barbiturates and oxidative phosphorylation. *Biochem J* 1960; 76:47–56.

70. Biaglow JE, Yau TM. Anaesthesia and efficacy of hyperbaric oxygen in radiation therapy. *Br J Radiol* 1980; 53:919–920.

71. Rockwell S, Loomis R. Effects of sodium pentobarbital on the radiation response of EMT6 cells in vitro and EMT6 tumors in vivo. *Radiat Res* 1980; 81:292–302.

72. Buelke-Sam J, Holson JF, Bazare JJ, Young JF. Comparative stability of physiological parameters during sustained anesthesia in rats. *Lab Anim Sci* 1978; 28:157–162.

73. van der Meer C, Versluys-Broers JA, Tuynman HA, Buur VA. The effect of ethylurethane on hematocrit, blood pressure and plasma-glucose. *Arch Int Pharmacodyn Ther* 1975; 217:257–275.

74. Volicer L, Loew CG. The effect of urethane anesthesia on the cardiovascular action of angiotensin II. *Pharmacology* 1971; 6:193–201.

75. Reinert H. Urethane hyperglycaemia and hypothalamic activation. *Nature* 1964; 204:889–891.

76. Hillebrand A, Meer C, van der, Ariens AT, Wijnans M. The effect of anesthetics on the occurrence of kidney lesions caused by hypotension. *Eur J Pharmacol* 1971; 14:217–237.

77. Field KJ, White WJ, Lang CM. Anaesthetic effects of chloral hydrate, pentobarbitone, and urethane in adult male rats. *Lab Anim* 1993; 27:258–269.

78. Sapru HN, Krieger AJ. Cardiovascular and respiratory effects of some anesthetics in the decerebrate rat. *Eur J Pharmacol* 1979; 53:151–158.

79. Alfaro V, Palacios L. Differential effects of hypothermia upon blood acid-base state and blood gases in sodium pentobarbital and urethane anesthetized rats. *Gen Pharmacol* 1992; 23:677–682.

80. Spriggs TLB, Stockham MA. Urethane anesthesia and pituitary adrenal function. *J Pharmacol Pharmac* 1964; 16:603–610.

81. Severs WB, Keil LC, Klase PA, Deen KC. Urethane anesthesia in rats. Altered ability to regulate hydration. *Pharmacology* 1981; 22:209–226.

82. Braun RD, Dewhirst MW, Hatchell DL. Quantification of erythrocyte flow in the choroid of the albino rat. *Am J Physiol* 1997; 272:H1444–H1453.

83. Boyland E, Rhoden E. The distribution of urethane in animal tissues, as determined by a microdiffusion method, and the effect of urethane treatment on enzymes. *Biochem J* 1949; 44:528–531.

84. Maggi CA, Meli A. Suitability of urethane anesthesia for physiopharmacological investigations in various systems. Part 1: General considerations. *Experientia* 1986; 42:109–114.

85. Pettinger WA, Tanaka K, Keeton K, Campbell WB, Brooks N. Renin release, an artifact of anesthesia and its implication in rats. *Proc Soc Exp Biol Med* 1975; 148:625–630.

86. Hamstra WN, Doray D, Dunn JD. The effect of urethane on pituitary-adrenal function of female rats. *Acta Endocrinol* 1984; 106:362–367.

87. Lincoln DW, Hill A, Wakerley JB. The milk ejection reflex in the rat: an intermittent function not abolished by surgical levels of anesthesia. *J Endocrinol* 1973; 57:459–476.

88. Johnson R, Fowler JF, Zanelli GD. Changes in mouse blood pressure, tumor blood flow, and core and tumor temperatures following nembutal or urethane anesthesia. *Radiology* 1976; 118:697–703.

89. Field KJ, Lang CM. Hazards of urethane (ethyl carbamate) a review of the literature. *Lab Anim* 1988; 22:255–262.

90. Kohrs R, Durieux ME. Ketamine: Teaching a old drug new tricks. *Anesth Analg* 1998; 87:1186–1193.

91. Cheney DH, Slogoff S, Allen GW. Ketamine-induced stress ulcers in the rat. *Anesthesiology* 1974; 40:531–535.

92. Schwartz DA, Horwitz LD. Effects of ketamine on left ventricular performance. *J Pharmacol Exp Ther* 1975; 194:410–414.

93. Stanley TH. Blood-pressure and pulse-rate responses to ketamine during general anesthesia. *Anesthesiology* 1973; 39:648–649.

94. Traber DL, Wilson RD, Priano LL. Blockade of the hypertensive effect to ketamine. *Anesth Analg* 1970; 49:420–426.

95. Miller ED, Jr, Kistner JR, Epstein RM. Whole-body distribution of radioactively labelled microspheres in the rat during anesthesia with halothane, enflurane, or ketamine. *Anesthesiology* 1980; 52:296–302.

96. Altura BM, Altura BT, Carella A. Effects of ketamine on vascular smooth muscle function. *Br J Pharmacol* 1980; 70:257–267.

97. Waterman AE, Livingston A. Effects of age and sex on ketamine anaesthesia in the rat. *Br J Anaesth* 1978; 50:885–889.

98. Aynsley-Green A, Biebuyck JF, Alberti KG. Anaesthesia and insulin secretion: the effects of diethyl ether, halothane, pentobarbitone sodium and ketamine hydrochloride on intravenous glucose tolerance and insulin secretion in the rat. *Diabetologia* 1973; 9:274–281.
99. Hsu WH, Hembrough FB. Intravenous glucose tolerance test in cats: influenced by acetylpromazine, ketamine, morphine, thiopental, and xylazine. *Am J Vet Res* 1982; 43:2060–2061.
100. Reyes Toso CF, Linares LM, Rodriguez RR. Blood sugar concentrations during ketamine or pentobarbitone anesthesia in rats with or without alpha and beta adrenergic blockade. *Medicina (B Aires)* 1995; 55:311–316.
101. Kawai N, Keep RF, Betz AL. Hyperglycemia and the vascular effects of cerebral ischemia. *Stroke* 1997; 28:149–154.
102. Hsu WH, Hummel SK. Xylazine-induced hyperglycemia in cattle: a possible involvement of alpha 2-adrenergic receptors regulating insulin release. *Endocrinology* 1981; 109:825–829.
103. Maze M, Buttermann AE, Kamibayashi T, et al. Alpha-2 adrenergic agonists: In: White PF, ed. *Textbook of Intravenous Anesthesia* Williams and Wilkins, London, 1997, pp. 433–445.
104. Steffey EP. Inhalation anesthetics: In Thurmon JC, Tranquilli WJ, Benson GJ, eds. *Lumb and Jones' Veterinary Anesthesia,* 3rd ed. Williams and Wilkins, Baltimore, MD, 1996, pp. 297–329.

VIII DISEASE AND TARGET-SPECIFIC MODELS

23

Tissue-Isolated Tumors in Mice

Ex Vivo Perfusion of Human Tumor Xenografts

Paul E.G. Kristjansen, MD, PhD

Contents

1. INTRODUCTION

The microenvironment surrounding cancer cells in vivo in a solid tumor exerts a profound influence on the tumor's growth and response to treatment. The heterogeneous blood flow and the complex exchange between vascular, interstitial, and cellular compartments govern the nutrient delivery, the metabolic activity, and the transport of agents in the neoplastic tissue. In vivo studies of whole tumors do not separate the relative contributions from various blood-borne metabolites, and in vitro studies are far from representative of tissue conditions in a solid tumor in vivo. The ex vivo perfused preparation represents a useful link between extremes. This chapter discusses these tumor-model types and demonstrates the type of information that can be obtained by such models.

In a series of investigations, we have found that the tumor-cell type is an important determinant of the overall steady-state metabolic status of the solid tumor tissue, regarded as a homogenous volume *(1–4)*. The uptake and distribution physiology of two low-mol-wt agents, a contrast agent *(5)* and gemcitabine, a cytostatic compound *(6,7)*, was different between tumor lines, despite similar anatomical tumor preparations. So important physiological differences, determined by the cell type, can be mediated through extracellular, microenvironmental factors. In the opposite direction, physiological factors such as hypoxia and other manifestations of hypoperfusion profoundly regulate both drug uptake and gene expression through several mechanisms, such as hypoxia-inducible factor *(HIF)* *(8–10)*. The emerging understanding of this process beautifully unifies tumor hypoxia, angiogenesis, and glycolytic predominance, i.e., metabolic adaptation. This illustrates the significance of linking cellular, or subcellular, levels to multi-compartmentalized in vivo systems.

From: *Tumor Models in Cancer Research*
Edited by: B. A. Teicher © Humana Press Inc., Totowa, NJ

The importance of tumor pathophysiology as a research discipline has increased in parallel to the continuous recognition of new subcellular targets for antineoplastic treatment. Genetically engineered compounds, gene vectors, antibodies, and modified cells all represent agents whose final delivery at an intratumoral target destination is heavily affected by physiological and microenvironmental factors. Future research into the interaction between tissue components and cancer cells, and between the solid tumor, viewed as an integrated organ, and therapeutic agents is important to ensure the ultimate benefit of therapeutic strategies developed in the test tube. Incessant refinement and specific adaptation of the experimental in vivo models are essential elements of progress in experimental oncology.

2. TISSUE-ISOLATED HUMAN TUMOR XENOGRAFTS

A tissue-isolated tumor grows with only a single artery-vein pair as its sole connection to the host vasculature. Therefore, complete ex vivo perfusion is feasible in contrast to spontaneous tumors or subcutaneous (sc) transplants, where the vascular network is variable and usually multifocal. Ex vivo perfusion of tumor xenografts permits several types of experiments, some of which are listed in Fig. 1 (top panel). In principle, the strategy is to establish growth of tumor tissue at an anatomically favorable site, where a distinct vascular pedicle can be established, and subsequently to avoid additional interaction with the surrounding host tissues. Various anatomical sites have been utilized in the rat—such as the kidney, the mammary glands, and the skin flaps—but foremost the left periovarium and the inguinal region. With the latter two anatomical regions, only minor volumes of nontumorous host tissue remain in the final preparation, whereas the kidney preparations contain a considerable amount of normal host parenchyma (11). The ovarian preparation, as pioneered by Gullino and Grantham (12) in rats, and later developed for nude mice (13), permits complete ex vivo perfusion of the tissue-isolated tumor. In SCID mice, the periovarian fat was considerably more difficult to dissect than in nudes, so in addition to their comfortable alopecia, the nude mice also possess other anatomical advantages.

This preparation was developed in mice to obtain a perfusable human xenograft model. The term "tissue-isolated" was coined by Gullino (11,12). Later, other investigators used tissue-isolated tumors in rats for various purposes: studies of blood flow and physiology (14–19), tumor metabolism (20–24), and pharmacokinetics (25–28).

2.1. Preparation of Tissue-Isolated Tumors in Mice

Tumor blocks are not an ideal transplantation material for this preparation. Alternatively, a tumor slurry is made from the donor tissue. For transplantation, the donor tumor is removed from the host animal upon euthanasia and washed in a salt solution, such as Hank's Balanced Salt Solution, (HBSS, Gibco, NY). After removal of macroscopically nonviable parts, the viable tissue is cut with scalpels and scissors and gradually minced into a thick slurry by adding a few drops of HBSS.

A 1-cm incision is made in the midcoronal plane of the left lumbar region of a properly anesthetized female nude mouse, and a sc space is created by blunt dissection. The left ovary, the mesovarium, and the left uterine horn are pulled out through a short incision in the abdominal wall (Fig. 2). The ovarian vessels are identified—i.e. the vein, since the artery is barely visible—and the perivascular connective tissue is detached

TISSUE-ISOLATED TUMORS

⇨ Ex vivo perfusion

Arterio-venous differences:
- Drugs and other agents ⇨ Tumor pharmacokinetics
- Nutrients & metabolites ⇨ Tumor metabolism

Tumor Blood Flow:
- Determinants (pressure, resistance)
- Modifiers ⇨ Tumor physiology

Corrosion casts
- Vascular 3-D morphology ⇨ Tumor vascular anatomy

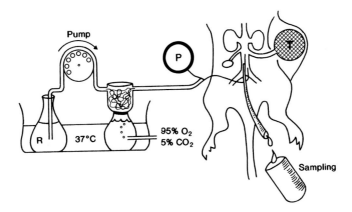

Fig. 1. Top: Types of experiments with *ex vivo* perfused human tumor xenografts. Bottom: Schematic of a perfusion experiments with a tissue-isolated tumor transplant. All vascular branches, except those draining or feeding the tissue-isolated tumor, are ligated. The abdominal aorta and the vena cava have been cannulated, and the vascular connection to the host is terminated by a ligature at the cranial side of the superior mesenteric artery. R = Perfusate reservoir; T = Tissue-isolated tumor in a sealed bag. (Adapted from ref. 7)

from the left kidney. The left uterine horn and the ovary are removed following proximal and distal ligatures. The remaining portions of the mesovarium are carefully removed, with care to observe and maintain the vascular integrity of the ovarian vessels, leaving a pedicle consisting of a reduced ovarian fat pad, some connective tissue, and the two ovarian vessels. Then the internal abdominal incision is closed with three sutures, and the pedicle is positioned in the sc space. A flat bag, made by an hourglass-shaped sterile parafilm sheet with a slit in the lower half, is tightened around the pedicle. Before closing the bag by pressing the edges of the two parafilm sheets together, 0.03 mL of tumor slurry is carefully injected into the fat pad and distal pedicle through a 20-gauge needle (0.9 mm internal diameter), without destroying the structure of the pedicle and carefully avoiding damage to the vessels. The bag is gently placed in the sc space in the flank of the mouse, and the skin is closed by a continuous suture, preferably intradermally. After 5–6 d the skin should be opened, upon anesthesia, and the bag

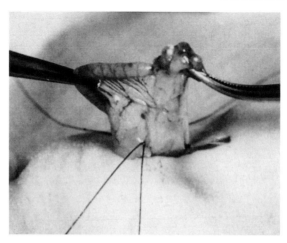

Fig. 2. The left uterine horn *(left side)* and the ovarian fat pad with the left ovarium *(right side)*. The ovarian vessels (mainly the vein) are seen as the vertical line at the right side.

should be opened and removed. Adherences between the pedicle and the abdominal wall should be loosened, if necessary, and the internal suture is checked. A new sterile bag should be placed, and the skin closed. Depending on the growth rate of the individual tumor, this procedure must be repeated after another 5–6 d.

The result of this procedure is a tissue-isolated tumor, which is only connected to the host organism through the vascular pedicle with one artery and one vein.

2.2. Ex Vivo Perfusion of Tissue-Isolated Tumors

Ex vivo perfusion provides complete control of the input concentration of any substance of interest, and no recirculation occurs. The major disadvantage is that the surgical preparation is technically demanding and quite laborious. Moreover, the ex vivo perfused tumor does not reveal information about interactions between the host organism and the tumor, since the tumor is exteriorized from the host organism. Any information obtained in such preparations may not hold true in an integrated physiological system, in which the tumor circulation is connected in parallel to intact organs, and where the adjoining tissue—and to an unknown extent the tumor itself—is under neural and endocrine regulation from the host organism. Finally, the ex vivo perfused tumor alone is a black box with regard to processes that take place inside it. Whether the inherent reductionism implied by this experimental model is advantageous or not is entirely dependent on the question posed and how its answer is interpreted.

2.3. Technical Aspects

The exteriorization of the tumors for ex vivo perfusion is obtained by a sequence of microsurgical procedures described in this section.

The strategy is to gain access to the tumor vasculature by cannulation as close as possible to the afferent and efferent tumor vessels. In the tissue-isolated preparation, the tumor artery is minute, and cannulation is difficult. If performed with sufficient microscopical technique, the flow resistance in a rigid catheter of minuscule dimensions is very high, which further complicates the perfusion. Instead, all aortic branches—except the former left ovarian artery—are ligated and the abdominal aorta is

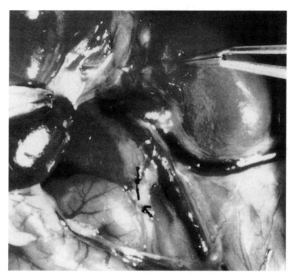

Fig. 3. The abdominal cavity of a female nude mouse with a tissue-isolated tumor at the right flank. The left kidney is seen at the upper right corner, held by the right forceps. The J-shaped vessel running horizontally along the lower kidney pole is the tumor vein, i.e., the former left ovarian vein. The tumor artery is not visible at this magnification, expect when a dye such as Evans blue is used.

cannulated. The tip of the arterial cannula is positioned close to the tumor (ovarian) artery without blocking it. Murine vessels are smaller than those of rats, and—more importantly—the vascular anatomy in nude mice differs from that of rats and humans, whose left ovarian vein enters the renal vein at some distance from the vena cava. In mice, the vein connects with vena cava at the angle between the renal and the caval vein (*see* Fig. 3). Therefore, in order to obtain access to the tumor effluent, the vena cava should be cannulated with the tip of the cannula positioned just caudally to the connection with the tumor vein. As on the arterial side, all other venous connections to the vena cava are ligated. The surgical field comprises all abdominal vascular branches between the coeliac truncus and the iliac bifurcation. The ligatures must be performed stepwise with great caution to avoid premature disturbance of the systemic circulation through the tumor *(7,13)*. Failure at any step immediately ruins the preparation, although in some instances a second chance is obtained by unhesitant and accurate application of a tiny drop of cyanoacrylate glue. The most critical steps during surgery are the separation of the tumor artery from the renal vessels prior to ligation of the latter, and the positioning of the final ligature between the coeliac truncus and the now ligated superior mesenteric artery. If this most cranial ligature is not placed at a sufficient distance from the entry of the tumor vein into the vena cava, the angle between the latter two vessels diminishes, creating a false valve that blocks the retrograde flow in the small section of the caval vein until the efferent catheter is reached. The ligation of the left superior suprarenal artery, which must be performed before ligation of the inferior suprarenal vessels, is a delicate step.

The perfusion set up is illustrated in Fig. 1 (bottom panel). When monitoring the perfusion pressure by the pressure transducer indicated in the figure, the particular contribution of the small aortic (afferent) catheter to the overall flow resistance should be

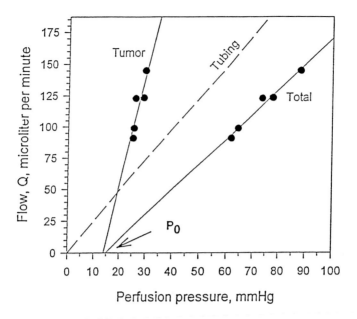

Fig. 4. The pressure-flow (p-Q plot) from a single perfusion experiment (a human SCLC xenograft, grown as a tissue-isolated tumor in a nude mouse). The curve at the right marked "Total" represent measured values of pressure and flow. The dashed line is the pressure-flow-relationship of the tubing system, obtained from calibration experiments. The left side curve, marked "Tumor," is the calculated tumor p-Q plot obtained by subtraction of baseline from total. The slopes of the curves represent the reciprocal flow resistances from which the geometric resistances are calculated. P0 is the zero-flow intercept. (Adapted from ref. 7)

kept in mind. With the very small PE-10 catheters (0.28 mm internal dimension (id) and 0.61 mm outside diameter (od), which are necessary in mice, a large fraction of the total pressure difference over the preparation will be caused by the afferent tube resistance. Therefore, standardized tubing dimensions, and baseline recordings of the pressure-flow relationship in every single experiment, are mandatory. The total flow resistance is the sum of the tubing resistance and the tumor-flow resistance, since they are connected in series (*see* Fig. 4). (Adapted from ref. 7)

2.4. Vascular Casts

Polymer casts of the tumor vasculature in tissue-isolated tumors can be prepared using commercially available methylmethacrylate-based mixtures. These preparations are undertaken in order to document the vascular integrity of the tissue-isolated tumors, or for visual analysis of the vascular morphology. Most commercially available kits are intended for casting of hollow structures larger than murine microvessels, through which the syrup-like casting agent can hardly be forced. So the procedure must usually be modified by dilution. Our experience is that a 45% dilution of the monomer base with additional methylmethacrylate, before adding promoter and catalyst, sufficiently balances the need for lower viscosity against an acceptable short time until curing and hardening of the cast. This mixture is functional only after clearing of the blood from the tumor by perfusion with heparinized saline containing 1.5 mM papaverine, before infusion of the casting mixture at a fixed perfusion pressure.

Table 1
Physiological Parameters in Human Colon Adenocarcinoma LS174T Xenografts
in Three Different Transplantation Sites in Athymic Nude Mice

	Tissue-isolated	Flank	Hind leg
IFP, mmHg	14.5[a]	9.0	9.3
range	(9–19.5)	(5–15)	(7.3–17)
Tumor volume, mm^3	542	475	405
range	(126–1080)	(205–706)	(108–1183)
Perfusion, % cardiac output x g^{-1}	1.25[b]	1.43[b]	1.58[b]
range	(0.60–1.44)	(0.97–2.22)	(0.33–2.36)
Tumor volume, mm^3	703	357	175
range	(473–1112)	(170–1054)	(57–475)
pO$_2$, mmHg	23[c]	14	18
Hypoxic fraction (<2.5 mmHg)	4%	7%	8%
Tumor volume, mm^3	250	225	230
range	(210–300)	(200–250)	(200–275)

IFP = interstitial fluid pressure. Perfusion rate was measured at d 21 after transplantation

[a] Significantly higher than both flank and leg tumors ($0.02 < p < 0.05$)

[b] No significant difference between transplantation groups

[c] Significantly higher than both flank and leg tumors ($p < 0.001$)

Values are medians. Statistical comparison between transplantation types is by the Wilcoxon test. Data from (13).

3. DEPENDENCE ON TRANSPLANTATION SITE AND TUMOR LINE

In the immune-incompetent mouse, all anatomical sites are potentially useful for transplantation. Some are more practical than others from a technical point of view, such as the sc space, and in other loci—such as bronchial mucosa or brain—growth of the transplant is lethal to the host animal. Some investigators believe that a particular match between the tissue of origin of the human tumor transplant and the corresponding murine recipient tissue, such as renal adenocarcinomas transplanted in the kidney and intradermal melanomas, is intradermal advantageous. Depending on which question is asked, the species difference may be of greater significance than the tissue or organ type. Different biological behavior of transplanted materials in different anatomical sites of the recipient animal also occurs as the result of topological differences in physiology and anatomy. In the human-colon adenocarcinoma LS174T, macroscopical tumor growth, tumor oxygen partial pressure (pO$_2$), tumor interstitial fluid pressure (IFP), and tumor-blood-perfusion rate were compared in three different transplantation sites in nude mice: tissue-isolated (ovarian), flank, and hind leg (13) (see Table 1. The growth functions in sc tumors in the flank and hind leg were compared with tissue-isolated tumors by a Gompertzian growth algorithm. The volume doubling time remained constant in the tissue-isolated preparation, whereas an exponential increase—corresponding to a gradual retardation of growth—was observed in the flank and hind leg tumors. These different growth patterns suggest that the presence of a superior nutrient supply in the tissue-isolated tumors, which is able to defer the usual retardation of tumor growth, is a prevalent characteristic of growing tumors (29).

The blood perfusion was not significantly different between transplantation modes, whereas the median pO_2 and the fraction of hypoxic readings (>2.5 mmHg) were. These findings are not contradictory. Rather, they are illustrative that global estimates of whole-organ (tumor) perfusion, in this case with ^{86}Rb uptake, do not yield information on the regional distribution of the flow within the tumors. In a steady-state situation with constant metabolism, the vascular density of the tissue and the overall endothelial surface area are the major determinants of tissue oxygenation (30). Correspondingly, increases in the adenosine triphosphate (ATP):P_i and ATP: adenosine diphosphate (ADP) + adenosine monophosphate (AMP), consistent with an improved oxygen availability, were found in a C3H murine mammary carcinoma grown in CDF1 mice, following treatment with nicotinamide. This occurred with no apparent modification of the tumor blood perfusion, as measured by the ^{86}Rb uptake method (31). The IFP of tissue-isolated tumors appeared somehow greater, compared with the two sc transplantation modes found. Since the tumor IFP is primarily maintained by microvascular pressure (32), the slightly higher IFP in tissue-isolates is believed to reflect the centrifugal branching pattern, and thus, the opposite directions of the vascular pressure drop in tissue-isolated vs sc tumors. This explanation is based on a schematic simplification, idealizing vascular morphologies into two different patterns: "central" and "peripheral" (33). From this perspective, the tissue-isolated tumors epitomize the central type. The different directions of tumor perfusion in tissue-isolated vs sc tumors were further documented in the small cell lung cancer (SCLC)-xenografts 54A and 54B, using an ultra-fast slip-ring computed tomography (CT)-scan technology with extremely high spatial resolution (5). The mice were prepared with a tissue-isolated tumor at their left flank and a conventional sc tumor at the right flank. Again, the perfusion distribution profiles of central vs peripheral tumor regions were opposite in sc vs tissue-isolated SCLC tumors, which was not surprising given the different vascular morphologies.

Interestingly, the pharmacokinetic parameters, describing the tissue uptake and elimination of the contrast agent, did not differ between transplantation types, whereas significant differences were found between the two SCLC lines. The intratumor tissue dispersion was influenced by tumor line ($p = 0.016$) more than by the transplantation mode ($p > 0.6$). Thus, the difference in physiological appearance between tissue-isolated and sc preparations, as demonstrated in the LS174T tumor line (13), was outweighed by intrinsic differences between the sublines 54A and 54B.

This observation raises interesting mechanistic questions as to how this difference is translated from the cellular to the organ level. On the other hand such data also fosters concern that physiological parameters obtained in spontaneous "unknown" tumors in patients would be extremely difficult to interpret because of their clonal heterogeneity.

4. PHYSIOLOGICAL AND PHARMACOKINETIC ASPECTS

Tumor blood perfusion is an important physiological parameter with pivotal influence on growth, metastasis, diagnosis, and treatment of solid tumors. The flow through any tissue is determined by the pressure drop over the vascular bed, the viscosity of the fluid, and the geometric resistance. (34,35).

4.1. Methodological Considerations

The constant that relates diffusive flux to the concentration gradient is called the vascular permeability, P (cm/s^{-1}); and the corresponding constant that relates fluid leakage to pressure gradients is referred to as the hydraulic conductivity, L_p ($cm\ mmHg^{-1}\ s^{-1}$). With this terminology, Starling's law of filtration can be expressed:

$$J_{fluid} = L_p\ [(MVP\text{-}IFP) - \sigma\ (\pi_v - \pi_i)]$$

where MVP and IFP are hydrostatic pressures in the microvasculature and in the interstitial fluid respectively, σ is the osmotic reflection coefficient, and π_v and π_i are the vascular and interstitial oncotic pressures. All examined tumors, murine, xenografts and clinical, have been shown to possess an abnormally high interstitial fluid pressure *(32,35–38)*. When analyzed from the point of view of Starling's law, this phenomenon seems to be explained by a lack of functional lymphatics in solid tumors. In normal tissues, the passage of fluids across vessel walls is governed by two counteracting forces: the hydrostatic and the oncotic pressures. These two forces are not balanced, and the net surplus filtrate is assumed to be drained by the lymphatics. When lymphatics are absent or insufficiently functional, an interstitial edema develops, which is likely to play a role in the pathophysiology of interstitial hypertension in solid tumors. In support of this theory, the interstitial space in tumors, estimated by tracer techniques, has been found to be larger than in normal tissues *(34)*. As demonstrated in a human colon adenocarcinoma, LS174T, *(39)*, systemic dexamethasone therapy decreases the tumor IFP, thus rendering support to an analogy of tumor interstitial hypertension to brain edema *(40)*.

In normal tissues, the IFP is close to 0 mmHg; thus, an interstitial fluid movement toward the periphery of the tumor would be expected to occur. This phenomenon has been observed *(41)* and predicted from mathematical modeling in various solid tumors to range from 5–10% of the plasma-flow rate through the tumor *(42)*. Correspondingly, a certain extent of fluid loss during ex vivo perfusion of tumors has occurred, at least according to those investigators who have looked for it. In series of perfusion experiments, with ex vivo perfused tissue-isolated SCLC tumors *(7)*, the fluid loss was estimated quantitatively by subtraction of the tumor-effluent flow rate from the input flow rate estimated on the basis of pump calibration curves. To which degree the oozing at the tumor periphery—and the resulting lack of complete recovery of the input—affects the outcome of a perfusion experiment depends entirely on the type and purpose of the experiment.

The flow rate Q is dependent on the geometric resistance *(Z)* and the viscous resistance (η), since the overall flow resistance FR = η Z:

$$Q = \Delta p/FR = \Delta p/(\eta\ Z)$$

At nonphysiologically high perfusion rates, visible oozing from the perfused tumor, associated with an estimated fluid loss of greater than 85%, is observed. This occurs accidentally when the study does not consider that what appears to be a physiological perfusion pressure is only so when the viscosity of the perfusate resembles that of blood. If a physiological arterial pressure of 100 mmHg is maintained as the Δp and the perfusate has a viscosity of less than 1.cP i.e., 5–6 times less than blood, the resulting five- to sixfold increase in perfusion rate might exceed the physiological capacity of parts of the vascular network.

As discussed here, it appears that some degree of peripheral fluid loss in solid tumors is a physiological phenomenon, and as such it should not call for rigorous avoidance in perfused tumor models. On the other hand, a limit must be drawn. My suggestion is a limit at 80% recovery—i.e., only perfusion experiments with an estimated fluid loss of less than 20% are included. In addition, all experiments in which macroscopically visible leakage occurred should be excluded.

There are morphological as well as physiological indications that the hydraulic conductivity, L_p, is greater than normal in tumor vessels (43). A high L_p *per se* would decrease the $(\pi_v - \pi_i)$ and the J/L_p, resulting in interstitial hypertension and convective fluid transport toward the tumor periphery. The ubiquitously elevated IFP in tumors is considered an obstacle to delivery of macromolecular agents because of the resulting decrease of the hydrostatic pressure difference, and thereby the convective transfer across the vessel wall (44). The observation that dexamethasone treatment reversibly decreases IFP relative to microvascular pressure (MVP) (39) is unfortunately unlikely, to be instrumental for improvements of the convective transfer of pharmaceutical compounds, since this effect is achieved at the expense of the hydraulic conductivity and the extravasation of both large and small molecules. Important aspects of these problems have been elegantly solved by Netti et al. (45) by utilizing the time delay in transfer of the MVP to the IFP to obtain windows of transvascular pressure gradients during pulsed infusion.

A linear dependence of flow rate on the perfusion pressure is found in various perfused, isolated tissues or organs. Upon extrapolation of the linear segment of such curves, an apparent pressure associated with zero flow, P_0, emerges (*see* Fig. 4). In normal physiology, this pressure has been termed the critical closing pressure. The value is interpreted as the minimal pressure needed to keep the vessels open, and the magnitude increases during sympathetic nerve stimulation. Values of P_0 less than 8–10 mmHg obtained with low-protein perfusates, such as Ringer's solution, have been attributed to tissue edema in perfused organs. However, the addition of albumin to the perfusate should diminish this problem, and furthermore, the values obtained in perfusion experiments (7,16,18) are higher than expected as a result of edema. An increased resistance to flow as the perfusion pressure is reduced towards the P_0 seems to occur in tumor vasculature (16,18). If the observation of larger-vessel diameters in the periphery than in central regions of solid tumors (46) is a general phenomenon, the result is a lower vascular resistance in the tumor periphery. In addition, the IFP is low in the outermost periphery of tumors (47). If an abnormal vascular leakiness is characteristic of all tumor vessels, a greater fraction of the inlet volume would be lost by peripheral leakage at lower perfusion pressures. Thus, the resulting apparent Δp-Q curve would be steeper than the true one. This constitutes an alternative—or additional—explanation for the magnitude of the apparent zero-flow intercept in Δp-Q curves obtained from perfused tumors.

5. INTRATUMOR PHARMACOKINETICS OF GEMCITABINE

Gemcitabine is 2,2-difluoro-deoxycytidine (dFdC). This compound, which is structurally related to 1-β-D-arabinofuranosylcytosine (Cytarabin, ara-C), has clinical activity in several solid-tumor types. The principal metabolic pathways of dFdC resemble those of ara-C. Deoxycytidine kinase (dCK) catalyzes the initial phosphorylation into dFdCMP, which is further phosphorylated twice into dFdCTP, the active metabolite. Cytidine deaminase (CDD) catalyzes the initial catabolism of dFdC into dFdU, an inactive metabolite. Although the latter pathway occurs in plasma and in several organs, dCK activity is believed to be present only intracellularly. In a resistant variant of a human ovarian-cancer cell line, dCK deficiency was found to be the primary mechanism of resistance (48).

Differences in the tumor accumulation of fluorine in 54 and 54B tumors following an ip injection bolus of gemcitabine were found using in vivo ^{19}F-MRS (6). The slightly more sensitive 54B tumors apparently accumulated more fluorine than did 54A. At that stage, the exact source of the observed fluorine signal from the tumors was unknown. That the fluorine originated from the drug is evident, but it is unknown to what extent the signals represent intracellular or extracellular fractions of the drug and/or its metabolites. In vitro studies showed that dFdC and its deaminated metabolite di-fluoro-deoxy-vidine (dFdU) are indistinguishable by ^{19}F MRS (6), and the active phosphorylated metabolite dFdCTP is present only in very small concentrations that would disappear completely in the NTP signals of a ^{31}P (MR)-spectrum. Based on the two previous studies (5,6), two questions were posed, and answers pursued in the ex vivo perfused tissue-isolated preparation (7). The questions were: Are there differences in the drug pharmacokinetic parameters during infusion of dFdC in 54A and 54B?, and how do simple physiological parameters influence the drug dispersion?

Like Hypaque, gemcitabine is a low-weight molecular agent with insignificant protein binding and rapid distribution throughout the body (49).

The following calculations were made (7):

The mass balance for the drug infusion into a tumor volume, V, was expressed using the principles of Fick's law, and a solution to the equation was:

$$C_{NORM}(t) = \alpha \, (1 - e^{-\beta t})$$

C_{NORM} is the normalized output drug concentrations. The parameter α contains information about the conversion/binding (sequestration) of the drug, and the rate constant β contains information about the passage of dFdC through the tumor—the initial distribution phase. The tumor:effluent partition coefficient, R, and the sequestration rate, k, can then be calculated:

$$R = \frac{Q}{\alpha \beta V} \quad \text{and} \quad k = \beta \, (1 - \alpha).$$

When $k = 0$, there is no conversion/binding: $\alpha = 1$. When $R = 1$ and $k = 0$, then $\beta = Q/V$. Finally, when $R > 1$, the drug partition in the tumor is greater than in the perfusate. The drug output function was best fitted by the simple monoexponential function, shown here, which indicates that the tumor uptake of parent drug is flow-limited (50). Correspondingly, a nonparametric correlation analysis identified the flow rate, Q, as the primary determinant of the initial dispersion phase, which on the contrary was not significantly influenced by the perfusion rate, q. Conversely, the drug partition coefficient, R, was significantly correlated to q, but not to Q, whereas the drug conversion rate, k, was independent on both q and Q. The early distribution phase was flow-dependent, the tissue accumulation was perfusion-dependent, and the metabolism or conversion appears to have been independent on both. A significant difference in the

Table 2
Physiological and Pharmacokinetic Parameters in Two Subpopulations
of the Same SCLC Tumor, Based on Ex Vivo Perfusion Experiments[a]

	SCCL 54A	SCCL 54B	54A vs 54B
W (g)	0.69 [0.41–1.24]	0.58 [0.13–1.4]	NS
Q (µL/min)	130 [100–300]	193 [140–330]	$p = 0.067$
q (µL/(min × g))	180 [143–322]	345 [200–643]	$p = 0.0095$
z_0 (10^8 g × cm^{-3})	15.85 [4.81–30.18]	3.86 [2.14–9.3]	$p = 0.0093$
Z_0 (10^8 cm^{-3})	22.8 [7.99–42.15]	6.35 [3.26–29.3]	$p = 0.053$
P_0 (mmHg	15 [10–33]	21 [8–38]	NS
β (min^{-1})	0.25 [0.16–0.35]	0.31 [0.28–0.42]	$p = 0.0251$
α	0.955 [0.88–0.99]	0.955 [0.79–1.0]	NS
R	1.04 [0.49–1.61]	1.15 [0.81–1.57]	NS
k (10^{-2} min^{-1})	1.13 [0.47–4.16]	1.36 [0.47–6.55]	NS
ΔpH	0.31 [0.12–0.48]	0.26 [0.16–0.41]	NS
Δlactate (µmol min^{-1} g^{-1})	1.044 [0.74–1.16]	1.342 [0.85–1.52]	$p = 0.035$
Δglucose (µmol min^{-1} g^{-1})	0.474 [0.1–0.702]	0.581 [0.28–0.89]	NS
ΔO_2 max (µL O_2 g^{-1} min^{-1})	28.33±8.5	10.50±2.16	

[a]Data from ref. 7.

Numbers are medians, ranges are given in brackets. Statistical comparison is performed by Mann-Witney's U test.

time constant, β, for the initial distribution phase in 54A and 54B tumors was found, whereas there was no significant difference in the tumor: effluent partition coefficient and the conversion (or binding) rate of parent drug. These data are summarized in Table 2. The conversion is likely to represent the intracellular phosphorylation into dFdCTP, since the magnitude is comparable with, and lower than, dFdC phosphorylation rates reported for mononuclear cell suspensions *(51)*. Furthermore, the constant levels of *k* at equilibrium, plus the fact that *k* was independent on *q,* is indicative that the reaction identified by its constant rate *k* is saturable. This finding also corresponds to observations in circulating mononuclear cells that the intracellular accumulation of dFdC levels off when the infusion concentrations exceed 20 µM, and that the intracellular half-life of dFdCTP is several hours long *(51,52)*.

5.1. Geometric Flow Resistance

Significantly different pharmacokinetic handling—or more specifically, a difference in intratumor disposition kinetics of low mol-wt nonprotein-bound agents—in 54A vs 54B tumors has been documented in different systems with normal blood *(5,6)* and with a perfusate of lower viscosity *(7)*. A key factor in this regard appears to be a significant difference in geometric resistance between 54A and 54B tumors. The vascular resistance to flow in idealized settings (i.e., a single nonrigid tube) is proportional to a constant $(8/\pi)$, a geometric component (L/r^4), and the viscosity (η). *L* represents vessel length, and *r*-vessel radius. When an acellular perfusate is used, the η can be assumed constant, which is documented by the linearity of the Δp-q curves above certain minimum pressures (Fig. 4). This flow equation can be divided by the tumor weight W (g), and thus expressed per unit weight:

$$q = \frac{Q}{W} = \frac{\Delta p}{\eta z}$$

where q (mL/min/g) is the perfusion rate and z (g/mL), which is the product of Z and W, is referred to as the extrinsic geometric resistance. In a perfused organ, the slope of the pressure-flow (Δp-Q) curve is equal to $1/FR = (\eta Z)^{-1}$. Thus, Z can be determined, since η is known. Above a certain perfusion pressure, the Z (or z) maintains a constant minimum value Z_0 (or z_0), corresponding to a linear Δp-Q curve.

As a consequence of the analogy to Ohm's law for electrical circuits, the total resistance of a system of parallel resistance components is less than the resistance of any single unit (vessel). Because of the distinct vascular branching pattern of tissue-isolated tumors, one could speculate that the total flow resistance in this preparation *per se* is lower than in spontaneous tumors with multifocal feeding vessels. Unfortunately, this hypothesis is difficult to test experimentally, since as yet only the tissue-isolated preparations permit determinations of Z (and z) in tumors. The global perfusion rate, which is averaged for the whole tumor, was not different when comparing tissue-isolated and SC LS174T tumors (*see* Table 1). But the intratumoral distribution of the flow is different (5). The vascular topology of tumors possess some general characteristics, despite great heterogeneity and a highly random organization (34). Using an intricate descriptional terminology developed on the basis of microscopical analysis of vascular casts of a tissue-isolated rodent mammary carcinoma (53), the presence of self-loops, venous convolutions, trifurcations, and polygonal-shaped meshworks in tumor vasculature have been recognized as more general characteristics. With intravital microscopy techniques—e.g., in the dorsal window preparation (54) or the cranial window (55)— flow parameters in small tumor transplants have been recorded.

In Table 3, literature values of geometric resistances z (or Z) and z_0 (or Z_0) in rodent solid tumors are compared with the only measurements obtained in human xenografts thus far (7). Interestingly, Sensky et al. found a significant difference in z values in a tissue-isolated rat tumor when growing as an ovarian or as an inguinal preparation (16). The geometric resistance was lower in tumors grown in the ovarian fat pad, indicating that the anatomical site plays a role in determining its magnitude. The mechanism underlying this difference is not clear, nor is it completely clear how to take different vessel and tubing dimensions in the nontumorous parts of the two preparations into account.

Thus far, we have determined values for geometric flow resistance in a human tumor, and concurrently demonstrated that this parameter is an important determinant for the initial distribution of drug in a solid tumor (7). At present, this is the only quantitative functional parameter representing the vascular morphology of intact solid tumors. This parameter is most likely to be of use in preclinical evaluation of drugs. More specifically, it constitutes a means of quantifying early effects in the preclinical setting of investigational therapeutic strategies directed at the tumor vasculature. This use was further documented in studies of the vascular effects of TNF-α (56).

5.2. Role of pH

In the SCLC tumor lines, 54A and 54B, a significant arteriovenous pH difference was found (7) during ex vivo perfusion. The 0.3 pH-unit drop was comparable to values reported in other human xenografts grown in nude rats by the inguinal preparation

Table 3
Comparison of Geometric Flow Resistance, z_0 or Z_0, Obtained from Linear Pressure-Flow
Behavior Measured in Normal Tissues and in Tumors

Host	Tissue	z_0 10^8 g cm^{-3}	Z_0 10^8 cm^{-3}	Author, year
Rat	Stomach	3.59		Flaim, 1987
	Jejunum	1.46		
	Ileum	1.78		
	Skeletal muscle	16.41		
	Kidney	0.48		
	Heart	0.82		
Dog	Hind limb		0.021	Whittaker, 1933
	Hind limb		0.021	Levy, 1953
	Paw		0.066	Benis, 1970
Rabbit	Heart		0.15	Sutera, 1988
Rat	Rat breast cancer R3230AC	1.65–17.29	2.09–5.48	Sevick, 1989
	P22 carcino-sarcoma (rat)	19.11 (inguinal) 8.53 (ovarian)		Sensky, 1993
Nude mouse	Human SCLC			
	54A	15.85	22.8	Kristjansen, 1995
	54B	3.86	6.35	

(21), and to those obtained in perfused normal tissues. In the study by Kallinowski et al. *(21)* a dependence of ΔpH on perfusion rate was found. This was not significantly present in the SCLC experiments *(7)*. The ΔpH across the tumor vasculature is indicative of the activity of metabolical processes in the perfused tumor, but does not translate directly into physiological conditions. Mixed venous blood from a tumor-bearing individual does not have a pH of 7.1. In an intact host organism with a spontaneous tumor, the venous blood recirculates, and the vascular morphology is usually multifocal rather than tree-like. Also the physiological buffers in the intact organism are minutely effective to a degree that is not necessarily met by a non-recirculating perfusate. The lactate production is not necessarily correlated to the ΔpH or to the ΔCO_2 *(7)*. When interpreting the ΔCO_2 readings, one should bear in mind that the bicarbonate buffer shifts its equilibrium towards CO_2 when the proton concentration increases. Thus, sources of H^+ other than lactate seem to have contributed to the acidity of the effluent. This is in harmony with the interesting observation that a glycolysis deficient subline of tumor cells can form tumors with an extracellular acidity comparable to that of the glycolysis-competent parental line *(57)*. Concordantly, using ^{13}C-MRS *(58)*, a corresponding lack of correlation between individual tumor pH and lactate derived from ^{13}C-labeled glucose was found. Hyperglycemia can induce decreases in tumor blood flow and tumor pH *(59,60)*, but this effect may be mediated through the surrounding tissues rather than by a tumor-specific metabolism *(61)*. Given the abundant heterogeneity between and within various tumor types, generalizations should be avoided. Further studies are indeed required before specific therapeutic modulation, based on pH gradients and other physiological parameters *(60,62,63)* can be fully

investigated in the clinical setting. Studies of the metabolic flux in the SCLC tumors, using ^{13}C MRS after addition of ^{13}C-enriched substrates, would clarify some of these aspects. Also, a combination of the ex vivo perfused tumor preparation and ^{31}P MRS, using metabolic inhibitors such as azide and 2-DG, would help to delineate these uncertainties.

Future studies with perfused tumor preparations should more fully explore the relationship between flow (or perfusion) and the arteriovenous lactate, pH, and glucose differences. In the perfusion experiments discussed here, the exact relationship between metabolic parameters and flow cannot be outlined from the data. This problem should be avoided in the planning of experiments. The much lower oxygen-carrying capacity of an acellular perfusate, compared with that of blood, is partly compensated by a flow rate that is five times greater (because of low viscosity) and ΔpO_2 approx 10 times greater. The ex vivo perfused tumor preparation would probably benefit from the use of specific oxygen-carrying perfusates (such as red blood cells, crosslinked hemoglobins, and perfluorocarbons), in order to approach the true physiology—if ever there was one.

REFERENCES

1. Kristjansen PEG, Pedersen EJ, Quistorff B, Elling F, Spang-Thomsen M. Early effects of radiotherapy in small cell lung cancer xenografts monitored by 31P magnetic resonance spectroscopy and biochemical analysis. *Cancer Res* 1990; 50:4880–4884.
2. Kristjansen PEG, Spang-Thomsen M, Quistorff B. Different energy metabolism in two human small cell lung cancer subpopulations examined by 31P magnetic resonance spectroscopy and biochemical analysis in vivo and in vitro. *Cancer Res* 1991; 51:5160–5164.
3. Kristjansen PEG, Pedersen AG, Quistorff B, Spang-Thomsen M. Different early effect of irradiation in brain and small cell lung cancer examined by in vivo 31P-magnetic resonance spectroscopy. *Radiother Oncol* 1992; 24:186–190.
4. Kristjansen PEG, Kristensen CA, Spang-Thomsen M, Quistorff B. Relationship between tumor response and the ratio of nucleotide triphosphates to inorganic phosphate in small cell lung cancer xenografts. *Int J Oncology* 1995; 7:127–131.
5. Hamberg LM, Kristjansen PEG, Hunter GJ, Wolf GL, Jain RK. Spatial heterogeneity in tumor perfusion measured with functional computed tomography at 0.05 microliter resolution. *Cancer Res* 1994; 54:6032–6036.
6. Kristjansen PEG, Quistorff B, Spang-Thomsen M, Hansen HH. Intratumoral pharmacokinetic analysis by 19F-magnetic resonance spectroscopy and cytostatic in vivo activity of gemcitabine (dFdC) in two small cell lung cancer xenografts. *Ann Oncol* 1993; 4:157–160.
7. Kristjansen PEG, Brown TJ, Shipley LA, Jain RK. Intratumor pharmacokinetics, flow resistance, and metabolism during gemcitabine infusion in *ex vivo* perfused human small cell lung cancer. *Clin Cancer Res* 1996; 2:359–367.
8. Dang CV, Semenza GL. Oncogenic alterations of metabolism. *Trends Biochem Sci* 1999; 24:68–72.
9. Wang GL, Jiang BH, Rue EA, Semenza GL. Hypoxia-inducible factor 1 is a basic-helix-loop-helix-PAS heterodimer regulated by cellular O_2 tension. *Proc Natl Acad Sci USA* 1995; 92:5510–5514.
10. Semenza GL. Hypoxia, clonal selection, and the role of HIF-1 in tumor progression. *Crit Rev Biochem Mol Biol* 2000; 35:71–103.
11. Gullino PM, Busch H, eds. Methods in cancer research. In: *Techniques for the Study of Tumor pathophysiology*. Academic Press, New York, NY, 1970; pp. 45–91.
12. Gullino PM, Grantham FH. Studies on the exchange of fluids between host and tumor. 1. A method for growing "tissue-isolated" tumors in laboratory animals. *J Natl Cancer Inst* 1961; 27:679–693.
13. Kristjansen PEG, Roberge S, Lee I, Jain RK. Tissue-isolated human tumor xenografts in athymic nude mice. *Microvasc Res* 1994; 48:389–402.
14. Vaupel P, Fortmeyer HP, Runkel S, Kallinowski F. Blood flow, oxygen consumption, and tissue oxygenation of human breast cancer xenografts in nude rats. *Cancer Res* 1987; 47:3496–3503.

15. Eskey CJ, Koretsky AP, Domach MM, Jain RK. 2H-Nuclear magnetic resonance imaging of tumor blood flow: spatial and temporal heterogeneity in a tissue-isolated mammary adenocarcima. *Cancer Res* 1992; 52:6010–6019.

16. Sensky PL, Prise VE, Tozer GM, Shaffi KM, Hirst DG. Resistance to flow through tissue-isolated transplanted rat tumours located in two different sites. *Br J Cancer* 1993; 67:1337–1341.

17. Sevick EM, Jain RK. Viscous resistance to blood flow in solid tumors: effect of hematocrit on intratumor blood viscosity. *Cancer Res* 1989a; 49:3513–3519.

18. Sevick EM, Jain RK. Geometric resistance to blood flow in solid tumors perfused ex vivo: effects of tumor size and perfusion pressure. *Cancer Res* 1989b; 49:3506–3512.

19. Tozer GM, Priese VE, Bell KM. The influence of nitric oxide on tumour vascular tone. *Acta Oncologica* 1995; 34:373–377.

20. Sauer LA, Stayman JW, Dauchy RT. Amino acids, glucose, and lactic acid utilization in vivo by rat tumors. *Cancer Res* 1982; 42:4090–4097.

21. Kallinowski F, Vaupel P, Runkel S, Berg G, Fortmeyer HP, Baessler KH, et al. Glucose uptake, lactate release, ketone body turnover, metabolic micromilieu, and pH distribution in human breast cancer xenografts in nude rats. *Cancer Res* 1988; 48:7264–7272.

22. Graham RA, Brown TR, Meyer RA. An *ex vivo* model for the study of tumor metabolism by nuclear magnetic resonance: characterization of the phosphorus-31 spectrum of the isolated perfused morris hepatoma 7777. *Cancer Res* 1991; 51:841–849.

23. Eskey CJ, Koretsky AP, Domach MM, Jain RK. Role of oxygen vs. glucose in energy metabolism in a mammary carcinoma perfused *ex vivo:* direct measurement by ^{31}P NMR. *Proc Natl Acad Sci USA* 1993; 90:2646–2650.

24. Sauer LA, Dauchy RT. Lactate release and uptake in hepatoma 7288CTC perfused in situ with L-[(U)-^{14}C] lactate or D-[(U)-^{14}C] glucose. *Metabolism* 1995; 43:1488–1497.

25. Jain RK, Wei J, Gullino PM. Pharmacokinetics of methotrexate in solid tumors. *J Pharmacokinet Biopharm* 1979; 7:181–194.

26. Ohkouchi K, Imoto H, Takakura Y, Hashida M, Sezaki H. Disposition of anticancer drugs after bolus arterial administration in a tissue-isolated tumor perfusion system. *Cancer Res* 1990; 50:1640–1644.

27. Imoto H, Sakamura Y, Ohkouchi K, Atsumi R, Takakura Y, Sezaki H, et al. Disposition characteristics of macromolecules in the perfused tissue-isolated tumor preparation. *Cancer Res* 1992; 52:4396–4401.

28. Eskey CJ, Wolmark N, McDowell CL, Domach MM, Jain RK. Residence time distributions of various tracers in tumors: implications for drug delivery and blood flow measurement. *J Natl Cancer Inst* 1994; 86:293–299.

29. Steel GG. *Growth Kinetics of Tumors.* Oxford University Press, Oxford, UK 1977.

30. Vaupel P, Kallinowski F, Okunieff P. Blood flow, oxygen and nutrient supply, and metabolic microenvironment of human tumors: a review. *Cancer Res* 1989a; 49:6449–6465.

31. Horsman MR, Kristjansen PEG, Mizuno M, Christensen KL, Chaplin DJ, Quistorff B, et al. Biochemical and physiological changes induced by nicotinamide in a C3H mouse mammary carcinoma and CDF1 mice. *Int J Radiat Oncol Biol Phys* 1992; 22:451–454.

32. Boucher Y, Jain RK. Microvascular pressure is the principal driving force for interstitial hypertension in solid tumors: implications for vascular collapse. *Cancer Res* 1992; 52:5110–5114.

33. Rubin P, Cassarett G. Microcirculation of tumors I. Anatomy, function, and necrosis. *Clin Radiol* 1966; 17:1640–1644.

34. Jain RK. Determinants of tumor blood flow: a review. *Cancer Res* 1988; 48:2641–2658.

35. Jain RK, Teicher B, eds. Physiological resistance to the treatment of solid tumors. In: *Durg Resistance in Oncology.* Marcel Dekker, new York, NY, 1993.

36. Boucher Y, Kirkwood JM, Opacic D, Desantis M, Jain RK. Interstitial hypertension in superficial metastatic melanomas in humans. *Cancer Res* 1991; 51:6691–6694.

37. Gutmann R, Leunig M, Feyh J, Goetz AE, Messmer K, Kastenbauer E, et al. Interstitial hypertension in head and neck tumors in patients: Correlation with tumor size. *Cancer Res* 1992; 52:1993–1995.

38. Tufto I, Rofstad EK. Interstitial fluid pressure in human melanoma xenografts. Relationship to fractional tumor water content, tumor size, and tumor volume-doubling time. *Acta Oncologica* 1995; 34:361–365.

39. Kristjansen PEG, Boucher Y, Jain RK. Dexamethasone reduces the interstitial fluid pressure in a human colon adenocarcinoma xenograft. *Cancer Res* 1993a; 53:4764–4766.

40. Neuwelt EA, Barnett PA, Ramsey FL, Hellström I, Hellström KE, McCormick CI. Dexamethasone decreases the delivery of tumor-specific monoclonal antibody to both intracerebral and subcutaneous tumor xenografts. *Neurosurgery* 1993; 33:478–484.

41. Butler TP, Grantham FH, Gullino PM. Bulk transfer of fluid in the interstitial compartment of mammary tumors. *Cancer Res* 1975; 35:3084–3088.
42. Jain RK. Vascular and interstitial barriers to delivery of therapeutic agents in tumors. *Cancer Metastasis Rev* 1990; 9:253–266.
43. Yuan F, Salehi HA, Boucher Y, Vasthare US, Tuma RF, Jain RK. Vascular permeability and microcirculation of gliomas and mammary carcinomas transplanted in rat and mouse cranial windows. *Cancer Res* 1994; 54:4564–4568.
44. Jain RK, Baxter LT. Mechanisms of heterogeneous distribution of monoclonal antibodies and other macromolecules in tumors: significance of elevated interstitial pressure. *Cancer Res* 1988; 48:7022–7032.
45. Netti PA, Baxter LT, Boucher Y, Skalak R, Jain RK. Time-dependent behavior of interstitial fluid pressure in solid tumors: implications for drug delivery. *Cancer Res* 1995; 55:5451–5458.
46. Vogel AW. Intratumoral vascular changes with increased size of mammary adenocarcinoma—new methods and results. *J Natl Cancer Inst* 1965; 34:571–578.
47. Boucher Y, Baxter LT, Jain RK. Interstitial pressure gradients in tissue-isolated and subcutaneous tumors: implications for therapy. *Cancer Res* 1990; 50:4478–4484.
48. Ruiz van Haperen VW, Veerman G, Eriksson S, Boven E, Stegmann AP, Hermsen M, et al. Development and molecular characterization of a 2′,2′-difluorodeoxycytidine-resistant variant of the human ovarian carcinoma cell line A2780. *Cancer Res* 1994; 54:4138–4143.
49. Shipley LA, Brown TJ, Cornpropst JD, Hamilton M, Daniels WD, Culp HW. Metabolism and disposition of gemcitabine, an oncolytic deoxycytidine analog, in mice, rats, and dogs. *Drug Metab Dispos* 1992; 20:849–855.
50. Gerlowski LE, Jain RK. Physiologically based pharmacokinetic modeling: principles and applications. *J Pharm Sci* 1983; 72:1103–1127.
51. Grunewald R, Abbruzzese J, Tarassoff P, Plunkett W. Saturation of 2′,2′-difluorodeoxycytidine 5′-triphosphate accumulation by mononuclear cells during a phase I trial of gemcitabine. *Cancer Chemother Pharmacol* 1991; 27:258–262.
52. Abbruzzese JL, Grunewald R, Weeks EA, Gravel D, Adams T, Nowak B, et al. A phase I clinical, plasma and cellular pharmacology study of gemcitabine. *J Clin Oncol* 1991; 9:491–498.
53. Less JR, Skalak TC, Sevick EM, Jain RK. Microvascular architecture in a mammary carcinoma: branching patterns and vessel dimensions. *Cancer Res* 1991; 51:265–273.
54. Leunig M, Yuan F, Menger MD, Boucher Y, Goetz AE, Messmer K, et al. Angiogenesis, microvascular architecture, microhemodynamics, and interstitial fluid pressure during early growth of human adenocarcinoma LS174T in SCID mice. *Cancer Res* 1992; 52:6553–6560.
55. Yuan F, Leunig M, Berk DA, Jain RK. Microvascular permeability of albumin, vascular surface area, and vascular volume measured in human adenocarcinoma LS174T using dorsal chamber in SCID mice. *Microvasc Res* 1993; 45:269–289.
56. Kristensen CA, Roberge S, Jain RK. Effect of tumor necrosisfactor alpha on vascular resistance, nitric oxide production, and glucose and oxygen consumption in perfused tissue-isolated human melanoma xenografts. *Clin Cancer Res* 1997; 3:319–324.
57. Newell K, Franchi A, Pouyssegur J, Tannock I. Studies with glycolysis-deficient cells suggest that production of lactic acid is not the only cause of tumor acidity. *Proc Natl Acad Sci USA* 1993; 90:1127–1131.
58. Bhujwalla ZM, Shungu DC, Chatham JC, Wehrle JP, Glickson JD. Glucose metabolism in RIF-1 tumors after reduction in blood flow: an in vivo ^{13}C and ^{31}P NMR study. *Magn Reson Med* 1994; 32:303–309.
59. Koutcher JA, Fellenz MP, Vaupel PW, Gerweck LE. FSaII mouse tumor metabolic changes with different doses of glucose measured by 31P nuclear magnetic resonance. *Cancer Res* 1988; 48:5917–5921.
60. Ross BD, Mitchell SL, Merkle H, Garwood M. In vivo ^{31}P and ^{1}H NMR studies of rat brain tumor pH and blood flow during acute hyperglycemia: differential effects between subcutaneous and intracerebral locations. *Magn Reson Med* 1989; 12:219–234.
61. Volk T, Jähde E, Fortmeyer HP, Glüsenkamp K-H, Rajewsky MF. pH in human tumour xenografts: effect of intravenous administration of glucose. *Br J Cancer* 1993; 68:492–500.
62. Anonymous. Tumour pH. *Lancet* 1992; 340:342–343.
63. Jensen PB, Sørensen BS, Sehested M, Grue P, Demant EJF, Hansen HH. Targeting the cytotoxicity of topoisomerase II-directed epipodophyllotoxins to tumor cells in acidic environments. *Cancer Res* 1994; 54:2959–2963.

24

Human Breast-Cancer Xenografts as Models of the Human Disease

Robert Clarke, PhD, DSc

Contents

1. INTRODUCTION

The generation of animal models for breast cancer has a long history, most notably since the attempts to produce models of human breast cancer by the administration of estrogens to male mice *(1)*. Subsequently, several significant events have given investigators the ability to reproducibly maintain human breast-cancer cells in vivo and to develop a series of human breast-cancer xenografts. These include the identification of the nude mutation in mice, and demonstration of both the accompanying immunodeficiency and ability of these mice to maintain tumor xenografts *(2,3)*. Another milestone was the isolation and characterization of a series of human breast-cancer-cell lines that could be maintained as xenografts. Among these cell lines was MCF-7 *(4)*, still the most widely used human breast-cancer-cell line available, which requires estrogenic supplementation for proliferation in vitro and successful establishment as xenografts.

Other significant developments in the use of animals to model various aspects of breast cancer include the demonstration by Huggins *(5)* of the ability of 7,12-dimethyl a benzanthracene to produce ovarian-dependent mammary adenocarcinomas in selected strains of rats. The viral etiology of spontaneous mammary tumors in some

From: *Tumor Models in Cancer Research*
Edited by: B. A. Teicher © Humana Press Inc., Totowa, NJ

mouse strains and the identification of the mouse mammary tumor virus (MMTV) have provided other rodent models for human breast cancer *(6)*. More recently molecular biological techniques have provided the ability to overexpress or eliminate the effects of single or multiple genes. The development of relatively mammary-gland-specific promoters can target molecular changes to the mammary gland, but expression is occasionally detected in other tissues. Although the majority of such models have been generated in mice, manipulation of the rat genome also has been demonstrated.

As with all animal models, the extent to which any single model can accurately reflect the entire disease is limited. Thus, it is important for investigators to select carefully, from among all available models, those that most closely mimic that aspect of the disease required by their hypothesis(es). This often requires selection of more than one model. Further considerations include specific aspects of an appropriate experimental design—one that is within the legal and ethical guidelines/requirements of any federal, local, and/or institutional mandates.

This chapter primarily focuses on human breast-tumor xenograft models. Brief discussions of issues relating to experimental design are also included, such as the immunobiologies of possible hosts, endocrinologic effects of treatments, and the choice of inoculation sites. A list of potentially useful websites is included, and citations to other reviews and resources are provided throughout the text.

1.1. Basic Biology and Management of Breast Cancer

An appreciation of available breast-cancer models requires a basic understanding of the biology underlying this disease. A detailed discussion is beyond the scope of this chapter; thus, only a brief and selective overview is presented. Breast cancer is among the most common cancers, and has the second highest cancer mortality rate among women in Western societies *(7)*. In recent years, the rate of mortality has seen a modest decline, but death remains a common outcome of the disease *(8)*.

Generally, management of the disease is related to its stage at diagnosis. For example, patients with high-risk benign lesions, including ductal carcinoma *in situ,* and many with Stage I disease ($T_{1<2cm} N_0 M_0$), are cured by local therapies (surgery and/or radiation). However, in approx 20% of patients with Stage I disease cancer will recur *(9)*. The use of adjuvant endocrine therapy for patients with hormone-receptor-positive tumors is common. Anti-estrogens, which are well-tolerated and can maintain bone-mineral density—thus reducing problems associated with osteoporosis—are frequently administered as first-line therapies. Many Stage I patients with tumors that do not express hormone receptors, and those presenting with more advanced disease, frequently receive more aggressive cytotoxic therapies following any appropriate surgery/radiotherapy *(10)*. Although combination chemotherapies are generally used, the Taxanes (e.g., taxol) and anthracycline antibiotics (such as, doxorubicin) are among the most effective single agents.

Many invasive breast cancers are believed to follow a predictable biological pattern. Initially confined within the breast, some tumors eventually disseminate to distant sites. This may occur by lymphatic spread to the axillary lymph nodes and/or hematologic spread to distant sites, including the lungs, bone, and brain. The biology of this progression has been described as following a path from benign breast disease to invasive cancer. Several benign lesions have premalignant potential, including the usual ductal hyperplasia, atypical ductal hyperplasia, ductal carcinoma *in situ,* and lobular carcinoma *in situ.* Since not all premalignant lesions will progress, a nonobligatory pathway has been described. Thus, some common hyperplasias first become atypical, followed by progression to *in situ* carcinoma and, finally, invasive breast cancer *(11).* Although it is generally believed that only invasive lesions will metastasize, 80% of Stage I lesions, which are invasive, will not recur *(9).*

Breast cancer has been considered to occur in one of two groups of women. One group is primarily composed of those cases with a family history of the disease, and who may inherit predisposing mutations in specific genes, e.g., BRCA1 and BRCA 2. The other group consists of high-risk women in whom the disease sporadically arises. This may be an oversimplification. Although high-risk populations can be identified, most breast cancers arise in women with few or none of the established risk factors.

Established risk factors for breast cancer—such as early age at menarche, and late age at both first full-term pregnancy and onset of menopause—clearly implicate hormones in the etiology of breast cancer. These events are expected to increase the lifetime exposure to estrogens and progesterone. The protective effects of a first full-term pregnancy, prolonged lactation, and multiparity *(12)* are consistent with the associated changes in the breast that may remove those cells that are the primary targets for neoplastic transformation.

Compelling evidence specifically implicates estrogens in the biology of breast cancer, with evidence supporting a role both as an initiator of the disease and as a promoter of initiated lesions *(13).* Although the former function remains controversial, few investigators dispute estrogen's promotional activities. Progesterone is also important. Mitogenic activity in the adult human breast is greatest during the luteal phase of the menstrual cycle, when elevated levels of both estrogens and progesterone are present. Hormone-replacement therapies also increase the risk of breast cancer, with estrogen+progesterone formulations producing a greater risk than those only containing estrogens *(14,15).* These observations likely reflect the promotional activities of estrogens and progestins.

The promotional activities of estrogens are further evidenced by the ability of ovariectomy, antiestrogens, and luteinizing hormone releasing hormone (LHRH) antagonists to induce responses in premenopausal patients. Anti-estrogens (primarily Tamoxifen; TAM) and inhibitors of estrogen metabolism (aromatase inhibitors), also have considerable utility in the management of postmenopausal breast cancer (16–18). Studies have also demonstrated the ability of TAM to produce at least a short-term reduction in the incidence of breast tumors in high-risk women *(19).* Whether this will produce a long-term reduction in survival is not fully established.

Although the endocrine responsiveness of some breast tumors is well-established, <10% of all breast tumors that do not express either estrogen receptors (ER) or progesterone receptors (PgR) respond to endocrine manipulations *(16,17).* ER-negative tumors, and tumors that have acquired resistance to one or more endocrine therapies, are frequently responsive to cytotoxic chemotherapies. However, relatively few patients with advanced breast cancer are cured by these systemic modalities, although statistically significant effects on overall survival are detected *(20).*

1.2. Overview of Human Breast-Cancer Xenografts

As the biology of the human disease has shown, hormones play a major role. Consequently, it is not surprising that the hormone responsiveness of human breast-cancer-cell lines and xenografts is a major determinant in model selection. Human breast-cancer xenografts can be considered to be either hormone- (generally estrogen-) responsive or-unresponsive. Estrogen-responsive xenografts may be either estrogen-dependent or estrogen-independent, but responsive. Generally, estrogen-dependent models will not form proliferating tumors in ovariectomized hosts. Such xenografts require estrogenic supplementation. Estrogen-independent but responsive xenografts will produce tumors without estrogenic supplementation (21). However, these models may respond by increasing their proliferative rate, and/or tumor take-rate, upon administration of estrogens (21). Tumor-growth inhibition, or regression of established estrogen-independent but responsive tumors, may occur either following antiestrogen treatment or other endocrine manipulations (22,23). In marked contrast, estrogen-unresponsive xenografts do not require endocrine supplementation, and rarely respond to either estrogen or anti-estrogen administration.

Most breast-cancer cells, whether or not they are useful as xenograft models and independent of the endocrine responsiveness of their phenotype, have been derived from cells obtained from malignant effusions in patients. Such effusions occur in advanced disease, and may be present in 20–50% of patients (24). Although most of the better-known cell lines have been available for 30 or more years, several new models have been described (25). However, this chapter primarily focuses on the most widely used xenografts.

2. ENDOCRINE-RESPONSIVE MODELS

MCF-7 cells, the most widely used of the estrogen-dependent cell lines, were derived from a pleural effusion in a woman who had already received radiotherapy and endocrine therapy (4,26). These cells express receptors for several steroid hormones and growth factors, including ER and PgR, and generally exhibit a typical estrogen-dependent phenotype. For example, maintenance of MCF-7 cell xenografts requires estrogenic supplementation, which can readily be accomplished by the subcutaneous (SC, interscapular) introduction of a 60-d-release 0.72-mg estrogen pellet (Innovative Research of America) (27,28). We and others have generated a series of variants of these cells/xenografts. These include estrogen-independent and-responsive (27,21), estrogen-independent and anti-estrogen-resistant (22,23,29), anti-estrogen-stimulated (30,31), retinoid-resistant (32), and cytotoxic drug-resistant (33–35) MCF-7 variants.

A widely used variant, MCF-7/ADR, was produced by selection against doxorubicin. These cells overexpress the P-glycoprotein product of the *mdr-1* gene, but are now estrogen-unresponsive (33). This multi-drug-resistance-membrane protein, which acts as an efflux pump, is expressed in breast tumors, and is associated with a worse than partial response to cytotoxic chemotherapy (36). A recent study failed to confirm the MCF-7 origin of some MCF-7/ADR cultures, which were recently redesignated NCI/ADR-RES (37). To provide a P-glycoprotein-positive MCF-7 model that retains estrogen-dependence, we overexpressed the *mdr 1* gene in these cells. The resulting CL10.3 cells express ER, and retain both a dependence upon estrogens and responsiveness to TAM (34). The latter effect is interesting because TAM is known to block the effects of P-glycoprotein (38). Other drug-resistant variants have been produced by selection against etoposide (VP-16). These cells overexpress the multidrug-resistance-related protein MRP (39), which also has been detected in some breast tumors (40,41).

There are two other endocrine-responsive human breast-cancer xenografts, which are used less frequently than MCF-7 but have a broadly comparable phenotype. T47D cells and ZR-75-1 cells produce xenografts in estrogen-supplemented nude mice. Variants of these cells also have been reported. The T47D$_{CO}$ variant is estrogen-unresponsive, and has lost expression of estrogen receptors. However, these retain expression of progesterone receptors, providing one model for the ER-negative but PgR-positive phenotype (42). BT474 cells also exhibit an ER-negative but PgR-positive phenotype (43). An ER-negative variant of the ER-positive ZR-75-1 cell line has been described. ZR-71-9a1 cells were generated by selecting against TAM, and re-express ER following removal of TAM and exposure to estrogens (44). The tumorigenicity of this cell line is unclear.

Although most estrogen-responsive xenografts perceive estrogens as mitogens, the T61 xenograft is inhibited by estrogens. Not surprisingly, estrogens are not required for maintenance of T61 xenografts (45). An estrogen-inhibited phenotype also has been described in cases when ER is overexpressed in some ER-negative breast-cancer cells.

Mutant ERs and ER splice variants are widely detected in breast tumors, but their precise biological relevance is uncertain (46). Various breast-cancer-cell lines also express mutant ER mRNAs, including some MCF-7 cells/variants (47). BT-20 cells, established in 1958 (48), express a mutant ER with an exon 5 deletion (49). These cells are effectively estrogen-unresponsive and tumorigenic in athymic nude mice (50).

Most ER-positive xenografts are nonmetastatic. However, we have described several MCF-7 variants that appear to have an increased metastatic potential. We have observed occasional lymphatic and hematogenous metastases, but the incidence is too low to provide a useful model of metastatic ER-positive breast cancer (51). Others have generated highly angiogenic MCF-7 variants by overexpressing fibroblast growth factors. These also produce a high incidence of detectable micrometastases (52). However, the most aggressive xenografts, and those that produce a reproducible incidence of micro- and macro-metastases, are ER-negative.

3. ENDOCRINE-UNRESPONSIVE MODELS

The estrogen-unresponsive phenotype involves xenografts that do not require or respond to hormonal or antihormonal manipulations. Currently, there are many more established ER-negative breast-cancer models than models expressing ER. The majority are tumorigenic, and many are locally invasive. A series of mostly ER-negative cell lines has been generated at MD Anderson Cancer Center (Houston, TX); the ER-positive MDA-MB-134 and MDA-MB-175 are among the exceptions (25). The best-characterized, and most widely used endocrine-unresponsive xenografts are obtained from inoculation of either MDA-MB-231 or MDA-MB-435 cells into nude mice. Transfection of ER into MDA-MB-231 cells produces a phenotype characterized by growth inhibition, rather than stimulation, in response to estrogens (53).

Xenografts generated by MDA-MB-435 cells, and to a lesser degree those from MDA-MB-231 cells, are metastatic when inoculated into the mammary fat pads of athymic nude mice (54). Although they are unresponsive to estrogens and anti-estrogens, MDA-MB-435 xenografts are responsive to specific dietary manipulations of their hosts (55,56). Unlike many breast-cancer-cell lines, MDA-MB-435 cells were derived from a patient before she had received systemic therapy (57). Perhaps not surprisingly, these cells exhibit a pattern of response to cytotoxic drugs in vivo that appears to closely reflect that seen in patients *(57)*. We have established an ascites variant of these cells (MDA435/LCC6), which is useful either as a solid-tumor or ascites model to screen cytotoxic agents. We also have transduced the MDA435/LCC6 cells with the *mdr 1* gene, providing a model of ER-negative, P-glycoprotein-mediated, multidrug resistance *(57)*.

While most human breast-cancer xenografts produce mammary adenocarcinomas of varying degrees of differentiation, the Hs578T cell line was derived from a carcinosarcoma *(58)*. These cells are tumorigenic, and can exhibit a somewhat higher metastatic potential than most human breast-cancer xenografts, although significantly lower than MDA-MB-435 cells.

4. COMMON RODENT HOSTS FOR HUMAN BREAST-CANCER XENOGRAFTS

The ability to maintain human breast-cancer cells in vivo requires the use of an immunodeficient host. Currently, the most widely used hosts are mice homozygous for the nude *(nu)* mutation. Many investigators also use immunodeficient mice because of the severe combined immunodeficiency (SCID) mutation. Combined immunodeficiency mutations also are available, including mice homozygous for three mutations: *nu,* beige *(bg),* and the X-linked immunodeficiency *(xid).* More recently, mutant mice combining the SCID with other mutations have been described, including the combination of SCID with the nonobese diabetes mutation (NOD). These various models exhibit both similarities and differences in their immunobiologies. Since the choice of model may be influenced by the immunobiology of the host, a brief description of the major models and their primary immunodeficiencies follows.

The nude mutation has been introduced into 70 mouse strains. Some differences in the ability of these strains to maintain xenografts have been described *(59,60),* but the relevance of these observations to breast-cancer xenografts are not well-established. Several of the more widely available strains, e.g., on the Balb/c, NCr, and Swiss backgrounds, appear to be good hosts. Other strains are likely to be as useful. A comparable mutation has been identified in rats, the rat nude mutation *(rnu),* which produces athymic nude rats with an immunobiology broadly comparable to that of nude mice *(61).*

Nude mice are functionally athymic, exhibiting major defects in B-cell maturation and the production of T-lymphocytes *(62).* Responses to T-cell-dependent antigens are either poor or absent, but can be restored by reconstitution with T-cells *(63,64).* Circulating IgG and IgA are rare, but may be detected in individual animals *(62,65).* Nude mice, like most immunodeficient hosts, are not fully immunocompromised. Many components of cell-mediated immunity remain intact. Thus, T-cell-independent antigen responses are often normal. Production of both lymphokine-activated killer (LAK) cells and tumoricidal macrophages are normal *(66,67).* Of particular importance may be the elevated levels of natural killer (NK) cells present in nude mice. These levels exceed those seen in wild-type animals, and may contribute to the poor take-rate of some primary human xenografts. Embedding xenografts in Matrigel, an artificial basement membrane *(68),* increases tumor take-rate. This type IV collagen-based matrix may protect cells from the elevated NK-cell activity, and/or the respective phagocytic and lytic activities of macrophages and LAK cells.

Elimination of the elevated NK activity in nude mice has been achieved by combining the *nu* and *bg* mutations *(69)*. The main immunodeficiency conferred by the *bg* mutation produces a block in NK function *(70,71)*. Defects in macrophages, granulocytes, and cytotoxic T-cells also are associated with this mutation *(72)*. Mice congenic for both the *nu* and *bg* mutation have NK-cell activities intermediate between animals bearing their respective single gene mutations *(73)*. Further reductions in immunocompetence are obtained by adding the *xid* mutation to that of the *nu/bg* genotype *(74)*. The major contribution of the *xid* mutation is an impaired development of B cells, probably because of their inability to respond to early activation signals *(75)*. Immunoglobulin levels, particularly IgM and IgG_3, are low *(65)*. One complication of models containing the *bg* mutation is a clotting disorder, which can be problematic when the experimental design requires surgery such as orthotopic implantation *(60)*.

The SCID mutation disrupts the process of rearrangement of genes encoding antigen-specific receptors on B- and T-cells *(76)*. This reflects an inability to effectively join the cleaved variable-region segments catalyzed by the immunoglobulin V(D)J recombinase. Null mutations in the Rag-1 and Rag-2 genes in humans also produce a severe immunodeficiency characterized by a lack of mature B and T cells (Omenn syndrome). The deficiency also produces a loss of V(D)J recombination. Young SCID mice exhibit defective differentiation/maturation of lymphocytes. Pre-B and B cells are absent, as are most IgGs *(77–79)*. Myeloid lineage cells, macrophages, NK cells, and LAK cells are normal. Functional B- and T-cells may become detectable in some individuals, particularly with age. These SCID mice are often referred to as "leaky." More recent SCID-based models, and those bearing the Rag mutations, do not become leaky with age. Some NOD/SCID mice have a sufficient lifespan to be useful as xenograft hosts. NOD/LtSz-rag1[null] mice have no mature B- or T-cells, and exhibit low levels of NK-cell activity *(80)*. Most of these more severely immunodeficient mice retain their coats, unlike models based on the *nu* mutation.

5. ENDOCRINE EFFECTS ON HOST IMMUNITY

Steroid hormones are well-known for their effects on immunity. Although this is perhaps most widely acknowledged for the glucocorticoids, estrogens and antiestrogens also exhibit significant effects on immune function. Often these effects are dose related, and biphasic responses have been reported. Pharmacological but not physiological concentrations of estradiol inhibit NK activity in nude mice *(81–84)*. The effect is clearly biphasic in many studies, with NK-cell levels rising for the first 30 d followed by an overall reduction in the longer term *(81–84)*.

Anti-estrogens also affect NK-cell function, stimulating NK activity both in vitro and in vivo *(30,85)*. For example, TAM stimulates NK activity in vivo *(30)*. We have demonstrated that TAM responsiveness can be restored to TAM-resistant MCF7/LCC2 xenografts by blocking their secreted TGFβ activity. This appears to reflect an inhibition of TGFβ's ability to block NK activity *(86)*. Thus, a TAM-induced stimulation of cell-mediated immunity may partly contribute to its effects in xenografts, and may be expected to have similar effects on some tumors in patients. Indeed, some breast tumors exhibit marked infiltration by reticuloendothelial cells *(13)*.

It should be considered that, since NK-cell activity has been implicated in restricting tumorigenesis and metastasis *(60)*, the growth of endocrine-responsive xenografts reflects perturbations in the host's immunity. This may not be the case for MCF-7 xenografts. In athymic nude mice, MCF-7 xenografts become readily palpable within 14 d following SC inoculation of $1–5 \times 10^6$ cells. (Clarke R. unpublished observations). During this period, NK-cell activity would be expected to be further increased above the already high levels present in these animals. Approximately 300 pg/mL/day of estradiol is released from the widely used 60–d-release 0.72-mg estrogen pellets (produced by Innovative Research of America, Toledo, OH) (87). This dosage appears to be below the concentration of estrogens required to suppress NK-cell activity significantly (81–84). Nonetheless, endocrinologic effects on immunity can influence response to anti-estrogens.

Other hormonal manipulations also affect various immunologic parameters. For example, the progestin lynestrenol stimulates active T-rosetting and phagocytosis by monocytes (88). Medroxyprogesterone acetate, which has both progestational and glucocorticoid activities, reduces the ratio of T4+/T8+ cells (89). Consistent with the effects of estrogens, the estrogen biosynthesis inhibitor aminoglutethimide, which blocks aromatization of androgens to estrogens, reduces serum estrogens and increases NK-cell activity in breast-cancer patients (90). Both medroxyprogesterone acetate and aminoglutethimide are effective as second-line endocrine therapies for breast tumors that have responded and then recurred while on TAM therapy (91,92). Toremiphene, an anti-estrogen structurally similar to TAM, increases pokeweed-mitogen-induced Ig synthesis of B-lymphocytes (93).

6. OTHER BREAST-CANCER ANIMAL MODELS

Although this article focuses upon xenograft models, it is important to note that other mammary-tumor models exist. These reflect various aspects of breast-cancer biology, but despite their nonhuman origin, have been widely and successfully used. These fall into three groups, the chemically induced models, those with a viral etiology, and models generated by genetic manipulations.

Mammary tumors can be induced in susceptible rat strains following exposure to either 7,12-dimethylbenz[a]anthracene (DMBA) or N-nitroso-N-methylurea (NMU). Generally, these models do not produce a significant or reproducible incidence of metastases. The basic biology of the two models is broadly similar. However, there is a higher incidence of Ha-*ras* mutations (≥80%) for NMU-induced tumors and ≤25% for those produced by DMBA (94). Depending upon the dosage, these carcinogens predominately produce mammary adenocarcinomas. Many are histologically similar to human ductal carcinoma *in situ,* or early invasive adenocarcinomas. The comparative biology of these rat models has been extensively reviewed (95). Some mouse strains also are susceptible to DMBA-induced mammary tumors. However, these can require pituitary isografts and different carcinogen-dose scheduling to produce a high tumor incidence (96,97).

There is little compelling evidence to support a viral etiology for human breast cancer, yet some mouse strains are readily infected with the mouse mammary-tumor virus (MMTV). The virus is passed vertically from dam to pups, and is transmitted through the mothers' milk. MMTV integration sites implicate several oncogenes that may be relevant to the human disease (6). However, there are differences between MMTV-driven tumors and those that spontaneously arise in many women. MMTV-driven tumors often have a histology that does not fully reflect the histology of human tumors. The highest incidence of mammary tumors arises after multiple pregnancies, but only in susceptible strains. Multiparity in humans, particularly beginning at a young age, is associated with a reduced lifetime risk of breast cancer *(12)*. However, there is now compelling evidence that pregnancy is associated with a short-term increased breast-cancer risk, even in younger women *(98,99)*. Callahan et al *(6)* have discussed the relevance and application of the MMTV models to the human disease. Other viruses that induce benign or malignant mammary lesions include the polyoma WTA2 virus and the human adenovirus type 9. The biology of these models has previously been described in detail *(100,101)*.

Many transgenic and gene knockout models of mammary cancer have been generated, and readers are referred to several reviews *(102–104)* and an excellent website maintained at http://www.mammary.nih.gov. Transgenic models that exhibit mammary tumorigenesis include those that overexpress growth factors and/or oncogenes. For example, mice transgenic for *c-myc* and transforming growth-factor alpha (TGFa) exhibit varying incidences of mammary tumors. These effects can be strain-or construct-dependent, and have been targeted to the gland through mammary-specific promoters, such as MMTV and whey-acidic promoter. As with all animal models, genetically manipulated models have both advantages and disadvantages. For example, such models may exhibit a high tumor incidence following the manipulation of a single gene. It is not clear whether the human disease is so readily generated—with multiple genetic and epigenetic changes evident—even in some benign breast lesions *(105,106)*. These models may more adequately reflect inherited breast cancers, since the altered genetic events are present from fetal life. Furthermore, the expressed transgene is generally expressed throughout the mammary epithelium, which probably does not occur in the majority of sporadic human breast cancers *(104)*.

7. SOME CONSIDERATIONS RELATING TO EXPERIMENTAL DESIGN

One of the most important aspects of any in vivo study is experimental design. Although this may seem obvious, many investigators who do not routinely use animal models fail to realize its central importance. When established and proven designs are available, this is not problematic. However, with the significant advances in molecular biology, many molecular biologists find themselves facing the prospect of attempting to determine gene function in vivo using cells that have been genetically manipulated in vitro.

General approaches to designing an appropriate animal experiment are, in principle, no different from other cellular, molecular, or biochemical experiments. However, the use of animals differs significantly from in vitro studies in several key aspects, such as specific animal welfare, animal husbandry, and ethical and legislative requirements, which must be adequately considered. In many ways, the use of animals is comparable to conducting a human clinical trial. For example, assessing the maximum tolerated dose (MTD) of an investigational agent may involve the use of escalating doses in a small number of animals bearing xenografts, until a dose-limiting toxicity is reached in one or two animals *(107)*. Essentially, this is similar in concept and design to a Phase I clinical trial in humans. Other experimental designs may be unique to in vivo models, reflecting hypotheses that cannot be tested in humans. This may include investigating gene function, or evaluating the preclinical safety and activity of a new experimental drug. Examples of several issues arising in the experimental design to test the latter have been previously discussed *(107)*.

A simple example can be used to illustrate several major issues in experimental design involving vertebrate species for breast-cancer research. A useful example may be one in which an investigator who has overexpressed an oncogene in nonmetastatic breast-cancer cells wishes to determine whether this confers a highly invasive or metastatic phenotype, or produces a tissue-specific pattern of metastasis.

Using this example, the initial hypothesis may be simply stated as: "we hypothesize that the overexpression of *gene a* confers an invasive and/or metastatic phenotype upon MCF-7 human breast-cancer cells." Clearly, the investigator will first perform the necessary in vitro gene manipulations, producing cells that appropriately overexpress *gene a's* mRNA and protein. However, before initiating any in vivo experiment, the investigator must first obtain formal institutional approval. In the United States, this requires approval from the investigator's Institutional Animal Care and Use Committee. These committees are required by law, and other countries have similar requirements. Readers in the United States may find useful information on how their Institutional Animal Care and Use Committee functions by consulting reference *(108)*. Several web sites also are available, and readers are encouraged to visit the following Internet sites as needed, and follow the additional links to other sites:

1. National Research Council, Institute of Laboratory Animal Resources.
   http://www.nap.edu/readingroom/books/labrats
2. U.S. Department of Agriculture, Animal and Plant Health Inspection Service.
   http://www.aphis.usda.gov
3. Home Office (U.K.), Animals, Bylaws & Coroners Unit.
   http://www.homeoffice.gov.uk/ccpd/abcu.htm
4. American Association for Laboratory Animal Science. http://www.aalas.org
5. Canadian Council on Animal Care. *http://www.ccac.ca*
6. Norwegian Reference Centre for Laboratory Science & Alternatives.
   http://oslovet.veths.no

Continuing with this example, the choice of MCF-7 as the target-cell line could be reasonable. These are well-characterized human breast-cancer cells, originally obtained from a postmenopausal patient with advanced disease *(4)*. MCF-7 cells express a relatively early phenotype, are tumorigenic, and produce poorly invasive and rarely metastatic xenografts in athymic nude mice *(51)*. However, these xenografts need supplemental estrogens. This will require consideration of how to best provide this supplementation, such as the use of slow-release estradiol pellets, the use of sterile silicon-tubing implants containing estradiol (if so, how much and in what vehicle?), the administration of sterile estrogen depots (at which site - ip, sc, im., in which vehicle, which dose of estrogen, and how often?).

The choice of dosage will be influenced by the choice of immunodeficient host species. For example, MCF-7 cells will grow in both athymic rats and mice. Adjusting the dose among species can be done using the conversions for drug dosage based on body surface area *(109)*. Assuming the choice of species is mouse, knowing that an immunodeficient host is required, the choice of recipient strain must be addressed: *nu, bg/nu, bg/nu/xid,* or *scid.*

The investigator may consider a *scid, bg/nu,* or *bg/nu/xid* host, avoiding any possible adverse effects on metastatic potential produced by the high NK-cell activity in athymic nude mice. However, the choice of host also will be influenced by the site of inoculation. Some experimental metastasis models use iv or intracardiac inoculation *(110,111).* This is a much less rigorous approach than requiring xenografts to metastasize from solid tumors. It is now apparent that human breast-tumor xenografts metastasize most effectively from mammary fat-pad inocula *(54,112).* This is not surprising, given the utility of orthotopic inoculation in other tumor models *(113).* If the investigator chooses mammary fat-pad inoculation, it is usually necessary to surgically expose the sites to ensure appropriate targeting of the xenograft. This will likely exclude models incorporating the *bg* mutation, since these animals have a clotting disorder that may result in the loss of several hosts to extensive hemorrhage during surgery.

Other considerations imposed by the choice of mammary fat-pad inoculation include training in the appropriate aseptic surgical techniques, and choice of anesthetic for surgery (dose, route of administration of anesthetic, and both the required depth and duration of anesthesia). The investigator also may need to consider postsurgical care—whether or not a heat source will be required, and if so, for how long. It also may be necessary to determine how any potential infections at the wound site might be treated, even though none are expected if the surgery has been appropriately performed.

The next issues for consideration are the number of animals required for the entire study, and the number of animals required per experimental group. The number of experimental groups will depend on how the investigator chooses to test her or his hypothesis. In this example, the investigator may choose to include control groups comprising xenografts of wild-type cells and one or two additional control cell lines, the latter containing "empty" expression vectors lacking only *gene a*. It is likely that two or more clones of cells expressing *gene a,* perhaps with different levels of expression, might be evaluated. If the investigator has used a regulable promoter, such as the tet on-off system, an appropriate dosage of the regulator in this case, doxycycline *(114)*—must be identified.

The number of animals required for each group is an important, and sometimes difficult, issue to address accurately. Like several other aspects of experimental design, arriving at a reasonable number is dependent upon several other features of the experimental design. Essentially, what is required is an estimate of the statistical power of the experimental design. This has been discussed in detail by Hanfelt *(115).* Briefly, the number of animals in each group should provide sufficient power to detect a significant difference among experimental groups where one exists. An underpowered study may lead to a rejection of our investigator's hypothesis for example the overexpression of *gene a* is not associated with conferring a metastatic phenotype. An overpowered study might conclude that *gene a* confers this phenotype the incidence of metastasis is statistically different among the control and experimental groups, while in reality the magnitude of this contribution has no true biological significance.

The determination of an investigator's statistical power is often best left to a collaborating biostatistician. In our example, the power estimates may need to include the possibility that some animals may die prematurely, perhaps reflecting undiagnosed but lethal metastases. The investigator may need to provide the biostatistician with some estimate of the likely magnitude of the effect, or how large an effect the investigator wishes to determine—some sense of what would reflect a meaningful or biologically relevant outcome. An integral component of this consideration is the choice of experimental end point—how sensitive is the measure of activity, in this case the detection of metastases.

The choice of a metastatic end point for assessing biological activity imposes additional considerations for experimental design. Evidence suggests that the incidence of metastasis is related to the size of the primary tumor. Most institutional animal care and use committee (IACUCs) impose an upper limit for tumor burden; for example, tumor burden might be restricted to ≤10% of each host's body wt. Tumor burden can readily be determined by following tumor size in a nonmetastatic model. However, our investigator must consider whether it may be necessary to attempt to obtain approval to allow the tumors to exceed the institutional requirement. An alternative may be to consider a debulking approach, in which a second surgery is required to either remove or debulk the primary tumor. This could increase the time available to allow the establishment of micrometastases.

How will tumor burden be assessed in a possible model of metastasis where palpation for metastases is unlikely to provide a useful measurement of total body tumor burden? The simple answer is that directly assessing tumor burden to a satisfactory degree may not be possible. Alternative indirect assessments may be necessary. If the genetically manipulated cells metastasize with a breast-cancer-specific tissue pattern, some hosts may experience problems reflecting lung, bone, liver, visceral, or brain metastases. Clearly, it will be necessary to carefully monitor animals for loss in rate of weight gain, reduced mobility, difficulty in breathing, and other behavioral changes.

The final consideration relates to analysis of the final data, which has been described in detail elsewhere *(115–118)*. Among the more obvious issues is the use of appropriate statistical tests to explore the data. For example, if the investigator wished to compare tumor growth, which would require the use of longitudinal data obtained on the same individuals, a repeated-measure analysis of variance may be required. This is likely to be preferable to the widely used comparison of tumor sizes at the end of an experiment, which places substantial weight on a single measurement from among a series of repeated measures. When one group has simply had smaller tumor sizes at the initiation of tumor measurements than the other, tumors growing at the same rate would be interpreted as growing more slowly if the single measurement was used. In contrast, analysis of the repeated measurement data for each tumor in each group, by Gompertzian or other appropriate transformations followed by a simple or multivariate analysis of variance *(115,117,119)*, would clearly show that the tumors in each group were growing at the same rate. If organ weights are to be compared, the analysis may need to consider the corresponding body wt data, since the two are related. Consequently, an analysis of covariance may be required *(116)*.

Clearly, many of the issues discussed here are fully appreciated by most experienced investigators. Nonetheless, it is evident from the literature that some investigators inadequately analyze their in vivo data. Not only is this problematic from a scientific perspective, but it also has implications for the use of animals. Inadequately analyzed studies may lead other investigators to perpetuate an inadequate design or analysis, thereby potentially using animals inappropriately and/or unnecessarily. The simplest way to avoid such problems would be for our investigator to return to the collaborating biostatistician for assistance in data analysis.

CONCLUSIONS AND FUTURE PROSPECTS

There is an urgent need to identify and fully characterize new xenograft models of breast cancer. For example, there are relatively few adequate metastatic models. Those that exist do not fully reflect the tissue-specific targeting of metastases seen in breast-cancer patients. There are few, if any, adequate endocrine-responsive or endocrine-dependent metastatic models. Indeed, the number of widely used and well-characterized estrogen-dependent models, or models of acquired anti-estrogen resistance, are relatively few. This is particularly true for models that are not derived from parental MCF-7 cells. The widespread use of MCF-7 cells is not surprising, but it is far from a perfect or universal model of estrogen-responsive breast cancer. For example, it is nonmetastatic, despite being derived from a metastatic effusion *(4)* and metastasis is the primary cause of mortality in patients bearing ER-positive tumors. MCF-7 cells also may also take different pathways for regulating apoptosis, since the cells have a truncated (nonfunctional) caspase-3 *(120)*. Whether this reflects signaling that also occurs in patients' tumors is unclear. These observations underscore the need to carefully select the appropriate model to address the hypothesis.

There are clear reservations, and widespread criticism, related to the use of cell-culture models in vitro and in vivo. Nonetheless, many properties of human breast-cancer-cell lines effectively and accurately reflect key aspects of the biology of breast cancer. For example, the histologies of these human breast-cancer xenografts frequently reflect those seen in tumors in patients. The inverse relationship between expression of the receptors for estrogen and epidermal growth factor in human tumors, is consistently demonstrated in most of the human breast-cancer-cell lines and xenografts. The patterns of responsiveness to many cytotoxic drugs are also broadly similar between several xenograft models and the human disease. When MCF-7 cells are exposed to in vivo selective pressures, comparable to several predicted to occur in patients, they apparently progress along an analogous pathway. Indeed, some phenotypes have first been observed in such models, only to be identified later in patients *(60)*. These observations clearly establish the utility and importance of human breast-cancer xenografts in pursing specific, but not all, breast-cancer-related hypotheses. They also illustrate the need to identify additional models for breast-cancer research.

ACKNOWLEDGMENTS

This work was supported by PHS awards R01-CA/AG58022, P30-CA51008. P50-CA58185, and Department of Defense (USAMRMC) awards BC980629 and BC990358.

REFERENCES

1. Lacassagne A. Apparition de cancers de la mammelle chez la souris male a des injections de folliculine. *C R Acad Sci (Paris)* 1932; 195:639–632. Lacassagne A. Apparition de cancers de la mammelle chez la souris male a des injections de folliculine. *C R Acad Sci (Paris)* 1932; 195:639–632.
2. Pantelouris EM. Absence of thymus in a mutant mouse. *Nature* 1968; 217:370–371.
3. Rygaard J, Povlsen CO. Heterotransplantation of a human malignant tumour to "nude" mice. *Acta Path Microbiol Scand* 1969; 77:758–760.
4. Soule HD, Vasquez J, Long A, Albert S, Brennan M. A human cell line from a pleural effusion derived from a human breast carcinoma. *J Natl Cancer Inst* 1973; 51:1409–1416.

5. Huggins C, Grand LC, Brillantes FP. Mammary cancer induced by a single feeding of polynuclear hyrocarbons, and its suppression. *Nature* 1961; 189:204.

6. Callahan R. MMTV induced mutations in mouse mammary tumors: their potential relevance to human breast cancer. *Breast Cancer Res Treat* 1995; 39:33–44.

7. Willett WC, Rockhill B, Hankinson SE, Hunter DJ, Colditz GA. Epidemiology and assessing and managing risk. In: Harris J, Lippman ME, Morrow M, Osborne CK, eds. *Diseases of the Breast.* Lippincott Williams & Wilkins, Philadelphia, PA, 2000, pp. 175–220.

8. Ingham JM. End-of-life considerations in breast cancer patients. In: Harris J, Lippman ME, Morrow M, Osborne CK, eds. *Diseases of the Breast.* Lippincott Williams & Wilkins, Philadelphia, PA, 2000, pp. 967–983.

9. Clark GM. Prognostic and predictive factors in node-negative breast cancer: results of long-term follow-up studies. In: Harris JR, Lippman ME, Morrow M, Hellman S, eds. *Diseases of the Breast.* Lippincott, Philadelphia, PA, 1996, pp. 461–485.

10. Ellis MJ, Hayes DF, Lippman ME. Treatment of metastatic breast cancer. In: Harris J, Lippman ME, Morrow M, Osborne CK, eds. *Diseases of the Breast.* Lippincott Williams & Wilkins, Philadelphia, PA, 2000, pp. 749–797.

11. Allred DC, Mohsin SK. Biological features of human premalignant disease. In: Harris JR, Lippman ME, Morrow M, Osborne CK, eds. *Diseases of the Breast.* Lippincott Williams & Wilkins, Philadelphia, PA, 2000, pp. 355–366.

12. Hulka BS, Stark AT. Breast cancer: cause and prevention. *Lancet* 1995; 346:883–887.

13. Clarke R, Dickson RB, Lippman ME. Hormonal aspects of breast cancer: growth factors, drugs and stromal interactions. *Crit Rev Oncol Hematol* 1992; 12:1–23.

14. Schairer C, Lubin J, Troisi R, Sturgeon S, Brinton L, Hoover R. Menopausal estrogen and estrogen-progestin replacement therapy and breast cancer risk. *J Am Med Assoc* 2000; 283:485–491.

15. Magnusson C, Baron JA, Correia N, Bergstrom R, Adami HO, Persson I. Breast-cancer risk following long-term oestrogen- and oestrogen-progestin-replacement therapy. *Int J Cancer* 1999; 81:339–344.

16. Early Breast Cancer Trialists Collaborative Group: Systemic treatment of early breast cancer by hormonal, cytotoxic, or immune therapy. *Lancet* 1992; 399:1–15.

17. Early Breast Cancer Trialists' Collaborative Group. Tamoxifen for early breast cancer: an overview of the randomized trials. *Lancet* 1998; 351:1451–1467.

18. Dowsett M. Future use of aromatase inhibitors in breast cancer. *J Steroid Biochem Mol Biol* 1997; 61:261–266.

19. Fisher B, Costantino JP, Wickerham DL, Redmond CK, Kavanah M, Cronin WM, et al. Tamoxifen for prevention of breast cancer: report of the National Surgical Adjuvant Breast and Bowel Project P-1 study. *J Natl Cancer Inst* 1998; 90:1371–1388.

20. Henderson IC. Chemotherapy for metastatic disease. In: Harris JR, Hellman S, Henderson IC, Kinne DW, JB, eds. *Breast Diseases.* Lippincott Co., Philadelphia, PA, 1991, pp. 604–665.

21. Brünner N, Boulay V, Fojo A, Freter C, Lippman ME, Clarke R. Acquisition of hormone-independent growth in MCF-7 cells is accompanied by increased expression of estrogen-regulated genes but without detectable DNA amplifications. *Cancer Res* 1993; 53:283–290.

22. Brünner N, Frandsen TL, Holst-Hansen C, Bei M, Thompson EW, Wakeling AE, et al. MCF7/LCC2: A 4-hydroxytamoxifen resistant human breast cancer variant which retains sensitivity to the steroidal antiestrogen ICI 182,780. *Cancer Res* 1993; 53:3229–3232.

23. Brünner N, Boysen B, Jirus S, Skaar TC, Holst-Hansen C, Lippman J, et al. MCF7/LCC9: an antiestrogen resistant MCF-7 variant where acquired resistance to the steroidal antiestrogen ICI 182,780 confers an early crossresistance to the non-steroidal antiestrogen tamoxifen. *Cancer Res* 1997; 57:3486–3493.

24. De Vita VT. Principles of chemotherapy. In: De Vita VT, Hellman S, Rosenberg SA, eds. *Cancer Principles and Practice of Oncology.* J.B. Lippincott, Philadelphia, PA, 1989, pp. 276–300.

25. Clarke R, Leonessa F, Brünner N, Thompson EW. *In vitro* models. In: Harris JR, Lippman ME, Morrow M, Hellman S, eds. *Diseases of the Breast.* Lippincott, Philadelphia, PA, 2000, pp. 335–354.

26. Levinson AS, Jordan VC. MCF-7 the first hormone-responsive breast cancer cell line. *Cancer Res* 1997; 57:3071–3078.

27. Clarke R, Brünner N, Katzenellenbogen BS, Thompson EW, Norman MJ, Koppi C, et al. Progression from hormone dependent to hormone independent growth in MCF-7 human breast cancer cells. *Proc Natl Acad Sci USA* 1989; 86:3649–3653.

28. Clarke R, Brünner N, Katz D, Glanz P, Dickson RB, Lippman ME, et al. The effects of a constitutive production of TGF-α on the growth of MCF-7 human breast cancer cells in vitro and in vivo. *Mol Endocrinol* 1989; 3:372–380.

29. Herman ME, Katzenellenbogen BS. Response-specific antiestrogen resistance in a newly characterized MCF-7 human breast cancer cell line resulting from long-term exposure to trans-hydroxytamoxifen. *J Steroid Biochem Mol Biol* 1996; 59:121–134.

30. Gottardis MM, Wagner RJ, Borden EC, Jordan VC. Differential ability of antiestrogens to stimulate breast cancer cell (MCF-7) growth in vivo and in vitro. *Cancer Res* 1989; 49:4765–4769.

31. Osborne CK, Coronado EB, Robinson JP. Human breast cancer in athymic nude mice: cytostatic effects of long-term antiestrogen therapy. *Eur J Cancer Clin Oncol* 1987; 23:1189–1196.

32. Butler WB, Fontana JA. Responses to retinoic acid of tamoxifen-sensitive and -resistant sublines of human breast cancer cell line MCF-7. *Cancer Res* 1992; 52:6164–6167.

33. Vickers PJ, Dickson RB, Shoemaker R, Cowan KH. A multidrug-resistant MCF-7 human breast cancer cell line which exhibits cross-resistance to antiestrogens and hormone independent tumor growth. *Mol Endocrinol* 1988; 2:886–892.

34. Clarke R, Currier S, Kaplan O, Lovelace E, Boulay V, Gottesman MM, et al. Effect of P-glycoprotein expression on sensitivity to hormones in MCF-7 human breast cancer cells. *J Natl Cancer Inst* 1992; 84:1506–1512.

35. Lee JS, Scala S, Matsumoto Y, Dickstein B, Robey R, Zhan Z, et al. Reduced drug accumulation and multidrug resistance in human breast cancer cells without associated P-glycoprotein or MRP overexpression. *J Cell Biochem* 1997; 65:513–526.

36. Trock BJ, Leonessa F, Clarke R. Multidrug resistance in breast cancer: a meta analysis of MDR1/gp170 expression and its possible functional significance. *J Natl Cancer Inst* 1997; 89:917–931.

37. Scudiero DA, Monks A, Sausville EA. Cell line designation change: multidrug-resistant cell line in the NCI anticancer screen. *J Natl Cancer Inst* 1998; 90:862–863.

38. Leonessa F, Jacobson M, Boyle B, Lippman J, McGarvey M, Clarke R. The effect of tamoxifen on the multidrug resistant phenotype in human breast cancer cells: isobologram, drug accumulation and gp-170 binding studies. *Cancer Res* 1994; 54:441–447.

39. Perez-Soler R, Neamati N, Zou Y, Schneider E, Doyle LA, Andreeff M, et al. Annamycin circumvents resistance mediated by the multidrug resistance- associated protein (MRP) in breast MCF-7 and small-cell lung UMCC-1 cancer cell lines selected for resistance to etoposide. *Int J Cancer* 1997; 71:35–41.

40. Nooter K, de la Riviere BG, Look NP, van Wingerden KE, Henzen-Logmans SC, Scheper RJ, et al. The prognostic significance of expression of the multidrug resistance-associated protein (MRP) in primary breast cancer. *Br J Cancer* 1997; 76:486–493.

41. Ito K, Fujimori M, Nakata S, Hama Y, Shingu K, Kobayashi S, et al. Clinical significance of the increased multidrug resistance-associated protein (MRP) gene expression in patients with primary breast cancer. *Oncol Res* 1998; 10:99–109.

42. Horwitz KB, Friedenberg GR. Growth inhibition and increase of insulin receptors in antiestrogen-resistant T47Dco human breast cancer cells by progestins: implications for endocrine therapies. *Cancer Res* 1985; 45:167–173.

43. Lasfargues EY, Coutinho WG, Redfield ES. Isolation of two human tumor epithelial cell lines from solid breast carcinomas. *J Natl Cancer Inst* 1978; 61:967–978.

44. van den Berg HW, Lynch M, Martin J, Nelson J, Dickson GR, Crockard AD. Characterization of a tamoxifen-resistant variant of the ZR-75-1 human breast cancer cell line (ZR-75-9a1) and stability of the resistant phenotype. *Br J Cancer* 1989; 59:522–526.

45. Brunner N, Bastert GB, Poulsen HS, Spang-Thomsen M. Characterization of the T61 human breast carcinoma established in nude mice. *Eur J Cancer Clin Oncol* 1985; 21:833–843.

46. Hopp TA, Fuqua SA. Estrogen receptor variants. *J Mammary Gland Biol Neoplasia* 1998; 3:73–83.

47. Poola I, Chatra S, Koduri S, Clarke R. Analysis of single-, double- and multiple-exon deletion transcripts of estrogen receptor in breast cancer cell lines and tumors by a novel approach. *J Steroid Biochem Mol Biol* 2000; 72:249–258.

48. Lasfargues EY, Ozzello L. Cultivation of human breast carcinomas. *J Natl Cancer Inst* 1958; 21:1131–1147.

49. Castles CG, Fuqua SA, Klotz DM, Hill SM. Expression of a constitutively active estrogen receptor variant in the estrogen receptor-negative BT-20 human breast cancer cell line. *Cancer Res* 1993; 53:5934–5939.

50. Ozzello L, Sordat B, Merenda C, Carrel S, Hurlimann J, Mach JP. Transplantation of a human mammary carcinoma cell line (BT 20) into nude mice. *J Natl Cancer Inst* 1974; 52:1669–1672.

51. Thompson EW, Brünner N, Torri J, Johnson MD, Boulay V, Wright A, et al. The invasive and metastatic properties of hormone-independent and hormone-responsive variants of MCF-7 human breast cancer cells. *Clin Exp Metastasis* 1993; 11:15–26.

52. McLeskey SW, Zhang L, Kharbanda S, Kurebayashi J, Lippman ME, Dickson RB, et al. Fibroblast growth factor overexpressing breast carcinoma cells as models for angiogenesis and metastasis. *Breast Cancer Res Treat* 1995; 39:103–117.

53. Jiang S-Y, Jordan VC. Growth regulation of estrogen receptor negative breast cancer cells transfected with estrogen receptor cDNAs. *J Natl Cancer Inst* 1992; 84:580–591.

54. Price JE, Polyzos A, Zhang RD, Daniels LM. Tumorigenicity and metastasis of human breast carcinoma cell lines in nude mice. *Cancer Res* 1990; 50:717–721.

55. Rose DP, Connolly JM, Meschter CL. Effect of dietary fat on human breast cancer growth and lung metastasis in nude mice. *J Natl Cancer Inst* 1991; 83:1491–1495.

56. Rose DP, Hatala MA, Connolly JM, Rayburn J. Effect of diets containing different levels of linoleic acid on human breast cancer growth and lung metastasis in nude mice. *Cancer Res* 1993; 53:4686–4690.

57. Leonessa F, Green D, Licht T, Wright A, Wingate-Legette K, Lippman J, et al. MDA435/LCC6 and MDA435/LCC6[MDR1]: ascites models of human breast cancer. *Br J Cancer* 1996; 73:154–161.

58. Thompson EW, Paik S, Brünner N, Sommers C, Zugmaier G, Clarke R, et al. Association of increased basement membrane-invasiveness with absence of estrogen receptor and expression of vimentin in human breast cancer cell lines. *J Cell Physiol* 1992; 150:534–544.

59. Maruo K, Ueyama Y, Hioki K, Saito M, Nomura T, Tamaoki N. Strain-dependent growth of a human carcinoma in nude mice with different genetic backgrounds: selection of nude mouse strains useful for anticancer agent screening system. *Exp Cell Biol* 1982; 50:115–119.

60. Clarke R. Human breast cancer cell line xenografts as models of breast cancer: the immunobiologies of recipient mice and the characteristics of several tumorigenic cell lines. *Breast Cancer Res Treat* 1996; 39:69–86.

61. Hougen HP, Klausen B. Effects of homozygosity of the nude (rnu) gene in an inbred strain of rats: studies of lymphoid and nonlymphoid organs in different age groups of nude rats of LEW background at a stage in the gene transfer. *Lab Anim* 1984; 18:7–14.

62. Weisz-Carrington P, Schrater AF, Lamm ME, Thorbecke GJ. Immunoglobulin isotypes in plasma cells of normal and athymic mice. *Cell Immunol* 1979; 44:343–351.

63. Kindred B. The inception of the response to SRBC by nude mice injected with various doses of congenic or allogeneic thymus cells. *Cell Immunol* 1975; 17:277–284.

64. De Sousa M, Pritchard H. The cellular basis of immunological recovery in nude mice after thymus grafting. *Immunology* 1974; 26:769–776.

65. Guy-Grand D, Griscelli C, Vassalli P. Peyer's patches, gut IgA, plasma cells and thymic function: study in nude mice bearing thymic grafts. *J Immunol* 1975; 115:361–364.

66. Hasui M, Saikawa Y, Miura M, Takano N, Ueno Y, Yachie A, et al. Effector and precursor phenotypes of lymphokine-activated killer cells in mice with severe combined immunodeficiency (Scid) and athymic (Nude) mice. *Cell Immunol* 1989; 120:230–239.

67. Johnson WJ, Balish E. Macrophage function in germ-free, athymic (nu/nu) mice and conventional flora (nu/+) mice. *J Reticuloendothel Soc* 1980; 28:55–66.

68. Fridman R, Kibbey MC, Royce LS, Zain M, Sweeney TM, Jicha DL, et al. Enhanced tumor growth of both primary and established human and murine tumor cells in athymic mice after coinjection with matrigel. *J Natl Cancer Inst* 1991; 83:769–774.

69. Karre K, Klein GO, Kiessling R, Klein G, Roder JC. In vitro NK-activity and in vivo resistance to leukemia: studies of beige, beige/nude and wild type hosts on C57BL background. *Int J Cancer* 1980; 26:789–797.

70. Roder JC. The beige mutation in the mouse. I. A stem cell predetermined impairment in natural killer cell function. *J Immunol* 1979; 123:2168–2173.

71. Roder JC, Duwe AK. The beige mutation in the mouse selectively impairs natural killer cell function. *Nature* 1979; 278:451–453.

72. Shultz LD. Single gene models of immunodeficieny diseases. In: Wu B, Zheng J, eds. *Immune-deficient animals in experimental medicine.* Karger, Basel, 1989, pp. 19–26.

73. Karre K, Klein GO, Kiessling R, Klein G, Roder JC. Low natural in vivo resistance to syngeneic leukemias in natural killer-deficient mice. *Nature* 1980; 284:624–626.

74. Andriole GL, Mule JJ, Hansen CT, Linehan WM, Rosenberg SA. Evidence that lymphokine-activated killer cells and natural killer cells are distinct based on an analysis of congenitally immunodeficient mice. *J Immunol* 1985; 135:2911–2913.

75. Kincade PW. Defective colony formation by B lymphocytes from CBA/N and C3H/HeJ mice. *J Exp Med* 1977; 145:249–263.

76. Bosma MJ, Carroll AM. The SCID mouse mutant: definition, characterization, and potential uses. *Annu Rev Immunol* 1991; 9:323–350.

77. Custer RP, Bosma GC, Bosma MJ. Severe combined immunodeficiency (scid) in the mouse. Pathology, reconstitution, neoplasms. *Am J Path* 1985; 120:464–477.

78. Bosma GC, Custer RP, Bosma MJ. A severe combined immunodeficiency mutation in the mouse. *Nature* 1983; 301:527–530.

79. Schuler W, Weiler IJ, Schuler A, Phillips RA, Rosenberg N, Mak TW, et al. Rearrangement of antigen receptor genes is defective in mice with severe combined immune deficiency. *Cell* 1986; 46:963–972.

80. Shultz LD, Lang PA, Christianson SW, Gott B, Lyons B, Umeda S, et al. NOD/LtSz-Rag1null mice: an immunodeficient and radioresistant model for engraftment of human hematolymphoid cells, HIV infection, and adoptive transfer of NOD mouse diabetogenic T cells. *J Immunol* 2000; 164:2496–2507.

81. Screpanti I, Santoni A, Gulino A, Herberman RB, Frati L. Estrogen and antiestrogen modulation of mouse natural killer activity and large granular lymphocytes. *Cell Immunol* 1987; 106:191–202.

82. Seaman WE, Blackman MA, Gindhart TD, Roubinian JR, Loeb JM, Talal N. β-Estradiol reduces natural killer cells in mice. *J Immunol* 1978; 121:2193–2198.

83. Hanna N, Schneider M. Enhancement of tumor metastases and suppression of natural killer cell activity by β-estradiol treatment. *J Immunol* 1983; 130:974–980.

84. Seaman WE, Talal N. The effect of 17β-estradiol on natural killing in the mouse. In: Herberman RB, ed. *Natural Cell-Mediated Immunity Against Tumors.* Academic Press, New York, NY, 1980, pp. 765–777.

85. Mandeville R, Ghali SS, Chausseau JP. In vitro stimulation of NK activity by an estrogen antagonist (Tamoxifen). *Eur J Cancer Clin Oncol* 1984; 20:983–985.

86. Arteaga CL, Koli KM, Dugger TC, Clarke R. Reversal of tamoxifen resistance of human breast carcinomas *in vivo* with neutralizing anti-transforming growth factor (TGF)-β antibodies involves paracrine mechanisms. *J Natl Cancer Inst* 1999; 91:46–53.

87. Blumenthal RD, Jordan JJ, McLaughlin WH, Bloomer WD. Animal modeling of human breast tumors: limitations in the use of estrogen pellet implants. *Breast Cancer Res Treat* 1988; 11:77–78.

88. Wyban J, Govaerts A, van Dam D, Appelbloom T. Stimulating properties of lynestrenol on normal human blood T-lymphocytes and other leucocytes. *Int J Immunopharmacol* 1979; 1:151–155.

89. Scambia G, Panci PB, Maccio A, Castelli P, Serri F, Mantovani G, et al. Effects of antiestrogen and progestin on immune functions in breast cancer patients. *Cancer* 1988; 61:2214–2218.

90. Berry J, Green BJ, Matheson DS. Modulation of natural killer cell activity in stage I postmenopausal breast cancer patients on low-dose aminoglutethide. *Cancer Immunol Immunother* 1987; 24:72–75.

91. Garcia-Giralt E, Ayme Y, Carton M, Daban A, Delozier T, Fargeot PFP, et al. Second and third line hormonotherapy in advanced post-menopausal breast cancer: a multicenter randomized trial comparing medroxyprogesterone acetate with aminoglutethimide in patients who have become resistant to tamoxifen. *Breast Cancer Res Treat* 1992; 24:139–145.

92. Canney PA, Priestman TJ, Griffiths T, Latief TN, Mould JJ, Spooner D. Randomized trial comparing aminoglutethimide with high-dose medroxyprogesterone acetate in therapy for advanced breast carcinoma. *J Natl Cancer Inst* 1988; 80:1147–1151.

93. Paavonen T, Andersson LC. The oestrogen antagonists tamoxifen, FC-1157a display oestrogen like effects on human lymphocyte functions in vitro. *Clin Exp Immunol* 1985; 61:467–474.

94. Clarke R. Animal models of breast cancer: their diversity and role in biomedical research. *Breast Cancer Res Treat* 1996; 39:1–6.

95. Russo J, Gusterson BA, Rogers AE, Russo IH, Wellings SR, van Zwieten MJ. Biology of disease: comparative study of human and rat mammary tumorigenesis. *Lab Investig* 1990; 62:244–278.

96. Medina D. Mammary tumorigenesis in chemical carcinogen-treated mice. II. Dependence on hormone stimulation for tumorigenesis. *J Natl Cancer Inst* 1974; 53:223–226.

97. Medina D. Mammary tumorigenesis in chemical carcinogen-treated mice. I. Incidence in BALB-c and C57BL mice. *J Natl Cancer Inst* 1974; 53:213–221.

98. Hsieh C, Pavia M, Lambe M, Lan SJ, Colditz GA, Ekbom A, et al. Dual effect of parity on breast cancer risk. *Eur J Cancer* 1994; 30A:969–973.

99. Williams EMI, Jones L, Vessey MP, McPherson K. Short term increase in risk of breast cancer associated with full pregnancy. *Br Med J* 1990; 300:578–579.

100. Fluck MM, Haslam SZ. Mammary tumors induced by polyoma virus. *Breast Cancer Res Treat* 1995; 45–56.

101. Javier R, Shenk T. Mammary tumors induced by adenovirus type-9:a role for the viral early region 4 gene. *Breast Cancer Res Treat* 1995; 39:57–67.

102. Humphreys RC, Hennighausen L. Transforming growth factor alpha and mouse models of human breast cancer. *Oncogene* 2000; 19:1085–1091.

103. Cardiff RD, Anver MR, Gusterson BA, Hennighausen L, Jensen RA, Merino MJ, et al. The mammary pathology of genetically engineered mice: the consensus report and recommendations from the Annapolis meeting. *Oncogene* 2000; 19:968–988.

104. Clarke R. Animal models. In: Harris JR, Lippman ME, Morrow M, eds. *Diseases of the Breast.* Lippincott, Philadelphia, PA, 2000, pp. 319–333.

105. Millikan R, Hulka B, Thor A, Zhang Y, Edgerton S, Zhang X, et al. p53 mutations in benign breast tissue. *J Clin Oncol* 1995; 13:2293–2300.

106. Dietrich CU, Pandis N, Teixeira MR, Bardi G, Gerdes AM, Andersen JA, et al. Chromosome abnormalities in benign hyperproliferative disorders of epithelial and stromal breast tissue. *Int J Cancer* 1995; 60:49–53.

107. Clarke R. Issues in experimental design and endpoint analysis in the study of experimental cytotoxic agents *in vivo* in breast cancer and other models. *Breast Cancer Res Treat* 1997; 46:255–278.

108. Silverman J, Suckow MA, Murthy S. *The IACUC Handbook.* CRC Press, Boca Raton, FL, 2000.

109. Freireich EJ, Gehan EA, Rall DP, Schmidt LH, Skipper HE. Quantitative comparison of toxicity of anticancer agents in mouse, rat, hamster, dog, monkey, and man. *Cancer Chemother Rep* 1966; 50:219–244.

110. Sung V, Gilles C, Murray A, Clarke R, Aaron AD, Azumi N, et al. The LCC15-MB human breast cancer cell line expresses osteopontin and exhibits an invasive and metastatic phenotype. *Exp Cell Res* 1998; 241:273–284.

111. Thompson EW, Sung V, Lavigne M, Baumann K, Azumi N, Aaron AD, et al. LCC15-MB: a human breast cancer cell line from a femoral bone metastasis. *Clin Exp Metastasis* 1999; 17:193–204.

112. Price JE. Metastasis from human breast cancer cell lines. *Breast Cancer Res Treat* 1995; 39:93–102.

113. Morikawa K, Walker SM, Nakajima M, Pathak S, Jessup JM, Fidler IJ. Influence of organ environment on the growth, selection, and metastasis of human colon carcinoma cells in nude mice. *Cancer Res* 1988; 48:6863–6871.

114. Gossen M, Bujard H. Tight control of gene expression in mammalian cells by tetracycline-responsive promoters. *Proc Natl Acad Sci USA* 1992; 89:5547–5551.

115. Hanfelt J. Statistical approaches to experimental design and data analysis of *in vivo* studies. *Breast Cancer Res Treat* 1997; 46:279–302.

116. Gad S, Weil CS. *Statistics and Experimental Design for Toxicologists.* Telford Press, New Jersey, 1988.

117. Heitjan DF, Manni A, Santen RJ. Statistical analysis of in vivo tumor growth experiments. *Cancer Res* 1993; 53:6042–6050.

118. Gart JJ, Krewski D, Lee PN, Tarone RE, Wahrendorf J. *The Design and Analysis of Long Term Animal Experiments.* International Agency for Research on Cancer, Lyon, France 1986.

119. Rygaard K, Spang-Thompsen M. Quantitation and gompertzian analysis of tumor growth. *Breast Cancer Res Treat* 1997; 46:303–312.

120. Pink JJ, Wuerzberger-Davis S, Tagliarino C, Planchon SM, Yang X, Froelich CJ, et al. Activation of a cysteine protease in MCF-7 and T47D breast cancer cells during beta-lapachone-mediated apoptosis. *Exp Cell Res* 2000; 255:144–155.

25 Animal Models of Melanoma

William E. Carson III, MD
and Michael J. Walker, MD

CONTENTS

1. INTRODUCTION

The worldwide incidence of malignant melanoma is rising faster than any other cancer, and in the United States alone, almost 50,000 new cases of melanoma were projected for the year 2000. While thin primary melanomas are highly curable with surgery, the prognosis for patients with advanced disease is poor: Over 70% of patients with primary melanomas thicker than 4 mm or metastasis to the regional lymph nodes will die of disseminated disease within 5 yr of diagnosis. The treatment of metastatic disease has undergone significant changes over the past two decades with the introduction of high-dose cytokine therapy (e.g., interferon-alpha and interleukin-2), biochemotherapeutic regimens, novel vaccination strategies, and sentinel lymph-node biopsy techniques. Despite these advances, and a better understanding of the molecular lesions underlying the development of the malignant phenotype, the therapeutic options for patients with metastatic disease remain limited. High-dose cytokine therapy infrequently produces durable responses and is often poorly tolerated by patients with advanced disease. Aggressive chemotherapeutic regimens have not consistently proved superior to therapy with single agents, and the improved response rates achievable with biochemotherapy come at the price of significant toxicity. Other approaches to the patient with advanced disease, such as peptide and anti-ganglioside vaccines, remain investigational. Thus, it is critical that novel regimens with favorable toxicity profiles enter into clinical development. In order to move new treatments rapidly into the clinic and to gain a better understanding of their mechanism of action, it is essential that

From: *Tumor Models in Cancer Research*
Edited by: B. A. Teicher © Humana Press Inc., Totowa, NJ

experiments be conducted in animal models of malignant melanoma. This chapter reviews those models that are currently in use and explores their strengths and disadvantages.

2. XIPHOPHORUS SPECIES

Central American freshwater fish of to the genus *Xiphophorus* do not normally develop pigmented tumors *(1)*. However, hybrids between different species of this genus may spontaneously develop melanomas in skin structures called "macromelanophores" that are formed by terminally differentiated melanocytes. Tumor development is markedly enhanced following treatments with ultraviolet radiation (UVR), X-rays, carcinogens, or differentiating agents (reviewed in ref. *2*). A series of studies in *Xiphophorus* hybrids has revealed that the development of melanomas is genetically determined *(2,3)*. The responsible genes (termed "Tu" for tumor) map to the sex chromosomes and are necessary for the formation of normal black spots within the skin as well as melanoma lesions. The Tu genes exhibit oncogenic potential in the absence of any moderating factors, and thus act in a dominant fashion. Tumor development is normally inhibited via the action of tumor-suppressor genes ("R" for regulating) which must be present in two copies in order to be fully functional. The R genes may or may not be linked to the Tu genes; however, R genes are not found in species that lack Tu genes. Melanoma results when the R genes of a Tu-bearing species are deleted from the genome by hybridization with a species lacking Tu genes *(2,4)*.

Wittebrodt et al. have cloned and characterized an important Tu gene (Xmrk) that is homologous to a number of other Tu alleles in *Xiphophorus (5–7)*. Xmrk apparently arose as the result of non-homologous recombination involving a highly related proto-oncogene that is present as a single copy in all species of *Xiphophorus (8)*. The recombination event resulted in a second copy of the gene that was placed under the control of a completely separate promoter region, and was thus was not subject to the same controls as the parent proto-oncogene. Overexpression of the Xmrk oncogene is necessary and sufficient for neoplastic transformation of pigment cells in *Xiphophorus*, and levels of Xmrk expression correlate with the malignancy of the melanoma tumor that eventually develops *(9)*. The protein encoded by the Xmrk gene is a novel receptor tyrosine kinase that is closely related to the receptor for human epidermal growth factor *(5)*. This kinase is constitutively autophosphorylated, and can induce tumor formation in the embryos of medakafish when driven by a strong promoter sequence *(10)*. There is evidence to suggest that transformation occurs in response to the binding of an unknown ligand to the extracellular domain of the Xmrk gene product *(10)*. Furthermore, activation of the Xmrk kinase induces tyrosine phosphorylation, nuclear translocation, and DNA binding of a STAT5 homolog. The STAT (signal transducer and activator of transcription) family of transcription factors are important mediators of cytokine signaling in mammalian cells. In fact, STAT1, 2, and 3 are activated in melanoma cells following exposure to IFN-α. *(11,12)*.

Certain hybrids and backcrosses are particularly sensitive to melanoma induction by carcinogens or tumor promoters, and others readily develop tumors following exposure to UVR wavelengths in the range of 290 to 304 nm. The mechanism involved appears to be inactivation of tumor-suppressor genes (such as the R gene), which are present in a single copy in these fish *(2)*. Malignant melanomas arise from the macromelanophore: a flattened, multinucleated, terminally differentiated cell that is 100–400 μm in diameter, contains a number of mature melanosomes, and is derived from the melanocyte population of the skin. Malignant lesions contain macromelanophores and small, spindle-shaped melanocytes with few melanosomes but numerous mitotic figures. Microscopic analysis reveals that these melanocytes differentiate from skin melanoblasts *(13)*. These tumors are locally aggressive, and invasion of the underlying muscle is common. Malignant melanomas are rapidly fatal to affected fish.

Xiphophorus are easily maintained, are possessed of a short generation time, and are genetically well-characterized. This system is therefore well-suited for the identification of oncogenes and tumor-suppressor genes involved in the development of malignant melanoma. However, the highly aggressive and invasive nature of these tumors and their genesis in pigmented structures unique to fish must be taken into account when interpreting any results obtained in this model.

3. SOUTH AMERICAN OPOSSUM

The South American opossum *Monodelphis domestica* possesses the photoreactivation pathway of pyrimidine dimer repair, and has been used extensively in photobiology studies. Pyrimidine dimers induced by UVR are recognized by the photolyase enzyme, which catalyzes the enzymatic monomerization of dimers using the energy of long-wavelength visible light. Thus, exposure of animals to photoreactivating light (PRL) can remove 80–90% of pyrimidine dimers induced by suberythemal doses of UVR *(14,15)*. In fact, exposure of UVR-treated *Monodelphis* to PRL reduces the incidence of melanoma from near 40% to well under 10%—clear evidence that UVR-induced DNA damage is important in the induction of melanoma *(16)*. Experimental comparisons can be made between UVR-exposed animals that have been treated with PRL and those that have received a control treatment of equal duration. In this manner, the effects of UVR-induced DNA damage can be specifically evaluated. UVR alone can induce melanoma tumors in *Monodelphis,* which makes this the only nontransgenic animal in which UVR alone acts as a complete carcinogen *(17)*. Interestingly, application of carcinogenic compounds such as 9,10-dimethyl-1,2-benz(a)anthracene are also highly effective in the induction of malignant melanoma in this species *(18)*.

Monodelphis is a small (approx 100 g), pouchless opossum that is easily maintained and has been well-characterized via numerous studies relating to the damaging effects of UVR *(19)*. It is clear that the development of tumors is not genetically determined. Melanomas do not arise spontaneously in this species with any great regularity; however, application of UVR (e.g., 125–250 J/m^2, three times per wk, for 70–80 wk) will induce tumors in 10–20% of animals, of which about one-third will metastasize to lymph nodes *(16)*. All tumors, regardless of their origin (e.g., naturally occurring, carcinogen-induced, and UVR-induced) possess the ability to metastasize to lymph-node basins, whereas only spontaneous and carcinogen-induced tumors can spread to visceral sites *(2)*. Melanomas arising in *Monodelphis* are dermal in location and have their origins in lesions of melanocytic hyperplasia *(17,18,20)*. Dendritic melanocytes enlarge during the development of malignant lesions, assume a more polygonal shape, and eventually give rise to clusters of infiltrative cells exhibiting deep pigmentation and epithelioid characteristics. The resulting lesions are characterized by cellular atypia, nuclear pleomorphism, and areas of depigmentation. Kusewitt et al. have also demonstrated the presence of S-100 immunoreactivity in the foci of melanocytic hyperplasia, UVR- and carcinogen-induced primary tumors, as well as in metastatic lesions (20). Tumors can be established in tissue culture and even implanted into immunodeficient mice for further analysis.

Older animals appear to be more susceptible to the effects of UVR exposure, and develop melanocytic lesions with much greater frequency than younger animals. Interestingly, approx 40% of newborn opossums exposed to UVR will later develop metastatic melanoma as adults. This suggests that early exposure to sunlight may act as an initiator in the progression to melanoma. The susceptibility to UVR-induced melanomas can be modulated by dietary factors. Animals receiving a diet high in saturated fat do not develop skin lesions following exposure to UVR, whereas no protection is observed in animals receiving high levels of unsaturated fat in their feed (2).

The susceptibility of *Monodelphis* to UVR, the ability to modulate DNA repair by photoreactivation, and the presence of large, easily characterized chromosomes makes this animal model attractive for studies of photobiology. Disadvantages include the dermal location of melanoma lesions, the infrequent rate of spontaneous regression, and the lack of information regarding the immune system of this species.

4. CANINE MELANOMA

Canine melanomas arising in the oral cavity, mucocutaneous junction, and distal extremities are highly aggressive tumors that grow rapidly, invade locally, and metastasize readily to lymph nodes and distant organs. Melanoma may arise in any breed, but it is especially prevalent in purebred dogs such as Golden Retrievers, Irish Setters, Scottish Terriers, Doberman Pinschers, and Schnauzers (21,22). Canine melanomas are difficult to control even with radical surgery, and chemotherapy and radiation therapy are not considered effective in the control of either primary tumors or metastatic disease, although significant palliation may occasionally be achieved. In the absence of distant metastases, the median survival following aggressive surgical resection of primaries located in the oral cavity or on the digits is approx 3–12 mo (23–26) Radiation treatments may be useful as an adjuvant to surgery, but not in the face of significant residual disease (27–29). Chemotherapeutic regimens employing dacarbazine (DTIC) with or without cyclophosphamide are employed most commonly in the setting of advanced disease, but generally yield only partial responses of short duration (22). The lungs are the most common site of metastasis, and spread to this organ is the usual cause of death. Thus, it should come as no surprise that 1-y survival rate for canine oral melanoma is just 25%. In the absence of distant disease, the size of the primary lesion and the ability to obtain local control are the most important determinants of survival (25). A high mitotic rate and presence of anueploidy may also possess prognostic significance; however, other factors such breed, age, sex, and anatomic location do not appear to affect prognosis (21).

Like their human counterparts, metastatic canine melanomas tend to be resistant to conventional therapies. Numerous in vitro studies have indicated that immunologic approaches to the treatment of this tumor may be effective (21). Therefore, canines with malignant melanoma have been employed in several large studies of biological response modifiers and other immunotherapeutic modalities. For example, administration of interleukin-2 (IL-2) in combination with recombinant tumor necrosis factor alpha resulted in tumor regression in 5 of 13 dogs bearing malignant melanoma tumors. One of the five dogs exhibited a complete response that persisted for greater than 3 yr *(30)*. In another study, MacEwan et al. compared surgical resection of malignant melanoma tumors to surgery followed by therapy with *Corynebacterium parvum.* The heat-killed bacteria act as a nonspecific immune stimulant, and it was hypothesized that this treatment might elicit an antitumor response. It was determined that the addition of this treatment led to a significant increase in overall survival (7.5 vs 12 mo) in animals with advanced-stage tumors (involvement of lymph nodes or distant organs) *(31)*. Other trials have targeted the monocyte/macrophage compartment with nonspecific stimulants, such as liposome-encapsulated muramyl tripeptide phosphatidylethanilamine (L-MTP-PE). L-MTP-PE stimulates the tumoricidal activity of canine macrophages and induces the secretion of proinflammatory factors. In a recently completed study it was found that the use of L-MTP-PE as an adjunct to surgical resection of Stage I oral melanomas resulted in a statistically significant increase in overall survival as compared to surgery alone, with 80% of the dogs treated with L-MTP-PE still alive at >2 yr *(32)*.

Canine oral melanomas also lend themselves to studies of gene therapy. Treatments that have been studied in this model include the intratumoral administration of a cDNA-encoding recombinant human GM-CSF and an autologous tumor vaccine composed of irradiated tumor cells transfected with the GM-CSF gene ex vivo *(33,34)*. Also, a recent study examined the efficacy of intratumoral injections of plasmid DNA-encoding staphylococcus enterotoxin B and either canine GM-CSF or IL-2 *(35)*. The overall response rate was 46%, although responses were more frequently seen in dogs with smaller tumors. Importantly, the survival times for animals bearing stage III tumors were significantly prolonged by the intratumoral administration of these genes as compared to animals receiving surgical treatment alone.

The results obtained in these trials serve to highlight the importance of this model and its utility in the investigation of novel immunotherapeutic modalities. Canine melanomas are locally aggressive and are resistant to systemic treatments, just like their human counterparts. Therefore, it is quite likely that this model will continue to be used in the analysis of innovative biologic treatments.

5. SINCLAIR SWINE

The Sinclair and Munich troll breeds of miniature pig exhibit a strong predisposition toward the development of cutaneous melanoma *(36)*. This is a genetic trait that can be enhanced through selective breeding, so that over 50% of swine will exhibit melanoma at birth and 85% will develop lesions by 1 yr of age *(37)*. Melanotic nevi are also observed in these species. Two separate loci appear to be involved in the development of tumors. One is the B haplotype located within the swine leukocyte antigen (SLA) complex. Animals homozygous for this gene exhibit a strong tendency toward the development of melanoma tumors. A second gene family, unlinked to the SLA complex, is fully expressed only in animals exhibiting the B haplotype *(38)*. The second locus may actually be related to the retinoblastoma (Rb) locus in humans. Susceptible animals have inherited either an inactive form of this allele or are missing it altogether. In this case, tumor development occurs following somatic mutation of the second allele *(39)*. Interestingly, animals that have undergone oophrectomy (but not orchiectomy) exhibit reduced tumor growth, which can be reversed via the administration of estradiol. Despite these observations, it is clear that melanoma inheritance is not sex-linked *(40)*.

Melanomas may develop *in utero* and animals are frequently born with congenital flat or raised black skin lesions, a proportion of which may represent malignant tumors. Malignant melanomas also arise throughout the life of the animal. These may develop from pre-existing pigmented lesion and may exhibit areas of ulceration. Malignant lesions are frequently large and exophytic. Metastasis to lymph nodes and vital organs occurs in up to 25% of animals, but is rarely a significant cause of morbidity because most primary and metastatic lesions eventually undergo significant regression characterized by shrinkage of tumors and loss of pigmentation *(40–42)*. Tumor development has been carefully characterized by several investigators, and occurs in five distinct stages *(2,41,42)*. Stage I lesions are flat black macules that contain heavily pigmented melanocytes. The melanocytes are located singly or in nests just superficial to the epidermal basement membrane. Stage II lesions are raised, pigmented nodules composed of melanocytes that have begun to invade the superficial dermal structures. Stage III lesions are exophytic and frequently ulcerated. These lesions are invasive and highly proliferative in nature. Melanocytes exhibit significant cellular atypia, and may exhibit an epithelioid or spindle-shaped morphology. Mitotic figures are commonly seen. These tumors are composed of pigmented melanocytes that deeply infiltrate the dermis and epidermis and give rise to metastatic lesions. Careful histologic analysis of these tumors reveals that approx 70% have features consistent with acral lentiginous melanoma of humans, with the remainder resembling superficial spreading melanomas (10%), or nodular melanomas (20%) *(43)*. The ultrastructure of tumor cells found in Sinclair swine melanomas is very similar to that of human tumors. Thus, it is not surprising that these cells stain positively for S100 *(43)*.

Stage IV represents the first stage of regression. Tumors are smooth and bluish in color, and may have a depigmented halo. T-laden macrophages invade the tumor mass. In the final phases of regression (Stage V), there is extensive infiltration of the tumor by lymphocytes and pigment-laden macrophages. Tumor cells disappear from the lesion, and depigmentation and dermal fibrosis become prominent histologic features. These findings suggest that tumor regression is largely mediated by immune mechanisms and may be related to increased activity of host immune effectors *(41)*. Indeed, those animals with malignant melanomas exhibit enhanced leukocyte reactivity to tumor-cell lysates *(44)*. Other studies suggest that the cytotoxic response to the melanoma is mediated in part by $\gamma\delta$ T cells *(36)*.

Advantages of the Sinclair swine melanoma model include the observed genetic tendency, the high level of spontaneous transformation, and pathologic parallels to human disease. This model also provides an interesting experimental system for the study of spontaneous tumor regression.

6. MURINE MODELS

There are a number of murine models of malignant melanoma, which may vary with respect to several parameters, such as the origin of the tumor line employed, the site of inoculation, and the genetic background of the host. Each model has distinct strengths and weaknesses, and these must be taken into consideration prior to the selection of a murine model for use in a specific experimental system. In the following section, we will review models which employ chemical and physical carcinogens, transgenic mice, naturally occurring murine melanoma cell lines, and immunodeficient mice.

6.1. Induction with Physical Agents

Melanoma tumors rarely develop spontaneously in rodents (e.g., mice, rats, hamsters, gerbils, or guinea pigs). Two general approaches are available to the researcher who wishes to induce the formation of melanomas or pigmented preneoplastic tumors in experimental animals. The first involves the repeated application of a carcinogen with or without subsequent applications of a tumor-promoter. Alternatively, animals may be exposed to UVR followed by applications of a reagent with the ability to promote tumor development (2). Carcinogens that have been employed in this fashion include 7,12-dimethylbenz(a)anthracene (DMBA), trimethylanthracene, nitrogen mustard, and nitrosurea compounds (2). Initially there is transient hyperpigmentation of the epidermis. This is followed by the development of lesions derived from the dermis that have little or no metastatic potential. Application of tumor promoters such as croton oil or TPA can markedly enhance the development of carcinogen-induced melanomas. In fact, a single application of DMBA can induce the formation of melanomas if animals are treated repeatedly with one of these tumor-promoters (2). A basic protocol involves the application of 100 µL of 0.4% DMBA in acetone to shaved skin followed by twice-weekly applications of 25 µL of 2.5% croton oil in acetone or dimethyl sulfoxide until the appearance of raised black skin lesions occurs (45). The resulting tumors are locally aggressive, metastasize to multiple organs, and may be transplanted to new hosts or established in culture. The ability to obtain nevi and malignant melanomas with the application of a simple chemical carcinogen implies that UVR-induced DNA damage is not an essential step in the development of this cancer (2,45).

This approach to tumor induction has been applied to multiple species, including transgenic murine strains, and has led to the development of several useful murine melanoma cell lines. The JB/MS and JB/RH melanomas were induced in C57BL/6 mice via a single application of DMBA to the scapular region of 4-d-old mice, followed by twice-weekly application of croton oil. These tumors arose at 16 wk and 23 wk, respectively. The tumors continued to display a melanotic phenotype following transplantation to normal C57BL/6 mice, and metastasized spontaneously in these new hosts (45). The K1735 cell line was induced in a C3H/HeN mouse via the application of UVR (ten 1-h exposures to a FS40 sunlamp over a 2-wk period) followed by 92 weekly treatments with croton oil (46). The K1735 cell line expresses MHC class I and class II molecules, and is capable of inducing a specific yet ineffective immune response in syngeneic mice (47). This cell line may be grown in culture and implanted via the subcutaneous (sc) injection of a single-cell suspension, or may be passaged via the (sc) implantation of tumor fragments derived from a solid tumor raised in a mouse. This line has been used to great effect in studies examining the role cell-surface molecules such as B7 and Fas ligand that are able to influence the host-immune response to tumor (47,48). Other investigators have applied these protocols to transgenic mice in the hopes of producing a murine melanoma cell line with a specific genetic alteration. For example, utilizing a DMBA protocol, melanomas were successfully induced in mice transgenic for an activated human H-RAS gene. Subsequent chromosomal analysis revealed translocations of chromosome 4 that led to reduced expression of the *p16* gene product, a situation similar to that reported for human melanomas *(49)*.

UVR may be employed in a variety of ways to induce melanoma formation. Interestingly, UVR can act as a promoter for carcinogen-induced melanoma in mice. Benign blue nevi induced with DMBA may be converted into malignant lesions via exposure of the pigmented areas to chronic low-dose UVR *(50)*. These results have been confirmed in other murine strains and UVA, UVB, and UVA plus UVB appear to be equally effective promoters *(51)*. UVR also increases the rate of melanoma induction following applications of DMBA plus croton oil *(52)*. In general, the effect of UVR appears to be a local one, since application of UVR to nontreated skin is ineffective in the induction of tumors *(52)*. Despite its reputation as a complete carcinogen in humans, UVR alone cannot induce malignant melanoma in normal murine strains *(53)*. However, UVR treatment of normal skin can induce the formation of malignant melanomas if the treatment is followed by the application of a standard tumor-promoter *(46)*. These observations tend to confirm the carcinogenic potential of UVR seen in sun-exposed human populations, and validate the use of these models to study malignant melanoma.

Chemically induced and UVR-induced melanomas of mice exhibit histologic features similar to those described for melanomas that arise spontaneously *(51)*. Hyperplasia of dermal melanocytes with dendritic characteristics is believed to be the first step in tumor development. Examination of benign tumors reveals the presence of large, polygonal cells that are heavily pigmented. Malignant lesions contain cells of similar morphology that in addition may exhibit nuclear atypia and variable pigmentation. Other rodent species (i.e., rat, chinese hamster, gerbil, and guinea pig) only rarely develop spontaneous melanoma. Rats and guinea pigs are relatively resistant to chemical carcinogens, whereas melanoma tumors can be reliably induced in chinese hamsters and gerbils using standard protocols *(2)*. In contrast, malignant melanomas develop spontaneously with some frequency in the Syrian hamster (*Mesocricetus auratus*) *(54)*. This species (especially the golden and white variety) is also quite susceptible to the induction of tumors by chemical carcinogens, although they appear to be resistant to the effects of UVR *(55)*.

Although the mouse is relatively resistant to the development of carcinogen-induced melanomas, there are several distinct advantages to the use of this laboratory animal in these protocols. There is a wealth of information relating to the murine immune system, immunologic and molecular reagents are widely available, and tumors may be induced in a variety of inbred and transgenic strains. The disadvantages of this approach are less obvious, but must be taken into consideration when contemplating this technique. Foremost, the tumors and cell lines obtained via DMBA treatments (e.g., JB/MS and JB/RH) are frequently nonpigmented, and this may represent a distinct phenotypical difference between these lesions and the majority of tumors that arise in humans. In addition, the incidence of melanoma formation following treatment with carcinogenic compounds appears to be strain- and species-dependent. This suggests that the mechanism responsible for carcinogenesis may not be fully generalizable to humans *(2)*.

6.2. Tumors Arising in Transgenic Mice

The limitations associated with the induction of melanoma tumors in mice via the use of carcinogens has led investigators to develop transgenic mice with the potential to develop these tumors. One such model employs mice transgenic for expression of the simian virus 40 (SV40) early region under the control of the melanocyte-specific tyrosinase gene. These mice express the small and large transforming (T) antigens and develop ocular melanomas, skin melanomas, and hyperplasia of neural-crest-derived pigmented cells *(56)*. The T antigen is expressed to a different degree in various inbred lines of mice derived from individual founders. Mice with light coats develop eye tumors that are rapidly growing and fatal at an early age, whereas mice with darker coats develop slow-growing eye tumors later in life. Thus, the cutaneous melanomas that do arise in susceptible transgenics are rare and usually benign at the time the animal dies because of the ocular lesions. To circumvent this problem, skin can be taken from the susceptible strains and grafted onto low-susceptibility transgenics with a longer lifespan. Interestingly, donor pigment cells in these grafts exhibited selective proliferation in those areas nearest the healing wound edges. This finding suggested that growth factors and cytokines produced at the site of wound repair are able trigger the growth and malignant conversion of melanocytes expressing the T-antigen *(56)*.

The T antigen functions to inactivate important tumor-suppressor genes (e.g., *p53* and Rb), and the results obtained with this model suggest that these well-studied pathways may be important in the development of melanoma in humans. Thus, the T antigens have powerful effects on a number of pathways that might influence cell proliferation. This explains why mice transgenic for the T antigens may develop melanoma, but this also makes it difficult to pinpoint key steps in the oncogenic process.

Interestingly, *p53* is infrequently inactivated in human melanomas *(57)*. In contrast, Rb function may be inhibited in melanoma via loss of specific regulatory pathways *(58)*. Cell-cycle entry and progression are regulated by the cyclin-dependent kinases (cdks). Cdk4 and cdk6 mediate the phosphorylation of Rb, which inactivates it and permits transcription factors to translocate to the nucleus, where they induce the transcription and expression of specific growth-related genes. The (INK)4a and INK4b gene products (*p16*^{INK4a} and *p16*^{INK4b}) are specific inhibitors of cdk4 and cdk6. In the absence of functional INK4 proteins, cdk4 and cdk6 are driven towards a more activated state. Rb becomes hyperphosphorylated, with subsequent dysregulation of the cell cycle. In addition, other cdk inhibitors (e.g., the Cip/Kip proteins encoding *p21* and *p27,* respectively) become sequestered from cdk2/cyclin E in an indirect manner following the loss of INK4a function *(59)*. Interestingly, the INK4a gene can code for an unrelated protein through the use of an alternate open reading frame. The resulting gene product (*p19*ARF) functions as a potent growth-suppressor via its ability to stabilize *p53 (58)*. Serrano et al. have developed a mouse model with a deletion of exons 2 and 3 of the INK4a gene that eliminates expression of both *p16*^{INK4a} and *p19*^{ARF}. These mice are essentially dysfunctional for both the Rb and *p53* pathways, and develop spontaneous cancers at an early age. Fibrosarcomas and B-cell lymphomas are the most common tumors that develop in these mice, yet despite the link between INK4a and melanoma, these transgenic mice fail to develop this particular tumor *(60)*.

One gene that can accentuate the oncogenic potential of cells expressing an inactivated INK4a gene is oncogenic *ras*. Mice transgenic for the activated H-*ras* gene (H-*ras*^{V12G}) under the control of the tyrosinase promoter develop cutaneous melanomas at a very low rate, and only after a long period of observation. Interestingly, both INK4a alleles become deleted in these rare tumors *(58)*. In contrast, INK4a$^{\Delta2/3}$ mice expressing activated H-*ras* develop large numbers of cutaneous melanomas spontaneously after only a few weeks. These tumors are amelanotic, highly vascular, and similar in many respects to nodular melanomas *(61)*. It was subsequently shown that melanoma genesis and maintenance in this model are strictly dependent upon expression of H-ras^{V12G}. These experiments were performed in INK4a-null mice that were transgenic for doxycycline-inducible H-ras^{V12G}. Withdrawal of doxycycline and downregulation of inducible H-*ras* led to the clinical and histologic regression of primary and explanted tumors in this murine model. The initial stages of regression were marked by extensive apoptosis of tumor cells and host-derived endothelial cells; however, enhanced expression of vascular endothelial growth factor (VEGF) could not substitute for the loss of activated H-*ras (62)*.

6.3. Spontaneously-Arising Murine Melanomas

Malignant melanomas are a rare occurrence in mice. There are three melanomas that arose in mice and could be propagated either as a cell line or as a transplantable tumor. The Harding-Passey cell line is derived from a dermal melanoma that developed on the ear of an ICR mouse and the S91 (or Cloudman) melanoma cell line developed in a DBA mouse. The transplantable B16 melanoma arose spontaneously in a C57BL/6J mouse in the 1950s, and several different subclones are now available *(63–65)*. These lines can be maintained either in vitro under standard culture conditions or can be passaged in vivo as sc tumors. Many innovative murine models of melanoma have been developed utilizing these three cell lines. Some of the most important ones are described here.

The Harding-Passey cell line has been utilized in numerous preclinical studies of novel anticancer therapies, including boron neutron capture therapy, hyperthermia, strategies employing attenuated herpes simplex virus I (HSV1), and radioiodinated antibodies *(66–69)*. This cell line can be implanted subcutaneously or intramuscularly *(66,70)*. It has also been used to generate a mouse brain-tumor model in which cells are injected intracranially into C57BL/6 mice *(68)*. Brain tumors develop in 100% of animals, and may be imaged in as few as 5 d. Melanotic and amelanotic variants of the Harding-Passey cell line also exist, thus it has been used in studies that correlate melanin content with biologic behavior *(71)*.

The Cloudman line can be used to generate sc tumors *(72)* for use in the evaluation of novel anticancer strategies *(72,73)*. In addition, these tumors can be harvested, mechanically disrupted (e.g., by forcing tissue fragments through a wire screen), cleared of cellular proteins and debris, and utilized as a single-cell suspension for injection *(74)*. An intracutaneous model of malignant melanoma was also developed using this cell line *(75)*.

6.3.1. MODELS EMPLOYING THE B16 CELL LINE

The B16 murine melanoma cell line arose spontaneously in the C57BL/6 mouse in 1954, and like most tumors, was probably monoclonal in origin. However, significant heterogeneity would likely have been generated within the primary tumor in a short period of time as the result of genetic instability and unique selective pressures (e.g., in vitro culture conditions and/or subsequent site of implantation). Subclones of the B16 line have been generated that exhibit an enhanced rate of proliferation, superior ability to colonize specific organs such as the lung following iv injection, and increased metastatic potential following sc implantation in a syngeneic host *(76)*. The ability to generate this variety of sublines suggested to some researchers that the B16 cell line may have accumulated a greater degree of hetereogeneity than more recently developed melanoma cell lines. However, newer murine melanoma lines appear to exhibit just as much phenotypic diversity as ones developed in the early portion of the twentieth century. Studies by Fidler et al. revealed that the K-1735 melanoma cell line (first isolated in 1979) is quite heterogeneous and contains subpopulations of cells exhibiting diverse biologic behavior. In fact, of the 22 subclones derived from the parental line, only two were indistinguishable from the original cell line *(77)*. Also, Stackpole et al. evaluated the phenotypic diversity of the B16 melanoma line using tumor fragments that had been kept in the frozen state for over 20 yr. They were able to isolate a large number of clones that varied widely in their potential for dissemination (e.g., growth rate, metastatic potential, and ability to colonize organs). Moreover, cells readily converted their phenotype during growth in vitro and in vivo *(78)*.

The subclones of the B16 cell line most commonly employed in murine experimental systems at the present time are B16F1 (low metastatic potential) and B16F10 (high metastatic potential. The differences in metastatic potential appear to relate to variations in cell-surface properties *(79)*. These clones were developed in experiments performed in the laboratory of J. Fidler in the 1970s *(80)*. The B16F0 tumor was obtained from Jackson Laboratories in 1970 and passaged in syngeneic mice as a sc tumor prior to being established in cell culture. After 4–5 in vitro passages, the tumor was frozen and stored in liquid nitrogen. Years later, the line was thawed, grown subcutaneously, and once again established in vitro. Two aliquots of cells were then prepared. One was further divided and used to inject a group of mice directly. The other was used to produce several clones. Aliquots of the unmanipulated cells and the distinct clones were then injected intravenously into syngeneic mice, and pulmonary metastases were counted at 18 d. The unmanipulated cells exhibited a metastatic potential similar to that of the parental line (median number of metastases = 40, range 8–131), whereas the clones differed markedly in their ability to colonize the lung (range 3–500). These experiments suggested that primary tumor-cell populations are enormously diverse with respect to their proclivity to disseminate to visceral organs. Another B16 variant with high metastatic potential is the BL6 subline *(81)*. The B16-BL6 cell line was generated by the injection of B16F10 cells into the urinary bladder of male C57BL/6 mice through the vas deferens. The bladder was then excised and cultured in vitro on semisolid agar (37°C, 5% CO_2). Tumor cells that invaded through the bladder wall into the agar were recovered and repassaged. This entire process was repeated six more times, and the resulting variant was designated BL6. As might be expected, the BL6 variant is highly invasive and highly tumorigenic, yet poorly immunogenic. In fact, this clone can invade through the bladder wall in just 24 h. Other variants that metastasize preferentially to the ovary (B16-O10), brain (B16-B15b), and liver have also been developed *(82,83)*.

The B16 variants—B16F1, B16F10, and B16-BL6—may be grown subcutaneously via the injection of 10^6 cells in a volume of 20–100 μL followed by therapeutic manipulation in 7–10 ds *(84)*. Alternatively, tumors may be treated after they have achieved a given size (e.g., 5–10 mm in diameter). The B16F1 cell line will not metastasize to visceral organs, whereas visceral spread (primarily to the lungs) can be expected uniformly in mice receiving sc implants of the B16F10 or B16 BL6 variants. Tumor volume may then be measured using calipers and standard formulas, or survival may be used as an end point. Antimetastatic therapies may be evaluated in mice that have been iv-injected (via the lateral tail vein) with 2×10^5 B16F10 cells *(84,85)*. Treatment may then be started 1 d later. Following a period of treatment (e.g., 3 wk), mice are euthanized, their lungs are harvested, and pulmonary surface colonies are enumerated with the aid of a dissecting microscope. Further metastasis to other visceral sites probably arise from the lung via hematogenous spread. In fact, most terminal-stage lung metastases themselves develop from lung lesions measuring only 1–2 mm in diameter *(86)*.

The generation of visceral metastases via the iv injection of tumor cells or sc implantation of unique subclones that metastasize directly to the lungs does not accurately reflect the normal sequence of events in the clinical setting, in which nodal metastases play a prominent role. To address this problem, several unique models have been developed that employ the B16 melanoma cell line. Nathanson et al. injected B16 cells subcutaneously into the left foot pad of 6–8-wk old C57BL/6 mice *(87)*. They used the F1, F10, and BL6 variants, injecting 5×10^4 viable cells in a volume of 0.05 mL. Animals were inspected daily for the development of tumors, which generally became visible approx 2 wk following inoculation. At 18 d, the affected limb was amputated and the popliteal lymph nodes were isolated. Visceral metastases were enumerated at d 18 or at the time of death from systemic disease. Analysis of tumor-bearing mice demonstrated a direct correlation between the development of lymph-node metastases and the size of the primary tumor. Pulmonary metastases also correlated with tumor size with the BL6 variant, exhibiting a greater tendency to spread to nodal basins and then to the lung than either the F1 or F10 strains. The incidence of pulmonary metastases in mice whose regional lymph nodes did not contain tumor also correlated with increased size of the primary tumor, an apparent indicator of hematogenous spread. A similar model was developed by Markovic et al. utilizing 1×10^6 B16F10L cells implanted as single-cell suspension into the right foot pad of mice *(88)*. The tumor-bearing limb was amputated when the tumors routinely measured 6–8 mm in diameter (approx 18 d). Animals with palpable inguinal lymphadenopathy were removed from the experimental group. In the absence of further therapy, mice characteristically died of metastatic pulmonary disease at about 35 d post surgery *(88)*. An alternative site of injection is the web space of the hind foot (10^6 cells/0.1 mL), which gives rise to tumors of similar behavior *(89)*.

Wanebo et al. have developed a variation of these models in which B16F10 tumor cells are injected subcutaneously in the mid-tail of syngeneic mice *(90)*. 5×10^5 cells are injected in a total vol, of 0.025 mL. Fully 100% of mice exhibit local tumor growth within 2–3 wk of inoculation, and the majority develop inguinal adenopathy caused by lymphatic spread by 5–7 wk. Mean survival time for tumor-bearing mice was found to be approx 54 d. At autopsy, inguinal lymph nodes were noted to be markedly enlarged, and multiple metastatic lesions were visible in the lungs. If desired, the tumor can be resected at 2 wk post inoculation via amputation of the tail 5–10 mm distal to the base. If tumors are allowed to grow, they will reach a diameter of 15–20 mm by 6 wk, displaying areas of necrosis and ulceration. This model is particularly useful for examining the effects of specific treatments on residual nodal disease following resection of the primary lesion. All of these local models of melanoma are valuable because they recreate the major clinical stages of malignant melanoma; local tumor growth, (Stage I), involvement of regional lymph nodes (Stage II), and metastases to distant organs such as the lungs (Stage III).

Several other models of B16 melanoma with unique characteristics have been described. B16 melanoma cells may also be injected subcutaneously into the dorsal surface of the ear *(91)*. This results in the formation of black tumor nodules that are visible within 3 d. Tumor growth proceeds rapidly in this site, and all mice are dead by d 22. An alternative site of tumor inoculation is the peritoneal cavity. Intraperitoneal (ip) injection of B16F1 melanoma cells ($10^6/0.1$ mL) into 6–8-wk-old C57BL/6 mice will give rise to tumor nodules that grow rapidly and develop into solid intra-abdominal tumors *(92)*. In the absence of treatment, mice succumb within 3 wk. Treatment with interferon-alpha consistently prolongs survival of tumor-bearing mice by 7–10 d. The B16F1 or the B16 F10 clones may be employed, depending on the need to induce the formation of distant metastases. This model has been used with success by Fleischmann et al. in the analysis of the effects of interferon-alpha on the growth of the B16 line. Cytotoxic treatments may given intraperitoneally beginning 1–5 d postinoculation and one obvious advantage of this model is the ability to deliver cytokines and chemotherapeutic agents directly to the site of tumor growth *(93)*. Another ip model involves the implantation of gelatin sponges containing B16F10 melanoma cells and recombinant human basic fibroblast growth factor (bF6F) onto the serosal surface of the left lateral hepatic lobe of syngeneic C57BL/6 mice. Initially, tumor growth is localized within the gelatin sponge. However, peritoneal implants eventually develop, giving rise to peritoneal carcinomatosis. This model permits the evaluation of the cellular infiltrate induced by cytokine combinations, as well as characterization of the pattern of vascularity before and after treatment *(94)*.

Induction of tumors in mice through the application of physical agents is a powerful approach to the study of melanoma, but is hampered by the long period of time required for the establishment of transplantable tumors. The use of transgenic approaches is gaining greater popularity, especially as we gain a better understanding of the molecular basis of malignant melanoma. The obvious disadvantage of this approach is the need to identify suitable molecular targets for manipulation and the requirement for transgenic capabilities. Spontaneously arising tumors represent an important resource for the animal researcher, and numerous models are available. Unfortunately, no one model precisely recapitulates the metastatic cascade observed in human tumors. Other concerns relating to models that employ murine cell lines involve the potential for alterations to occur following prolonged in vitro culture or in vivo passage.

6.4. Tumor Models That Employ Immunodeficient Mice

It has long been a goal of cancer researchers to propagate human tumors in other species in order to facilitate the study of tumor biology and evaluation of novel therapeutic modalities. Early attempts focused on the implantation of tumors into privileged sites, such as the anterior chamber of the eye, the hamster cheek pouch, and the parenchyma of the brain. Tumors have also been implanted into fetuses and newborn animals which are naturally immunocompromised, as well as adult animals that have been rendered immune-deficient via thymectomy and total body irradiation (TBI) *(95)*. An alternative approach became available in the mid-1960s with the description of the congenitally athymic nude mouse, which arose on Balb/c background as the result of a mutation in a winged helix protein gene on chromosome 11 *((Hfh11) (96)*. The thymus is almost totally absent in nude mice because of failure of development of the thymic anlage, which arises from the ectoderm of the third pharyngeal pouch *(97)*. Functional

T cells cannot develop to maturity in the absence of the thymic microenvironment, and therefore the nude mouse cannot efficiently reject human xenografts consisting of normal or neoplastic tissue. Another mouse that is equally useful is the severe combined immunodeficiency (SCID) mouse which arose as the result of a mutation in the C.B-17 strain. This syndrome is characterized by a complete lack of functional T cells and B cells in the adult mouse. It was later determined that the SCID phenotype resulted from an inactivating (non-sense) mutation in the gene encoding DNA-activated protein kinase (*Prkdc*) located on mouse chromosome 16. DNA-activated protein kinase functions in double-stranded DNA break repair and in recombination among the variable, diversity, and joining segments of immunoglobulin and T-cell-receptor genes. Loss of this gene results in arrested development of T and B cells.

Immunodeficient mice may be injected intracranially, intradermally, subcutaneously, intraperitoneally, or intravenously with cultured melanoma cell lines or cell suspensions derived from primary melanoma tumors or experimental tumors. Fragments of human tumors may also be implanted in various anatomic sites, with the expectation that engraftment will occur in a significant percentage of cases. The histological, molecular, and biochemical characteristics for human tumor xenografts are generally maintained in the nude mouse. Melanomas and colon carcinomas grow well in the nude mouse, whereas prostate carcinomas and leukemic tumors often fail to engraft *(95)*. Previous work by Fogh et al. has demonstrated that xenografts derived from recurrent tumors or metastatic lesions are more likely to engraft (50% and 39%, respectively) than are primary tumors (approx 20%) *(98)*. A large number of cells or a large volume of primary tumor are generally required in order to ensure successful tumor take in the sc position, however, sc xenografts rarely metastasize unless special techniques are employed *(95)*. Most human tumors grown in nude mice exhibit a proliferative pattern similar to that seen in the original tumor, especially if the cells are grown orthotopically (i.e., within the same organ from which they originated). The SCID mouse has been useful for studies of human tumor specimens and tumor-cell lines that grow with difficulty in other strains. This system also provides a much-needed mechanism for developing improved models of tumor metastasis. In addition, SCID mice may be reconstituted with immune cells from syngeneic mice or with human hematologic tissues (adult peripheral blood lymphocytes) to generate the so-called hu-PBL-SCID model *(99)*. Human immune cells can survive and remain functional for a considerable period of time, as measured by the production of human immunoglobulin by implanted B cells. PBL and tumor-infiltrating lymphocytes derived from cancer patients may be engrafted along with the primary tumor to create a host-tumor model *(100)*. This model is complicated by the potential for reactivation of latent Epstein-Barr virus (EBV) infection if EBV+ donors are employed, and EBV-induced human B-cell lymphomas routinely develop unless specific measures are employed *(101)*.

6.4.1. NUDE MOUSE MODELS

Numerous nude mouse models of malignant melanoma have been described. These vary primarily according to the nature of the tumor inoculum and the details of the implantation procedure (e.g., sc or iv injection, or orthotopic implantation). Recent reviews of this topic offer a comprehensive survey of this topic *(95,102)*. Of particular interest are nude mouse models, which closely approximate specific clinical entities, and models which accurately reflect the metastatic cascade that progresses from primary lesion to sc sites and nodal basins and then on to visceral organs.

Most melanoma cell lines, such as the MeWo human melanoma cell line, will grow subcutaneously only if large numbers of cells are injected. However, tumor-take and lethality were markedly enhanced when mice received sc implants of lung cubes that had become impregnated with small numbers of MeWo cells as a result of prior in vitro coincubation. Numerous, large lung nodules were found in one mouse receiving such implants and sc transfer of the metastatic lung nodule to new recipients led to formation of tumors with increased potential for metastatic spread to the lungs. Cell lines from such metastases or from primary tumors that arose from implanted lung cubes were remarkable for their ability to colonize the lung following iv injection *(103)*. Also, iv injection of MeWo sublines derived from metastatic lesions consistently gave rise to extrapulmonary metastases. Other investigators have isolated sublines of parental tumors that exhibit a distinct tendency toward pulmonary metastasis following sc implantation or iv inoculation. Examples of these lines include the HSR+ MeWo variant, MM-RU, 451Lu, and CRML *(104–107)*.

Another approach to the development of metastatic models in nude mice involves the use of cells derived from particularly aggressive human tumors. The (BRO) human melanoma cell line was derived from a tumor that exhibited very rapid growth, a distinct tendency for local recurrence, and rapidly fatal metastasis to visceral organs. Nude mice inoculated intraperitoneally with 10^6 BRO cells survived only 14 d. BRO cells metastasized to the lung and diaphragm following ip or sc injection, and exhibited a doubling time of just 2.3 d *(108)*. Cell lines with increased metastatic potential may also be established via the iv-injected human tumor cells and selection of tumor deposits that have colonized visceral sites. The LOX-L amelanotic human melanoma cell line was established in this fashion from the LOX parental line normally, which does not spread to visceral sites after sc inoculation *(109)*. LOX-L cells metastasize rapidly to the lungs following ip or sc injection and have been used to evaluate novel chemotherapeutic regimens in vivo. Fodstad *et al.* utilized this same general strategy to develop the FEMX-1 human melanoma cell line that preferentially metastasizes to sc sites *(110)*.

Other investigators have determined that orthotopic (i.e., intradermal) injection of human melanoma-cell lines increases the likelihood that the xenografted tumors will behave in a manner similar to the parent tumor. Rofstad established cell lines from sc deposits obtained from four different patients *(111)*. These cells were injected intradermally and evaluated for several parameters. It was found that the growth rate, histopathologic character, and angiogenic potential of the parent tumors were maintained in the orthotopically located xenografts. In addition, the organ-specific metastatic pattern of the xenografts closely resembled that seen in the donor patients. Lines with organ-specific metastatic patterns may also be generated via in vitro manipulations. Human melanoma cells with the propensity to metastasize to the brain following iv inoculation were developed by culturing the parental melanoma line in increasing concentrations of wheat germ agglutinin (a toxic lectin compound). The resulting subline (70-W) consistently gave rise to brain and sc metastases as well as to lesions in the bone marrow, ovaries, muscle, and intra-abdominal organs *(112)*. Other models of interest include cell lines that induce severe cancer cachexia in nude mice when grown subcutaneously *(113)*, and a cell line that induces a syndrome of diffuse hyperpigmentation (melanosis) caused by the release of pigment granules from the xenografted tumor and uptake of the structures by macrophages throughout the body *(114)*.

6.4.2. SCID MOUSE MODELS

Human melanoma tumors engraft readily into SCID mice, and exhibit a tendency to metastasize more readily and grow more rapidly than when implanted into nude mice. As with the nude mouse, various cell lines have been adapted to this model, and a variety of ingenious methods for the inoculation of tumor have been devised *(102)*. SCID mouse models have been used extensively in the analysis of basic tumor biology as well as the evaluation of various therapeutic modalities *(115,116)*. It was discovered early on that cell lines that metastasize spontaneously from sc tumors in nude mice will do so more rapidly and with greater frequency when implanted into SCID mice *(102)*. Other investigators have evaluated the behavior of freshly isolated tumor specimens obtained from metastatic lesions *(117)*. 100% tumor take (9 of 9) was observed when cell suspensions were injected subcutaneously into SCID mice, and two-thirds of these tumors could be transplanted successfully into new hosts. As few as 5×10^5 cells were required to yield a 100% incidence of tumor formation. Interestingly, 7 of 9 tumors metastasized to distant sites on the first or second passage. The lungs were the primary site of metastasis, but spread to the abdominal viscera, and thoracic lymph nodes was also noted. The expression of specific surface antigens was found to be maintained over the course of passaging in SCID mice. Tumor-associated lymphocytes were identified in the original tumor inoculum, but the presence of these immune cells did not appear to influence the outgrowth or metastatic potential of sc tumors.

A more extensive study conducted by Taylor et al. investigated the engraftment and dissemination of human melanoma cells obtained from various sources *(118)*. They examined two cell lines, four early-passage cell lines, and fresh or cryopreserved cells from nine patient biopsies. SCID mice were inoculated via the ip, sc, and iv routes. The take-rate was highest for established cell lines (77%), and early-passage cell lines and fresh tumor cells engrafted in 65% and 53% of mice, respectively. Administration of tumor cells via the ip route resulted in tumor growth in 77% of mice, as compared to 41% for sc injection and 48% for iv injections. A distinct correlation was noted to exist between the number of cells injected and the percent of mice developing tumor: Only 26% engraftment was obtained when 1×10^6 cells were injected, whereas 69% take could be achieved with an injection of $2–5 \times 10^6$ cells. 100% engraftment was only achieved with the injection of very large numbers of cells (50×10^6). Each tumor engrafted in at least one animal. Dissemination of tumor cells to distant organs via hematogenous or lymphatic spread was common and reproducible, with the number of metastases per animal averaging 16.3. The lung, liver, spleen, abdomen (viscera and peritoneum), and kidneys were the most common sites of spread. Moreover, the histologic character of the patient biopsy specimens was maintained after extensive passage in SCID hosts.

A very sophisticated orthotopic model was reported by Juhasz et al. in 1993 (119). SCID mice and nude mice were given full-thickness human skin grafts measuring approx 1.5 cm in diameter. After the grafts were completely healed, 2×10^6 melanoma cells were injected intradermally in a volume of 50 μL into the skin transplants. It was theorized that the human skin grafts would provide the melanoma cells with the unique dermal environment necessary for optimal engraftment. The skin grafts themselves were successful in over 90% of mice. Seven different cell lines were employed in this study, and all seven engrafted without difficulty. Interestingly, several of the melanoma lines (WM164, WM9, and 451Lu) grew as multiple nodules that infiltrated the grafts without effecting major changes in the overall architecture of the dermis. Other cell lines (WM582, WM793, and 1205Lu) appeared to infiltrate the human dermis along collagen fibrils, and seemed to have induced the formation of endothelial vessels. In each case, the overall pattern of invasion was found to be quite similar to that of the original patient biopsy. Moreover, cell lines that produced metastases when implanted subcutaneously in SCID mice also formed metastases in this model. For example, the metastatic cell lines 1205Lu and 405Lu possessed the ability to invade human dermis and disseminated to the lungs in the majority of animals.

Immunodeficient mice provide an important model for the study of melanoma in which human tumors may be studied directly. Tumors with different clinical behaviors may be employed, and the effect of novel treatments may be assessed prior to the initiation of clinical trials. The use of human skin grafts and intradermal injections of tumor cells is a novel approach that may help us to understand the earliest stages of tumor invasion. It is important to remember that these mice are not entirely immune-deficient, and the effects of the remaining effector cells (e.g., macrophages and NK cells in SCID mice) cannot be completely ignored. The cost of acquiring and housing immunodeficient mice is another limitation that prevents these models from being more widely employed.

SUMMARY

A wide variety of animal models of malignant melanoma are currently available to the researcher interested in this disease process. The *Xiphophorus* fish represents a genetic form of melanoma in which tumor formation is tied to the activity of a tyrosine kinase and specific tumor-suppressor genes. The South American opossum *Monodelphis domestica* possesses the photoreactivation pathway of pyrimidine dimer repair, and has been used extensively in photobiology studies of melanoma. Melanomas arise spontaneously in dogs, and this model has been used to evaluate novel cytokine combinations and gene-therapy protocols. The Sinclair swine also develops melanoma tumors, and the tumor regressions seen in this model provide a unique model for the study of interactions between tumor cells and immune effectors. Murine models are by far the most widely employed animal model of melanoma, and include the induction of tumors via application of physical agents or transgenic manipulations as well as the inoculation of mice with tumor-cell lines such as the spontaneously occurring Harding-Passey, Cloudman, and B16 cell lines. Finally, the more recently described models which employ immunodeficient mice provide a method for studying human tumors under controlled conditions.

REFERENCES

1. Schartl A, Malitschek B, Kazianis S, Borowsky R, and Schartl M. Spontaneous melanoma formation in non-hybrid Xiphophorous. *Cancer Res* 1995; 55:159–165.
2. Kusewit DF, Ley RD. Animal models of melanoma. *Cancer Surv* 1996; 26:35–70.
3. Schartl A, Pagany M, Engler M, Schartl M. Analysis of genetic factors and molecular mechanisms in the development of hereditary and carcinogen-induced tumors of Xiphophorus. *Recent Results Cancer Res* 1997; 143:225–235.

4. Anders F, Schartl M, Barnekow A, Anders A. Xiphophorus as an in vivo model for studies on normal and defective control of oncogenes. *Adv Cancer Res* 1984; 42:191–275.

5. Wittbrodt J, Adam D, Malitschek B, Maueler W, Raulf F, Telling A, et al. Novel putative receptor tyrosine kinase encoded by the melanoma-inducing Tu locus in Xiphophorus. *Nature* 1989; 341:415–421.

6. Wittbrodt J, Lammers R, Malitschek B, Ullrich A, Schartl M. The Xmrk receptor tyrosine kinase is activated in Xiphophorus malignant melanoma. *EMBO J* 1992; 11:4239–4246.

7. Malitschek B, Wittbrodt J, Fischer P, Lammers R, Ullrich A, Schartl M. Autocrine stimulation of the Xmrk receptor tyrosine kinase in Xiphophorus melanoma cells and identification of a source for the physiological ligand. *J Biol Chem* 1994; 269:10423–10430.

8. Adam D, Dimitrijevic N, Schartl M. Tumor suppression in Xiphophorus by an accidentally acquired promoter. *Science* 1993; 259:816–819.

9. Maueler W, Schartl A, Schartl M. Different expression patterns of oncogenes and proto-oncogenes in hereditary and carcinogen-induced tumors of Xiphophorus. *Int J Cancer* 1993; 55:288–296.

10. Winkler C, Wittbrodt J, Lammers R, Ullrich A, Schartl M. Ligand-dependent tumor induction in medakafish embryos by a Xmrk receptor tyrosine kinase transgene. *Oncogene* 1994; 9:1517–1525.

11. Baudler M, Schartl M, Altschmied J. Specific activation of a STAT family member in Xiphophorus melanoma cells. *Exp Cell Res* 1999; 249:212–220.

12. Carson WE. Interferon-alpha-induced activation of signal transducer and activator of transcription proteins in malignant melanoma. *Clin Cancer Res* 1998; 4:2219–2228.

13. Ozato K, Wakamatsu Y. Multi-step genetic regulation of oncogene expression in fish hereditary melanoma. *Differentiation* 1983; 24:181–190.

14. Ley RD. Photoreactivation in mammalian skin: mouse, marsupial and man. *Photodermatol* 1987; 4:173–175.

15. Ley RD, Applegate LA, Fry RJ, Sanchez AB. Photoreactivation of ultraviolet radiation-induced skin and eye tumors of Monodelphis domestica. *Cancer Res* 1991; 51:6539–6542.

16. Ley RD, Applegate LA, Padilla RS, Stuart TD. Ultraviolet radiationinduced malignant melanoma in Monodelphis domestica. *Photochem Photobiol* 1989; 50:1–5.

17. Kusewitt DF, Applegate LA, Ley RD. Ultraviolet radiation-induced skin tumors in a South American opossum (Monodelphis domestica). *Vet Pathol* 1991; 28:55–65.

18. Kusewitt DF, Miska KB, Ley RD. S-100 immunoreactivity in melanomas of the South American opossum Monodelphis domestica. *Vet Pathol* 1997; 34:346–350.

19. Robinson ES, VandeBerg JL, Hubbard GB, Dooley TP. Malignant melanoma in ultraviolet irradiated laboratory opossums: initiation in suckling young, metastasis in adults, and xenograft behavior in nude mice. *Cancer Res* 1994; 54:5986–5991.

20. Kusewitt DF, Applegate LA, Bucana CD, Ley RD. Naturally occurring malignant melanoma in the South American opossum (Monodelphis domestica). *Vet Pathol* 1990; 27:66–68.

21. Modiano JF, Ritt MG, Wojcieszyn J. The molecular basis of canine melanoma: pathogenesis and trends in diagnosis and therapy. *J Vet Intern Med* 1999; 13:163–174.

22. MacEwan EG. Spontaneous tumors in dogs and cats: models for the study of cancer biology and treatment. *Cancer Metastasis Rev* 1990; 9:125–136.

23. Marino DJ, Matthiesen DT, Stefanacci JD, Moroff SD. Evaluation of dogs with digit masses: 117 cases (1981–1991). *J Am Vet Med Assoc* 1995; 207:726–728.

24. Carpenter JL, Arohnson MG. Distal extremity melanocytic nevi and malignant melanoma in dogs. *J Am Anim Hosp Assoc* 1990; 26:605–612.

25. Todoroff RJ, Brodey RS. Oral and pharyngeal neoplasia in the dog: a retrospective survey of 361 cases. *J Am Vet Med Assoc* 1979; 175:567–571.

26. Kurzman ID, MacEwan EG. Effect of extent of surgery on survival in canine oral melanomas. *Proc Annu Mtg Vet Cnacer Soc* 1997; 17:85 (abstract).

27. Theon AP, Rodriguez C, Griffey S, Madewell BR. Analysis of prognostic factors and patterns of failure in dogs with periodontal tumors treated with megavoltage irradiation. *J Am Vet Med Assoc* 1997; 210:785–788.

28. Blackwood L, Dobson JM. Radiotherapy of oral malignant melanomas in dogs. *J Am Vet Med Assoc* 1996; 209:98–102.

29. Bateman KE, Catton PA, Pennock PW, Kruth SA. 0-7-21 radiation therapy for the treatment of canine oral melanoma. *J Vet Intern Med* 1994; 8:267–272.

30. Moore AS, Theilen GH, Newell AD, Madewell BR, Rudolf AR. Preclinical study of sequential tumor necrosis factor and interleukin 2 in the treatment of spontaneous canine neoplasms. *Cancer Res* 1991; 51:233–238.

31. MacEwen EG, Patnaik AK, Harvey HJ, Hayes AA, Matus R. Canine oral melanoma: comparison of surgery versus surgery plus Corynebacterium parvum. *Cancer Invest* 1986; 4:397–402.

32. MacEwen EG, Kurzman ID, Vail DM, Dubielzig RR, Everlith K, Madewell BR, et al. Adjuvant therapy for melanoma in dogs: results of randomized clinical trials using surgery, liposome-encapsulated muramyl tripeptide, and granulocytemacrophage colony-stimulating factor. *Clin Cancer Res* 1999; 5:4249–4258.

33. Hogge GS, Burkholder JK, Culp J, Albertini MR, Dubielzig RR, Yang NS, et al. Preclinical development of human granulocyte-macrophage colony-stimulating factor-transfected melanoma cell vaccine using established canine cell lines and normal dogs. *Cancer Gene Ther* 1999; 6:26–36.

34. Hogge GS, Burkholder JK, Culp J, Albertini MR, Dubielzig RR, Keller ET, et al. Development of human granulocyte-macrophage colony-stimulating factor-transfected tumor cell vaccines for the treatment of spontaneous canine cancer. *Hum Gene Ther* 1998; 9:1851–1861.

35. Dow SW, Elmslie RE, Willson AP, Roche L, Gorman C, Potter TA. In vivo tumor transfection with superantigen plus cytokine genes induces tumor regression and prolongs survival in dogs with malignant melanoma. *J Clin Investig* 1998; 101:2406–2414.

36. Misfeldt ML, Grimm DR. Sinclair miniature swine: an animal model of human melanoma. *Vet Immunol Immunopathol* 1994; 43:167–175.

37. Hook RR Jr, Aultman MD, Adelstein EH, Oxenhandler RW, Millikan LE, Middleton CC. Influence of selective breeding on the incidence of melanomas in Sinclair miniature swine. *Int J Cancer* 1979; 24:668–672.

38. Tissot RG, Beattie CW, Amoss MS Jr, Williams JD, Schumacher J. Common swine leucocyte antigen (SLA) haplotypes in NIH and Sinclair miniature swine have similar effects on the expression of an inherited melanoma. *Anim Genet* 1993; 24:191–193.

39. Hook RR Jr, Berkelhammer J, Oxenhandler RW. Melanoma: sinclair swine melanoma. *Am J Pathol* 1982; 108:130–133.

40. Amoss MS Jr, Ronan SG, Beattie CW. Growth of Sinclair swine melanoma as a function of age, histopathological staging, and gonadal status. *Cancer Res* 1988; 48:1708–1711.

41. Greene JF Jr, Townsend JS 4th, Amoss MS Jr. Histopathology of regression in Sinclair swine model of melanoma. *Lab Investig* 1994; 71:17–24.

42. Flatt RE, Nelson LR, Middleton CC. Melanotic lesions in the internal organs of miniature swine. *Arch Pathol* 1972; 93:71–75.

43. Das Gupta TK, Ronan SG, Beattie CW, Shilkaitis A, Amoss MS Jr. Comparative histopathology of porcine and human cutaneous melanoma. *Pediatr Dermatol* 1989; 6:289–299.

44. Aultman MD, Hook RR Jr. In vitro lymphocyte reactivity to soluble tumor extracts in Sinclair melanoma swine. *Int J Cancer* 1979; 24:673–678.

45. Berkelhammer J, Oxenhandler RW, Hook RR, Hennessy JM. Development of a new melanoma model in C57BL/6 mice. *Cancer Res* 1982; 42:3157–3163.

46. Kripke ML. Speculations on the role of ultraviolet radiation in the development of malignant melanoma. *J Natl Cancer Inst* 1979; 63:541–548.

47. Townsend SE, Allison JP. Tumor rejection after direct costimulation of CD8+ T cells by B7-transfected melanoma cells. *Science* 1993; 259:368–370.

48. Owen-Schaub LB, van Golen KL, Hill LL, Price JE. Fas and Fas ligand interactions suppress melanoma lung metastasis. *J Exp Med* 1998; 188:1717–1723.

49. Gause PR, Lluria-Prevatt M, Keith WN, Balmain A, Linardopolous S, Warneke J, et al. Chromosomal and genetic alterations of 7,12-dimethylbenz[a]anthracene-induced melanoma from TP-ras transgenic mice. *Mol Carcinogenesis* 1997; 20:78–87.

50. Epstein JH, Epstein JL, Nakai T. Production of melanomas from DMBA-induced "blue nevi" in hairless mice with ultraviolet light. *J Natl Cancer Inst* 1967; 38:19–30.

51. Husain Z, Viola MV. Role of ultraviolet radiation in the induction of melanocytic tumors in hairless mice following 7,12-dimethyl(a)benzanthracene application and ultraviolet irradiation. *Cancer Res* 1991; 51:4964–4970.

52. Donawho CK, Kripke ML. Photoimmunology of experimental melanoma. *J Immunotherapy* 1991; 10:177–188.

53. van Weelden H, van der Putte SCJ, Toonstra J, van der Leun JC. Ultraviolet B-induced tumors in pigmented hairless mice, with an unsuccessful attempt to induce cutaneous melanoma. *Photodermatol Photoimmunol Photomed* 1990; 7:68–72.

54. Pour P, Althoff J, Salmasi SZ, Stephan K. Spontaneous tumors and common diseases in three types of hamsters. *J Natl Cancer Inst* 1979; 63:797–811.

55. Pawlowski A, Lea PJ. Nevi and melanoma induced by chemical carcinogenesis in laboratory animals: similarities and differences with human lesions. *J Cutaneous Path* 1983; 10:81–110.

56. Mintz B, Silvers WK. Transgenic mouse model of malignant skin melanoma. *Proc Natl Acad Sci USA* 1993; 90:8817–8821.

57. Saenz-Santamaria MC, McNutt NS, Bogdany JK, Shea CR. p53 expression is rare in cutaneous melanomas. *Am J Dermatopathol* 17:344–349.

58. Chin L. Modeling malignant melanoma in mice: pathogenesis and maintenance. *Oncogene* 1999; 18:5304–5310.

59. Sherr CJ, Roberts JM. CDK inhibitors: positive and negative regulators of G1-phase progression. *Genes Dev* 1999; 13:1501–1512.

60. Serrano M, Lee H, Chin L, Cordon-Cardo C, Beach D, DePinho R. Role of the INK4a locus in tumor suppression and cell mortality. *Cell* 1996; 85:27–37.

61. Chin L, Pomerantz J, Polsky D, Jacobson M, Cohen C, Cordon-Cardo C, et al. Cooperative effects of INK4a and ras in melanoma susceptibility in vivo. *Genes Dev* 1997; 11:2822–2834.

62. Chin L, Tam A, Pomerantz J, Wong M, Holash J, Bardeesy N, et al. Essential role for oncogenic Ras in tumour maintenance. *Nature* 1999; 400:468–472.

63. Harding HE, Passey RD. A transplantable melanoma of the mouse. *J Pathol Bacteriol* 1930; 33:417–427.

64. Cloudman AM. The effect of an extra-chromosomal influence upon transplated spontaneous tumors in mice. *Science* 1941; 93:380–381.

65. Stackpole CW. Generation of phenotypic diversity in the B16 mouse melanoma relative to spontaneous metastasis. *Cancer Res* 1983; 43:3057–3065.

66. Setiawan Y, Moore DE, Allen BJ. Selective uptake of boronated low-density lipoprotein in melanoma xenografts achieved by diet supplementation. *Br J Cancer* 1996; 74:1705–1708.

67. Lopez Ballester JA, Penafiel R, Cremades A, Valcarcel MM, Solano F, Lozano JA. Effects of treatments with alpha-difluoromethylornithine and hyperthermia on the growth and polyamine metabolism of Harding-Passey murine melanoma. *Anticancer Res* 1991; 11:691–696.

68. Randazzo BP, Kesari S, Gesser RM, Alsop D, Ford JC, Brown SM, et al. Treatment of experimental intracranial murine melanoma with a neuroattenuated herpes simplex virus 1 mutant. *Virology* 1995; 211:94–101.

69. Fand I, Sharkey RM, Goldenberg DM. Use of whole-body autoradiography in cancer targeting with radiolabeled antibodies. *Cancer Res* 1990; 50:885s–891s.

70. Yong JH, Barth RF, Wyzlic IM, Soloway AH, Rotaru JH. In vitro and in vivo evaluation of o-carboranylalanine as a potential boron delivery agent for neutron capture therapy. *Anticancer Res* 1995; 15:2033–2038.

71. Watts KP, Fairchild RG, Slatkin DN, Greenberg D, Packer S, Atkins HL, et al. Melanin content of hamster tissues, human tissues, and various melanomas. *Cancer Res* 1981; 41:467–472.

72. Knight GD, Laubscher KH, Fore ML, Clark DA, Scallen TJ. Vitalethine modulates erythropoiesis and neoplasia. *Cancer Res* 1994; 54:5623–5635.

73. Horton HM, Anderson D, Hernandez P, Barnhart KM, Norman JA, Parker SE. A gene therapy for cancer using intramuscular injection of plasmid DNA encoding interferon alpha. *Proc Natl Acad Sci USA* 1999; 96:1553–1558.

74. Nordlund JJ, Ackles A, Gershon RK. Quantitative factors which determine the effect of the immune response on the growth rate of the Cloudman Melanoma in the DBA/2 mice. *Cell Immunol* 1980; 56:258–272.

75. Gehlsen KR, Hadley ME, Levine N, Ray CG, Hendrix MJ. Effects of a melanotropic peptide on melanoma cell growth, metastasis, and invasion. *Pigment Cell Res* 1992; 5:219–223.

76. Alterman AL, Fornabaio DM, Stackpole CW. Metastatic dissemination of B16 melanoma: pattern and sequence of metastasis. *J Natl Cancer Inst* 1985; 75:691–702.

77. Fidler IJ, Gruys E, Cifone MA, Barnes Z, Bucana C. Demonstration of multiple phenotypic diversity in a murine melanoma of recent origin. *J Natl Cancer Inst* 1981; 67:947–956.

78. Stackpole CW. Generation of phenotypic diversity in the B16 mouse melanoma relative to spontaneous metastasis. *Cancer Res* 1983; 43:3057–3065.

79. Poste G, Nicolson GL. Arrest and metastasis of blood-borne tumor cells are modified by fusion of plasma membrane vesicles from highly metastatic cells. *Proc Natl Acad Sci USA* 1980; 77:399–403.

80. Fidler IJ, Kripke ML. Metastasis results from preexisting variant cells within a malignant tumor. *Science* 1977; 197:893–895.

81. Hart IR. The selection and characterization of an invasive variant of the B16 melanoma. *Am J Pathol* 1979; 97:587–600.

82. Nicolson GL, Dulski K, Basson C, Welch DR. Preferential organ attachment and invasion in vitro by B16 melanoma cells selected for differing metastatic colonization and invasive properties. *Invasion Metastasis* 1985; 5:144–158.

83. Nathanson SD, Nelson LT, Lee M. A spontaneous subcutaneous tumor in C57BL/6 mice that metastasizes to the liver. *Clin Exp Metastasis* 1993; 11:45–54.

84. Brunda MJ, Luistro L, Warrier RR, Wright RB, Hubbard BR, Murphy M, et al. Antitumor and antimetastatic activity of interleukin 12 against murine tumors. *J Exp Med* 1993; 178:1223–1230.

85. Kobayashi M, Kobayashi H, Pollard RB, Suzuki F. A pathogenic role of Th2 cells and their cytokine products on the pulmonary metastasis of murine B16 melanoma. *J Immunol* 1998; 160:5869–5873.

86. Stackpole CW. Intrapulmonary spread of established B16 melanoma lung metastases and lung colonies. *Invasion Metastasis* 1990; 10:267–280.

87. Nathanson SD, Haas GP, Mead MJ, Lee M. Spontaneous regional lymph node metastases of three variants of the B16 melanoma: relationship to primary tumor size and pulmonary metastases. *J Surg Oncol* 1986; 33:41–45.

88. Markovic SN, Murasko DM. Role of natural killer and T cells in interferon induced inhibition of spontaneous metastases of the B16F10L murine melanoma. *Cancer Res* 1991; 51:1124–1128.

89. Dyce M, Sharif SF, Whalen GF. Search for anti-metastatic therapy: effects of phenytoin on B16 melanoma metastasis. *J Surg Oncol* 491992; 49:107–112.

90. Shrayer DP, Bogaars H, Wolf SF, Hearing VJ, Wanebo HJ. A new mouse model of experimental melanoma for vaccine and lymphokine therapy. *Int J Oncol* 1998; 13:361–374.

91. Shiohara T, Moellman G, Jacobson K, Kuklinska E, Ruddle NH, Lerner AB. Anti-tumor activity of class II MHC antigen-restricted cloned autoreactive T cells. II. Novel immunotherapy of B16 melanomas by local and systemic adoptive transfer. *J Immunol* 1987; 138:1979–1986.

92. Fleischmann CM, Stanton GJ, Fleischmann WR Jr. Enhanced in vivo sensitivity to interferon with in vitro resistant B16 tumor cells in mice. *Cancer Immunol Immunother* 1994; 39:148–154.

93. Fleischmann WR Jr, Masoor J, Wu TY, Fleischmann CM. Orally administered IFN-alpha acts alone and in synergistic combination with intraperitoneally administered IFN-gamma to exert an antitumor effect against B16 melanoma in mice. *J Interferon Cytokine Res* 1998; 18:17–20.

94. Watanabe M, McCormick KL, Volker K, Ortaldo JR, Wigginton JM, Brunda MJ, et al. Regulation of local host-mediated anti-tumor mechanisms by cytokines: direct and indirect effects on leukocyte recruitment and angiogenesis. *Am J Pathol* 1997; 150:1869–1880.

95. Giovanella BC, Fogh J. The nude mouse in cancer research. *Adv Cancer Res* 1985; 69–120.

96. Nehls M, Pfeifer D, Schorpp M, Hedrich H, Boehm T. New member of the winged-helixprotein family disrupted in mouse and rat nude mutations. *Nature* 1994; 372:103–107.

97. Pantelouris EM. Absence of thymus in a mouse mutant. *Nature* 1968; 217:370–371.

98. Fogh J, Orfeo T, Tiso J, Sharkey FE, Fogh JM, Daniels WP. Twenty-three new human tumor lines established in nude mice. *Exp Cell Biol* 1980; 48(3):229–239.

Fogh J, Dracopoli N, Loveless JD, Fogh H. Cultured human tumor cells for cancer research: assessment of variation and stability of cultural characteristics. *Prog Clin Biol Res* 1982; 89:191–223.

99. Mosier DE, Gulizia RJ, Baird SM, Wilson DB. Transfer of a functional human immune system to mice with severe combined immunodeficiency. *Nature* 1988; 335:256–259.

100. Bankert RB, Umemoto T, Suguyama Y, Chen FA, Repasky E, Yokota S. Human lung tumors, patients' peripheral blood lymphocytes and tumor infiltrating lymphocytes propagated in scid mice. *Curr Topics Micobiol Immunol* 1989; 152:201–210.

101. Baiocchi RA, Caligiuri MA. Low-dose interleukin 2 prevents the development of Epstein-Barr virus (EBV)-associated lymphoproliferative disease in scid/scid mice reconstituted i.p. with EBV-seropositive human peripheral blood lymphocytes. *Proc Natl Acad Sci USA* 1994; 91:5577–5581.

102. Rofstad EK, Lyng H. Xenograft model systems for human melanoma. *Mol Med Today* 1996; 2:394–403.

103. Kerbel RS, Man MS, Dexter D. A model of human cancer metastasis: extensive spontaneous and artificial metastasis of a human pigmented melanoma and derived variant sublines in nude mice. *J Natl Cancer Inst* 1984; 72:93–108.

104. Gitelman I, Dexter DF, Roder JC. DNA amplification and metastasis of the human melanoma cell line MeWo. *Cancer Res* 1987; 47:3851–3855.

105. Gattoni-Celli S, Byers RH, Calorini L, Ferrone S. Organ-specific metastases in melanoma: experimental animal models. *Pigment Cell Res* 1993; 6:381–384.

106. Herlyn D, Adachi K, Koprowski H, Herlyn M. In vitro properties of human melanoma cells metastatic in nude mice. *Cancer Res* 1990; 50:2296–2302.

107. Herlyn D, Adachi K, Koprowski H, Herlyn M. Experimental model of human melanoma metastases. In: *Melanoma Research: Genetics, Growth factors, Metastases*. Kluwer Academic Publishers, Boston, MA, 1991, pp. 105–118.

108. Lockshin A, Giovanella BC, De Ipolyi PD, Williams LJ Jr, Mendoza JT, Yim SO, et al. Exceptional lethality for nude mice of cells derived from a primary human melanoma. *Cancer Res* 1985; 45:345–350.

109. Shoemaker RH, Dykes DJ, Plowman J, Harrison SD Jr, Griswold DP Jr, Abbott BJ, et al. Practical spontaneous metastasis model for in vivo therapeutic studies using a human melanoma. *Cancer Res* 1991; 51:2837–2841.

110. Fodstad O, Kjonniksen I, Aamdal S, Nesland JM, Boyd MR, Pihl A. Extrapulmonary, tissue-specific metastasis formation in nude mice injected with FEMX-I human melanoma cells. *Cancer Res* 1988; 48:4382–4388.

111. Rofstad EK. Orthotopic human melanoma xenograft model systems for studies of tumour angiogenesis, pathophysiology, treatment sensitivity and metastatic pattern. *Br J Cancer* 1994; 70:804–812.

112. Ishikawa M, Fernandez B, Kerbel RS. Highly pigmented human melanoma variant which metastasizes widely in nude mice, including to skin and brain. *Cancer Res* 1988; 48:4897–4903.

113. Mori M, Yamaguchi K, Honda S, Nagasaki K, Ueda M, Abe O, et al. Cancer cachexia syndrome developed in nude mice bearing melanoma cells producing leukemia-inhibitory factor. *Cancer Res* 1991; 51:6656–6659.

114. Spremulli EN, Bogaars HA, Dexter DL, Matook GM, Jolly GA, Kuhn RE, et al. Nude mouse model of the melanosis syndrome. *J Natl Cancer Inst* 1983; 71:933–939.

115. Jansen B, Schlagbauer-Wadl H, Brown BD, Bryan RN, van Elsas A, Muller M, et al. bcl-2 antisense therapy chemosensitizes human melanoma in SCID mice. *Nat Med* 1998; 4:232–234.

116. Naramura M, Gillies SD, Mendelsohn J, Reisfeld RA, Mueller BM. Therapeutic potential of chimeric and murine anti-(epidermal growth factor receptor) antibodies in a metastasis model for human melanoma. *Cancer Immunol Immunother* 1993; 37:343–349.

117. Hill LL, Korngold R, Jaworsky C, Murphy G, McCue P, Berd D. Growth and metastasis of fresh human melanoma tissue in mice with severe combined immunodeficiency. *Cancer Res* 1991; 51:4937–4941.

118. Taylor CW, Grogan TM, Lopez MH, Leong SP, Odeleye A, Feo-Zuppardi FJ, et al. Growth and dissemination of human malignant melanoma cells in mice with severe combined immune deficiency. *Lab Invest* 1992; 67:130–137.

119. Juhasz I, Albelda SM, Elder DE, Murphy GF, Adachi K, Herlyn D, et al. Growth and invasion of human melanomas in human skin grafted to immunodeficient mice. *Am J Pathol* 1993; 143:528–537.

26 Experimental Animal Models for Renal Cell Carcinoma

Gilda G. Hillman, PhD

CONTENTS

1. INTRODUCTION

The incidence of renal-cell carcinoma (RCC) has increased in recent years with approximately 31,200 new cases each year in the United States *(1)*. This increased RCC incidence may be linked to certain risk factors, including smoking, obesity, high-protein diets, and hypertension *(2,3)*. The disease is responsible for an estimated 12,000 deaths each year *(1)*. Nearly one-half of patients present only with localized disease that can be treated by surgical removal *(2,4,5)*. However, one-third of the patients also present with metastatic disease, and one-half of the patients treated for localized carcinomas subsequently develop metastatic disease *(2,4)*. The median survival of patients with metastases is only 8 mo, with a 5-yr survival rate of less than 10% *(2,4)*. Patients with metastatic RCC frequently present with pulmonary metastases that are poorly responsive to conventional treatment, including most chemotherapeutic drugs, hormones, and radiation therapy *(2,4,5)*. The treatment of metastatic disease has been and remains a difficult clinical challenge. To develop new and alternative therapeutic modalities for metastatic disease and to investigate the metastatic progression and the molecular genetics of RCC, various preclinical animal models have been established.

The properties of an ideal tumor model for RCC are: spontaneous origin, histologically proven adenocarcinoma, predictable growth rate, and ability to metastasize similarly to human RCC in a reasonable time frame *(6,7)*. This chapter reviews several experimental models, including the murine Renca renal adenocarcinoma in Balb/c

From: *Tumor Models in Cancer Research*
Edited by: B. A. Teicher © Humana Press Inc., Totowa, NJ

mice, the rat kidney carcinoma in the Wistar-Lewis rat, the Eker rat model of hereditary RCC, and the human RCC tumor xenograft models in athymic nude mice. These models have been well-characterized and extensively used to study the pathogenesis of RCC disease, and to assess the efficacy and safety of novel treatment modalities.

2. MURINE SYNGENEIC RENAL ADENOCARCINOMA: THE RENCA MODEL

In the early 1970s, the (Renca) murine renal adenocarcinoma model was isolated and characterized by Murphy and Hrushesky *(8)*. The Renca tumor arose spontaneously in the kidney of a Balb/c mouse, and was found to induce metastatic kidney tumors when injected under the renal capsule of Balb/c mice *(8)*. Renca was histologically characterized as a poorly differentiated renal cortical adenocarcinoma of the granular type—pleomorphic with large nuclei *(6,8)*. Renca can be maintained by either in vitro culture or in vivo passage by intraperitoneal (ip) injection, or by subcapsular renal injection in syngeneic Balb/c mice. The progression of the Renca tumor following subcapsular implantation mimics that of human RCC because of the formation of a primary tumor mass on the kidney followed by the development of spontaneous metastases *(8–10)*. Metastases develop in the regional lymph nodes, lung, liver and peritoneum; thus, Renca can be staged similarly to human RCC (8–10). The renal Renca model allows evaluation of the therapy, on the primary tumor as well as on metastatic deposits. A nephrectomy of the tumor-bearing kidney can be performed *(10);* therefore, the model is applicable for the development of therapeutic protocols for advanced metastatic disease similarly to the clinical situation of postnephrectomy metastatic RCC patients. The mean survival time of Renca-bearing mice is approx 46 d when 10^5 cells are implanted intrarenally, thus allowing for a therapeutic evaluation in a reasonable time frame.

Based on these properties, Renca does represent an ideal RCC tumor model, and indeed has been used extensively as a preclinical model to investigate various therapeutic approaches for metastatic RCC. In the 1970s, early studies of this model have included hormonal therapy, and chemotherapy with single or combined drugs that were found of limited efficacy (reviewed in ref. 6). The immunogenicity of this tumor is relatively low, although some protection to rechallenge with viable Renca cells following immunization with crude membrane preparations from Renca cells has been reported *(11)*. This model is a valuable tool in the evaluation of immunotherapy approaches. Immunotherapy is a novel therapeutic approach developed in the 1980s for the treatment of disseminated cancers refractory to conventional treatments. This approach utilizes Biological Response Modifiers (BRMs)/cytokines, and immune cells capable to of enhancing immune mechanisms directed against the tumor that may be present, although ineffective in cancer-bearing hosts *(12)*. The most commonly used BRMs are interferons and the lymphokine interleukin 2 (IL-2). In the 1980s, Wiltrout has developed chemoimmunotherapy combining the administration of chemotherapeutic agents (doxorubicin hydrochloride or flavone acetic acid) with adoptive immunotherapy (IL-2 and lymphokine-activated killer cells) for the treatment of Renca that resulted in significant antitumor responses *(6,9,10,13)*. These preclinical studies were translated into clinical trials for RCC patients *(14)*. Other cytokines such as IL-7, IL-1, or a combination of cytokines including IFNα/IL-2 or IFNα/IFNγ were tested (reviewed in refs.

6,13). Gregorian and Battisto have demonstrated the existence of immunosuppressive effects induced by the tumor cells in Renca-bearing mice (15,16). Generation of specific cytotoxic T-lymphocytes to Renca cells is particularly difficult when using irradiated Renca cells in in vitro assays because of their immunosuppressive activity (personal communications).

In the 1990s, we have further developed the Renca model to address the efficacy and mechanism of action of cytokine therapy alone or in combination with radiation therapy (17–27). We have defined the kinetics of the tumor model following Renca-cell implantation in various sites. A concentration of 10^5 cells can be administered in 0.1 mL Hank's Balanced Salt Solution (HBSS) for intraperitoneal (ip) or flank subcutaneous (sc) injections or in 0.5 mL HBSS for iv injection via a tail vein. For kidney implantation, the right kidney of anesthetized mice is exposed through a right-flank incision and injected subcapsularly with 10^5 Renca cells in 50 μL HBSS using a 27-gauge needle. Intraperitoneal (ip) injection of Renca induced metastases in the mesenteric lymph nodes starting on d 16, and progressing to carcinomatosis (19). Liver metastases were observed in 38% of the mice, and lung metastases were detected in 5%. (19). Following sc injections of Renca cells in the right flank, small tumors were detectable by d 14, and grew progressively, reaching a size of 1–1.5 cm^3 (19). Large tumors showed a tendency to become ulcerative and necrotic. Tumors remained localized at the site of injection, and metastases were not detectable in other organs (19).

Following kidney implantation, a macroscopic primary tumor was detectable by d 7–10, which then grew progressively to 1–2 cm^3 by d 20–21 (17). Large tumors of 7–8 cm^3 were present by d 25–35. Pulmonary metastases were first noted by d 15–20 following renal implantation. However, large variations in the number of lung metastases were observed from mouse to mouse. Metastases to the liver, hemorrhagic ascites, and/or carcinomatosis were also observed in most animals after 21 d, confirming previous studies. Similar to previous reports, mice began to die on d 21, with a 50% survival rate by d 37, and less than 10% mice survived more than 45 d (17). To increase the incidence and number of pulmonary metastases, we have iv-injected Renca cells and observed visible tumor nodules of <1 mm diameter by d 15. By d 20, numerous lung metastases (100–200) were consistently enumerated by d 20 in both lobes, and increased in size (18,19,21). Tumor was not detectable in other organs. Mice became moribund by d 30, and a median survival of 38 d was observed. This more predictable model of lung metastases was essential for quantitative evaluation of new therapeutic approaches for the treatment of lung metastases (18,21,22,25,27), thus mimicking the clinical situation of postnephrectomy patients presenting with lung metastases.

Using these various Renca models, we have studied the interaction between local tumor irradiation and systemic (ip) IL-2 immunotherapy. In the kidney-tumor model, a greater therapeutic effect was demonstrated on the primary tumor and distant metastases by local irradiation of the tumor-bearing kidney followed by IL-2 therapy than with each modality by itself (17). In the pulmonary metastases model, irradiation of the left tumor-bearing lung followed by systemic IL-2 therapy resulted in increased tumor reduction in both lungs, suggesting that radiation enhances the systemic effect of IL-2 (18,21). We demonstrated the requirement for T-cell and natural killer (NK)-cell functions in the mechanism of action of the combined therapy (21). In histological studies of lung-tumor nodules, we found that radiation caused tumor-cell apoptosis, but also vascular damage, allowing for an influx of macrophages and mononuclear cells in the tumor nodules and surrounding tissues *(21,22)*. The combination of both therapies induced a greater vascular damage and massive infiltration of immune cells that may play a role in tumor destruction *(21,22)*. Our data in the Renca models suggest that radiation therapy causes changes in the tumor cells and the tumor environment, which increases the tumor susceptibility to destruction by the immune system activated by IL-2. The Renca system was an ideal animal model to investigate these complex issues, and these studies were translated into a clinical trial for metastatic RCC *(23)*. The Renca kidney model and lung metastases model were also helpful for evaluation of IL-4 and IFNγ *(25–27)*. Following in vitro studies on human RCC-cell lines demonstrating growth inhibition induced by IL-4 and IFNγ *(24)*, we have tested the therapeutic effect of these cytokines in the Renca models in vivo. We found that systemic treatment of either cytokine-induced regression of pulmonary metastases in a dose-dependent manner and increased mouse survival *(25,27)*. We showed that IL-4 and IFNγ have different antitumor mechanisms of action, consequently we found that sequential administration of IFNγ followed by IL-4 resulted in a greater therapeutic effect *(27)*. During these studies, we developed a new treatment approach of intratumoral injection of IL-4 in Renca kidney tumors *(26)*. On d 16 following Renca-cell renal implantation, the tumor-bearing kidney was re-exposed through a midline abdominal incision, and the kidney tumor (of 4–6 mm diameter) was injected with 50 μL IL-4. This treatment was safely performed, and resulted in a marked inhibition of tumor growth in the kidney, with minimal effect on the progression of metastases in other sites *(26)*. Thus, the Renca kidney model can be adapted to therapeutic manipulations. Other studies used IL-4 for transfection of Renca tumor cells and showed that IL-4 transduced Renca cells injected subcutaneously caused systemic immunity *(6,13,28)*.

In the 1990s, the newly discovered cytokine IL-12 seemed to be the most promising, because it was found to be particularly effective at mediating a specific immune antitumor response in various tumor models, including the Renca model *(29,30)*. Subsequently, the Renca model was extensively used to study IL-12 combination with other cytokines, the IL-12 mechanism of action, and IL-12 gene therapy. IL-12 antitumor effects were shown to be increased by tumor irradiation *(30)*, similar to our findings with IL-2 and tumor irradiation *(17–22)*. Using the Renca kidney model, Wiltrout et al. showed that IL-12 administered with pulse IL-2 was safe, and induced a rapid and complete regression of primary and metastatic Renca tumors that was greater than with each cytokine alone *(31)*. This effect was found to be related to enhanced macrophage production of nitric oxide following studies in the sc Renca model *(32)*. Furthermore, in the same sc Renca model, the mechanism of IL-12 antitumor activity was found to depend on induced expression of IFNγ by T- and NK cells, leading to IFNγ induced expression of chemokines IP-10 and Mig within tumor tissue. These chemokines act as chemoattractants for activated T-lymphocytes *(33,34)*. IL-12 was also found to potentiate the cytolytic effector function of recruited CD8+ T cells *(33)*. These studies in the Renca model led to monitoring IFNγ, IP-10, and Mig mRNA in biopsies of RCC tumors and peripheral-blood mononuclear cells from IL-12 treated patients, demonstrating augmented levels of those molecules after therapy *(35)*. Thus, the Renca model is helpful for testing new treatments for translational purpose, and it also allows the investigation of mechanism of these treatments and determination of response parameters for patient monitoring.

Recently, a novel Fas-mediated antitumor pathway also involving IFNγ was discovered in studies performed with the Renca model *(36,37)*. Renca cells express low levels of Fas that can be enhanced by IFNγ and TNFα, making the cells susceptible to apoptosis induced by Fas ligand (FasL)-expressing hybridomas (dIIS), crosslinking of anti-Fas antibodies or soluble Fas (FasL) *(36)*. The Fas/FasL pathway was found to be involved in cell-mediated killing of Renca cells by activated T-cells, whereas a granule-mediated pathway predominated in killing of Renca cells by activated NK cells *(36)*. When Fas-overexpressing Renca cells (post IFNγ and TNFα treatment) were injected into mice, there was a consistent and significant delay in tumor progression, reduced metastasis, and prolonged survival *(37)*. These novel findings show that therapeutic manipulation of Fas expression may represent a means of tumor treatment, as well as a novel mechanism for IFNγ mediated antitumor effect.

The Renca model was also very useful for addressing various approaches of cytokine gene therapy, mostly using IL-2 and IL-12 cytokines. A recent approach involves the use of plasmids containing cytokine cDNA inserts. Intradermal injections of murine IL-12 plasmid DNA induced systemic biological effects characteristic of IL-12, including enhanced NK activity and IL-12-inducible IFNγ genes *(38,39)*. Pretreatment of mice with IL-12 plasmid DNA-induced tumor growth delay when mice were rechallenged with sc Renca *(38)*. A different approach used IL-2 plasmid DNA complexed with a cationic lipid for intratumoral injection of Renca tumors and showed antitumor activity and induction of specific immunity *(40)*. Alternatively, an IL-12 adenovirus construct, administered intravenously, could also inhibit Renca hepatic metastases in a Renca hepatic metastasis tumor model induced by intrasplenic Renca-cell injection followed by splenectomy *(41)*. This effect seemed to be mediated by macrophages and neutrophils *(41)*. In another gene-therapy approach, Renca cells transfected with cytokine genes showed efficacy when used as cancer vaccines. Renca cells transfected with IL-2, IFNγ granulocyte-macrophage colony-stimulating factor (GM-CSF), or IL-12 failed to produce sc tumors *(42,43)*. We found that sc vaccination with cytokine-transfected Renca cells combined with lung radiation significantly reduced the number of pulmonary metastases in the Renca lung metastases model *(43)*. Others showed that IL-12 transfected Renca cells used as a cancer vaccine inhibited the growth of parental Renca cells injected at a distant site, and were synergistic with systemic IL-18 treatment *(42)*.

In conclusion, the Renca system has been of great value in the testing of multiple new therapeutic approaches for RCC—including novel gene therapies—and in the investigation of their mechanism of action, as well as the role of several components of the immune system in the antitumor response.

Other issues related to the progression and angiogenesis of RCC were recently addressed in the Renca system, including ways to inhibit these processes. Transfection of Renca cells with basic fibroblast growth factor (bFGF) gene increased their metastatic potential when injected intravenously, or intrarenally probably through the production of metalloproteinase 2 (MMP-2) *(44)*. The ratio of MMP-2 and tissue of inhibitor of metalloproteinase-2 (TIMP-2) was found to be a critical factor in the invasion and metastases of RCC, based on Renca studies *(45)*. The absence of expression of TGFβ type II receptor in Renca was also associated with an aggressive growth pattern *(46)*. Transfection of Renca cells with this receptor conferred tumor-suppressive activity, emphasizing the role of TGFβ type II receptor as a mediator in Renca tumorigenicity

(47). Transfection of mouse endostatin into Renca cells decreased the rate of tumor growth when these cells were injected subcutaneously or intravenously, suggesting that gene delivery of the angiogenetic inhibitor endostatin may be an effective strategy to prevent progression of RCC disease *(48)*.

3. RAT RENAL CARCINOMA MODELS

3.1. The Wistar-Lewis Rat Renal Adenocarcinoma

The Wistar-Lewis rat renal adenocarcinoma, like murine Renca, also arose spontaneously in the kidney of a Wistar-Lewis rat and originated in the renal cortical tubules. Its growth and expansion were characterized by White and Olsson and found to be non-hormonal-dependent *(49)*. This tumor is maintained by transplantation in the flank of syngeneic rats. The sc tumor takes 3 wk to develop and does not metastasize, and the mean survival is unpredictable *(49)*. To induce metastases, rats were first splenectomized. Then, 24 h later, a tumor fragment was placed into the peritoneal cavity. Nine weeks later, all animals displayed ascites and metastatic disease into the diaphragm, bowel, and muscle throughout the abdominal cavity *(49)*. Alternatively, the rat-cancer cells could be injected into the renal capsule, resulting in 80% tumor occurrence. However, the time required for widespread metastases was unpredictable. Chemotherapeutic studies were performed on sc tumors as well as on the ip metastatic tumors, and showed selective responses to drugs *(6,49)*. Thus, although this rat RCC tumor model was less predictable and required a longer time-frame study than Renca, it was useful to test chemotherapeutic agents.

Renal implantation of the rat tumor showed a rapid growth rate of the primary kidney tumor, and within 90 d metastasized to the lungs, even when the primary tumor was resected. Electron-microscopic studies in this model revealed that the rat RCC cells shared many ultrastructural features with human RCC cells, such as the presence of large nuclei, abundant glycogen granules, and numerous large vacuoles *(50)*. The primary tumor was used to study the tumor cholesterol metabolism, and also showed some similarity with human RCC tumors in its accumulation of an excess of esterified cholesterol caused by an increased rate of cholesterol synthesis *(50)*.

3.2. The Eker Rat Model

In 1954 and 1961, Eker and Mossige described a dominantly inherited cancer syndrome in Wistar rats in which bilateral multicentric RCC develops at an early age *(51,52)*. The hereditary tumors that develop in the Eker rat model have many parallels with their human counterparts. They have similar histology, are bilateral, overexpress transforming growth factor (TGFα), and do not exhibit a high frequency of *ras* oncogene activation *(53,54)*. Loss of sequences on rat chromosomes 4 (q11 through qter), 5 (monosomy), and 6 (q24) occur in these tumors and tumor-derived cell lines. Animals carrying the Eker mutation develop hemangiosarcomas in the spleen (males and females) and uterine leiomyosarcomas as second primary tumors later in life *(53,54)*. Vascular neoplasms (hemangioblastomas) and second primary tumors are also associated with RCC in human von Hippel-Lindau (VHL) disease *(54)*. Genetic analysis of Eker rats showed that the familial tumors were caused by an alteration in a single gene, which caused heterozygote carriers of the mutation to develop spontaneous RCCs between 4 and 12 mo of age, whereas rats that are homozygous for the wild-type allele rarely develop spontaneous RCC (<0.5%) *(53)*. When homozygous, the mutation is lethal prenatally at 9–10 d of gestation *(53)*. Eker rats were found to have a 70-fold increase in susceptibility to chemical carcinogenesis *(54)* and increased sensitivity to radiation *(53,55)*, resulting in greater cancer incidence. A carcinogen that targeted both renal-epithelial and mesenchymal cells caused an increase in tumors of epithelial origin in susceptible animals; the number of carcinogen-induced mesenchymal tumors was unaffected by the presence of the mutation at the susceptibility locus *(54)*. The cancer susceptibility gene was identified in the 1990s as the rat homolog of the tuberous sclerosis gene 2 *(Tsc2)*, and the mutation involved a 6.3-kb insertion within an intron of the gene on chromosome 10q *(56,57)*. This region was found to be homologous with human chromosome band 16p13.3, the site of human *Tsc 2* gene *(56)*. Rat *Tsc2* functions as a tumor-suppressor gene as normal kidneys of heterozygote carriers express both normal and abnormal *Tsc2* mRNA, whereas primary tumors and tumor-derived cell lines exhibit only the mutant transcript *(53)*. Tumor-suppressor genes represent a class of cancer susceptibility genes in humans. Inheritance of a mutation in one allele of a tumor-suppressor gene predisposes individuals to develop tumors after sustaining an additional spontaneous mutation in the remaining normal allele of this gene. In humans, several tumor-suppressor genes including the *VHL* gene, the *WTI* gene and the *Tsc2* gene have been implicated in the development of sporadic as well as hereditary tumors in the kidney *(2)*. In the Eker rats, a single gene mutation *(Tsc2)* predisposes to multiple bilateral RCCs with an autosomal dominant pattern of inheritance. Therefore, animals carrying the Eker mutation serve as a model for hereditary RCC.

In the 1990s, the Eker rat model was extensively studied to identify key genetic components in the pathogenesis of RCC and to dissect the molecular mechanisms underlying tubular epithelial carcinogenesis. Very early preneoplastic stages in tubular transformation in hereditary RCC can be identified in Eker rats. By laser microdissection procedure, loss of heterozygosity (LOH) was detected in the region of *Tsc2* locus on rat chromosome 10 in preneoplastic renal tubular lesions in Eker rats *(58)*. These studies suggested that, in heterozygotes, at least two events (one inherited and one somatic) are necessary to produce large adenomas and carcinomas *(58)*. Studies on patients with tuberous sclerosis complex (TSC) documented that it is an autosomal dominant disorder characterized by seizures, mental retardation, and hamartomas. These TSC patients have an increased frequency for developing RCC at an early age, similar to Eker rats *(59)*. The role of the *Tsc2* gene was further elucidated using the Eker rat model. This gene encodes a large membrane-associated GTPase-activated protein (GAP) designated tuberin, and its biological activity was determined by transfection of Eker rat-derived RCC cells with wild-type *Tsc2* gene. These cells demonstrated a decreased ability to form colonies in vitro and tumors in vivo, providing evidence for the tumor-suppressor function of the *Tsc2* gene *(60)*. The *Tsc2* gene may also contribute to regulation of the cell cycle and cell survival *(61)*. Recently, a *Tsc2* knockout mouse was generated to further characterize the tuberin function in vivo *(62)*. *Tsc2* heterozygous mice developed renal carcinomas, and *Tsc2* homozygous mice died at d 10 embryonic age, similar to the observations made in Eker rats *(62)*. These studies emphasize an essential function for tuberin in mouse and rat embryonic development, as well as in RCC incidence. Other recent studies have investigated the role of the *VHL* gene in the rat RCC pathogenesis. The rat *VHL* gene was identified and found to be

90% homologous to the human *VHL* gene *(63)*. However, alterations were not detected in the rat *VHL* gene in Eker rat RCC cell lines, suggesting that RCC development in the rat is independent of *VHL* mutation or deletion in contrast to human sporadic RCC *(63)*. The influence of hormonal and dietary factors on RCC incidence was also investigated in the Eker rat model. Estrogen treatment was found to enhance the development of renal tumors in Eker rats *(64)* and a high-fat diet increased renal preneoplasia *(65)*.

In conclusion, the Eker rat model is an excellent example of a Mendelian dominant predisposition to RCC in an experimental animal that allows the study of genes and molecular events involved in the development of hereditary RCC and secondary tumors.

4. XENOGRAFTS OF HUMAN TUMOR-CELL LINES IN IMMUNODEFICIENT MICE

Athymic nude mice are deficient in immune T-cell functions, and do not reject xenografts. Thus, they are used for implantation of human tissues. In the beginning of the 1990s, human RCC cells have been successfully heterotransplanted in nude mice, and grew locally as a solid tumor after sc injection *(66)*. The tumorigenicity of tumor cells in nude mice is used as a criterion for characterizing the malignancy of the cells isolated from a tumor specimen *(66)*. In addition, human RCC xenografts established by sc or ip injection in nude mice have been tested for their responsiveness to therapy. Human RCC tumors growing in nude mice were studied for localization and treatment by monoclonal antibodies (MAbs), including the G250 and DAL K29 MAbs directed specifically against human renal-tumor lines. Dijk et al. have demonstrated that G250 MAb or the bispecific MAb CD3/G250, injected intravenously, preferentially localized in human renal tumors transplanted subcutaneously in nude mice *(67)*. In a subsequent study, G250 administered intraperitoneally induced a significant growth inhibition of this tumor, and this effect was enhanced by intratumoral injection of IFNα and TNFα, resulting in macrophage infiltrates into the tumor stroma. Singh et al. found that human RCC cells administered intraperitoneally in nude mice developed into an ascites tumor, and could be targeted by specific MAb DAL K29 linked to liposomes containing methotrexate, resulting in a higher drug uptake *(68)*.

At the same time, other groups explored the subcapsular renal implantation of human RCC cells in the nude mouse kidneys. Based on the concept that neoplasms are heterogeneous and contain subpopulations of cells with different biological behavior patterns, including metastatic potential, Fidler has demonstrated the usefulness of orthotopic-implantation human RCC in the kidneys of nude mice *(69)*. Fidler has implanted human RCC cells obtained from surgical specimens into different organs of nude mice, and showed that growth at different organs selected for different subpopulations of human RCC cells. However, the cells did not metastasize unless they were implanted orthotopically in the kidney *(69)*. The injection of human RCC cells into the kidney produces the highest incidence of tumorigenicity, suggesting that the kidney is a better environment than the skin, spleen, or peritoneum. Some of these tumors spontaneously metastasize to the lung, pancreas, diaphragm, and mesenteric lymph nodes *(69)*. Tumor cells were isolated from the kidney tumors to establish RCC cell lines in culture to study their biological activity in vitro and in vivo *(69)*. Other studies have confirmed the tumorigenicity and metastatic potential of human RCC cells obtained from cell lines or surgical specimens

(70,71). Not every cell line or cells from different surgical specimens are tumorigenic. However, established human RCC tumors in the mouse kidney usually showed histological characteristics of the original primary tumor, including positivity to cytokeratins and vimentin *(71)*. Orthotopic xenograft RCC models were recently used to test new anticancer drugs (BCH-4556) or gene therapy *(72–74)*. Human RCC cells transfected with IFNβ did not induce localized tumors, kidney tumors, and spontaneous lung metastases when injected subcutaneously or intravenously in the kidney *(73)*. These IFNβ transfected RCC tumor cells stimulated a high level of nitric oxide production by murine macrophages in vitro and in vivo that was cytotoxic to tumor cells *(73)*. This study led to testing retroviral vectors encoding murine macrophage-inducible nitric oxide synthase *(iNOS)* gene for the treatment of RCC *(74)*. Infection of metastatic human RCC cells with iNOS retrovirus decreased their tumor growth and metastasis when injected intravenously or in the kidney of nude mice by producing nitric oxide that enhanced the rate of apoptosis of the tumor cells *(74)*.

We have recently developed a new xenograft RCC experimental tumor model in nude mice. We have established a tumor-cell line designated KCI-18 RCC from a primary renal-tumor specimen obtained from a patient with papillary *RCC* (nuclear grade III/IV) *(75)*. Chromosome analysis of KCI-18 RCC cell line (passage 8 in vitro) revealed a hypertriploid karyotype with multiple clonal aberrations: 75–85, XX, –X, add (1) *(p36)* ×2, +2, +3, +5, +i (5) (q10), +6, +del *(7)* (q11), +8, der (9,14) (q10;q10), –9, +10, +12, –14, add (15) (q26), +16, +17, +21, +mar, ace [cp6]. Cells were injected into the kidney of Balb/c nude mice. Renal tumors were resected, recultured in vitro, and repassaged in the kidney in vivo to produce KCI-18/IK cell lines *(75)*. Cells from the KCI-18/IK lines preserved the karyotype of the original KCI-18 RCC cell line. The KCI-18/IK lines were highly tumorigenic, and grew in the kidney with faster kinetics than the original KCI-18 RCC cell line. Tumor nodules of 0.2 cm were detectable on the kidney by d 11 post-cell-injection, and grew to large tumors of 2–2.5 cm, invading the kidney by d 44. Metastases were detectable by d 37, and observed mostly in the lungs and occasionally in the liver *(75)*. Mouse survival was about 44–50 d. The tumor presence in the kidney and lungs was histologically confirmed and defined as a high-grade carcinoma with a sinusoidal vascular pattern. Tumor cells were characterized by large pleiomorphic nuclei, prominent nucleoli, and abundant eosinophilic cytoplasm. Tumor cells co-expressed cytokeratin and vimentin. These features resembled those of the original human tumor specimen *(75)*. Thus, we have developed a reproducible RCC tumor model in nude mice, in which human tumor cells metastasize from the primary renal tumor to the lungs, similar to human RCC. These studies demonstrate that orthotopic models of heterotransplanted human RCC cells are representative of human RCC progression, and preserve the karyotypic and histological characteristics of the human primary tumor. These models can be used to study human RCC progression and metastasis, and responsiveness in vivo of human RCC tumors to treatment.

The disadvantages of using heterotransplants in nude mice reside in their deficient immune system, which allows the study of NK cell and macrophage responses, but not T-cell responses that are significant in antitumor responses. This system may be more appropriate for direct testing of novel chemotherapeutic drugs or gene therapy on human RCC tumors in vivo *(72–74)*. Moreover, because of their deficient immune system, nude mice are extremely sensitive to infections, and are expensive to use because they require housing and handling in sterile conditions.

ACKNOWLEDGMENTS

We thank Dr. J. Forman and the Patricia and E. Jan Hartmann Cancer Fund for supporting our studies. We thank Johanna Rubio, Andrey Layer and Jennifer Wright for technical assistance.

REFERENCES

1. Greenlee RT, Murray T, Bolden S, Wingo PA. Cancer statistics 2000. *CA Cancer J Clin* 2000; 50:7–33.
2. Mulders P, Figlin R, deKernion JB, Wiltrout R, Linehan M, Parkinson D, et al. Renal cell carcinoma: recent progress and future directions. *Cancer Res* 1997; 57:5189–5195.
3. Chow WH, Gridely G, McLaughlin JK, Mandel JS, Wacholder S, Blot WJ, et al. Protein intake and risk of renal cell cancer. *J Natl Cancer Inst* 1994; 86:1131–1139.
4. Haas GP, Hillman GG. Update on the role of immunotherapy in the management of kidney cancer. *Cancer Control* 1996; 3:66–71.
5. Motzer RJ, Bander NH, Nanus DM. Renal-cell carcinoma. *N Engl J Med* 1996; 335:865–875.
6. Hillman GG, Droz JP, Haas GP. Experimental animal models for the study of therapeutic approaches in renal cell carcinoma. *In Vivo* 1994; 8:77–80.
7. van Moorselaar RJA, Schalken JA, Oosterhof GON, Debruyne FMJ. Use of animal models in diagnosis and treatment of renal cell carcinoma. An overview. *World J Urol* 1991; 9:192–197.
8. Hrushesky WJ, Murphy GP. Investigation of a new renal tumor model. *J Surg Res* 1973; 15:327–332.
9. Salup RR, Wiltrout RH. Adjuvant immunotherapy of established murine renal cancer by interleukin 2 stimulated cytotoxic lymphocytes. *Cancer Res* 1986; 46:3358–3363.
10. Salup RR, Back TC, Wiltrout RH. Successful treatment of advanced murine renal cancer by bicompartmental adoptive chemoimmunotherapy. *J Immunol* 1987; 138:641–647.
11. Huben RP, Connelly RC, Goldrosen MH, Murphy GP, Pontes JE. Immunotherapy of a murine renal cancer. *J Urol* 1983; 129:1075–1078.
12. Hillman GG, Haas GP, Wahl W, Callewaert DM. Adoptive immunotherapy of cancer: biological response modifiers and cytotoxic cell therapy. *Biotherapy* 1992; 5:119–129.
13. Wiltrout RH, Gregorio TA, Fenton RG, Longo DL, Ghosh P, Murphy WJ, et al. Cellular and molecular studies in the treatment of murine renal cancer. *Semin Oncol* 1995; 22:9–16.
14. Holmlund JT, Kopp WC, Wiltrout RH, Longo DL, Urba WJ, Janik JE, et al. A phase I clinical trial of flavone-8-acetic acid in combination with interleukin 2. *J Natl Cancer Inst* 1995; 87(2):134–136.
15. Gregorian SK, Battisto JR. Immunosuppression in murine renal cell carcinoma: I. Characterization of extent, severity and sources. *Cancer Immunol Immunother* 1990; 31:325–334.
16. Gregorian SK, Battisto JR. Immunosuppression in murine renal cell carcinoma: II. Identification of responsible lymphoid cell phenotypes and examination of elimination of suppression. *Cancer Immunol Immunother* 1990; 31:335–341.
17. Dybal EJ, Haas GP, Maughan RL, Sud S, Pontes JE, Hillman GG. Synergy of radiation therapy and immunotherapy in murine renal cell carcinoma. *J Urol* 1992; 148:1331–1337.
18. Chakrabarty A, Hillman GG, Maughan RL, Ali E, Pontes JE, Haas GP. Radiation therapy enhances the therapeutic effect of immunotherapy on pulmonary metastases in a murine renal adenocarcinoma model. *In Vivo* 1994; 8:25–32.
19. Chakrabarty A, Hillman GG, Maughan RL, Visscher D, Ali E, Pontes JE, et al. Influence of tumor site on the therapy of murine kidney cancer. *Anticancer Res* 1994; 14:373–378.
20. Younes E, Haas GP, Dezso B, Ali E, Maughan RL, Montecillo EJ, et al. Radiation induced effects on murine kidney tumor cells: role in the interaction of local irradiation and immunotherapy. *J Urol* 1995; 153:2029–2033.
21. Younes E, Haas GP, Dezso B, Ali E, Maughan RL, KuKuruga MA, et al. Local tumor irradiation augments the response to IL-2 therapy in a murine renal adenocarcinoma. *Cellular Immunol* 1995; 165:243–251.
22. Dezso B, Haas GP, Hamzavi F, Kim S, Montecillo EJ, Benson PD, et al. Insights into the mechanism of local tumor irradiation combined with IL-2 therapy in murine renal carcinoma: histological evaluation of pulmonary metastases. *Clin Cancer Res* 1996; 2:1543–1552.
23. Redman BG, Hillman GG, Flaherty L, Forman J, Dezso B, Haas GP. Phase II trial of sequential radiation and interleukin-2 in the treatment of patients with metastatic renal cell carcinoma. *Clin Cancer Res* 1988; 4:283–286.

24. Hillman GG, Puri RK, KuKuruga MA, Pontes JE, Haas GP. Growth and major histocompatibility antigen expression regulation by interleukin-4, interferon gamma and tumor necrosis factor α on human renal cell carcinoma tumor cell lines. *Clin Exp Immunol* 1994; 96:476–483.

25. Hillman GG, Younes E, Visscher D, Ali E, Montecillo EJ, Pontes JE, et al. Systemic treatment with interleukin-4 induces regression of pulmonary metastases in a murine renal cell carcinoma model. *Cellular Immunol* 1995; 160:257–263.

26. Younes E, Haas GP, Visscher D, Pontes JE, Puri RK, Hillman GG. Intralesional treatment of established murine primary renal tumor with interleukin-4: localized effect on primary tumor with no impact on metastases. *J Urol* 1995; 153:490–493.

27. Hillman GG, Younes E, Visscher D, Hamzavi F, Kim S, Lam JS, et al. Pontes JE, Puri RK, Haas GP. Inhibition of murine renal carcinoma pulmonary metastases by systemic administration of interferon gamma: mechanism of action and potential for combination with IL-4. *Clin Cancer Res* 1997; 3:1799–1806.

28. Golumbek PT, Lazenby AJ, Levitsky HI, Jaffee LM, Karasuyama H, Baker M, et al. Treatment of established renal cancer by tumor cells engineered to secrete interleukin-4. *Science* 1991; 254:713–716.

29. Brunda MJ, Luistro L, Warrier RR, Wright RB, Hubbard BR, Murphy M, et al. Antitumor and antimetastatic activity of interleukin 12 against murine tumors. *J Exp Med* 1993; 178:1223–1230.

30. Teicher BA, Ara G, Menon K, Schaub RG. *In vivo* studies with interleukin-12 alone and in combination with monocyte colony-stimulating factor and/or fractionated radiation treatment. *Int J Cancer* 1996; 65:80–84.

31. Wigginton JM, Komschlies KL, Back TC, Franco JL, Brunda MJ, Wiltrout RH. Administration of interleukin 12 with pulse interleukin 2 and the rapid and complete eradication of murine renal carcinoma. *J Natl Cancer Inst* 1996; 88:38–43.

32. Wigginton JM, Kuhns DB, Back TC, Brunda MJ, Wiltrout RH, Cox GW. Interleukin 12 primes macrophages for nitric oxide production *in vivo* and restores depressed nitric oxide production by macrophages from tumor-bearing mice: implications for the antitumor activity of interleukin 12 and/or interleukin 2. *Cancer Res* 1996; 56:1131–1136.

33. Tannenbaum CS, Wicker N, Armstrong D, Tubbs R, Finke J, Bukowski RM, et al. Cytokine and chemokine expression in tumors of mice receiving systemic therapy with IL-2. *J Immunol* 1996; 156:693–699.

34. Tannebaum CS, Tubbs R, Armstrong D, Finke JH, Bukowski RM, Hamilton TA. The CXC chemokines IP-10 and Mig are necessary for IL-12-mediated regression of the mouse RENCA tumor. *J Immunol* 1998; 161:927–932.

35. Bukowski RM, Rayman P, Molto L, Tannenbaum CS, Olencki T, Peereboom D, et al. Interferon-gamma and CXC chemokine induction by interleukin 12 in renal cell carcinoma. *Clin Cancer Res* 1999; 5:2780–2789.

36. Sayers TJ, Brooks AD, Lee J, Fenton RG, Komschilies KL, Wigginton JM, et al. Molecular mechanisms of immune-mediated lysis of murine renal cancer: differential contributions of perforin-dependent versus fas-mediated pathways in lysis by NK and T cells. *J Immunol* 1998; 161:3957–3965.

37. Lee J, Sayers TJ, Brooks AD, Back TC, Young HA, Komschilies KL, et al. IFN-γ-dependent delay of *in vivo* tumor progression by fas overexpression on murine renal cancer cells. *J Immunol* 2000; 164:231–239.

38. Tan J, Newton CA, Djeu JY, Gutsch DE, Chang AE, Yang NS, et al. Injection of complementary DNA encoding interleukin-12 inhibits tumor establishment at a distant site in a murine renal carcinoma model. *Cancer Res* 1996; 56:3399–3403.

39. Watanabe M, Fenton RG, Wigginton JM, McCormick KL, Volker KM, Fogler WE, et al. Intradermal delivery of IL-12 naked DNA induces systemic NK cell activation and Th1 response *in vivo* that is independent of endogenous IL-12 production. *J Immunol* 1999; 163:1943–1950.

40. Saffran DC, Horton HM, Yankauckas MA, Anderson D, Barnhart KM, Abai AM, et al. Immunotherapy of established tumors in mice by intratumoral injection of interleukin-2 plasmid DNA: induction of CD8+ T-cell immunity. *Cancer Gene Ther* 1998; 5:321–330.

41. Siders WM, Wright PW, Hixon JA, Alvord WG, Back TC, Wiltrout RH, et al. T cell-and NK cell-independent inhibition of hepatic metastases by systemic administration of an IL-12-expressing recombinant adenovirus. *J Immunol* 1998; 160:5465–5474.

42. Hara I, Nagai H, Miyake H, Yamanaka K, Hara S, Micallef MJ, et al. Effectiveness of cancer vaccine therapy using cells transduced with the interleukin-12 gene combined with systemic interleukin-18 administration. *Cancer Gene Ther* 2000; 7:83–90.

43. Nishisaka N, Maini A, Kinoshita Y, Yasumoto R, Kishimoto T, Jones RF, et al. Immunotherapy for lung metastases of murine renal cell carcinoma: synergy between radiation and cytokine-producing tumor vaccines. *J Immunother* 1999; 22:308–314.

44. Miyake H, Hara I, Yoshimura K, Eto H, Arakawa S, Wada S, et al. Introduction of basic fibroblast growth factor gene into mouse renal cell carcinoma cell line enhances its metastatic potential. *Cancer Res* 1996; 56:2440–2445.

45. Miyake H, Hara I, Gohji K, Yamanaka K, Hara S, Arakawa S, et al. Relative expression of matrix metalloproteinase-2 and tissue inhibitor of metalloproteinase-2 in mouse renal cell carcinoma cells regulates their metastatic potential. *Clin Cancer Res* 1999; 5:2824–2829.

46. Kundu SD, Kim IY, Zelner D, Janulis L, Goodwin S, Engel JD, et al. Absence of expression of transforming growth factor-beta type II receptor is associated with an aggressive growth pattern in a murine renal carcinoma cell line, Renca. *J Urol* 1998; 160:1883–1888.

47. Engel JD, Kundu SD, Yang T, Lang S, Goodwin S, Janulis L, et al. C. Transforming growth factor-beta type II receptor confers tumor suppressor activity in murine renal carcinoma (Renca) cells. *Urology* 1999; 54:164–170.

48. Yoon SS, Eto H, Lin CM, Nakamura H, Pawlik TM, Song SU, et al. Mouse endostatin inhibits the formation of lung and liver metastases. *Cancer Res* 1999; 59:6251–6256.

49. deVere White R, Olssen CA. Renal adenocarcinoma in the rat: new tumor model. *Investig Urol* 1980; 17:405–412.

50. Clayman RV, Bilhartz LE, Buja LM, Spady DK, Dietschy JM. Renal cell carcinoma in the Wistar-Lewis rat: a model for studying the mechanisms of cholesterol acquisition by a tumor *in vivo*. *Cancer Res* 1986; 46:2958–2963.

51. Eker R. Familial renal adenomas in Wistar rats. *Acta Pathol Microbiol Scand* 1954; 34:554–562.

52. Eker R, Mossige J. A dominant gene for renal adenomas in the rat. *Nature* 1961; 189:858–859.

53. Everitt JI, Goldsworthy TL, Wolf DC, Walker CL. Hereditary renal cell carcinoma in the Eker rat: a unique animal model for the study of cancer susceptibility. *Toxicol Lett* 1995; 82/83:621–625.

54. Walker C, Goldsworthy TL, Wolf DC, Everitt J. Predisposition to renal cell carcinoma due to alteration of a cancer susceptibility gene. *Science* 1992; 255:1693–1695.

55. Hino O, Klein-Szanto AJ, Freed J, Testa JR, Brown DQ, Vilensky M, et al. Spontaneous and radiation-induced renal tumors in the Eker rat model of dominantly inherited cancer. *Proc Natl Acad Sci USA* 1993; 90:327–331.

56. Yeung RS, Xiao GH, Jin F, Lee WC, Testa JR, Knudson AG. Predisposition to renal carcinoma in the Eker rat is determined by germ-line mutation of the tuberous sclerosis 2 *(Tsc2)* gene. *Proc Natl Acad Sci USA* 1994; 91:11,413–11,416.

57. Kobayashi T, Hirayama Y, Kobayashi E, Kubo Y, Hino O. A germline insertion in the tuberous sclerosis *(Tsc2)* gene gives rise to the Eker rat model of dominantly inherited cancer. *Nat Genet* 1995; 9:70–74.

58. Kubo Y, Klimek F, Kikuchi Y, Bannasch P, Hino O. Early detection of Knudson's two-hits in preneoplastic renal cells of the Eker rat model by the laser microdissection procedure. *Cancer Res* 1995; 55:989–990.

59. Bjornsson J, Short MP, Kwiatkowski DJ, Henske EP. Tuberous sclerosis-associated renal cell carcinoma. Clinical, pathological, and genetic features. *Am J Pathol* 1996; 149:1201–1208.

60. Jin F, Wiennecke R, Xiao GH, Maize JC Jr, DeClue JE, Yeung RS. Suppression of tumorigenicity by the wild-type tuberous sclerosis 2 *(Tsc2)* gene and its C-terminal region. *Proc Natl Acad Sci USA* 1996; 93:9154–9159.

61. Orimoto K, Tsuchiya H, Sakurai J, Nishizawa M, Hino O. Identification of cDNAs induced by the tumor suppressor Tsc2 gene using a conditional expression system in Tsc2 mutant (Eker) rat renal carcinoma cells. *Biochem Biophys Res Commun* 1998; 247:728–733.

62. Kobayashi T, Minowa O, Kuno J, Mitani H, Hino O, Noda T. Renal carcinogenesis, hepatic hemangiomatosis, and embryonic lethality caused by a germ-line *Tsc2* mutation in mice. *Cancer Res* 1999; 59:1206–1211.

63. Walker C, Ahn YT, Everitt J, Yuan X. Renal cell carcinoma development in the rat independent of alteration at the VHL gene locus. *Mol Carcinog* 1996; 15:154–161.

64. Wolf DC, Goldsworthy TL, Donner EM, Harden R, Fitzpatrick B, Everitt JI. Estrogen treatment enhances hereditary renal tumor development in Eker rats. *Carcinog* 1998; 19:2043–2047.

65. Miki S, Miki Y, Mitani H, Sato B, Yamamoto M, Hino O. Hyperlipidemia enhancement of renal preneoplasia but not tumor formation is due to elevated apoptosis in the Eker rat. *Cancer Res* 1997; 57:4673–4676.

66. Ebert T, Bander NH, Finstad, Ramsawak RD, Old LJ. Establishment and characterization of human renal cancer and normal kidney cell lines. *Cancer Res* 1990; 50:5531–5536.

67. Dijk JV, Zegveld S, Fleuren GJ, Warnaar SO. Localization of monoclonal antibody G250 and bispecific monoclonal antibody CD3/G250 in human renal cell carcinoma xenografts: relative effects of size and affinity. *Int J Cancer* 1991; 48:738–743.

68. Singh M, Ghose T, Mezei M, Belitski P. Inhibition of human renal cancer by monoclonal antibody targeted methotrexate containing liposomes in an ascites tumor model. *Cancer Letters* 1991; 56:97–102.

69. Fidler IJ, Naito S, Pathak S. Orthotopic implantation is essential for the selection, growth and metastasis of human renal cell cancer in nude mice. *Cancer Met Rev* 1991; 9:149–165.

70. Grossi FS, Zhao X, Romijn JC, ten Kate FWJ, Schroder FH. Metastatic potential of human renal cell carcinoma: experimental model using subrenal capsule implantation in athymic nude mice. *Urol Res* 1992; 20:303–306.

71. Beniers AJMC, Peelen WP, Schaafsma HE, Beck JLM, Ramaekers FCS, Debruyne FMJ et al. Establishment and characterization of five new human renal tumor xenografts. *Amer J Path* 1992; 140:483–495.

72. Kadhim SA, Bowlin TL, Waud WR, Angers EG, Bibeau L, DeMuys JM, et al. Potent antitumor activity of a novel nucleoside analogue, BCH-4556 (β-L-dioxolane-cytidine), in human renal cell carcinoma xenograft tumor models. *Cancer Res* 1997; 57:4803–4810.

73. Xie K, Bielenberg D, Huang S, Xu L, Salas T, Juang SH, et al. Abrogation of tumorigenicity and metastasis of murine and human tumor cells by transfection with the murine IFN-beta gene: possible role of nitric oxide. *Clin Cancer Res* 1997; 3:2283–2294.

74. Juang S, Xie K, Xu L, Shi Q, Wang Y, Yoneda J, et al. Suppression of tumorigenicity and metastasis of human renal carcinoma cells by infection with retroviral vectors harboring the murine inducible nitric oxide synthase gene. *Human Gene Ther* 1998; 9:845–854.

75. Hillman GG, Grignon DJ, Mohamed AN, Kocheril SV, Montecillo EJ, Talati B, et al. Establishment of a new renal experiment tumor model. *J Urol* 1998; 159:766.

27 Animal Models of Mesothelioma

Harvey I. Pass, MD, Orlin Hadjiev, BS,
and Michele Carbone, MD, PhD

CONTENTS

INTRODUCTION
ASBESTOS-INDUCED MESOTHELIOMA IN ANIMAL MODELS
SPONTANEOUS MODELS OF MESOTHELIOMA
OTHER AGENTS FOR ANIMAL PRODUCTION OF MESOTHELIOMA
VIRAL-INDUCED MODELS OF MESOTHELIOMA
ORTHOTOPIC TRANSPLANTS AND XENOGRAFTS
CONCLUSIONS
REFERENCES

1. INTRODUCTION

Mesotheliomas are tumors that originate from the serosal lining of the pleural, pericardial, and peritoneal cavities *(1)*. Malignant pleural mesotheliomas (MPM) are among the most aggressive human tumors, with a survival after diagnosis of less than 1 yr. None of the current therapeutic approaches has been shown to alter the natural history of this disease *(2)*.

This continued rise in the incidence of mesotheliomas in the United States and abroad (2000–3000 cases per year in the United States) has been related to the widespread commercial use of asbestos during the last 50 yr *(3–5)*. The exact biochemical mechanism that causes asbestos to induce mesothelioma is unclear *(6–10)*. In tissue culture, asbestos fibers can cause mutagenic events, including DNA-strand breaks and deletion mutations through the production of hydroxyl radicals and superoxide anions. They can also alter chromosome morphology and ploidy by mechanically interfering with their segregation during mitosis. Furthermore, macrophages produce DNA-damaging oxyradicals following phagocytosis of asbestos fibers, and will elaborate lymphokines that may depress the host immune response.

Although the association between asbestos and mesothelioma is indisputable, less than 10% of the people exposed to high doses of asbestos will develop mesotheliomas. Moreover, approx one-half of the reported cases of mesothelioma have *no* documented exposure to asbestos *(10)*. In areas where asbestos mines exist, more than 70% of mesothelioma patients have a positive exposure history, but in areas with no substantial

From: *Tumor Models in Cancer Research*
Edited by: B. A. Teicher © Humana Press Inc., Totowa, NJ

asbestos-using industries, as few as 10% of patients with mesothelioma have a positive exposure history. These findings, and reports of mesothelioma developing in child-hood—or even in utero—as well as the continued description of the disease in individuals too young to have the usual latency period (25–40 yr) from asbestos exposure to MPM development suggest that there are probably other *unknown factors* involved in the pathogenesis of mesothelioma. Thus, researchers have long sought additional car-cinogens that may be responsible for mesotheliomas in non-asbestos-exposed individuals, or that could render particular individuals more susceptible to the carcinogenic effect of asbestos.

This chapter focuses on the development of animal models for mesothelioma. Since conventional wisdom dictates that the etiology of most mesotheliomas is asbestos, a large part of the discussion will focus on animal models of mesothelioma using asbestos fibers. However, since there is interest in viral-induced mechanisms for mesothelioma in humans, particularly because of the series of papers that describe the presence of SV40-like sequences in human mesothelioma, viral-induced mesothe-liomas in hamster models are also discussed. Finally, orthotopic transplantation of established mesothelioma cell lines in various positions in immunocompromised ani-mals are described.

The individual sections of the chapter discuss the individual means by which the tumor can be produced or propogated in the animal. Routes of delivery, as well as dif-ferences among species, are highlighted.

2. ASBESTOS-INDUCED MESOTHELIOMA IN ANIMAL MODELS

2.1. Types of Asbestos Fibers

There are two families of asbestos fibers: *serpentine* (chrysotile), which is curly and pliable, and the rod-like *amphiboles,* which include Crocidolite, Amosite, and Anthro-phylite, Tremolite, and Actinolyte *(11).* The size and thickness of these fibers will vary considerably, and the carcinogenic effects are related to their physical characteristics, with greater tumor promotion seen in the long, thin fibers that are readily phagocytosed and are stable in tissue *(12).* Inhaled fibers are cleared from the tracheobronchial tree by macrophages and ciliary action, and the remaining fibers accumulate in the lower one-third of the lungs, adjacent to the visceral pleura *(13).* As opposed to crocidolite and other amphiboles, the serpentine fibers break down into smaller subunits that dete-riorate or dissolve in the lung, and are then eliminated by lymphatics.

The relative carcinogenicity of the fibers remains controversial. It is safe to say that in humans there seems to be a "gradient" from crocidolite to crysotile in potency in order to induce mesothelioma and—despite the ability of crysotile to induce mesothe-lioma in laboratory animals—it is generally agreed that crocidolite is of greater car-cinogenicity in humans *(14).* Nevertheless, crysotile constitutes the majority (90%) of the asbestos used worldwide, and there are marked differences in the disease incidence in crysotile workers *(15–17).* Brake-lining workers chiefly exposed to crysotile fibers and other automobile maintenance workers are estimated to represent 20,000 deaths from asbestos-related cancer over the next 40 years. This finding may be a function of difference in fiber size or contamination with crocidolite fibers. The necessity to delin-eate the risk of crysotile-induced mesothelioma is even clearer when one considers that most buildings use this fiber for cement products and insulation.

Attempts at delineating the *dose intensity* and *relation of fiber type* to mesothelioma development has been performed using fiber analysis of tissues. This fiber content, measured by light and electron microscopic techniques, depends on the amount of fiber deposition (a function of the duration and dose intensity) as well as fiber clearance. Recent data suggests that the fiber concentration exceeding 1 million fibers per g of dried tissue may be associated with increased mesothelioma risk. Moreover, epithelial mesothelioma may be associated with significantly lower fiber content than sarcomatoid mesothelioma *(18)*.

2.2. Asbestos-Induced Animal Models of Mesothelioma: General Comments

Animal models for mesothelioma have been developed using all types of asbestos fibers *(19–22)*. There have been many similarities between these models of malignant mesothelioma, and the human situation in that fiber length, diameter, shape, and durability have been found to be of greater importance than the type of fiber.

All types of asbestos can induce tumor formation in animals through intraperitoneal (ip), intrathoracic, or intratracheal inoculation. The observation that some fibers are more mesotheliomatogenic than other is not coincidental. There seems to be a relationship between the carcinogenicity of a specific fiber and the proportion of long, thin fibers it contains. The general consensus is that long, thin fibers over 8 µm in length and thinner than 1 µm have the strongest carcinogenic effects because they cannot be readily phagocytized by alveolar macrophages for mechanical clearance via the mucociliary escalator. However, a threshold toxicity has yet to be defined, because asbestos dust comes in variety of particle lengths and it is almost impossible to administer a fiber of some precise length (e.g., 5 µm, 10 µm) without also injecting fibers of other lengths. As a result, most studies have attempted to characterize carcinogenic potential as a function of number of particles over or under a certain length.

2.3. Intraperitoneal Asbestos Injection

Intraperitoneal (ip) injections with asbestos have the disadvantage of introducing foreign material into the body in an unnatural manner. It has been argued that the conclusions drawn from carcinogenic studies are not applicable to humans because the physiological route of entry into the respiratory tract via the conducting airways is effectively bypassed. Thus, mesothelial cells are exposed to massive local doses of fiber that are not relevant for human exposure. Advocates of this method of induction point to it as being less labor-intensive than inhalation studies, and view it as an excellent opportunity to test the carcinogenic potential and potency of a fiber. Studies using the peritoneal mode of induction also offer the advantage of producing tumors in a large number of the injected animals.

2.4. Intraperitoneal Asbestos Injection: Rats

Tumor induction rates vary between 56% and 97.5% in the rat mesothelioma model. A variety of naturally occurring asbestos fibers—such as crocidolite, standard chrysotile, Canadian chrysotile, Rhodesian chrysotile, and amosite—have been studied for their ability to induce mesothelioma *(23,24)*. In these studies, where a fixed, non-adjusted-for-fiber-length dose in mg of a fiber has been administered, there is conflicting evidence as to whether standard chrysotile or standard crocidolite is more tumorigenic. Davis found chrysotile and amosite to be more carcinogenic than crocidolite *(24)*. However, a study by Minardi and Maltoni suggests that standard crocidolite is the most hazardous material used in the study, inducing mesothelioma in 97.5% of animals tested, followed by amosite (90%), Rhodesian chrysotile (82.5%), Canadian chrysotile (80%), and Californian chrysotile (72.5%) *(23)*.

Davis suggested that the hazard of a particular fiber (e.g., chrysotile, amosite, crocidolite) is related to the number of long fibers it contains *(24)*. Thus, chrysotile with over 60 million fibers >10 μm produced mesothelioma in 68% of injected animals at the 2.5-mg dose. By contrast, amosite with only 10 million fibers >10 μm induced mesothelioma in 59.4% and crocidolite with 9 million fibers >10 μm in 56.3% of animals at the same dose. Wagner similarly showed that the length of the crocidolite fiber is directly proportional to its tumorigenic ability *(21)*. Samples that were milled for 4 h and 8 h, and as a result contained far fewer crocidolite fibers >6.5 μm than 1-h and 2-h milled fibers, induced mesothelioma in 34% of the animals compared to 80% for the 1-h and 2-h group. A rat study by Miller found that injecting a dose containing 10^9 amosite particles >5 μm led to an incidence of mesothelioma in 88% of the animal group, confirming that a dose containing a large number of long fibers will be successful in promoting tumor growth *(25)*.

In the rat species, the appearance of effusions and solid-tumor nodules after inoculation is often associated with the development of mesothelioma. When these are present, the tumors have been characterized as predominantly biphasic and spindle-shaped (sarcomatous), but few reports indicate that all the patterns observed in humans—including tubular, papillary, solid, and spindle-cell—are possible *(23,25)*. In addition, several different patterns have been seen in the same tumor, and metastases are common.

Intraperitoneally injected rats had a mean survival time between 509 d and 1002 d. In general, there is a direct relationship between administered dose, the ability of the fiber to induce mesothelioma, and average survival time *(i.e., high doses and very toxic fiber administration resulted in a decrease of the life span of the animal)*. Amosite administration resulted in an average survival time between 462 and 889 d, crocidolite in 416–1002 d, and chrysotile in 476–903 d—all depending on the administered dose, type of chrysotile, and milling time *(23,27)*.

2.5. Intraperitoneal Asbestos Injection: Mice

Various rates of tumor induction have been reported in the murine mesothelioma model, ranging from 25–45% *(20,28)*. Davis reported tumor growth in 25% of Balb/c mice and 45% of CBA mice treated with Wittenoon George crocidolite *(28)*. A study on the carcinogenic potential of amosite, chrysotile, and calindra chrysotile by Suzuki *(20)* showed amosite to be the most mesotheliomatogenic fiber, inducing tumors in 40.5% of Balb/c mice, followed by Calidria chrysotile (25%) and standard chrysotile (0%) at the administered dose.

The relationship between fiber toxicity and number of long fibers contained, which has been observed in the rat mesothelioma model, holds true for the murine model as well. In the Suzuki study discussed here, amosite was the most mesotheliomatogenic fiber—causing tumors in 40% of the treated group—presumably because it had the highest percentage of long fibers (6% >7.5 μm). Calindra chrysotile, with the second highest percentage of long fibers (4.6% >5 μm), induced mesothelioma in just 25% of animals, and chrysotile with only 2% of fibers >3 μm was found to be nontumorigenic at the given dose *(20)*.

In the murine animal model, the latency period has been established at 7 mo *(20,28)*. It has been speculated that this period is shorter in the mouse than in many other species, because of the animal's relative short life span.

Ultrastructural analysis of mesothelioma in the mouse species provides a blurred picture on the predominant cell type. Davis reports that while all three histological forms of human malignant mesothelioma were present, as with the human disease, the majority of malignant cells identified in the ascites were epithelial tumors exhibiting typical mesothelial differentiation, with long, thin microvilli, intermediate filaments, numerous microscopic vesicles, and much glycogen *(28)*. No evidence of metastases was noted. Suzuki similarly notes the presence of ascites in most mesothelioma cases, but the vast majority of fibrous tumors and the small minority of biphasic tumors reported is in stark contrast with both the history of human disease and Davis' findings *(20)*. Tumors grew preferentially in the omentum, mesentery, serosae of the gastrointestinal and genital organs, the diaphragm, the capsule of liver and spleen, and the abdominal wall peritoneum.

Mesothelioma cell lines from rats and mice have been established in vitro, with the majority established in mice as described by Davis *(28)*. Mesothelial tumors of the Balb/c strain were more likely to be established than tumors of the CBA strain of mouse. All cell lines achieved greater than 32 passages, were in culture for at least 7 mo, and exhibited a wide range of morphologies ranging from stellate-shaped cells to fibroblast-like cells. No correlation was found between morphology and doubling time, which ranged from 16 h to 30 h. The tumorigenicity of all cell lines was tested by inoculation in syngeneic mice. The kinetics of tumor development varied substantially among cell lines, with the most tumorigenic lines (AB1 and AC29) producing ascites in 27 and 24 d, respectively, and solid tumors 34 and 25 d after subcutaneous (sc) inoculation. All cell lines produced solid-tumor growth, at times without concurrent ascite formation. In vivo aggressiveness did not correlate with in vitro morphology or growth rate.

2.6. Intrapleural Asbestos Injection

Because most human mesothelioma is manifested in the pleural cavity, the intrapleural mode of induction is cited as being more relevant to the human disease than studies done in the peritoneum. However, its applicability to the human disease fibers introduced in this manner still bypasses the body's natural defenses, and subjects mesothelial cells to doses of fiber that would not be encountered under normal circumstances with the human cases.

2.7. Intrapleural Asbestos Injection: Rat

Tumor induction rates appear to be somewhat lower in the pleura than the peritoneum, with chrysotile viewed as a more potent tumor initiator than crocidolite, inducing mesothelioma in 65% of injected animals compared to 45% induction for crocidolite *(23)*. Whitaker reports successful induction rates in 56% of the animals inoculated with Western Australian crocidolite *(26)*. Although few analyses have been performed to link the carcinogenicity of a fiber to its length, it is logical to assume that the same relationship holds true as with peritoneal studies. The time it takes to develop tumor in the pleura of rats is relatively long. Whitaker reports a latency of 56 wk in animals treated with Western Australia crocidolite asbestos. The average survival time is longer in animals afflicted with pleural mesothelioma than in their peritoneal counterparts, with pleurally injected rats surviving between 105 and 111 wk (23). Crocidolite administration resulted in an average survival time of 105 wk, and animals injected with Canadian chrysotile lived an average of 111 wk (23).

Malignant cell lines have been developed from rat pleural ascites. Whitaker reports establishing cell cultures in two of five pleural effusions for 2 and 8 mo (26). The presence of collagen fibers using using Gieson's stain. Examination of the cell junctions, profuse microvillous borders, and intermediate filaments further confirmed the mesothelial nature of the culture.

2.8. Inhalation of Asbestos in Animal Models

Inhalation studies offer the advantage of introducing the carcinogen through the only significant pathway for humans, because almost all exposure to asbestos in our species occurs through breathing. However, these studies are often expensive, pose a hazard to the researchers conducting them, and have a very low incidence of mesothelioma induction, which makes them impractical for discriminating the fibers' potential for mesothelioma production.

2.8.1. INHALATION STUDIES IN THE RAT

It has been known for some time that inhalation studies are not as efficient in producing mesothelioma as intracavital injections. Miller reported mesothelioma induction in 2 of 42 (5%) of animals, yet a study by Botham in which rats were exposed to high concentrations of Northwest Cape crocidolite failed to induce any mesothelioma in the animal group (25,29). In the Miller study, amosite asbestos with, a significant proportion of fibers >25 µm, was used to induce mesothelioma in 5% of the treated group.

2.8.2. INHALATION STUDIES: GUINEA PIG

A study by Botham et al. shows that West Cape crocidolite and Transvaal crocidolite are capable of producing mesothelioma in albino Guinea pigs (29).

2.8.3. INTRATRACHEAL ASBESTOS ADMINISTRATION

Intratracheal instillations are considered to be nonphysiological and unsuitable for risk characterization because of the frequent, uneven distribution of fibers within the different lobes. One common result of this mode of introduction is the formation of areas of greater deposition leading to high local doses and acute inflammatory responses. However, like intracavital injections, this method can be considered for comparative risk assessment among different fiber types.

2.8.4. INTRATRACHEAL ASBESTOS ADMINISTRATION: SYRIAN GOLDEN HAMSTER

There is some evidence that long fibers (i.e., fibers > 8 µm) are not required for the induction of mesothelioma in intratracheal insitllations. Mohr et al. reported an incidence of mesothelioma of 5.6% (8 of 142) in the Syrian golden hamsters after intratracheal instillations of crocidolite fibers, with 50% <2.1 µm and <0.2 µm in diameter (19).

Light microscopy observation has revealed tumors consisting of large, polyhedral cells of the epitheloid type, with abundant amphophylic cytoplasm and sharply defined cell contours (19). Areas of papillary formations have also been observed. Scanning electron microscopy analysis has shown individual, minute polypoid alterations, with surfaces composed of normal mesothelial cells, and polymorphic cells which varied in size and shape. The microvilli of these cells displayed clear pleomorphism.

3. SPONTANEOUS MODELS OF MESOTHELIOMA

Spontaneous mesotheliomas are generally rare in experimental animals. However, Fisher 344 rats have been reported to have a 3–4% natural occurrence of tumors by a number of investigators, and it is generally accepted that spontaneously occurring tumors are quite similar to those induced by asbestos. Tanigawa reported that sponta-neously induced mesothelial tumors were specific to males, with an incidence of 4.3%, or 17 of 395 *(30)*. The majority of tumors (16 of 17) were confined to the geni-tal serosa and peritoneum, with one tumor occurring in the pleural cavity. Expansion of the peritoneal cavity caused by ascites is typical in this disease, as is protrusion of the scrotum. Microscopically, the tumors are notable for complex papillary growth and sessile nodular growths resembling sarcomas. Immunohistochemical localization of keratin proteins and histological patterns of the tumors examined suggest that spontaneous mesothelioma essentially resembles the epithelial type of human mesothelioma.

4. OTHER AGENTS FOR ANIMAL PRODUCTION OF MESOTHELIOMA

4.1. Chemical

Although most cases of mesothelioma can be linked to asbestos exposure, some have not been linked to known asbestos exposure, which raises the question of whether mesothelioma can be caused in humans by agents other than asbestos, and whether other environmental agents can augment the effect of asbestos *(31)*.

Rice reports that the polycyclic aromatic hydrocarbon carcinogen 3-methylcholan-threne (MC) is capable of inducing mesothelioma when injected intragastrically in cer-tain strains of mice. The C3H strain was the most susceptible of the six strains tested, with a mesothelioma incidence of 39% (12 of 31 treated animals) and an average sur-vival time of 8.3 mo. The Balb/c strain had an incidence of 28% (9 of 32) and average survival of 10.4 mo. Because both groups of animals sustained high rates of peritoneal injury, there is some uncertainty as to whether the mesothelial proliferation was caused primarily by the mechanical insult caused by the 12 injections received by each group. A few of the mesotheliomas were predominantly mesothelial. However, most were mixed and fibrous in nature with epithelial elements. The neoplasms grew within the peritoneal cavity over the surfaces of the viscera, and were frequently invasive of other organs, including the diaphragm.

Methyl (acetoxymethyl) nitrosamine (DMN-OAc) has been established as an agent capable of inducing mesothelioma in male Sprague-Dawley and Buffalo rats. Berman and Rice report the induction of 25 testicular mesotheliomas in 78 treated rats (32%) *(32)*. It was notable that intraperitoneal (ip) administration of the chemical agent did not produce mesotheliomas in any other location except the testes, and there was no evidence of metastases or local invasion. Although some tumors contained massive amounts of stroma, there were no examples of the sarcomatoid variant of tumor found in humans among the examined mesotheliomas. All tumors examined stained positive by the colloidal iron method.

4.2. Man-Made Fibers

Experimental studies suggest that certain man-made fibers have a greater toxicity than naturally occurring asbestos fibers. This greater mesotheliomatogenic effect is believed to be a result of the greater proportion of long fibers contained in these materials and their long durability. In intracavital injection studies in rats, erionite-induced mesothelioma at rates of 54.5–93% of treated animals percentages considerably higher than the incidence produced by either amosite, crocidolite, or chrysotile (20,28). Suzuki suggests that erionite's toxicity is linked to its higher content of long fibers (4% >9.5 μm)—more than any of the tested asbestos fibers. The median survival time for the animals treated with erionite, which can be indicative of the toxicity of a fiber, was also sigificantly shorter (513) days for animals treated with erionite than for rats treated with crocidolite, chrysotile, and amosite (28). Davis suggests that doses of less than 160,000 fibers >8 μm seldom produce mesothelioma, and that about 600,000 fibers of this length are needed to produce substantial levels of mesothelioma. Ultrastructural and histological characteristics of erionite-induced mesothelioma were similar to those of asbestos fibers

Man-made vitreous fiber 21 (MMVF 21), or stonewool, has similarly been shown to be very mesotheliomatogenic. Miller reports a 95% incidence of mesothelioma in rats treated with MMVF 21 (vs 88% for amosite), and a mean survival time of 284 d (vs 509 d for amosite) (25). The results correlate well with the hypothesis that long fibers are more toxic than shorter ones—MMVF 21 contains more than seven fold more fibers >10 μm than amosite.

5. VIRAL-INDUCED MODELS OF MESOTHELIOMA

An association between mesothelioma and viruses is not new. Malignant mesotheliomas, immunohistochemically and architecturally identical to those seen in humans, have been induced in chickens when a DNA fragment of the oncogene of the rous sarcoma virus was introduced intraperitoneally (33). Most recently, however, our group was the first to report that 60% (25 of 48) of human mesotheliomas contain DNA for the amino terminus region of T-antigen a protein associated with various DNA viruses, including simian virus 40 (SV40), which is capable of causing malignant transformation (34). Humans were at least "exposed" to SV40 through the administration of SV40-contaminated polio vaccines between 1955 and 1963.

Simian virus 40 (SV40) is a DNA-tumor virus that infects monkeys and causes malignant transformation of hamster cells. SV40 produces two transforming proteins: the large T antigen, which is responsible for binding and inhibiting cellular pS3, and RB, and the small T antigen, which binds and inhibits cellular phosphatase (1A). In nonpermissive hosts, SV40 has been shown to be oncogenic (35). No productive infection and virions result in nonpermissive hosts. SV40 is capable of transforming a number of different mammalian cells in vitro. Murine cells transformed by SV40 infection in vitro are capable of producing lethal tumors in vivo when transplanted back into the syngeneic host. Thus, SV40 murine transformed cells can be oncogenic in syngeneic hosts, and the tumors induced in vivo express SV40 tumor-specific transplantation antigens. These transplantation antigens include SV40 large T-antigen and small T-antigen, both of which are derived from a single early gene-product transcript (36).

Newborn hamsters are also extremely susceptible to SV40-induced tumors. In 1962, Gerber and Kirschstein reported that SV40 induced ependymomas in hamsters and since that discovery, it has been known that wild-type SV40 is highly oncogenic in hamsters *(37)*. Newborn animals are particularly susceptible, and will develop fibrosarcomas at the injection site following sc inoculation of a low dose of SV40 *(38)*. When newborn hamsters are inoculated with intracerebral SV40, they develop ependymomas *(37)*. Weanling and adult animals may develop fibrosarcomas if injected subcutaneously with a high dose of virus ($>10^9$ plaque-forming units (pfu), but only with a low tumor incidence and after prolonged incubation periods *(39)*. When SV40 ($>10^{8.5}$ pfu) is injected *intravenously* into weanling hamsters, subjecting many cell types to high concentrations of virus, lymphocytic leukemia, lymphoma, and osteosarcoma will develop at sites distant from the injection *(40)*. Carcinomas—the most common tumors in humans—never develop following SV40 injection, suggesting that epithelial cells may be resistant to SV40 transformation.

These data indicate that only specific types of cells are susceptible to SV40 transformation: mesothelial cells, osteoblasts/osteocytes, macrophages, and B-lymphocytes, and that the specific routes of SV40 inoculation used apparently plays a key role in the induction of specific hamster tumors.

It is actually fortuitous that a *relationship between SV40 and mesothelioma was discovered in the hamster.* Lipotich reported the use of an SV40-induced hamster mesothelioma-cell line (800TU) *(41)*. Before this study, mesotheliomas were not observed following sc, intracerebral, and intravenous inoculation of SV40 in the hamster. Indeed, the development of the 800 TU line was an inoculation accident, for newborn hamsters in these experiments were injected between the scapulae with SV40, and all of the other animals in the experiment developed *in situ* fibrosarcomas. The development of the mesothelioma was caused by accidental pleural injection of the SV40 (Moyer RC, personal communication).

Stimulated by these isolated yet intriguing pieces of data, Carbone investigated the oncogenicity of wild-type SV40 and SV40 small t-deletion mutants when injected into the hearts, pleura, or peritoneum of 21-d-old hamsters *(42)*. Mesotheliomas that could be characterized as macroscopically, microscopically, ultramicroscopically, and histochemically identical to those seen in humans, developed within a 3-mo period in 30 of the 43 hamsters injected with wild-type SV40. All ($n=34$) the hamsters injected with the small t-mutant SV40 developed true histiocytic or B-cell lymphomas, yet only 1 developed a mesothelioma. The decreased oncogenicity in the deletion mutant group was puzzling, because small T-antigen binds and inhibits the activity of the cellular phosphatase 2A that will subsequently prevent dephosphorylation of large T-antigen and the *p53* protein product *(43,44)*. It is theorized, therefore, that in addition to physical binding between large T-antigen and the products of *p53* and retinoblastoma (Rb), alteration of the Rb and *p53* phosphorylation state by small T-antigen may be required to completely inactivate their function, and thus allow the cell to progress to S phase during which transformation could occur. Mesothelial cells may have a very low cycling rate, possibly making their transformation dependent on small t.

The SV40-induced hamster mesotheliomas spread along the pleural, pericardial, and peritoneal surfaces obliterating the cavities and infiltrating the diaphragm and the chest wall in the absence of distant metastases. Histologically, epithelial, spindle-cell, and more often mixed-type mesotheliomas are seen. Ultramicroscopically, the tumors and derived cell lines showed long, branching microvilli without core filaments, basal lamina, intracellular lumens, perinuclear tonofilaments, intercellular junctions, absence of secretory granules, and limited cytoplasmic organelles, especially rough endoplasmic reticulum. These mesotheliomas are associated with hyaluronic acid, contain cytokeratins, and are immunohistochemically similar to human mesotheliomas. Southern blot hybridization of the DNAs extracted from the tumors reveals SV40 DNA sequences, and the cell lines derived from these tumors contain and express the early region of SV40 DNA. Immunohistochemical staining of the cell lines and tumors reveals the presence of intranuclear T-antigen.

6. ORTHOTOPIC TRANSPLANTS AND XENOGRAFTS

Xenografts offer the advantage of producing mesothelial tumors in the animal model at a faster rate and with a higher success rate than asbestos animal models. Furthermore, the resulting tumors are of a similar histological type as their human counterparts and retain their functional and morphological features during several generations, and can therefore provide accurate information on the chemosensitivity of the human tumor.

The mouse species has been successfully used to replicate human malignant pleural mesothelioma. Chahinian reports the original transplant of human mesothelial tumor from two patients into nude mice of the Balb/c strain (45). Intraperitoneal (ip) transplants did not grow, but sc xenografts/implants were able to produce tumor in an average of 46 d in the animal. The tumor transplants of the first generation grew in 6 of 20 mice (30%), with a take-rate of implants of 53%. Overall, tumors grew in 52 of 80 mice (65%) in a total of 169 of 266 implants (multiple implants were made on the same animal). Tumor examination of the first- and second-generation xenografts confirmed their histological similarity to the original epithelial tumors.

Colt et al. commented on the implantation of intact human mesothelial tissue in the pleural space of four athymic nude mice and subcutaneously in another mouse (46). The sc implantation resulted in progressive tumor growth, with the tumor reaching a size of 10×12 mm. Of the four ip. mice, one died early, another at 162 d, and the remaining two mice were sacrificed at 180 d after implantation. Both of the sacrificed animals demonstrated tumor growth at the implantation site as well as at the visceral, diaphragmatic, and mediastinal pleural surfaces. No metastases to distant organs were noted a feature similar to the natural history of human malignant mesothelioma. In the human tumor, sections of pleural biopsies showed malignant neoplasms composed of epitheloid cells, which on immunohistochemical study demonstrated diffuse and strong positive stainings for cytokeratin, vimentin, and epithelial-membrane antigen, but tested negative for carcinoembryonic antigen and Leu M1. As a result, the neoplasm was classified as monophasic epithelial-type mesothelioma. In the mouse, the immunohistochemical profile characterized by positive stainings for vimentin and cytokeratin, and negative CEA and Leu M1 stainings, strongly pointed to the similarity between the human and animal tumor.

Rats have also been a species of choice for mesothelioma-cell transplants. Linden successfully inoculated athymic Rowett rats subcutaneously with a coarse cell suspension of mesothelioma cells from a human patient (47). The take-rate was 93% (13 of 14) in the initial passages (P) and 100% (192/192) in P3-P9. There was a decrease in the tumor-volume doubling (TD) time during the serial passage of rats from 6 d in P2 to 3 d in P9, with no further reduction noted in later passages. The average latency, measured by the time needed to reach a specified tumor volume, was found to decrease sharply from P2 to P12, but not thereafter. It took 36 d in P2 to reach a volume of 2cm3, and only 11–12 d in P10-P12. Morphological examination of the tumors revealed mesothelioma of an epithelial type. The histological pattern of the original tumor was retained in all xenograft generations of rats, with no differentiation noted.

Prewitt describe the orthotopic implantation of the tumor-cell line H-Meso 1 in pneumonectomized Fischer *nu/nu* rats (48). Tumor reproducibly filled the chest cavity 6 wk after implantation with 10^6 tumor cells, and were identical in histologic pattern to epithelioid mesothelioma.

There have been reports of transplants of mesothelioma cells from rat to rat (49). After the successful induction of mesothelioma in F344 rats with crocidolite fibers, the cell lines were cultured in vitro in RPMI-1640 and inoculated intrapleurally in F344 rats. The mesothelial origin of the cells was confirmed by the co-expression of keratin and vimentin, using an alkaline and anti-alkaline phosphatase. Polyclonal rabbit antibodies directed against human 56-kDa cytokeratin and monoclonal mouse anti-swine vimentin 57-kDa were also used.

There was a clear-cut dose-response relationship when several concentrations of cells were inoculated, with the largest dose of mesothelioma cells administered (5×10^6) able to induce the most tumors, as determined by chest radiographs performed on 15 and 30 d postinoculation. No rats showed abnormalities at 15 d postinoculation but by 30 d, most animals showed features suggesting massive tumor volumes. Most tumors predominantly invaded the mediastinum and pericardium, with diaphragm involvement, but no metastasis was noted.

Transplants of mesothelioma cells from hamster to hamster have been performed (50). In a study designed to test the usefulness of various chemotherapeutic agents against mesothelioma, Smith reports successfully transplanting mesothelioma induced by intrapleural injection of tremolite asbestos in one golden Lak:LVG Syrian hamster to others (50). Ascites were noted 76 d after transplant in the first generation of three hamsters that had received intraperitoneal injections of peritoneal effusions from the original animal, with two of the animals sacrificed on d 76 and the third dying on d 90. The tumor was carried through 39 serial transplant generations by ip injections. The average survival time was found to decrease with continuous passage, leading to the death of new hosts within 21–38 d, and an average survival time of 28–32 d days depending on the generation examined. The transplantable tumor line was defined as mesothelioma 10–24. Tumors of animals bearing transplants continued to resemble the epithelial nature of the mesothelioma in the original animal.

CONCLUSIONS

A number of animal models for the investigation of mesothelioma are now available. These models have been used in a number of preclinical models for the treatment of mesothelioma, including gene therapy with suicide genes (51–54), anti-sense gene therapy (55), re-expression gene therapy (56), photodynamic therapy (57,58), immunotherapy (59–64), and in vivo chemosensivity (65–68). Many cell lines are available, and the models are reproducible.

REFERENCES

1. Antman KH, Pass HI, Schiff PB. Benign and malignant mesothelioma. In: De Vita VT Jr, Hellman S, Rosenberg SA, eds. *Cancer: Principles and Practice of Oncology,* 5th ed. Lippincott-Raven, Philadelphia, PA, 1997, pp. 1853–1878.
2. Kaiser LR. New therapies in the treatment of malignant pleural mesothelioma. *Semin Thorac Cardiovasc Surg* 1997; 9:383–390.
3. Mark EJ, Yokoi T. Absence of evidence for a significant background incidence of diffuse malignant mesothelioma apart from asbestos exposure. In: Landrigen J, Kazemi H, eds. The Third Wave of Asbestos Disease: Exposure to Asbestos in Place. *Ann NY Acad Sci* 1960; pp. 196–204.
4. Wagner JC, Sleggs CA, Marchand P. Diffuse pleural mesothelioma and asbestos exposure in the North Western Cape Province. *Br J Ind Med* 1960; 17:260–271.
5. Selikoff IJ, Hammond EC, Seidman H. Latency of asbestos disease among insulation workers in the United States and Canada. *Cancer* 1980; 46:2736–2740.
6. Weitzman SA, Graceffa P. Asbestos catalyzes hydroxyl and superoxide radical generation from hydrogen peroxide. *Arch Biochem Biophys* 1984; 228:373–376.
7. Jaurand MC, Fleury J, Monchaux G, Nebut M, Bignon J. Pleural carcinogenic potency of mineral fibers (asbestos attapulgite) and their toxicity on cultured cells. *J Natl Cancer Inst* 1987; 79:797–804.
8. Weissman LB, Antman KH. Incidence, presentation and promising new treatments for malignant mesothelioma. *Oncology* 1989; 3:67–72.
9. Mossman BT, Bignon J, Corn M, Seaton A, Gee JBL. Asbestos: scientific developments and implications for public policy. *Science* 1990; 247:294–301.
10. Roggli VL, Santillppo F, Shelburne J. Mesothelioma. In: Roggli VL, Greenberg SD, Pratt PC, eds. Pathology of Asbestos and Associated Diseases. Little Brown Co., Boston, MA, 1995, pp. 383–391.
11. Mossman B, Light W, Wei E. Asbestos: mechanisms of toxicity and carcinogenicity in the respiratory tract. *Annu Rev Pharmacol Toxicol* 1983; 23:595–615.
12. Stanton MF, Layard M, Tegeris A, Miller E, May M, Morgan E, et al. Relation of particle dimension to carcinogenicity in amphibole asbestoses and other fibrous minerals. *J Natl Cancer Inst* 1981; 67:965–975.
13. Leveston SA, McKeel DW Jr, Buckley PG, et al. Acromegaly and Cushing's syndrome associated with a foregut carcinoid. *J Clin Endocrinol Met* 1981; 53:682–689.
14. Huncharek MD. Changing risk groups for malignant mesothelioma. *Cancer* 1992; 69:2704–2711.
15. Leigh J, Ferguson DA, Ackad M, Thompson R. Lung asbestos fiber content and mesothelioma cell type, site, and survival. *Cancer* 1991; 68:135–141.
16. Rogers AJ, Leigh J, Berry G, Ferguson DA, Mulder HB, Ackad M. Relationship between lung asbestos fiber type and concentration and relative risk of mesothelioma. *Cancer* 1991; 67:1912–1920.
17. Murai Y, Kitagawa M. Asbestos fiber analysis in 27 malignant mesothelioma cases. *Am J Ind Med* 1992; 22:193–207.
18. Mowé G, Gylseth B, Hartveit F, Skaug V. Fiber concentration in lung tissue of patients with malignant mesothelioma. *Cancer* 1985; 56:1089–1093.
19. Mohr U, Potts F, Vonnahme F.-J. Morphological aspects of mesotheliomas after intratracheal instillations of fibrous dusts in Syrian golden hamsters. *Exp Pathol* 1984; 26:179–183.
20. Suzuki Y, Kohyama M. Malignant mesothelioma induced by asbestos and zeolite in the mouse peritoneal cavity. *Environ Res* 1984; 35:277–292.
21. Wagner JC, Griffiths DM, Hill RJ. The effect of fibre size on the *in vivo* activity of UICC crocidolite. *Br J Cancer* 1984; 49:453–458.
22. Hill RJ, Edwards RE, Carthew P. Early changes in the pleural mesothelium following intrapleural inoculation of the mineral fibre erionite and the subsequent development of mesotheliomas. *J Exp Pathol* 1990; 71:105–118.
23. Minardi F, Maltoni C. Results of recent experimental research on the carcinogenicity of natural and modified asbestos. *Ann Acad Sci* 1988; 534:754–761.
24. Davis J, Bolton R, Miller B, Niven K. Mesothelioma dose response following intraperitoneal injection of mineral fibres. *Int J Exp Pathol* 1991; 72:263–274.
25. Miller G, Searl A, Davis J, Kenneth D. Influence of fibre length, dissolution and biopersistence on the production of mesothelioma in the rat peritoneal cavity. *Ann Occup Hyg* 1999; 43:155–166.
26. Whitaker D, Shilkin KB, Walters MN. Cytologic and tissue culture characteristics of asbestos-induced mesothelioma in rats. *Acta Cytol* 1984; 28:185–189.

27. Wagner JC, Griffiths DM, Hill RJ. The effect of fibre size on the in vivo activity of UICC crocidolite. *Br J Cancer* 1984; 48:453–458.

28. Davis MR, Manning LS, Whitaker D, Garlepp MJ, Robinson BW. Establishment of a murine model of malignant mesothelioma. *Int J Cancer* 1992; 52:881–886.

29. Botham S, Holt P. The effects of inhaled crocidolites from Transvaal and North-west Cape mines on the lungs of rats and guinea-pigs. *Br J Exp Pathol* 1972; 53:612–620.

30. Tanigawa H, Onodera H, Maekawa A. Spontaneous mesotheliomas in Fischer rats—a histological and electron microscopic study. *Toxicol Pathol* 1987; 15:157–163.

31. Rice JM, Kovatch RM, Anderson LM. Intraperitoneal mesotheliomas induced in mice by a polycyclic aromatic hydrocarbon. *J Toxicol Environ Health* 1989; 27:153–160.

32. Berman J, Rice J. Mesotheliomas and proliferative lesions of the testicular mesothelium produced in Fischer, Sprague-Dawley and Buffalo rats by methyl(acetoxymethyl)nitrosamine (DMN-OAc). *Vet Pathol* 1979; 16:574–582.

33. England JM, Panella MJ, Ewert DL, Halpern MS. Induction of a diffuse mesothelioma in chickens by intraperitoneal inoculation of v-*src* DNA. *Virology* 1991; 182:423–429.

34. Carbone M, Pass HI, Rizzo P, Marinetti M, Di Muzio M, Mew DJY et al. Simian virus 40-like DNA sequences in human pleural mesothelioma. *Oncogene* 1994; 9:1781–1790.

35. Eddy BE. Simian virus 40: an oncogenic virus. *Prog Exp Tumor Res* 1964; 4:1–26.

36. Tevethia SS. Immunology of simina virus 40. In: Klein G, ed. Viral Oncology. Raven Press, New York, NY, 1980, pp. 581–601.

37. Gerber P, Kirschstein RL. SV40-induced ependymomas in newborn hamsters. *Virology* 1962; 18:582–588.

38. Lewis AM Jr, Martin RG. Oncogenicity of simian virus 40 deletion mutants that induce altered 17-kilodalton t-proteins. *Proc Natl Acad Sci USA* 1979; 76:4299–4302.

39. Allison AC, Chesterman FC, Baron S. Induction of tumors in adult hamsters with simian virus 40. *J Natl Cancer Inst* 1967; 38:567–577.

40. Diamandopoulous GT. Leukemia, lymphoma and osteosarcoma induced in the Syrian Golden hamster by simian virus 40. *Science* 1972; 176:73–75.

41. Lipotich G, Moyer MP, Moyer RC. Rescue of SV40 following transfection of TC7 cells with cellular DNAs containing complete and partial SV40 genomes. *Mol Gen Genet* 1982; 186:78–81.

42. Cicala C, Pompetti F, Carbone M. SV40 induces mesotheliomas in hamsters. *Am J Pathol* 1993; 142:1524–1533.

43. Scheidtmann KH, Mumby MC, Rundell K, Walter G. Dephosphorylation of simian virus 40 large-T antigen and *p53* protein by protein phosphatase 2A: inhibition by small-t antigen. *Mol Cell Biol* 1991; 11:1996–2003.

44. Carbone M, Hauser J, Carty MC, Rundell K, Dixon K, Levine AS. Simian virus 40 small t antigen inhibits SV40 DNA replication in vitro. *J Virol* 1992; 66:1804–1808.

45. Chahinian AP, Beranek JT, Suzuki Y, Bekesi JG, Wisniewski L, Selikoff IJ, et al. Transplantation of human malignant mesothelioma into nude mice. *Cancer Res* 1980; 40:181–185.

46. Colt H, Astoui P, Wang Xiaoen, Yi E, Boutin C. Clinical course of human epithelial-type malignant pleural mesothelioma replicated in an orthotopic-transplant nude mouse model. *Anticancer Res* 1996; 16:633–639.

47. Linden C.-J. Progressive growth of a human pleural mesothelioma xenografted to athymic rats and mice. *Br J Cancer* 1988; 58:614–618.

48. Prewitt TW, Lubensky IA, Pogrebniak HW, Pass HI. Orthotopic implantation of mesothelioma in the pneumonectomized immune-deficient rat: a model for innovative therapies [letter]. *Int J Cancer* 1993; 55:877–880.

49. Le Pimpec-Barthes, Bernard I, Alsamad Abd. Pleuro-pulmonary tumours detected by clinical and chest X-ray analyses in rats transplanted with mesothelioma cells. *Br J Cancer* 1999; 81:1344–1350.

50. Smith W, Huhert DD, Holiat SM, Sobel HJ, and Davis S. An experimental model for treatment of mesothelioma. *Cancer* 1981; 47:658–663.

51. Smythe WR, Kaiser LR, Hwang HC, Amin KM, Pilewski JM, Eck et al. Successful adenovirus-mediated gene transfer in an in vivo model of human malignant mesothelioma. *Ann Thorac Surg* 1994; 57:1395–1401.

52. Smythe WR, Hwang HC, Elshami AA, Amin KM, Eck SL, Davidson BL et al. Treatment of experimental human mesothelioma using adenovirus transfer of the herpes simplex thymidine kinase gene. *Ann Surg* 1995; 222:78–86.

53. Hwang HC, Smythe WR, Elshami AA, Kucharczuk JC, Amin KM, Williams JP, et al. Gene therapy using adenovirus carrying the herpes simplex-thymidine kinase gene to treat in vivo models of human malignant mesothelioma and lung cancer. *Am J Respir Cell Mol Biol* 1995; 13:7–16.

54. Kucharczuk JC, Elshami AA, Zhang HB, Smythe WR, Hwang HC, Tomlinson JS, et al. Pleural-based mesothelioma in immune competent rats: a model to study adenoviral gene transfer. *Ann Thorac Surg* 1995; 60:593–597.

55. Pass HI, Mew DJ, Carbone M, Matthews WA, Donington JS, Baserga R, et al. Inhibition of hamster mesothelioma tumorigenesis by an antisense expression plasmid to the insulin-like growth factor-1 receptor. *Cancer Res* 1996; 56:4044–4048.

56. Frizelle SP, Grim J, Zhou J, Gupta P, Curiel DT, Geradts J, et al. Re-expression of p16INK4a in mesothelioma cells results in cell cycle arrest, cell death, tumor suppression and tumor regression. *Oncogene* 1998; 16:3087–3095.

57. Feins RH, Hilf R, Ross H, Gibson SL. Photodynamic therapy for human malignant mesothelioma in the nude mouse. *J Surg Res* 1990; 49:311–314.

58. Foster TH, Gibson SL, Raubertas RF. Response of Photofrin-sensitised mesothelioma xenografts to photodynamic therapy with 514 nm light. *Br J Cancer* 1996; 73:933–936.

59. Christmas TI, Manning LS, Garlepp MJ, Musk AW, Robinson BW. Effect of interferon-alpha 2a on malignant mesothelioma. *J Interferon Res* 1993; 13:9–12.

60. Leong CC, Marley JV, Loh S, Milech N, Robinson BW, Garlepp MJ. Transfection of the gene for B7-1 but not B7-2 can induce immunity to murine malignant mesothelioma. *Int J Cancer* 1997; 71:476–482.

61. Caminschi I, Venetsanakos E, Leong CC, Garlepp MJ, Scott B, Robinson BW. Interleukin-12 induces an effective antitumor response in malignant mesothelioma. *Am J Respir Cell Mol Biol* 1998; 19:738–746.

62. Astoul P, Boutin C. [An experimental model of pleural cancer. Value of orthotopic implantation of human tumor tissue in nude mice]. *Rev Mal Respir* 1997; 14:355–362.

63. Bielefeldt-Ohmann H, Fitzpatrick DR, Marzo AL, Jarnicki AG, Musk AW, Robinson BW. Potential for interferon-alpha-based therapy in mesothelioma: assessment in a murine model. *J Interferon Cytokine Res* 1995; 15:213–223.

64. Ohnuma T, Szrajer L, Holland JF, Kurimoto M, Minowada J. Effects of natural interferon alpha, natural tumor necrosis factor alpha and their combination on human mesothelioma xenografts in nude mice. *Cancer Immunol Immunother* 1993; 36:31–36.

65. Chahinian AP, Norton L, Holland JF, Szrajer L, Hart RD. Experimental and clinical activity of mitomycin C and *cis*-diamminedichloroplatinum in malignant mesothelioma. *Cancer Res* 1984; 44:1688–1692.

66. Sklarin NT, Chahinian AP, Feuer EJ, Lahman LA, Szrajer L, Holland JF. Augmentation of activity of cis-diamine-dichloroplatinum (II) and mitomycin-C by interferon in human malignant mesothelioma xenografts in nude mice. *Cancer Res* 1988; 48:64–67.

67. Roboz J, Chahinian AP, Holland JF, Silides D, Azrajer L. Early diagnosis and monitoring of transplanted human malignant mesothelioma by serum hyaluronic acid. *J Natl Cancer Inst* 1989; 81:924–928.

68. Chahinian AP, Mandeli JP, Gluck H, Naim H, Teirstein AS, Holland JF. Effectiveness of cisplatin, paclitaxel, and suramin against human malignant mesothelioma xenografts in athymic nude mice. *J Surg Oncol* 1998; 67:104–111.

28 SCID Mouse Models of Human Leukemia and Lymphoma as Tools for New Agent Development

Fatih M. Uckun, MD, PhD
and Martha G. Sensel, PhD

CONTENTS

1. INTRODUCTION

The severe combined immunodeficiency (SCID) CB-17 mouse, which lacks functional B- and T-cells and is therefore unable to reject allogeneic or xenogeneic tumor-cell grafts, provides a unique model system for investigating the engraftment and proliferation of normal and neoplastic human cells. *(1)*. Early studies by Kamel-Reid et al. *(2)* and Cesano et al. *(3)* demonstrated that human leukemia cells could cause overt leukemia in SCID mice. In a subsequent study by Kamel-Reid et al. *(4)*, leukemic cells obtained at diagnosis from patients who remained relapse-free did not engraft or were detected only in low numbers in SCID mice, whereas leukemic cells from patients who relapsed engrafted in multiple organs and caused the SCID mice to die within 4 mo. These data provided the first evidence that the ability of a leukemic cell to grow in the SCID mouse may be correlated with patient prognosis. SCID mice have now been used extensively to examine biological characteristics of neoplastic human hematopoietic cells. For example, engraftment and proliferation in SCID mice has been demonstrated for primary cells and cell lines derived from subsets of patients with various forms of leukemia, including acute lymphoblastic leukemia (ALL), acute myeloblastic leukemia

From: *Tumor Models in Cancer Research*
Edited by: B. A. Teicher © Humana Press Inc., Totowa, NJ

(AML), chronic lymphocytic (CLL), and chronic myelocytic leukemia (CML) *(6–10)*, as well as various forms of lymphoma, including Burkitt's lymphoma, T-cell lymphoma, non-Hodgkin's B-cell lymphoma, and CD30[+] anaplastic large-cell lymphoma *(11–17)*. The SCID mouse model therefore provides a system for studying biological heterogeneity of leukemias, for predicting patient outcome, and for assessing the toxicity and efficacy of new treatment modalities.

2. SCID MOUSE MODELS OF PEDIATRIC ALL

ALL is the most common form of childhood cancer, accounting for approx 19% of all cancers in children less than 20 yr of age *(18)*. ALL is a biologically heterogeneous disease marked by a plethora of immunophenotypic, cytogenetic, and molecular genetic features. Leukemic cells from the majority (approx 85%) of pediatric ALL patients express the B-lineage-associated lymphoid differentiation antigens CD19 and CD24 *(19–22)*. Leukemic cells from approx 15% of pediatric ALL patients express the T-lineage associated lymphoid differentiation antigens CD2, CD5, and CD7. According to National Cancer Institute (NCI) risk criteria *(23)*, approx 60% of children are designated as having standard risk ALL (age 1–9 yr and white blood cell (WBC) <50,000/μL) and nearly 40% of patients are designated as having poor-risk ALL (≥10 yr of age with WBC count ≥50,000/μL). Infants <1 yr of age represent approx 3% of all patients, and form a distinct classification category *(23)*. Recurrent chromosomal translocations that define subsets of patients with increased risk of treatment failure include t(9;22)(q34;q11), t(4;11)(q21;q23), or t(1;19)(q23;p13) *(24–27)*. The intensive risk-adjusted therapies of the children's cancer group (CCG) have resulted in favorable 5-yr event-free survival (EFS) outcomes approximating 75% for standard risk B-lineage patients and 65% for poor-risk B-lineage patients *(28)*. Despite the gains achieved with contemporary therapy programs, relapse continues to be the major cause of treatment failure for the remaining 25–35% of ALL patients. Thus, a major current challenge is the identification of biologically defined subsets of patients currently designated as lower risk, whose outcome may be improved by assignment to more intensive treatment programs or introduction of alternative treatment modalities.

As a first step in using the SCID mouse model for these goals, we developed several SCID mouse models of higher risk B-lineage leukemia *(9,10,29,30)*. In brief, the methods utilized for these experiments involved intravenous (iv) tail-vein injection of leukemic cells into pathogen-free 7–10-wk-old CB-17 SCID mice, followed by close monitoring of animals for signs of tumors and death *(9,10)*. Confirmation of the human origin of the leukemic-cell infiltrate was accomplished using multiparameter flow cytometry with an anti-CD19 monoclonal antibody (MAb) and polymerase chain reaction (PCR) using a human β-globin gene probe *(9,10)*. Necropsies were performed at the time of death to assess the extent of leukemic engraftment. Initially, we used the highly aggressive CD10[+] cytoplasmic (IgM)[+] NALM-6 human pre-B ALL cell line to establish the feasibility of the model, and to carry out preliminary in vivo testing of novel immunotoxins directed against specific forms of leukemia *(10)*. These experiments showed that injection of 1×10^6 (NALM)-6 cells caused paraplegia in the majority of mice followed by disseminated and fatal leukemia in all mice. Histopathologic and immunohistochemical analyses indicated the presence of diffuse leukemic infiltrates in multiple organs, including bone marrow, bone, lymph nodes, spleen, liver, bladder, colon, skeletal muscle, and brain.

In subsequent experiments, we demonstrated that primary human leukemia cells from children with the higher risk t(1;19)(q23;p13)$^+$ ALL or t(4;11)(q21;q23)$^+$ ALL could engraft and cause disseminated leukemia in SCID mice. In the case of t(1;19)$^+$ leukemia, there was heterogeneity in the pattern and extent of engraftment. Primary blast cells from 6 of 10 patients caused disseminated leukemia in SCID mice, whereas cells from four patients either did not engraft or only partially engrafted *(30)*. Interestingly, outcome appeared to be worse for the patients whose leukemic cells caused disseminated disease in SCID mice compared with that of patients whose cells did not cause disseminated disease in SCID mice. Similarly, in the case of t(4;11)$^+$ leukemia, blast cells from eight of twelve patients caused overt disseminated leukemia, and cells from four patients caused only occult leukemia that was detectable only by PCR assays *(29)*. Outcome appeared to be worse for the eight patients whose leukemia caused overt disease, compared with that of the patients whose leukemia caused occult disease in SCID mice.

We then demonstrated that the ability of leukemic cells to grow in SCID mice predicted relapse for a group of 42 very high-risk {age <1 yr or ≥10 yr; WBC count ≥50,000/µL; or presence of a t(9;22); a t(4;11), or a t(1;11)} B-lineage ALL patients *(31)*. Although interpatient variation existed with respect to extent of leukemic-cell engraftment and outgrowth, 5-yr EFS outcome was significantly worse for patients whose cells caused overt leukemia in SCID mice, compared to those whose cells did not cause histopathologically detectable disease (29.5% vs 94.7%, respectively: *p* <0.0001).

More recently, we have used the SCID mouse model to investigate whether in vivo engraftment and proliferation of primary leukemic cells from larger cohorts of children with ALL could predict outcome and identify patients who might benefit from more or less intensive or alternative therapy. Primary leukemic cells from 681 children with newly diagnosed B-lineage ALL treated on Children's Cancer Group protocols were evaluated for their ability to cause overt leukemia in SCID mice *(32)*. The majority of patients (66%) studied were classified as NCI standard risk. Leukemic blasts from 104 of 681 patients (15%) engrafted and proliferated in one or more SCID mouse organs, whereas primary cells from the remaining patients failed to engraft. Among mice with overt human B-lineage leukemia, the primary organs affected were the bone marrow, liver, spleen, thymus, lung, and kidney. Disseminated disease involving six or more organs was observed in 22 cases. Interestingly, patients whose cells caused overt leukemia in SCID mice (SCID$^+$ patients) were more likely to be classified as NCI poor-risk than patients whose leukemic blasts did not cause overt leukemia (SCID$^-$) mice, but other presenting features, including early response to therapy and a highly significant prognostic factor in childhood ALL *(33)*, were similar for SCID$^+$ and SCID$^-$ patients. Overall, EFS outcome 3 yr from study entry was similar for SCID$^+$ and SCID$^-$ patients (*p* = 0.24). Interestingly, poorer EFS was observed for SCID$^+$ patients whose cells caused leukemic infiltration into skeletal muscle (*p* = 0.0003), or kidney (*p* = 0.05), compared with EFS of SCID$^-$ patients. These findings suggested that infiltration of skeletal muscle by primary leukemia from adjacent bone marrow may reflect a biologically more aggressive form of the disease. The lack of overall difference in outcome in this study contrasts with the data reported for the very high-risk subset of ALL patients. This difference could be attributable to the lower numbers of patients with very high-risk features in the more recent study, and to the overall improved outcome achieved by both standard and higher-risk patients on the more recent CCG studies *(34–38)*. T-lineage ALL was previously shown to predict poorer outcome compared with that of pediatric B-lineage ALL patients *(19,20,39–49)*. Therefore, we also developed a SCID mouse model of human T-lineage ALL and examined the prognostic significance of engraftment primary leukemic cells from T-lineage ALL patients *(50)*. Among 88 T-lineage ALL patients, 24 (27%) were SCID$^+$. The SCID$^+$ patients were similar to SCID$^-$ patients with respect to presenting clinical features. SCID$^+$ and SCID$^-$ patients had similar 2-yr EFS ($p = 0.2$) and overall survival ($p = 0.36$). Notably, however, among the subset of T-lineage patients with a rapid early marrow response to treatment (<25% blasts in the marrow at d 7 of induction), those who were SCID$^+$ had significantly worse outcome than those who were SCID$^-$ ($p = 0.06$; relative risk = 3.06). These data suggest that engraftment into SCID mice may identify a subset of T-lineage ALL patients who are at increased risk of treatment failure. The lack of overall difference in outcome for SCID$^+$ vs SCID$^-$ T-lineage ALL patients may be a result of the improved outcome now achieved by T-lineage patients enrolled on CCG and other cooperative group trials *(28,51–56)*.

Infants with ALL represent a unique disease category with a very poor outcome *(55,57–60)*. Most infants have unfavorable cytogenetic features, particularly, a t(4;11)(q21;q23), and are more susceptible to therapy-induced toxicity than older children. We recently established a SCID mouse model for infant ALL *(61)*. Primary leukemic blasts from 13 infants were tested for their ability to cause overt leukemia in SCID mice. Nearly all patients had chromosomal translocations, including five cases with a t(4;11)(q21;q23) and two with t(11;19)(q23;p13). Nine of the 13 patients had the unfavorable CD10$^-$ immunophenotype and most had WBC counts ≥150,000/μL. Eight of 13 patients were found to be SCID$^+$. Among these eight, nearly all were either CD10$^-$ or had an 11q23 rearrangement. Six of the 8 SCID$^+$ patients relapsed, and of the two who remained in remission, one received a bone-marrow transplant. There were also two relapses among the five SCID$^-$ patients. These data establish the feasibility of the SCID mouse model of infant leukemia, but larger numbers of infants must be studied to determine the true prognostic significance of infant leukemic-cell growth in this system.

The SCID mouse model also provides a means for comparing biologically distinct forms of leukemia. For example, we have found distinct engraftment and growth patterns in for primary leukemic cells from children with either t(1;19)$^+$/E2A-PBX1$^+$ or t(9;22)$^+$/BCR-ABL$^+$ ALL.[62] Leukemic cells from 13 of 24 t(1;19)+/E2A-PBX1+ patients caused overt leukemia in SCID mice. All 13 mice had microscopic lesions; organs involved were bone marrow, brain, heart, gut, liver, kidney, lung, ovary, pancreas, skeletal muscle, spleen, and thymus. Six of the 13 cases had macroscopic lesions, with involvement of multiple sites, including the liver, spleen, thymus, kidney, and abdomen in some mice. By comparison, leukemic cells from only 5 of 20 t(9;22)$^+$/BCR-ABL$^+$ patients caused overt leukemia in SCID mice. All five mice had microscopic lesions in the bone marrow, whereas only one mouse had evidence of macroscopic lesions. Thus, the engraftment of (1;19)$^+$/E2A-PBX1$^+$ leukemic cells differed markedly from that of t(9;22)$^+$/BCR-ABL$^+$ leukemic cells because of the lack of involvement of major organs with the latter. These data illustrate the biological heterogeneity of pediatric ALL and suggest that differential engraftment and proliferation in vivo may contribute to the prognosis of patients with (1;19)$^+$/E2A-PBX1$^+$ or t(9;22)$^+$/BCR-ABL$^+$ ALL.

Fewer studies have examined SCID models of adult ALL. Jeha et al. *(63)* reported that engraftment and proliferation in SCID mice of leukemic cells from 10 of 13 adults with ALL-engrafted cells retained the immunophenotype or cytogenetic feature of the injected cells, and transplantation of engrafted human leukemia cells into recipient mice resulted in consistent engraftment. In contrast to our studies with pediatric ALL, leukemic-cell engraftment in the studies of Jeha et al. required 10-fold more leukemic cells and pretreatment of mice with cyclophosphamide. Steele et al. *(64)* reported engraftment of T-lineage ALL cells for 12 of 19 patients (16 adults and 3 children). Survival was shorter for patients whose cells engrafted compared with that of patients whose cells did not engraft ($p < 0.01$), suggesting that the SCID model may identify a subset of higher risk T-lineage ALL patients. Interestingly, however, leukemic blasts from all 19 patients were able to engraft in a nonobese diabetic (NOD)-SCID mouse, which is more immunocompromised than the SCID mouse. Palucka et al. reported that mice inoculated with primary ALL blasts obtained from patients at the time of relapse had a shorter survival than mice inoculated with primary blasts obtained from the same patients at diagnosis ($p = 0.0002$) *(65)*.

Taken together, the collective data described here suggest that the SCID mouse provides a unique model that can identify subsets of ALL patients with increased risk of treatment failure, and can provide clues to the biological heterogeneity of ALL. Reliable data on the prognostic significance of the growth of human leukemias in SCID mice must be obtained, however, using large cohorts of patients.

3. SCID MOUSE MODELS OF HUMAN MYELOID LEUKEMIA

Acute and chronic forms of myeloid leukemia (AML, CML, and CLL) occur in significant numbers of adults and children, and AML represents the most common leukemia in adults and the second most common from of leukemia in children *(18,66)*. Despite recent gains in the treatment of pediatric AML, multi-agent chemotherapy regimens remain unable to cure more than one-half of all AML patients *(67–71)*. The use of myeloablative chemotherapy and bone-marrow transplantation has resulted in only modest improvement in survival *(72–74)*. Development of SCID mouse models of these forms of leukemia, therefore, would provide a powerful tool for in vivo testing of novel drug combinations and new therapeutic agents. Initial studies that sought to develop a SCID mouse model of human AML suggested that AML cell lines—but not primary leukemic cells from AML patients—could engraft and cause disseminated disease in SCID mice *(75–79)*. Primary AML blasts failed to engraft in SCID mice, even when immunosuppressive regimens or sublethal irradiation were used *(75,77,78,80)* Sawyers et al *(79)* reported growth of primary AML cells inoculated into the kidney capsule of SCID mice, but only local growth, not disseminated disease, was observed. In a few studies, primary leukemic cells from some patients with newly diagnosed or relapsed AML were able to cause disseminated disease *(76,81)*. Subsequently, Lapidot et al. *(82)* reported that iv injection coupled with administration of a fusion protein consisting of granulocyte-macrophage colony-stimulating factor (GM-CSF) and interleukin (IL)-3 allowed reproducible engraftment and proliferation of primary AML cells in sublethally irradiated SCID mice. Additional experiments indicated that CD34$^+$CD38$^-$ AML cells,—termed AML-initiating cells—were required for engraftment and proliferation (82). In contrast to these studies, we have established a SCID mouse model of pediatric AML without the use of cytokines (83). In our studies, primary blasts from children with newly diagnosed t(8;21)⁺, inv(16)⁺, or t(9;11)⁺ AML that were intravenously injected into sublethally irradiated SCID mice engrafted and proliferated in multiple organs, including the bone marrow and thymus.

Namikawa et al. (84) have employed a distinct model, the SCID-hu mouse, (85) to overcome the poor engraftment and proliferation of AML cells in SCID mice. In this system, human fetal long-bone fragments are implanted into SCID mice 6–8 wk prior to inoculation with leukemic cells. Leukemic cells then are injected directly into the human fetal bone grafts. In the studies by Namikawa et al. myeloid leukemias from 7 of 8 patients engrafted and proliferated within the human fetal bone grafts of SCID-hu mice, but did not spread to the mouse bone marrow (84). The human leukemias grown in these SCID-hu mice could be transferred to a secondary SCID-hu donor and still retain their original phenotypic and morphologic features.

Leukemic cell lines established from patients with CML in blast crisis (76,79,80,86–88), as well as primary leukemic cells from patients with CML in blast crisis (76,89,90), have been shown to cause disseminated disease in sublethally irradiated SCID mice. In contrast, leukemic cells from patients in chronic phase CML are much less likely to engraft and cause disseminated disease (79,87,88,91). For example, Sawyers et al. observed that whereas leukemic cells from two of two patients in blast crisis exhibited invasive growth with infiltration of the bone marrow, peripheral blood, and other organs, cells from only two of six patients in chronic phase of CML caused myeloid tumors and both were localized to the site of injection without spreading to surrounding tissues (79). Sirard et al. reported that bone marrow or peripheral blood cells obtained from 9 of 12 patients in chronic phase CML were able to engraft in sublethally irradiated SCID mice (91). Notably, however, the majority of engrafted cells obtained during the chronic phase were Philadelphia chromosome-negative normal cells, implying that normal myeloid-precursor proliferation was favored, whereas engrafted cells from CML in blast crisis were exclusively leukemic. The administration of exogenous cytokines had no effect on engraftment of cells obtained from patients in chronic-phase CML. Both Dazzi et al. and McGuirk et al. reported that blast-phase CML-cell lines grew rapidly in bone marrow and spleen and caused disseminated disease in SCID mice, whereas chronic-phase cell lines grew only transiently and failed to cause disseminated disease (87,88). These models appeared to recapitulate the kinetics of CML in patients and provide a model for studying CML biology in vivo.

Lewis et al (92) established a mouse model of chronic phase CML using the NOD-SCID mouse. Peripheral blood cells from patients with newly diagnosed chronic-phase CML were infused into the tail vein of sublethally irradiated NOD-SCID mice. CML cells engrafted in the bone marrow of 84% of the mice; 60% of these mice also showed engraftment of CML cells in the spleen. Administration of recombinant stem-cell factor, but not granulocyte colony-stimulating factor (G-CSF) or GM-CSF, enhanced engraftment. As was the case in the study by Sirard et al. (91), engrafted human cells were both normal and leukemic cells, with a median of 35% leukemic cells. Additional experiments showed that engraftment was restricted to CD34⁺ cells.

SCID models of other myeloid diseases also have been described. Lapidot et al. (89) observed disseminated human leukemia in SCID mice inoculated with primary cells from patients with juvenile chronic myelogenous leukemia (JCML). Bone marrow, peripheral blood, or spleen cells obtained from eight patients, either at diagnosis or during treatment, all showed bone-marrow engraftment and extensive proliferation after injection into sublethally irradiated SCID mice. Consistent engraftment and proliferation required the use of required approx 10^7 leukemic cells and administration of exogenous GM-CSF. Zhang et al. *(93)* established a SCID mouse-ascites model of human acute promyelocytic leukemia (APL) in which NB4 human APL cells initially transplanted into the SCID mouse peritoneum engrafted, resulting in development of ascites cells. Serially transplanted NB4-ascites cells induced tumors in recipient SCID mice and caused death at a median of 22 d. NB4 ascites cells retained the morphological, immunological, cytogenetic, and molecular characteristics of the parent-cell line after nine passages.

4. SCID MOUSE MODELS OF HUMAN LYMPHOMA

SCID mouse models of human lymphoma have been difficult to establish from primary tumor cells. In one of the few SCID mouse models developed using primary human lymphoma tissue, *(94)*, the origin of the tumors was unclear. These investigators transplanted tumor biopsy samples from 13 patients with Hodgkin's disease into the renal capsule or liver of SCID mice. Tumors were observed after 3–5 mo in mice transplanted with tissue from three of the 13 patients. Sites of tumor growth included the site of transplantation, as well as spleen, lymph nodes, thymus, and liver. Lesions in mice transplanted with tissue from all three patients contained mixed histological tumor subtypes, including lymphoproliferative disease, anaplastic large-cell lymphoma, and Hodgkin's-like lesions. In all mice that showed tumor growth, more than 80% of tumor cells were Epstein-Barr Virus (EBV)$^+$, whereas primary tumor cells from only one patient were EBV+. Furthermore, all had abnormal karyotypes that were different from those of the transplanted tumors. These findings suggest that tumors were derived from either EBV-infected Hodgkin's or Reed Sternberg cells or from EBV-infected bystander cells. Another SCID mouse model of human lymphoma was developed by intraperitoneal (ip) injection into SCID mice of Epstein-Barr virus human peripheral-blood lymphocytes (PBL) from EBV$^+$ individuals *(95)*. Injection of these EBV$^+$ PBLs results in development of EBV$^+$ tumors that resemble the EBV$^+$ large-cell lymphomas observed in immunocompromised individuals.

By comparison, numerous SCID mouse models of lymphoma have been developed using human lymphoma cell lines. For example, Kawata et al. *(96)* developed a SCID mouse model of human B-cell lymphoma using a subclone (BALL-1a) of the B-cell leukemia/lymphoma cell line BALL-1 that was pre-adapted for transplantation by serial passages in newborn and nude mice. Intraperitoneal injection of BALL-1a cells resulted in disseminated tumors in all SCID mice tested, and the cell-surface markers of the BALL-1a cells were retained on the tumor cells recovered from the SCID mice. Myers et al. *(15)* developed a model of human Burkitt's lymphoma by injection of the Ramos-BT lymphoma cell line into SCID mice. These mice developed large abdominal tumors that extended into abdominal organs. Lymphoma cells also infiltrated the bone marrow, spleen, abdominal lymph nodes, brain, kidneys, lung, heart, and liver. An additional SCID mouse model of Burkitt's lymphoma was established by Abe et al. *(97)* using the HBL-7 and HBL-8 Burkitt's lymphoma-derived cell lines, and by Schnell et al. using BL-38 Burkitt's lymphoma cells. Other B-cell lymphoma models in

SCID mice were developed using the t(14;18)$^+$ B-cell lymphoma-cell lines SUDHL-4, OCI-Ly8, and DoHH2 *(98–100)*. In the case of the DoHH2 SCID mouse model *(100)* subcutaneous (sc) or iv inoculation resulted in disseminated disease in hematopoietic and lymphoid organs, including the bone marrow, peripheral blood, peripheral lymph nodes, and liver, without involvement of the gut or mesenteric lymph nodes—a pattern similar to that observed in human B-cell non-Hodgkin's lymphoma.

Other investigators *(101–104)* demonstrated in vivo growth in SCID mice of Hodgkin's disease cell lines, including L428, L540, L591, DEV, HD-LM2, KM-H2, and HD-MyZ. In all cases, engrafted tumor cells in these mice retained the immunophenotype and karyotype of the injected cells. SCID mouse models of other types of lymphoma, including anaplastic large-cell lymphoma, *(13,105,106)* disseminated large-cell lymphoma *(107)*, and T-cell lymphoma *(108)* also have been created using lymphoma-derived cell lines.

5. USE OF SCID MOUSE MODELS OF LEUKEMIA AND LYMPHOMA FOR DEVELOPMENT OF NEW AGENTS AND TREATMENT STRATEGIES

The various SCID mouse models of human leukemia and lymphoma described here have proven useful for evaluating new chemotherapy drugs, new drug combinations, immunotoxins, and other novel treatment strategies for these diseases. In the following section, various treatment modalities evaluated in SCID mouse models are described according to disease type.

5.1. ALL

Using the NALM-6 SCID mouse model of human B-lineage leukemia, Uckun et al. *(10)* demonstrated that treatment with 15 µg or 30 µg of the B43 (anti-CD19)-poke-weed antiviral protein (PAP) immunotoxin *(109,110)* reduced the incidence of both paraplegia and death compared to control mice treated with either PBS or PAP conjugated to a nonspecific antibody. Survival of the B43-PAP-treated SCID mice was estimated to be 60–65% at 7 mo following inoculation of NALM-6 cells. Analysis of tissues in survivor mice killed at 7 mo showed no histopathological or immunological evidence of overt leukemia, although occult leukemia in organs of mice treated with 15 µg of B43-PAP was suggested by PCR detection of human β-globin gene sequences in various organs. Subsequent experiments showed that treatment of SCID mice inoculated with NALM-6 leukemia with the combination of B43-PAP and cyclophosphamide resulted in 70% survival 6 mo after inoculation of leukemic cells *(9)*. Studies by Jansen et al. demonstrated that the B43-PAP/cyclophosphamide combination resulted in a 5-mo survival estimate of 90% for SCID mice inoculated with the t(4;11)$^+$ ALL cell line RS4 *(111)*. Other investigators *(112)* have reported that an anti-CD19 antibody conjugated to the protein synthesis inhibiting plant toxin saporin *(113)* also was effective for prolonging survival of SCID mice inoculated with doses of NALM6 cells that caused disseminated and fatal leukemia in sham-treated controls.

Gunther et al. *(114)* demonstrated that intrathecal administration of B43-PAP was highly effective in eradicating central nervous system (CNS) leukemia in SCID mice injected with NALM-6 cells. In this model system, leukemia first develops in the bone marrow, with occult (PCR-detectable) CNS leukemia appearing by d 8 and overt (histopathologically detectable) CNS leukemia appearing by d 23. Intrathecal injection of 4 weekly doses of 2.5 μg B43-PAP starting at d 14 following inoculation with NALM-6 cells increased median survival to 68 d, compared with 41 d for PBS-treated control mice. Two mice treated with intrathecal B43-PAP survived with no evidence of disease for the entire 111 d of the study. Interestingly, as described here, intra peritoneal injection of B43-PAP was equally effective at prolonging survival, but mice subsequently died of CNS leukemia.

More recent investigations have shown that treatment of NALM-6 B-lineage leukemia in SCID mice with B43-PAP was more effective than the standard three-drug combination of vincristine, prednisone, and L-asparaginase (VPL), whereas the combination of VPL and B43-PAP was more effective than either treatment agent alone, resulting in 100% survival of SCID mice challenged with 5×10^6 NALM-6 leukemia cells *(115)*. Similarly, the combination of B43-PAP and the new agent ZD1694 (Tomudex) *(116)* and the combination of B43-PAP and cytarabine[117] were more effective than either agent alone in the SCID mouse model of human B-lineage ALL, resulting in 100% survival of SCID mice inoculated with NALM-6 leukemia cells. Addition of the new chemotherapy agent temozolomide to the B43-PAP regimen, however, provided no additional benefit *(117)*. Thus, the B43-PAP immunotoxin may prove most effective when used as a component of multi-agent therapy with standard drugs. These preclinical studies have led to a Phase I trial of B43-PAP given in conjunction with VPL and daunomycin for induction therapy in children with refractory CD19+ ALL *(118)*.

Immunotoxins directed against the T-cell-associated cell-surface antigen CD7 have also shown promise in treatment of SCID mice engrafted with human T-lineage leukemia. Gunther et al. *(119)* have shown that an anti-CD7 antibody conjugated to PAP improves survival of SCID mice challenged with 1×10^7 MOLT3 human T-lineage ALL cells. Whereas all MOLT3-injected SCID mice treated with PBS or anti-CD19 PAP-died at a median of 33 or 36 d, five of nine mice treated with anti-CD7-PAP survived long-term (median > 172 d). Interestingly, disseminated disease was present in some anti-CD7-PAP-treated survivors, but the tissue distribution, morphology, and immunophenotypic features of these mice were distinct from that of MOLT3-injected, PBS-treated SCID mice. In particular, anti-CD7-PAP-treated mice had evidence in organs that were not involved in disease in the majority of control mice (heart, pancreas, spleen, thymus, and lung), whereas, PBS-treated mice had evidence of leukemia in organs that were not involved in disease in the majority of mice treated with anti-CD7-PAP (bone marrow, liver, kidney, brain, and adrenals). Moreover, leukemic cells recovered from bone marrow of mice that survived after anti-CD7-PAP treatment had an undifferentiated immunophenotype, lacking cell-surface expression of CD2, CD3, CD5, or CD7) and showing partial expression of CD45. In contrast, leukemic cells recovered from the bone marrow of PBS-treated controls exhibited a CD5+, CD7+, CD45+ immunophenotype similar to that of cells from patients with T-lineage ALL. These findings suggested that anti-CD7-PAP eliminated a subpopulation of MOLT-3 cells that preferentially engrafted in the bone marrow, adrenal cortex, brain, and kidney of SCID mice. In subsequent studies, Waurzyniak et al. *(120)* reported that cardiotoxicity was the dose-limiting toxicity at cumulative doses of 25 to 50 μg of anti-CD7-PAP in Balb-c mice, whereas doses up to 1 mg/kg were tolerated without significant clinical side effects in cynamolgous monkeys. The elimination plasma half-life of anti-CD7-PAP in monkeys was approx 8 h at a dose of

0.1 mg/kg. Initial trials of anti-CD7-PAP in children and adults with relapsed T-lineage ALL are forthcoming.

The plant toxin ricin, a potent protein synthesis inhibitor *(121)* has also been used as a fusion partner for creation of anti-CD7 immunotoxins. Jansen et al. *(111)* reported that SCID mice inoculated with a T-lineage ALL cell line established from a patient with refractory disease had significantly improved survival following treatment with an anti-CD7-deglycosylated ricin A (ricin A_{dg}) immunotoxin. Administration of anti-CD7-ricin A_{dg} (10 µg/mouse/day) for 5 d was administered starting 8 d following inoculation of leukemic cells into the SCID mice. All immunotoxin-treated mice survived 216 d postinoculation, representing a significant improvement over control treated mice ($p < 0.001$). Similarly, Morland et al. *(122)* and Flavell et al. *(123)* observed significantly prolonged survival of SCID mice inoculated with T-lineage ALL HSB-2 cells following treatment with a single iv dose of an anti-CD7-saporin immunotoxin. Interestingly, other investigators reported that SCID mice injected with MOLT16 T-lineage ALL cells that developed a tumor burden of approx 2g responded to treatment with an anti-CD7 antibody alone: 83% of mice showed complete remission 10 d after treatment. The anti-CD7 antibody treatment also prolonged survival of mice with advanced disease. The effects of the anti-CD7 antibody were later attributed to antibody-dependent cell-mediated cytotoxicity via host natural killer (NK) cells *(124)*.

5.2. Myeloid Diseases

Novel chemotherapeutic agents evaluated in SCID mouse models of myeloid leukemias include the alkylating agent tallimustine, the 3-hydroxy-3-methylglutaryl coenzyme A inhibitor simvastin, and the topoisomerase inhibitor 9-aminocamptothecin (9-AC). Beran et al. *(125)* reported that the tallimustine induced remission in SCID mice engrafted with myeloid leukemia, whereas Clutterbuck et al. *(126)* showed that simvastin reduced the number of human leukemic cells in the bone marrow and spleen of SCID mice engrafted with HL60 cells. Jeha et al. *(127)* reported that either oral or iv administration of 9-AC prevented development of leukemia in 11 of 20 mice injected with KBM-3 human AML cells. Thus, these agents show promise as combination chemotherapeutic agents for myeloid leukemia.

The high-affinity GM-CSF receptors expressed on the surface of leukemic cells from most patients with AML *(128–131)* provide a target for novel biotherapeutic agents, such as the fusion products consisting of GM-CSF and the catalytic and translocation domains of diptheria toxin (DT). Terpstra et al. *(132)* initially demonstrated that pretreatment of primary leukemic blasts from two of three AML patients with such a DT-GM-CSF fusion protein resulted in a reduction in the number of engrafted cells in SCID mice. In vitro colony-forming assays showed that normal hematopoietic cells were unaffected by this treatment, suggesting that the DT-GM-CSF fusion protein had significant potential as a biotherapeutic agent. Perentesis et al. reported that administration of a nontoxic dose of the DT-GM-CSF fusion protein 24 h following inoculation with an otherwise fatal dose of human HL-60 myeloid leukemia cells resulted in 60% survival of SCID mice at 6 mo *(133)*. Rozemuller et al. found that four of seven AML cases engrafted into SCID mice were sensitive to DT-GM-CSF; in three of the four cases, PCR assays demonstrated the absence of human leukemia cells *(134)*. Hall et al. reported that a DT-GM-CSF fusion injected intraperitoneally in SCID mice on d 2–6 following challenge with 1×10^7 HL-60 cells significantly improved survival compared with controls or cytarabine-treated mice *(135)*. An IL-6-pseudomonas exotoxin (PE) conjugate was tested for use as an ex vivo purging agent for autologous stem-cell transplant *(136)*. In these experiments, pre-incubation of the IL-6-PE conjugate with primary AML cells that expressed IL-6 receptors prior to leukemic-cell inoculation of SCID mice completely prevented leukemic-cell engraftment. Neither overt nor occult disease was detected 185 d after inoculation. These preclinical studies suggest a role for immunotoxins in adjuvant treatment of AML or for stem-cell/bone-marrow purging.

SCID mouse models of AML also have proven useful for initial testing of immunological strategies involving cytotoxic T-cells. As described here, CD38$^+$CD34$^-$ leukemic precursors were identified as the initiating cells required for engraftment of human primary AML cells in SCID mice *(82)*. Bonnet et al. found that CD8$^+$ cytotoxic T-lymphocytes (CTLs) specific for minor histocompatibility antigens effectively prevented engraftment of human AML in NOD/SCID mice by direct recognition and killing of the leukemia-initiating cell *(137)*. This NOD/SCID AML model therefore may provide a system for identifying and selecting CTL clones with immunotherapeutic potential for treatment of AML. In addition, a novel method of adoptive transfer of cellular cytotoxicity that utilized a potent major histocompatibility complex (MHC) nonrestricted human killer T-cell clone (TALL-104) was described by Cesano et al. *(138)*. In these experiments, repeated injections of TALL-104 cells, together with either IL-2 or IL-12 after inoculation of U937 myeloid leukemia cells into SCID mice, were effective in prolonging survival and in some cases curing mice of leukemia.

SCID mouse models of human myeloid leukemias also have been used for evaluation of anti-sense oligonucleotide-based therapy. Skorski et al. reported that SCID mice inoculated with 1×10^7 leukemic cells and treated 21 d later with anti-sense phosphorothioate oligonucleotides to both c-myc and bcr-abl resulted in reduced engraftment of leukemic cells and prolonged survival, although all mice eventually succumbed to disease *(139)*. In a subsequent study, these investigators reported that 50% of SCID mice inoculated with Ph$^+$ CML cells 20 d prior to treatment with a combination of a bcr-abl anti-sense phosphorothioate oligonucleotide and cyclophosphamide appeared to be cured of leukemia *(140)*. These data must be interpreted with caution, because of the reported nonspecific effects associated with anti-sense therapy *(141–145)*.

5.3. Lymphoma

Numerous SCID mouse models of human B-cell lymphoma and Hodgkin's disease have been used for the evaluation of new drug strategies. For example, treatment with an immunotoxin consisting of an anti-CD19 MAb (B43) conjugated to genistein (Gen), a naturally occurring protein-tyrosine-kinase inhibitor, was effective in preventing development of disseminated lymphoma in SCID mice injected with Ramos-BT cells *(15)*. In these experiments, B43-Gen, control unconjugated B43 antibody, unconjugated Gen, PBS, or an anti-CD7-Gen immunoconjugate were injected for three consecutive days starting 24 h after inoculation with 5×10^6 Ramos-BT cells. Control mice died of disseminated disease with a median survival of 48 d, whereas 7 of 10 mice treated with B43-Gen survived for more than 4 mo with no clinical evidence of lymphoma.

In other studies *(11,96)*, survival of SCID mice inoculated with 1×10^6 B-ALL lymphoma cells was increased by treatment with an anti-B-cell lymphoma antibody (SN7) conjugated to ricin A_{dg} compared with sham PBS treatment: all control animals died within 35 d of tumor inoculation, whereas immunotoxin-treated animals as well as unconjugated antibody-treated animals survived for the duration of the 250-d study, although the unconjugated antibody was less effective than the immunotoxin in mice inoculated with larger numbers of lymphoma cells. Other cell-surface antigens that appear to be useful targets for immunotherapy in SCID mouse models of human B-cell lymphoma include CD45 and CD52 *(146)*, CD24 *(147)*, CD25 *(103)*, and CD22 *(148,149)*.

Anti-CD30 antibodies, either alone or conjugated to an immunotoxin such as saporin, ricin, or momordin, have been evaluated for treatment of both ALCL and Hodgkin's disease. For example, Pfiefer et al. observed that treatment with anti-CD30 1 d following anaplastic large-cell lymphoma (ALCL) transplantation in SCID mice prevented tumor growth, and later treatment caused growth arrest and prevented development of disseminated disease. Pasqualucci et al. observed lasting complete remission in 80% of mice treated with three doses of an anti-CD30/saporin immunotoxin 24 h following ALCL inoculation. Lower remission induction rates were achieved when the immunotoxin was given at later time-points, suggesting that the immunotoxin may be most effective when used as adjuvant therapy. Schnell et al. reported development of a high affinity anti-CD30-ricin A_{dg} immunotoxin that prolonged survival time of SCID mice bearing disseminated human Hodgkin's disease to 132 d compared with 42 d in untreated controls *(150)*.

Bispecific antibodies, consisting of one variable region directed against a tumor antigen and the second variable region directed against an effector-cell triggering molecule, also have been investigated in the context of SCID models of human lymphoma. These agents represent a unique class of anticancer therapeutic agents that have the potential to recruit and target host-effector functions specifically to tumor cells. A bispecific antibody directed against both the CD30 cell-surface antigen, as well as CD16 (FcRγIII), has been evaluated against tumor cells in a SCID mouse model of human Hodgkin's disease. Hombach et al. reported complete tumor regression in all of 10 animals treated with the bispecific antibody together with human PBLs. Arndt et al. observed that a modified anti-CD30/CD16 diabody, containing only the immunoglobulin variable-region domains, was equally effective in causing tumor regression *(17)*. The diabody may be a more efficacious agent, because it is expected to be less allergenic and immunogenic in vivo. Renner et al. utilized a two different bispecific antibodies, anti-CD3/CD30 and anti-CD28/CD30, together with patient-donor T-lymphocytes for treatment of xenotransplanted Hodgkin's disease in SCID mice *(105)*. In these experiments, mice were inoculated with 2×10^7 L540cy cells, and only animals with increasing soluble CD30 levels at d 5—which was shown to be indicative of tumor engraftment—were used to evaluate effects of the bispecific antibodies. All such mice treated on d 7 with anti-CD3/CD30, anti-CD28/CD30, and human donor T-cells survived for the duration of the study (150 d) and had undetectable soluble CD30 levels by d 20. Initiation of therapy on d 11 or d 14 after inoculation of tumor cells resulted in 60% and 20% survival, respectively. Initiation of therapy on d 21 did not result in cure, but prolonged survival compared with treatment initiated later. Similarly, a bispecific antibody directed against CD3 and CD19 used in conjunction with an anti-CD28 antibody prevented B-cell lymphoma growth in SCID mice *(152)*.

Cellular-based anticancer strategies also have been investigated in SCID mice. Katsanis et al. used a SCID mouse model of B-cell lymphoma for evaluating the cellular-based therapy *(98)*. These investigators obtained peripheral-blood mononuclear cells (PBMNC) obtained from patients who underwent autologous stem-cell transplant followed by IL-2 treatment. B-cell lymphoma-bearing animals infused with these autografted, IL-2-stimulated human PBMNC had significantly prolonged survival compared with untreated controls.

CONCLUSIONS

The studies described here demonstrate the utility of the SCID mouse for evaluating a myriad of new therapeutic strategies for the treatment of human leukemia and lymphoma. However, these studies represent only an initial step in the quest for new and improved anticancer agents. In the majority of studies described here, efficacy was demonstrated by prolonged SCID mouse survival when an agent(s) was given shortly after inoculation with neoplastic cells—in essence, before massive infiltration of mouse tissues had occurred. While these studies prove that the agent in question has a specific antitumor effect, equivalent efficacy in humans cannot be presumed, since in human disease these agents will need to be effective against established or disseminated tumors. In addition, drug concentrations required for therapeutic efficacy in humans may be substantially higher, and lead to increased toxicity, than those observed in the SCID mouse-model system. In particular, the toxicity and immunogenicity of an immunotoxin consisting of murine immunoglobulin domains would be expected to be low in the SCID mouse, but may be significant in humans. In summary, the SCID mouse has proven to be a valuable tool for distinguishing biological features of disease and for initial preclinical in vivo evaluations of novel anticancer agents, including antisense oligonucleotides and immunotoxins, as well as novel cellular-based immune-response therapies. Future studies in SCID mice should test the most promising agents at different stages of disease progression, as models more closely approximating human disease and toxicity must continue to be evaluated in nonhuman primates as well as Phase I and Phase II human trials.

REFERENCES

1. Bosma MJ, Carroll AM. The SCID mouse mutant: definition, characterization, and potential uses. *Annu Rev Immunol* 1991; 9:323–350.
2. Kamel Reid S, Letarte M, Sirard C, et al. A model of human acute lymphoblastic leukemia in immune-deficient scid mice. *Science* 1989; 246:1597–1600.
3. Cesano A, O'Connor R, Lange B, et al. Homing and progression patterns of childhood acute lymphoblastic leukemias in severe combined immunodeficiency mice. *Blood* 1991; 77:2463–2474.
4. Kamel Reid S, Letarte M, Doedens M, et al. Bone marrow from children in relapse with pre-B Acute Lymphoblastic Leukemia proliferates and disseminates rapidly in scid mice. *Blood* 1991; 78:2973–2981.
5. Uckun FM. Severe combined immunodeficient mouse models of human leukemia. *Blood* 1996; 88:1135–1146.
6. Dick JE, Lapidot T, Pflumio F. Transplantation of normal and leukemic human bone marrow into immune-deficient mice: development of animal models for human hematopoiesis. *Immunol Rev* 1991; 124:25–43.
7. McCune JM, Namikawa R, Kaneshima H, et al. The SCID-hu mouse: murine model for the analysis of human hematolymphoid differentiation and function. *Science* 1988; 241:1632–1639.

8. Mosier DE, Gulizia RJ, Baird SM, et al. Transfer of a functional human immune system to mice with severe combined immunodeficiency. *Nature* 1988; 335:256–259.

9. Uckun FM, Chelstrom LM, Finnegan D, et al. Effective immunochemotherapy of CALLA+C mu+ human pre-B acute lymphoblastic leukemia in mice with severe combined immunodeficiency using B43 (anti-CD19) pokeweed antiviral protein immunotoxin plus cyclophosphamide. *Blood* 1992; 79:3116–3129.

10. Uckun FM, Manivel C, Arthur D, et al. In vivo efficacy of B43 (anti-CD19)-pokeweed antiviral protein immunotoxin against human pre-B cell acute lymphoblastic leukemia in mice with severe combined immunodeficiency. *Blood* 1992; 79:2201–2214.

11. Yoshida M, Rybak RJ, Choi Y, et al. Development of a severe combined immunodeficiency (SCID) mouse model consisting of highly disseminated human B-cell leukemia/lymphoma, cure of the tumors by systemic administration of immunotoxin, and development/application of a clonotype-specific polymerase chain reaction-based assay. *Cancer Res* 1997; 57:678–685.

12. Weimar IS, Weijer K, van den Berk PC, et al. HGF/SF and its receptor c-MET play a minor role in the dissemination of human B-lymphoma cells in SCID mice. *Br J Cancer* 1999; 81:43–53.

13. Pasqualucci L, Wasik M, Teicher BA, et al. Antitumor activity of anti-CD30 immunotoxin (Ber-H2/saporin) in vitro and in severe combined immunodeficiency disease mice xenografted with human CD30+ anaplastic large-cell lymphoma. *Blood* 1995; 85:2139–2146.

14. Pfeifer W, Levi E, Petrogiannis-Haliotis T, et al. A murine xenograft model for human CD30+ anaplastic large cell lymphoma. Successful growth inhibition with an anti-CD30 antibody (HeFi-1). *Am J Pathol* 1999; 155:1353–1359.

15. Myers DE, Jun X, Waddick KG, et al. Membrane-associated CD19-LYN complex is an endogenous p53-independent and Bcl-2-independent regulator of apoptosis in human B-lineage lymphoma cells [published erratum appears in Proc Natl Acad Sci USA 1996 Feb 6;93(3):1357]. Proc Natl Acad Sci USA 1995; 92:9575–9579.

16. Daniel PT, Kroidl A, Kopp J, et al. Immunotherapy of B-cell lymphoma with CD3×19 bispecific antibodies: costimulation via CD28 prevents "veto" apoptosis of antibody-targeted cytotoxic T cells. *Blood* 1998; 92:4750–4757.

17. Arndt MA, Krauss J, Kipriyanov SM, et al. A bispecific diabody that mediates natural killer cell cytotoxicity against xenotransplanted human Hodgkin's tumors. *Blood* 1999; 94:2562–2568.

18. Ries L, Smith M, Gurney J, et al. Cancer Incidence and Survival Among Children and Adolescents: United States SEER Program 1975–1995, vol. NIH Pub. No. 99–4649. Bethesda, MD: National Cancer Institute, 1999.

19. Pui CH, Behm FG, Singh B, et al. Heterogeneity of presenting features and their relation to treatment outcome in 120 children with T-cell acute lymphoblastic leukemia: *Blood* 1990; 75:174–179.

20. Pui CH, Behm FG, Crist WM. Clinical and biologic relevance of immunologic marker studies in childhood acute lymphoblastic leukemia. *Blood* 1993; 82:343–362.

21. Uckun FM, Gajl Peczalska KJ, Provisor AJ, et al. Immunophenotype-karyotype associations in human acute lymphoblastic leukemia. *Blood* 1989; 73:271–280.

22. Uckun FM, Ledbetter JA. Immunobiologic differences between normal and leukemic human B-cell precursors. *Proc Natl Acad Sci USA* 1988; 85:8603–8607.

23. Smith M, Arthur D, Camitta B, et al. Uniform approach to risk classification and treatment assignment for children with acute lymphoblastic leukemia. *J Clin Oncol* 1996; 14:18–24.

24. Raimondi SC. Current status of cytogenetic research in childhood acute lymphoblastic leukemia. *Blood* 1993; 81:2237–2251.

25. Uckun FM, Nachman JB, Sather HN, et al. Clinical significance of Philadelphia chromosome positive pediatric acute lymphoblastic leukemia in the context of contemporary intensive therapies: a report from the Children's Cancer Group. *Cancer* 1998; 83:2030–2039.

26. Uckun FM, Sensel MG, Sather HN, et al. Clinical significance of translocation t(1;19) in childhood acute lymphoblastic leukemia in the context of contemporary therapies: a report from the Children's Cancer Group. *J Clin Oncol* 1998; 16:527–535.

27. Heerema N, Sather H, Reaman G, et al. Cytogenetic studies of Acute Lymphoblastic Leukemia: clinical correlations results from the Children's Cancer Group. *J Assoc Genetic Technol* 1998; 24:206–212.

28. Uckun F, Reaman G, Steinherz P, et al. Improved outcome for children with T-lineage Acute Lymphoblastic Leukemia after contemporary chemotherapy: a Children's Cancer Group study. *Leuk Lymphoma* 1996; 24:57–70.

29. Uckun FM, Downing JR, Chelstrom LM, et al. Human t(4;11)(q21;q23) acute lymphoblastic leukemia in mice with severe combined immunodeficiency. *Blood* 1994; 84:859–865.

30. Uckun FM, Downing JR, Gunther R, et al. Human t(1;19)(q23;p13) pre-B acute lymphoblastic leukemia in mice with severe combined immunodeficiency. *Blood* 1993; 81:3052–3062.

31. Uckun FM, Sather H, Reaman G, et al. Leukemic cell growth in SCID mice as a predictor of relapse in high-risk B-lineage acute lymphoblastic leukemia. *Blood* 1995; 85:873–878.

32. Uckun FM, Sather HN, Waurzyniak BJ, et al. Prognostic significance of B-lineage leukemic cell growth in SCID mice: a Children's Cancer Group study [In Process Citation]. *Leuk Lymphoma* 1998; 30:503–514.

33. Gaynon PS, Bleyer WA, Steinherz PG, et al. Day 7 marrow response and outcome for children with Acute Lymphoblastic Leukemia and unfavorable presenting features. *Med Pediatr Oncol* 1990; 18:273–279.

34. Nachman JB, Sather HN, Sensel MG, et al. Augmented post-induction therapy for children with high-risk acute lymphoblastic leukemia and a slow response to initial therapy. *N Engl J Med* 1998; 338:1663–1671.

35. Nachman J, Sather H, Cherlow J, et al. Response of children with high risk Acute Lymphoblastic Leukemia treated with and without cranial irradiation: a report from the Children's Cancer Group. *J Clin Oncol* 1998; 16:920–930.

36. Nachman J, Sather HN, Gaynon PS, et al. Augmented Berlin-Frankfurt-Munster therapy abrogates the adverse prognostic significance of slow early response to induction chemotherapy for children and adolescents with Acute Lymphoblastic Leukemia and unfavorable presenting features: a report from the Children's Cancer Group. *J Clin Oncol* 1997; 15:2222–2230.

37. Hutchinson R, Bertolone S, Cooper H, et al. Early marrow response predicts outcome for patients with low risk ALL: results of CCG-1881. *Proc Amer Soc Clin Oncol* 1994; 13:319.

38. Lange B, Sather H, Weetman R, et al. Double delayed intensification improves outcome in moderate risk pediatric acute lymphoblastic leukemia (ALL): a Children's Cancer Group study, CCG-1891. *Blood* 1997; 90:559a.

39. Greaves MF, Janossy G, Peto J, et al. Immunologically defined subclasses of acute lymphoblastic leukaemia in children: their relationship to presentation features and prognosis. *Br J Haematol* 1981; 48:179–197.

40. Crist W, Boyett J, Pullen J, et al. Clinical and biologic features predict poor prognosis in acute lymphoid leukemias in children and adolescents: a Pediatric Oncology Group review. *Med Pediatr Oncol* 1986; 14:135–139.

41. Crist WM, Shuster JJ, Falletta J, et al. Clinical features and outcome in childhood T-cell leukemia-lymphoma according to stage of thymocyte differentiation: a Pediatric Oncology Group study. *Blood* 1988; 72:1891–1897.

42. Pullen DJ, Sullivan MP, Falletta JM, et al. Modified LSA2-L2 treatment in 53 children with E-rosette-positive T-cell leukemia: results and prognostic factors (a Pediatric Oncology Group study). *Blood* 1982; 60:1159–1168.

43. Pullen DJ, Boyett JM, Crist WM, et al. Pediatric Oncology Group utilization of immunologic markers in the designation of acute lymphocytic leukemia subgroups: influence on treatment response. *Ann NY Acad Sci* 1984; 428:26–48.

44. Dowell BL, Borowitz MJ, Boyett JM, et al. Immunologic and clinicopathologic features of common acute lymphoblastic leukemia antigen-positive childhood T-cell leukemia. A Pediatric Oncology Group study. *Cancer* 1987; 59:2020–2026.

45. Falletta JM, Shuster JJ, Crist WM, et al. Different patterns of relapse associated with three intensive treatment regimens for pediatric E-rosette positive T-cell leukemia: a Pediatric Oncology Group study. *Leukemia* 1992; 6:541–546.

46. Garand R, Vannier JP, Bene MC, et al. Comparison of outcome, clinical, laboratory, and immunological features in 164 children and adults with T-All. The Groupe D'Etude Immunologique Des Leucemies. *Leukemia* 1990; 4:739–744.

47. Kubiczek K, Rytlewska M, Pituch Noworolska A (Treatment results of T-cell acute lymphoblastic leukemia therapy in children from 1983–1985). *Pol Tyg Lek* 1994; 49:273–275.

48. Henze G, Langermann HJ, Kaufmann U, et al. Thymic involvement and initial white blood count in childhood acute lymphoblastic leukemia. *Am J Pediatr Hematol Oncol* 1981; 3:369–376.

49. Shuster JJ, Falletta JM, Pullen DJ, et al. Prognostic factors in childhood T-cell acute lymphoblastic leukemia: a Pediatric Oncology Group study. *Blood* 1990; 75:166–173.

50. Uckun FM, Waurzyniak BJ, Sather HN, et al. Prognostic significance of T-lineage leukemic cell growth in SCID mice: a Children's Cancer Group study. *Leuk Lymphoma* 1999; 32:475–487.

51. Uckun F, Sensel M, Sun L, et al. Biology and treatment of childhood T-lineage Acute Lymphoblastic Leukemia. *Blood* 1998; 91(3):735–746.

52. Uckun FM, Gaynon P, Sensel M, et al. Clinical features and treatment outcome of childhood T-lineage Acute Lymphoblastic Leukemia according to the apparent maturational stage of T-lineage leukemic blasts: a Children's Cancer Group study. *J Clin Oncol* 1997; 15:2214–2221.

53. Clavell LA, Gelber RD, Cohen HJ, et al. Four-agent induction and intensive asparaginase therapy for treatment of childhood acute lymphoblastic leukemia. *N Engl J Med* 1986; 315:657–663.

54. Gaynon P, Steinherz P, Bleyer WA, et al. Intensive therapy for children with acute lymphoblastic leukemia and unfavorable presenting features. *Lancet* 1988; 2:921–924.

55. Schorin MA, Blattner S, Gelber RD, et al. Treatment of childhood acute lymphoblastic leukemia: results of Dana-Farber Cancer Institute/Children's Hospital Acute Lymphoblastic Leukemia Consortium Protocol 85-01. *J Clin Oncol* 1994; 12:740–747.

56. Steinherz PG, Gaynon P, Miller DR, et al. Improved disease-free survival of children with acute lymphoblastic leukemia at high risk for early relapse with the New York regimen—a new intensive therapy protocol: a report from the Children's Cancer Study Group. *J Clin Oncol* 1986; 4:744–752.

57. Pui CH. Acute leukemias with the t(4;11)(q21;q23). *Leuk Lymphoma* 1992; 7:173–179.

58. Pui CH, Kane JR, Crist WM. Biology and treatment of infant leukemias. *Leukemia* 1995; 9:762–769.

59. Reaman G, Zeltzer P, Bleyer WA, et al. Acute Lymphoblastic Leukemia in infants less than one year of age: a cumulative experience of the Children's Cancer Study Group. *J Clin Oncol* 1985; 3:1513–1521.

60. Heerema NA, Arthur DC, Sather H, et al. Cytogenetic features of infants less than 12 months of age at diagnosis of acute lymphoblastic leukemia: impact of the 11q23 breakpoint on outcome: a report of the Children's Cancer Group. *Blood* 1994; 83:2274–2284.

61. Uckun FM, Waurzyniak BJ, Sensel MG, et al. Primary blasts from infants with acute lymphoblastic leukemia cause overt leukemia in SCID mice [In Process Citation]. *Leuk Lymphoma* 1998; 30:269–277.

62. Waurzyniak BJ, Heerema N, Sensel MG, et al. Distinct in vivo engraftment and growth patterns of t(1;19)+/E2A-PBX1+ and t(9;22)+/BCR-ABL+ human leukemia cells in SCID mice [In Process Citation]. *Leuk Lymphoma* 1998; 32:77–87.

63. Jeha S, Kantarjian H, O'Brien S, et al. Growth and biologic properties of karyotypically defined subcategories of adult acute lymphocytic leukemia in mice with severe combined immunodeficiency. *Blood* 1995; 86:4278–4285.

64. Steele JP, Clutterbuck RD, Powles RL, et al. Growth of human T-cell lineage acute leukemia in severe combined immunodeficiency (SCID) mice and non-obese diabetic SCID mice. *Blood* 1997; 90:2015–2019.

65. Palucka AK, Scuderi R, Porwit A, et al. Acute lymphoblastic leukemias from relapse engraft more rapidly in SCID mice. *Leukemia* 1996; 10:558–563.

66. Schiffer CA, McIntyre OR. Age related changes in adults with acute leukemia. *Adv Exp Med Biol* 1993; 330:215–229.

67. Katano N, Tsurusawa M, Hirota T, et al. Treatment outcome and prognostic factors in childhood acute myeloblastic leukemia: a report from the Japanese Children's Cancer and Leukemia Study Group (CCLSG) [published erratum appears in *Int J Hematol* 1997 Oct;66(3):395–6]. *Int J Hematol* 1997; 66:103–110.

68. Sartori PC, Taylor MH, Stevens MC, et al. Treatment of childhood acute myeloid leukaemia using the BFM-83 protocol. *Med Pediatr Oncol* 1993; 21:8–13.

69. Wells RJ, Woods WG, Lampkin BC, et al. Impact of high-dose cytarabine and asparaginase intensification on childhood acute myeloid leukemia: a report from the Children's Cancer Group. *J Clin Oncol* 1993; 11:538–545.

70. Woods WG, Kobrinsky N, Buckley JD, et al. Timed-sequential induction therapy improves postremission outcome in acute myeloid leukemia: a report from the Children's Cancer Group. *Blood* 1996; 87:4979–4989.

71. Stevens RF, Hann IM, Wheatley K, et al. Marked improvements in outcome with chemotherapy alone in paediatric acute myeloid leukemia: results of the United Kingdom Medical Research Council's 10th AML trial. MRC Childhood Leukaemia Working Party. *Br J Haematol* 1998; 101:130–140.

72. Vignetti M, Rondelli R, Locatelli F, et al. Autologous bone marrow transplantation in children with acute myeloblastic leukemia: report from the Italian National Pediatric Registry (AIEOP-BMT). *Bone Marrow Transplant* 1996; 18(Supp. 2):59–62.

73. Wells RJ, Woods WG, Buckley JD, et al. Treatment of newly diagnosed children and adolescents with acute myeloid leukemia: a Children's Cancer Group study. *J Clin Oncol* 1994; 12:2367–2377.

74. Woods WG, Kobrinsky N, Buckley J, et al. Intensively timed induction therapy followed by autologous or allogeneic bone marrow transplantation for children with acute myeloid leukemia or myelodysplastic syndrome: a Children's Cancer Group pilot study. *J Clin Oncol* 1993; 11:1448–1457.

75. Beran M, Pisa P, Kantarjian H, et al. Growth of sensitive and drug-resistant human myeloid leukemia cells in SCID mice. *Hematol Pathol* 1994; 8:135–154.

76. Cesano A, Hoxie JA, Lange B, et al. The severe combined immunodeficient (SCID) mouse as a model for human myeloid leukemias. *Oncogene* 1992; 7:827–836.

77. De Lord C, Clutterbuck R, Powles R, et al. Growth of primary human acute lymphoblastic and myeloblastic leukemia in SCID mice. *Leuk Lymphoma* 1994; 16:157–165.

78. De Lord C, Clutterbuck R, Titley J, et al. Growth of primary human acute leukemia in severe combined immunodeficient mice. *Exp Hematol* 1991; 19:991–993.

79. Sawyers CL, Gishizky ML, Quan S, et al. Propagation of human blastic myeloid leukemias in the SCID mouse. *Blood* 1992; 79:2089–2098.

80. Beran M, Pisa P, O'Brien S, et al. Biological properties and growth in SCID mice of a new myelogenous leukemia cell line (KBM-5) derived from chronic myelogenous leukemia cells in the blastic phase. *Cancer Res* 1993; 53:3603–3610.

81. Lapidot T, Sirard C, Vormoor J, et al. AML blast cells obtained from newly diagnosed patients engraft and proliferate in SCID mice in response to cytokines. *Blood* 1992; 80(Suppl. 1):32a.

82. Lapidot T, Sirard C, Vormoor J, et al. A cell initiating human acute myeloid leukaemia after transplantation into SCID mice. *Nature* 1994; 367:645–648.

83. Chelstrom LM, Gunther R, Simon J, et al. Childhood acute myeloid leukemia in mice with severe combined immunodeficiency. *Blood* 1994; 84:20–26.

84. Namikawa R, Ueda R, Kyoizumi S. Growth of human myeloid leukemias in the human marrow environment of SCID-hu mice. *Blood* 1993; 82:2526–2536.

85. Kyoizumi S, Baum CM, Kaneshima H, et al. Implantation and maintenance of functional human bone marrow in SCID-hu mice. *Blood* 1992; 79:1704–1711.

86. Skorski T, Nieborowska-Skorska M, Calabretta B. A model of Ph' positive chronic myeloid leukemia-blast crisis cell line growth in immunodeficient SCID mice. *Folia Histochem Cytobiol* 1992; 30:91–96.

87. Dazzi F, Capelli D, Hasserjian R, et al. The kinetics and extent of engraftment of chronic myelogenous leukemia cells in non-obese diabetic/severe combined immunodeficiency mice reflect the phase of the donor's disease: an in vivo model of chronic myelogenous leukemia biology. *Blood* 1998; 92:1390–1396.

88. McGuirk J, Yan Y, Childs B, et al. Differential growth patterns in SCID mice of patient-derived chronic myelogenous leukemias. *Bone Marrow Transplant* 1998; 22:367–374.

89. Lapidot T, Grunberger T, Vormoor J, et al. Identification of human juvenile chronic myelogenous leukemia stem cells capable of initiating the disease in primary and secondary SCID mice. *Blood* 1996; 88:2655–2664.

90. De Lord C, Clutterbuck RD, Powles RL, et al. Human Philadelphia chromosome-positive chronic myeloid leukemia: a potential model for antisense therapy. *Exp Hematol* 1993; 21:826–828.

91. Sirard C, Lapidot T, Vormoor J, et al. Normal and leukemic SCID-repopulating cells (SRC) coexist in the bone marrow and peripheral blood from CML patients in chronic phase, whereas leukemic SRC are detected in blast crisis. *Blood* 1996; 87:1539–1548.

92. Lewis ID, McDiarmid LA, Samels LM, et al. Establishment of a reproducible model of chronic-phase chronic myeloid leukemia in NOD/SCID mice using blood-derived mononuclear or CD34+ cells. *Blood* 1998; 91:630–640.

93. Zhang SY, Zhu J, Chen GQ, et al. Establishment of a human acute promyelocytic leukemia-ascites model in SCID mice. *Blood* 1996; 87:3404–3409.

94. Kapp U, Wolf J, Hummel M, et al. Hodgkin's lymphoma-derived tissue serially transplanted into severe combined immunodeficient mice. *Blood* 1993; 82:1247–1256.

95. Rowe M, Young LS, Crocker J, et al. Epstein-Barr virus (EBV)-associated lymphoproliferative disease in the SCID mouse model: implications for the pathogenesis of EBV-positive lymphomas in man. *J Exp Med* 1991; 173:147–158.

96. Kawata A, Yoshida M, Okazaki M, et al. Establishment of new SCID and nude mouse models of human B leukemia/lymphoma and effective therapy of the tumors with immunotoxin and monoclonal

antibody: marked difference between the SCID and nude mouse models in the antitumor efficacy of monoclonal antibody. *Cancer Res* 1994; 54:2688–2694.

97. Abe M, Suzuki O, Tasaki K, et al. Establishment and characterization of new human Burkitt's lymphoma cell lines (HBL-7 and HBL-8) that are highly metastatic in SCID mice: a metastatic SCID mouse model of human lymphoma lines. *Pathol Int* 1996; 46:630–638.

98. Katsanis E, Weisdorf DJ, Miller JS. Activated peripheral blood mononuclear cells from patients receiving subcutaneous interleukin-2 following autologous stem cell transplantation prolong survival of SCID mice bearing human lymphoma. *Bone Marrow Transplant* 1998; 22:185–191.

99. Schmidt-Wolf IG, Negrin RS, Kiem HP, et al. Use of a SCID mouse/human lymphoma model to evaluate cytokine-induced killer cells with potent antitumor cell activity. *J Exp Med* 1991; 174:139–149.

100. de Kroon JF, Kluin PM, Kluin-Nelemans HC, et al. Homing and antigenic characterization of a human non-Hodgkin's lymphoma B cell line in severe combined immunodeficient (SCID) mice. *Leukemia* 1994; 8:1385–1391.

101. von Kalle C, Wolf J, Becker A, et al. Growth of Hodgkin cell lines in severely combined immunodeficient mice. *Int J Cancer* 1992; 52:887–891.

102. Kapp U, Dux A, Schell-Frederick E, et al. Disseminated growth of Hodgkin's-derived cell lines L540 and L540cy in immune-deficient SCID mice. *Ann Oncol* 5 (Suppl. 1):1994; 121–126.

103. Winkler U, Gottstein C, Schon G, et al. Successful treatment of disseminated human Hodgkin's disease in SCID mice with deglycosylated ricin A-chain immunotoxins. *Blood* 1994; 83:466–475.

104. Bargou RC, Mapara MY, Zugck C, et al. Characterization of a novel Hodgkin cell line, HD-MyZ, with myelomonocytic features mimicking Hodgkin's disease in severe combined immunodeficient mice. *J Exp Med* 1993; 177:1257–1268.

105. Renner C, Bauer S, Sahin U, et al. Cure of disseminated xenografted human Hodgkin's tumors by bispecific monoclonal antibodies and human T cells: the role of human T-cell subsets in a preclinical model. *Blood* 1996; 87:2930–2937.

106. Terenzi A, Bolognesi A, Pasqualucci L, et al. Anti-CD30 (BER=H2) immunotoxins containing the type-1 ribosome-inactivating proteins momordin and PAP-S (pokeweed antiviral protein from seeds) display powerful antitumour activity against CD30+ tumor cells in vitro and in SCID mice. *Br J Haematol* 1996; 92:872–879.

107. Mohammad RM, Pettit GR, Almatchy VP, et al. Synergistic interaction of selected marine animal anticancer drugs against human diffuse large cell lymphoma. *Anticancer Drugs* 1998; 9:149–156.

108. Biondi A, Motta T, Garofalo A, et al. Human T-cell lymphoblastic lymphoma expressing the T-cell receptor gamma/delta established in immune-deficient (bg/nu/xid) mice. *Leukemia* 1993; 7:281–289.

109. Uckun FM, Ramakrishnan S, Houston LL. Immunotoxin-mediated elimination of clonogenic tumor cells in the presence of human bone marrow. *J Immunol* 1985; 134:2010–2016.

110. Uckun FM, Ramakrishnan S, Houston LL. Increased efficiency in selective elimination of leukemia cells by a combination of a stable derivative of cyclophosphamide and a human B-cell-specific immunotoxin containing pokeweed antiviral protein. *Cancer Res* 1985; 45:69–75.

111. Jansen B, Kersey JH, Jaszcz WB, et al. Effective immunochemotherapy of human t(4;11) leukemia in mice with severe combined immunodeficiency (SCID) using B43 (anti-CD19)-pokeweed antiviral protein immunotoxin plus cyclophosphamide. *Leukemia* 1993; 7:290–297.

112. Flavell DJ, Flavell SU, Boehm DA, et al. Preclinical studies with the anti-CD19-saporin immunotoxin BU12-SAPORIN for the treatment of human-B-cell tumours. *Br J Cancer* 1995; 72:1373–1379.

113. Stirpe F, Gasperi-Campani A, Barbieri L, et al. Ribosome-inactivating proteins from the seeds of Saponaria officinalis L. (soapwort), of Agrostemma githago L. (corn cockle) and of Asparagus officinalis L. (asparagus), and from the latex of Hura crepitans L. (sandbox tree). *Biochem J* 1983; 216:617–625.

114. Gunther R, Chelstrom LM, Tuel-Ahlgren L, et al. Biotherapy for xenografted human central nervous system leukemia in mice with severe combined immunodeficiency using B43 (anti-CD19)-pokeweed antiviral protein immunotoxin. *Blood* 1995; 85:2537–2545.

115. Ek O, Gaynon P, Zeren T, et al. Treatment of human B-cell precursor leukemia in SCID mice by using a combination of the anti-CD19 immunotoxin B43-PAP with the standard chemotherapeutic drugs vincristine, methylprednisolone, and L-asparaginase. *Leuk Lymphoma* 1998; 31:143–149.

116. Ek O, Reaman GH, Crankshaw DL, et al. Combined therapeutic efficacy of the thymidylate synthase inhibitor ZD1694 (Tomudex) and the immunotoxin B43 (anti-CD19)-PAP in a SCID mouse model of human B-lineage acute lymphoblastic leukemia. *Leuk Lymphoma* 1998; 28:509–514.

117. Messinger Y, Reaman GH, Ek O, et al. Evaluation of temozolomide in a SCID mouse model of human B-cell precursor leukemia [In Process Citation]. Leuk *Lymphoma* 1999; 33:289–293.
118. Siebel NL, Krailo M, O'Neill K, et al. Phase I study of B43-PAP immunotoxin in combination with standard 4-drug induction for patients with CD19⁺ Acute Lymphoblastic Leukemia (ALL) in relapse: a Children's Cancer Group study. *Blood* 1998; 92:400a.
119. Gunther R, Chelstrom LM, Finnegan D, et al. In vivo anti-leukemic efficacy of anti-CD7-pokeweed antiviral protein immunotoxin against human T-lineage acute lymphoblastic leukemia/lymphoma in mice with severe combined immunodeficiency. *Leukemia* 1993; 7:298–309.
120. Waurzyniak B, Schneider EA, Turner N, et al. In vivo toxicity, pharmacokinetics, and antileukemic activity of TXU (Anti-CD7)-pokeweed antiviral protein immunotoxin. *Clin Cancer Res* 1997; 3:881–890.
121. Neville DM Jr, Youle RJ. Monoclonal antibody-ricin or ricin A chain hybrids: kinetic analysis of cell killing for tumor therapy. *Immunol Rev* 1982; 62:75–91.
122. Morland BJ, Barley J, Boehm D, et al. Effectiveness of HB2 (anti-CD7)—saporin immunotoxin in an in vivo model of human T-cell leukaemia developed in severe combined immunodeficient mice. *Br J Cancer* 1994; 69:279–285.
123. Flavell DJ, Boehm DA, Okayama K, et al. Therapy of human T-cell acute lymphoblastic leukaemia in severe combined immunodeficient mice with two different anti-CD7-saporin immunotoxins containing hindered or non-hindered disulphide cross-linkers. *Int J Cancer* 1994; 58:407–414.
124. Flavell DJ, Warnes S, Noss A, et al. Host-mediated antibody-dependent cellular cytotoxicity contributes to the in vivo therapeutic efficacy of an anti-CD7-saporin immunotoxin in a severe combined immunodeficient mouse model of human T-cell acute lymphoblastic leukemia. *Cancer Res* 1998; 58:5787–5794.
125. Beran M, Jeha S, O'Brien S, et al. Tallimustine, an effective antileukemic agent in a severe combined immunodeficient mouse model of adult myelogenous leukemia, induces remissions in a phase I study. *Clin Cancer Res* 1997; 3:2377–2384.
126. Clutterbuck RD, Millar BC, Powles RL, et al. Inhibitory effect of simvastatin on the proliferation of human myeloid leukaemia cells in severe combined immunodeficient (SCID) mice. *Br J Haematol* 1998; 102:522–527.
127. Jeha S, Kantarjian H, O'Brien S, et al. Activity of oral and intravenous 9-aminocamptothecin in SCID mice engrafted with human leukemia. *Leuk Lymphoma* 1998; 32:159–164.
128. Young DC, Wagner K, Griffin JD. Constitutive expression of the granulocyte-macrophage colony-stimulating factor gene in acute myeloblastic leukemia. *J Clin Investig* 1987; 79:100–106.
129. Onetto-Pothier N, Aumont N, Haman A, et al. Characterization of granulocyte-macrophage colony-stimulating factor receptor on the blast cells of acute myeloblastic leukemia. *Blood* 1990; 75:59–66.
130. Park LS, Waldron PE, Friend D, et al. Interleukin-3, GM-CSF, and G-CSF receptor expression on cell lines and primary leukemia cells: receptor heterogeneity and relationship to growth factor responsiveness. *Blood* 1989; 74:56–65.
131. Budel LM, Touw IP, Delwel R, et al. Granulocyte colony-stimulating factor receptors in human acute myelocytic leukemia. *Blood* 1989; 74:2668–2673.
132. Terpstra W, Rozemuller H, Breems DA, et al. Diphtheria toxin fused to granulocyte-macrophage colony-stimulating factor eliminates acute myeloid leukemia cells with the potential to initiate leukemia in immunodeficient mice, but spares normal hemopoietic stem cells. *Blood* 1997; 90:3735–3742.
133. Perentesis JP, Gunther R, Waurzyniak B, et al. In vivo biotherapy of HL-60 myeloid leukemia with a genetically engineered recombinant fusion toxin directed against the human granulocyte macrophage colony-stimulating factor receptor. *Clin Cancer Res* 1997; 3:2217–2227.
134. Rozemuller H, Terpstra W, Rombouts EJ, et al. GM-CSF receptor targeted treatment of primary AML in SCID mice using Diphtheria toxin fused to huGM-CSF. *Leukemia* 1998; 12:1962–1970.
135. Hall PD, Willingham MC, Kreitman RJ, et al. DT388-GM-CSF, a novel fusion toxin consisting of a truncated diphtheria toxin fused to human granulocyte-macrophage colony-stimulating factor, prolongs host survival in a SCID mouse model of acute myeloid leukemia. *Leukemia* 1999; 13:629–633.
136. Boayue KB, Gu L, Yeager AM, et al. Pediatric acute myelogenous leukemia cells express IL-6 receptors and are sensitive to a recombinant IL6-Pseudomonas exotoxin. *Leukemia* 1998; 12:182–191.
137. Bonnet D, Warren EH, Greenberg PD, et al. CD8(+) minor histocompatibility antigen-specific cytotoxic T lymphocyte clones eliminate human acute myeloid leukemia stem cells. *Proc Natl Acad Sci USA* 1999; 96:8639–8644.

138. Cesano A, Visonneau S, Cioe L, et al. Reversal of acute myelogenous leukemia in humanized SCID mice using a novel adoptive transfer approach. *J Clin Investig* 1994; 94:1076–1084.

139. Skorski T, Nieborowska-Skorska M, Wlodarski P, et al. Antisense oligodeoxynucleotide combination therapy of primary chronic myelogenous leukemia blast crisis in SCID mice. *Blood* 1996; 88:1005–1012.

140. Skorski T, Nieborowska-Skorska M, Wlodarski P, et al. Treatment of Philadelphia leukemia in severe combined immunodeficient mice by combination of cyclophosphamide and bcr/abl antisense oligodeoxynucleotides. *J Natl Cancer Inst* 1997; 89:124–133.

141. O'Brien SG, Kirkland MA, Melo JV, et al. Antisense BCR-ABL oligomers cause non-specific inhibition of chronic myeloid leukemia cell lines. *Leukemia* 1994; 8:2156–2162.

142. Flanagan WM. Antisense comes of age. *Cancer Metastasis Rev* 1998; 17:169–176.

143. Smetsers TF, Linders EH, van de Locht LT, et al. An antisense Bcr-Abl phosphodiester-tailed methylphosphonate oligonucleotide reduces the growth of chronic myeloid leukaemia patient cells by a non-antisense mechanism. *Br J Haematol* 1997; 96:377–381.

144. White JR, Gordon-Smith EC, Rutherford TR. Phosphorothioate-capped antisense oligonucleotides to Ras GAP inhibit cell proliferation and trigger apoptosis but fail to downregulate GAP gene expression. *Biochem Biophys Res Commun* 1996; 227:118–124.

145. Vaerman JL, Moureau P, Deldime F, et al. Antisense oligodeoxyribonucleotides suppress hematologic cell growth through stepwise release of deoxyribonucleotides. *Blood* 1997; 90:331–339.

146. de Kroon JF, de Paus RA, Kluin-Nelemans HC, et al. Anti-CD45 and anti-CD52 (Campath) monoclonal antibodies effectively eliminate systematically disseminated human non-Hodgkin's lymphoma B cells in Scid mice. *Exp Hematol* 1996; 24:919–926.

147. Schnell R, Katouzi AA, Linnartz C, et al. Potent anti-tumor effects of an anti-CD24 ricin A-chain immunotoxin in vitro and in a disseminated human Burkitt's lymphoma model in SCID mice. *Int J Cancer* 1996; 66:526–531.

148. Van Horssen PJ, Preijers FW, Van Oosterhout YV, et al. Highly potent CD22-recombinant ricin A results in complete cure of disseminated malignant B-cell xenografts in SCID mice but fails to cure solid xenografts in nude mice. *Int J Cancer* 1996; 68:378–383.

149. Ghetie MA, Tucker K, Richardson J, et al. The antitumor activity of an anti-CD22 immunotoxin in SCID mice with disseminated Daudi lymphoma is enhanced by either an anti-CD19 antibody or an anti-CD19 immunotoxin. *Blood* 1992; 80:2315–2320.

150. Schnell R, Linnartz C, Katouzi AA, et al. Development of new ricin A-chain immunotoxins with potent anti-tumor effects against human Hodgkin cells in vitro and disseminated Hodgkin tumors in SCID mice using high-affinity monoclonal antibodies directed against the CD30 antigen. *Int J Cancer* 1995; 63:238–244.

151. Hombach A, Jung W, Pohl C, et al. A CD16/CD30 bispecific monoclonal antibody induces lysis of Hodgkin's cells by unstimulated natural killer cells in vitro and in vivo. *Int J Cancer* 1993; 55:830–836.

152. Bohlen H, Manzke O, Titzer S, et al. Prevention of Epstein-Barr virus-induced human B-cell lymphoma in severe combined immunodeficient mice treated with CD3×CD19 bispecific antibodies, CD28 monospecific antibodies, and autologous T cells. *Cancer Res* 1997; 57:1704–1709.

29

Models for Studying the Action of Topoisomerase-I Targeted Drugs

Joyce Thompson, MD,
Clinton F. Stewart, PHARMD,
and Peter J. Houghton, PhD

CONTENTS

1. INTRODUCTION

Many of the cytotoxic drugs that are active in the curative or palliative treatment of human cancers are now known to mediate their effects through interaction with DNA topoisomerases stabilizing covalent DNA-protein intermediates. The epipodophylotoxins, anthracyclines, anthrapyrazoles, and actinomycins appear to target topoisomerase II, whereas drugs of the camptothecin class work specifically through their interaction with topoisomerase I. Some, such as actinomycin D, certain rebeccamycin analogs, and a new class of ethylidene glucoside-epipodophyllotoxins, may be dual-topoisomerase inhibitors *(1)*. The clinical utility of the epipodophyllotoxin, etoposide, and the anthracyclines doxorubicin, daunorubicin, and actinomycin D have been well-established *(2)*. The spectrum of utility of camptothecin drugs in treatment of human cancer also remains to be determined. However, current results from clinical trials suggest that drugs that target topoisomerase I may represent novel agents with considerable activity in a relatively broad spectrum of malignancies.

As with other drugs, the agents that target topoisomerases that are currently in clinical trials, or approved for use in particular indications, have proceeded through preclin-

From: *Tumor Models in Cancer Research*
Edited by: B. A. Teicher © Humana Press Inc., Totowa, NJ

Table 1
Activity of Camptothecin against Various Mouse Tumors

Tumor	Optimal dose (mg/kg) and schedule*	Increase in median Survival time over controls (%)	Long-term survivors (%)†
Leukemia L1210	40, q,4.d.	265	0
Leukemia L5178Y	40, 1,5,9	>1000‡	90
Leukemia K1964	40, 1,5,9	>1000	70
Leukemia P388	40, q.4.d.	185	0
Plasma cell YPC-1	40, 1,5,9	136	0
Mast cell P815	30, 1,5,9	65	0
Reticulum cell sarcoma A-RCS	40, q,4.d.	50	0

* Mice were treated ip with 30, 40, or 50 mg/kg on days 1, 5 and 9 after tumor inoculation or with 40 mg/kg every 4 ds for as long as 6 mo.

† Survivors 6 mo or longer after death of all controls.

‡ Where there were over 50% survivors, long-term survivors' increase in median survival time was not calculated beyond 1000%.

From Gallo et al (5)

ical stages of identifying cytotoxic potency, and confirmation of in vivo antitumor activity. Acceptable toxicity in both rodents and other species, as mandated by regulatory agencies, has been studied prior to clinical evaluation. However, despite remarkable activity against animal models (3), similar activity has not been reported in clinical trials, resulting in discontinuation of at least one agent, 9-aminocamptothecin.

This chapter examines this preclinical-clinical interface with respect to understanding the value and limitations of preclinical models, and potential lessons that can be applied to future development of drugs that induce cytotoxicity through their interactions with topoisomerase-I. The chapter focuses on preclinical models to assess antitumor activity and toxicity for this class of compounds, and how information derived from valid models may be used to direct the design of clinical trials.

2. EARLY STUDIES

Camptothecin was studied extensively in the Cancer Chemotherapy National Service Center (CCNSC) of the National Cancer Institute during the 1960s. In early in vivo testing, camptothecin as the base was formulated in carboxymethylcellulose, and administered by intraperitoneal (ip) injection using the Walker 256 rat carcinosarcoma model as the test system. Of interest was the relatively low therapeutic activity of camptothecin, relative to other drugs evaluated (4). Yet further studies, using the sodium salt of camptothecin, demonstrated significant activity in increasing survival time in several lymphocytic leukemias (5), including L1210, L5178Y, K1964, and P388, with a high proportion of long-term survivors in mice bearing L5178Y and K1964, (Table 1). Based on a lack of cross-resistance to dichloromethotrexate, carmustine (BCNU), cytosine arabinoside (ara-C), 6-mercaptopurine, and other agents in these models, it was proposed that camptothecin had a novel mechanism of action. Contrary to the activity in tumor model systems, camptothecin, evaluated as the sodium salt, was found to be ineffective in patients with advanced disseminated

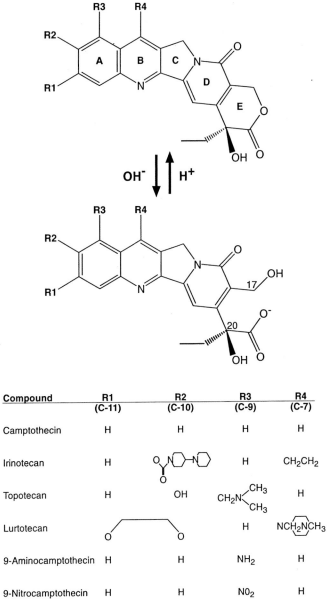

Fig. 1. Chemical structures of camptothecin analogs in clinical trials. Each analog exists in a pH-dependent equilibrium between lactone (active) and hydroxy-acid (inactive) forms.

Compound	R1 (C-11)	R2 (C-10)	R3 (C-9)	R4 (C-7)
Camptothecin	H	H	H	H
Irinotecan	H	(O,N piperidino-piperidine carbamate)	H	CH_2CH_2
Topotecan	H	OH	$CH_2N(CH_3)_2$	H
Lurtotecan	(O—CH₂CH₂—O)		H	NCH_2NCH_3
9-Aminocamptothecin	H	H	NH_2	H
9-Nitrocamptothecin	H	H	NO_2	H

melanoma or gastrointestinal malignancies *(6,7)*. Unpredictable and severe toxicities included myelosuppression, vomiting, diarrhea, and hemorrhagic cystitis that resulted in discontinuation of clinical trial of sodium camptothecin. Other studies in China, however, demonstrated activity of 10-hydroxycamptothecin in treatment of head and neck and bladder cancers (reviewed in ref. 8).

The motivation to pursue the development of these compounds followed studies that defined topoisomerase I as the target for camptothecin, and the observation that camptothecins caused trapping of topoisomerase I on DNA and induced single-strand breaks *(9,10)*. Camptothecin inhibits the religation step, effectively trapping topoisomerase I on DNA after a single-strand nick has been made by the enzyme. In cells replicating DNA, this could result in a collision between an advancing replication fork and the covalently linked enzyme-DNA complex, leading to a double-strand DNA break. Generation of this break is believed to initiate a cascade, leading to apoptosis. Although outside the scope of this chapter, it is important to understand that camptothecins induce toxicity by converting a normal cellular enzyme into a cellular poison *(11)*. Increased levels of topoisomerase I would favor increased formation of DNA-topoisomerase I-drug complexes, which would increase the probability of a collision with the advancing replication fork, and generation of a double-strand DNA break. In the absence of DNA replication, the reversibly stabilized DNA-topoisomerase-I-covalent complexes do not appear to be toxic. This has significance in the design of therapeutic trials, as one would anticipate predominantly or exclusively S-phase cells would be sensitive to camptothecins *(12)*. Many tumors are characterized by relatively low-growth fractions, and consequently, protracted infusions or repeated exposures to drug over a long period should optimize cell killing. The structures of camptothecin and analogs under clinical investigation are shown also in Fig. 1.

3. RODENT TUMOR MODELS

Traditionally, syngeneic transplanted rodent tumors have been used as the primary in vivo screen for activity of camptothecin analogs. Increase in lifespan (ILS) of mice bearing L1210 or P388 lymphocytic leukemias, inoculated intraperitoneally, have been used when the drug is also administered intraperitoneally. Although such tests have been described as "in vivo test tubes," one objective of these screens is to avoid elimination of active compounds (i.e., false negatives). In the development of topotecan, several in vivo criteria were established for selecting analog for further development. These included being as active as camptothecin in a panel of preclinical models, and demonstration of potency in vivo (i.e., a maximally tolerated dose, MTD) at similar or lower levels than camptothecin in order to minimize the requirements for camptothecin as a starting material *(8)*. Topotecan (9-dimethylaminomethyl, 10-hydroxycamptothecin) demonstrated superior ILS in mice bearing L1210 leukemia compared to that achieved by camptothecin at their respective MTD (173 ± 16 vs 118 ± 6% ILS). Because of the potential to kill only cells during DNA replication, protracted therapy with topoisomerase I inhibitors should theoretically prove most efficacious. Thus, oral administration may prove to be most practical in therapy of human cancer. Secondary evaluation of topotecan compared the efficacy of oral and intravenous (iv)-administered drug in syngeneic mice bearing advanced systemic (iv-inoculated) L1210, advanced systemic (iv-inoculated) Lewis Lung Carcinoma (LLC). subcutaneous (sc)-implanted LLC, systemic (iv) B16 melanoma, and ip-implanted M5076 reticulum-cell sarcoma *(13)*. The drug was administered every 3 h four times per day at 4- or 7-d intervals. Administered by oral gavage topotecan was comparable in efficacy to parenteral treatment in four of five tumor models tested. The M5076 sarcoma ip-implanted responded to topotecan administered intraperitoneally or subcutaneously, but not when given orally. Irinotecan (CPT-11; 7-ethyl-10-(4-[1-piperidino]-1-piperidino)-carbonyloxy-(20S)camptothecin) is a prodrug that is activated in rodents by plasma car-

Table 2
Evaluation of Antitumor Activity of CPT-11 against sc-Implanted Tumors

Tumor	Drug route	Total dose (mg/kg)[a]		Dose for cure[b] (mg/kg)	No. of cured mice/total (dose, mg/kg)
		ID_{58}	ID_{90}		
S180	iv	50	180	200	4/10 (200)
	po	100	365	400	3/10 (400), 6/10 (800)
Meth A	iv	61	195	>400	6/10 (1,000)
	po	140	420	1000	7/7 (1,600)
Lewis lung ca.	ip	72	118	200	5/6 (200), 6/6 (400)
	po	215	410	400	1/6 (400), 4/6 (600), 5/6 (800), 6/6 (1,600)
Ehrlich	ip	32	92	50	1/6 (50), 3/6 (100), 3/6 (200)
	po	110	450	400	2/6 (400), 3/5 (800)
MH134	ip	66	200	200	1/6 (200), 1/6 (400)
	po	215	620	600	1/6 (600), 4/6 (800)
Mammary ca.	ip	96	>400	200	1/6 (200)
	po	600	>800	800	1/6 (800)

[a] Total dose for 58% or 90% inhibition of tumor growth. The values were obtained graphically on a probit scale. Tumor-free mice were excluded from the calculation of 90% inhibition.

[b] The minimum total dose for incidence of total regression of the tumor.

From Kunimoto et al. (14)

boxylesterases, and has been extensively studied in syngeneic tumors (14–16). The activity of irinotecan against a panel of tumors transplanted subcutaneously is presented in Table 2. Irinotecan demonstrated significant activity by both parenteral and oral routes against disseminated models following iv inoculation systemic (iv-inoculated highly metastatic B16-F10 melanoma), or in spontaneous metastases from SC implants (murine colon 26). The most comprehensive study reported (16) evaluated irinotecan in 10 murine tumors and one human xenograft. All 11 tumors responded to irinotecan—eight were responsive at the Decision Network-2 level (DN-2, where treated/control volumes were <10%), which is the criteria used by the NCI to justify further development. This work also showed no cross-resistance in vivo in P388/VCR leukemic cells resistant to vincristine or human breast-carcinoma cells selected for resistance to docetaxel (taxotere). However, the limited pharmacokinetic data reported showed that significantly higher levels of SN-38, (7-ethyl,10-hydroxy-(20S)camptothecin) the active metabolite of irinotecan, were achieved in the mouse compared to that achieved in patients.

4. HUMAN XENOGRAFT MODELS

Human-tumor xenografts, growing in immune-incompetent mice, are now established as predictive models for many human cancers. Minimum requirement for validation of these models is that they should parallel the chemosensitivity-chemoresistance profile of the clinical disease. The most frequent approach taken is to heterograft surgical specimens of tumor into congenitally immune deficient (athymic nude mice, or severe combined immunodeficiency (SCID) mice), or mice that have been immune-deprived to prevent graft rejection. Alternatively, cells initially propagated in vitro from human tumors may be injected into the mice subcutaneously, or intravenously if disseminated disease is required. In certain circumstances it may be important to assess the preclinical activity of a new drug under conditions that mimic the clinical situation (i.e., metastatic disease), in which case the development of orthotopic models can be attempted by injecting cells into the natural occurring site within the host. Of importance is that cell lines retain their sensitivity to chemotherapeutic agents. A number of lines representing a tumor type are generally required to accurately recapitulate the clinical situation and to conduct "preclinical phase II evaluation." However, conditions for tumor growth in the mouse may differ from patients, and differences in drug disposition and metabolism in the mouse may significantly influence tumor responses.

The curative activity of 9-aminocamptothecin (9-AC) against chemorefractory colon cancers focused considerable attention on this class of anticancer agent (3). Interestingly, while SC administration of drug was highly active, subsequent studies with iv administration were relatively disappointing. Activity of camptothecin analogs has been confirmed against an extensive panel of human-tumor xenografts possessing a broad pattern of biological properties and chemosensitivities (17–31), Table 3. The growth of all tumors was significantly inhibited by administration of the respective analog, with a high percentage of complete and partial tumor regressions. In contrast, standard agents used for clinical treatment of the appropriate tumor type, showed considerably less activity. 9-AC induced complete remissions in mice bearing xenografts of colon adenocarcinoma and malignant melanoma (BRO) xenografts. 9-Nitrocamptothecin (9-NC), is converted to 9-AC, and is currently under clinical investigation. 9-NC has shown superior therapeutic efficacy over 9-AC or camptothecin in a large number of human xenograft models (18). Topotecan also demonstrated good antitumor activity when administered intravenously, intraperitoneally, and orally, against xenografts derived from various childhood solid tumors, with a high percentage of complete regressions against rhabdomyosarcomas, neuroblastomas, and some brain tumors. In contrast, reduced activity was found against colon-carcinoma xenografts (19).

Irinotecan appears to be the most efficacious analog in preclinical studies, and has been investigated most extensively. When administered by iv, ip, or oral routes, irinotecan showed substantial activity against a broad spectrum of human tumor enografts, including human-cancer xenograft lines unresponsive to many cytotoxic agents. High cure rates were obtained against MX-1 mammary tumor, rhabdomyosarcomas, neuroblastomas, colon cancers, and brain tumors. Activity was also retained against tumors selected for resistance to topotecan, vincristine, melphalan, busulphan, procarbazine, and cyclophosphamide. However, mice readily activate irinotecan to SN-38, and plasma systemic exposure to SN-38 in mice greatly exceeds that achieved in patients. Thus, exposures to SN-38 associated with tumor regressions in mice, may far exceed exposures achievable in patients.

Two water-soluble analog of camptothecin—GI147211, and GI149893, 10,11-methylenedioxy, 7-substituted compounds—have been assessed in preclinical models of colon and mammary carcinoma. Their antitumor effects were dose- and schedule-dependent, with a greater reduction in tumor volume achieved by protracted dosing. Concurrent experiments demonstrated that they were more effective than topotecan in

Table 3

Responsiveness of Human Tumor Xenografts to Treatment with Camptothecin Analogues

Drug	Xenograft tumor	Dose (mg/kg) and schedule	Comment	Reference
9-AC	Colon HT-29	10–12.5 mg/kg × 2/wk for 5–6 wk sc	Highly effective	(3)
	Colon CASE Colon SW48		ADR, 5 FU, MTX, nitrosoureas, ALK, less effective/ineffective	
CPT-11	Mammary MX-1	200 mg (TD) i.v.	Very significant antitumor activity against all tumors Curative against MX-1	(17)
	Gastric St-15	400–800 mg (TD) q (4dX3) po	ADR, 5FU, CDDP less effective	
	Gastric SC-6		CPT-11 more effective as three injections than one single injection for same total dose	
	Lung QG56 Colon Co-4			
CAM, 9-AC, 9-NC	Melanoma BRO	4 mg X2/wk im	Growth inhibition and tumor regression	(18)
			BRO tumors unresponsive to ADR, 5FU, VCR, VBL, MTX, nitrosourea, ALK	
Topotecan	6 rhabdomyo-sarcoma lines	1.5–2.0 mg (dX5)3 iv/po	Complete regression in rhabdo-myosarcomas. Significant activity in osteosarcomas. Growth	(19)
	7 colon lines	12.5 mg q (4dX4) ip	inhibition in several colon lines Results suggest significant schedule dependence	
	3 osteosarcoma lines			

(continues)

Table 3 (continued)

Drug	Xenograft tumor	Dose (mg/kg) and schedule	Comment	Reference
9-AC, 9-NC, 9-CL-AM	Breast carcinoma		9-AC effective — Short infusions (72 h every 21 d) not effective; Long infusions (5 d every 7 days) very effective 9-NC effective 9-CL-CAM not effective — Results were dose-, schedule- and route of administration-dependent	(20)
CPT-11	6 rhabdomyo-sarcoma lines	10–40 mg (dX5)2 iv and [(dX5)2]3 iv	All tumors very sensitive — CPT-11 effective against 2 xenografts selected for resistance to topotecan and rhabdomyosarcoma lines resistant to VCR and melphalan	(21)
	7 colon lines		Complete and partial regressions in 5/8 colon lines; Complete responses in 5/6 rhabdomyosarcoma lines	
CPT-11	TNB9 Neuroblastoma	15–59 mg q (4dX3) ip	Growth inhibition — VCR, aclarubicin, VP-16 5F-U, THP-ADR, ineffective	(22)
CPT-11, topotecan	6 rhabdomyo-sarcoma lines	CPT-11: 2.5–10 mg [(dX5)2]3 iv	CPT-11 highly active (complete regressions) against colon lines — CPT-11 and topotecan active against tumors selected for resistance to VCR	(23)
	8 colon lines	Topotecan: 0.5–1.5 mg (dX5) 12 po	Both drugs similar high activity against rhabdomyosarcomas and brain tumors — CPT-11 active against tumor selected for resistance to melphalan	
	3 brain tumors		Concluded: low dose protracted scheduling of daily administration is equi-efficacious as shorter more intense schedules	

Drug	Tumor model	Dose/schedule	Result	Comments	Ref.
Topotecan, G1147211, G1149893	Colon HT-79 Colon SW-48 Mammary MX-1 Prostate PC-3	MTD divided into 3 doses infused q 4 hourly in 24 h X2/wk for 5 wk	G1147211 and G1149893: Regressions >50% in HT79 and SW-48 Complete regressions in MX-1, growth inhibition in PC3 Topotecan: Growth inhibition only		(24)
CPT-11	PNET SKNMC Neuroblastomas N835 NB8 NB3	27–40 mg (dX5) iv and q (4dX3) iv	Very effective, high complete response rates		(25)
CPT-11	6 neuroblastoma lines	10–40 mg (dX5) iv 5–10 mg [(dX5)2]3 iv 25–50 mg (dX5)12 po	Highly efficacious Complete regression of all tumors on the protracted iv schedule and all tumors using oral schedule		(26,27)
CPT-11	9 brain tumor lines Gliomas Medulloblastomas Ependymomas	40 mg (dX5)2 ip	Tumor regression in every treated tumor line	CPT-11 active against tumors resistant to busulfan, procarbazine, cyclophosphamide and melphalan	(28)
9-AC	Prostate PC3	2 mg X2/wk for 3 wk sc 0.35–1 mg (dX5)3 po	Inhibition and regression of tumor growth	PC3 is a hormone refractory prostate line	(29)
Topotecan	6 neuroblastoma lines	0.36–2 mg [(dX5)2]3 i.v.	Highly effective	Minimum daily systemic exposure related to to objective response	(30)

Complete regressions in all tumors

CAM, camptothecin; 9-AC, 9-aminocamptothecin; 9-NC, 9-nitrocamptothecin; 9-CL–CAM, 9-chlorocamptothecin suppressing tumor growth, although optimal schedules for topotecan were not compared in these studies *(24)*. As a liposomal formulation GI147211 (designated NX211) has demonstrated good antitumor activity against more than 20 lines of tumor xenografts, with minimal toxic effects.

For camptothecin analogs, evaluation of the antitumor efficacy requires schedules in the mouse that produce drug exposures similar to those achievable in patients. For many of the experiments reported in Table 3, systemic exposures in the mouse to lactone forms of the camptothecin used far exceed exposures that can be achieved in patients at tolerated dose levels. The data presented demonstrate the relative sensitivity of a given tumor to a series of analogs administered to their maximum tolerated dose (MTD) levels in the mouse. Such data may overpredict activity in patients. Without knowing the relative toxicity-systemic exposure relationship in humans, such data may have limited predictive value for selecting analogs for further development.

5. SCHEDULE-DEPENDENT ANTITUMOR ACTIVITY

Animal models may also be useful for examining alternative schedules of drug administration. Indeed, obtaining information about the schedule-dependency in relation to both the antitumor activity and host toxicity of an agent is one of the goals of preclinical studies. Topoisomerase I inhibitors exert their activity potentially during the S phase of the cell cycle. Therefore, it is assumed that once a cytotoxic threshold is achieved, exposure time—rather than further dose escalation—is the important parameter for determining the tumor response. Consequently, protracted drug administration could increase antitumor activity.

The importance of scheduling was first reported by Kawato *(17)*, and confirmed subsequently in additional models *(18–20)*. These studies showed that for similar total dosages administered, protracted schedules were more effective than more intense treatments of shorter duration. Several groups have reported schedule-dependent activity of camptothecin analogs, although this finding does not appear to have been used in design of the initial clinical trials. Schedule-dependency is illustrated in Fig. 2, where the responses of individual rhabdomyosarcoma xenografts have been measured in mice receiving drug vehicle (control) or irinotecan treatment. Both treatment groups received the same total dose of drug, the only difference being that drug was given over 5 d or 10 d. Clearly, irinotecan administered over 10 d was significantly more active than the same dose given over 5 d. In xenograft models, at least, drugs such as irinotecan appear to be "self-limiting". Above some dose level, further increases in dose per administration does not result in further antitumor activity. This is illustrated in Fig. 3, where mice received irinotecan for two 5-d courses [(dx5)2] for a single cycle, or where lower doses were administered every 21 d for three cycles on the (dx5)2 schedule *(21)*. In this colon tumor, increasing the dose from 10 to 40 mg/kg per administration did not result in enhanced antitumor activity. Three cycles of (dx5)2 therapy (5 mg/kg/administration, total dose administered: 150 mg/kg) over 8 wk resulted in significantly greater activity compared to drug administratd over 12 days (40 mg/kg/administration, total dose administered: 400 mg/kg). Similar results have been obtained with 9-AC and other camptothecin analogs in various tumor models. Interestingly, administration of irinotecan using the (dx5)2 schedule every 21 d has demonstrated significant antitumor activity in a Phase I clinical trial in children with tumors resistant to conventional therapy *(32)*.

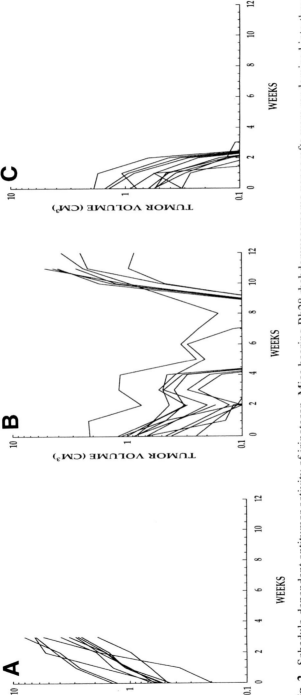

Fig. 2. Schedule-dependent antitumor activity of irinotecan. Mice bearing Rh28 rhabdomyosarcoma xenografts were randomized into three groups of seven mice. Group A received no treatment (Controls), group B received irinotecan daily for 5 d at a dose of 5 mg/kg/d. Mice in group C received 2.5 mg/kg daily for 5 d on 2 consecutive wk. Courses of treatment were repeated ever 21 d over 8 wk for groups B and C. The total dose per 21-d course was 25 mg/kg for both treatment groups. Each curve shows the growth of an individual tumor. In group B irinotecan caused regressions, but most tumors had recurred by wk 12. In contrast, delivering the same dose of irinotecan over 10 ds induced complete responses without regrowth during the period of observation (12 wk).

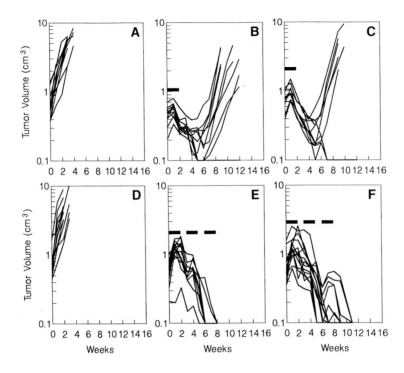

Fig. 3. Efficacy of repeated courses of therapy relative to more intense treatment schedules against VRC$_5$ colon xenografts. *Top:* A, control; B, irinotecan 40 mg/kg/dose; C, 10 mg/kg/dose given (dx5)2 intravenously. *Bottom:* D, control; E, irinotecan 10 mg/kg/dose; F, 5 mg/kg/dose given (dx5)2 repeated every 21 d for 3 cycles (treatment periods marked by heavy horizontal bars). Each curve represents the growth of an individual tumor. Total doses administered were 400, 100, 300, and 150 mg/kg in groups B,C,E and F, respectively. (From ref. *21,* with permission).

6. MODELS OF RESISTANCE TO TOPOISOMERASE-I INHIBITORS

Two camptothecin analogs, topotecan and irinotecan, are approved for treatment of refractory ovarian carcinoma and 5-fluorouracil (5-Fu) refractory colon carcinoma, respectively. Thus, new agents should demonstrate clear superiority over these established drugs to justify full development—for example, demonstration of significant activity against tumors that have intrinsic or acquired resistance to topotecan or irinotecan. Irinotecan is highly active against certain tumors that are intrinsically resistant to topotecan, and against some xenografts selected *in situ* for acquired resistance to topotecan *(21).* Several cell lines selected for resistance to camptothecin have been reported. In one line (CEM/C2) resistance is mediated by a mutation (Asn722Ser) in topoisomerase-I *(33).* In yeast, several mutations in topoisomerase-I yield camptothecin resistance *(34).* However, it is less certain in clinical tumors whether intrinsic or acquired resistance is caused by topoisomerase-I mutations. Thus, establishing xenograft models from cell lines in which resistance is caused by mutant enzyme may not necessarily recapitulate clinical resistance. At this time, mechanisms that confer camptothecin resistance in clinical cancers remain uncharacterized. Potentially, resistance could be complex and analog-specific, and involve

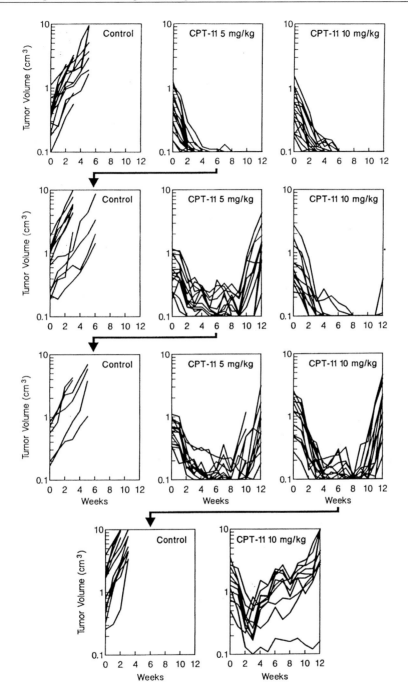

Fig. 4. Selection *in situ* of NB-1691 neuroblastoma with acquired resistance to irinotecan. Mice bearing sc NB-1691 xenografts were treated intravenously using an optimal schedule of irinotecan (daily × 5 on 2 consecutive wk), with cycles of therapy repeated every 21 d over 8 wk. A single tumor that regrew in the 5 mg/kg dose group, was retransplanted into recipient hosts, and treatment was repeated. Retransplantation and treatment at 5 and 10 mg/kg yielded tumors that regrew after treatment with 10 mg/kg. Subsequent treatment showed only minor responses to irinotecan (unpublished data).

mechanisms proximal to DNA damage (i.e., accumulation/efflux), at the target level (mutation or activity of topoisomerase-I) or distal to damage (repair processes). In several xenograft models, selection *in situ* for resistance to topotecan did not result in cross-resistance to irinotecan *(21)*. However, relatively few models of acquired resistance to camptothecin analogs have been reported. Relatively rapid development of an irinotecan-resistant neuroblastoma xenograft (NB-1691/CPT) is depicted in Fig. 4. As shown, the parent tumor is highly sensitive to irinotecan, with complete regressions at the dose level and optimal schedules of drug administration used. To develop resistance, a single tumor that recurred (wk 20) following treatment (5 mg/kg/administration) was transplanted into new host mice. The same treatment produced less response, a single tumor was retransplanted, and treatment was repeated. A single tumor was transplanted from mice receiving the higher dose of irinotecan. After four rounds of treatment/transplantation, a stable irinotecan-resistant line was derived. This tumor is partially resistant to topotecan. Although the mechanism of resistance has not been characterized, this tumor may represent a useful model for identifying novel topoisomerase-I targeted agents with characteristics that significantly differ from either irinotecan or topotecan.

7. TOXICITY

7.1. Hematopoietic Toxicity

The often dramatic preclinical activity of camptothecin analogs in xenograft models contrasts with the clinical activity observed in many Phase II studies. As would be predicted from their S-phase activity, topoisomerase I inhibitors cause dose-limiting toxicity to rapidly renewing tissues, such as hematopoietic tissues in humans and animals. However, dose-limiting toxicity occurs at far lower systemic exposures in humans than in mice. Humans can tolerate only 11% as much topotecan per day as mice. This differential may be greater for irinotecan. Based on pharmacokinetic estimates of SN-38 systemic exposure at the MTD in patients receiving irinotecan every 7 d, it was estimated that the systemic exposure represented only 6% of the MTD in mice *(35)*. For myelosuppressive camptothecin analogs, the failure to achieve drug exposures in patients that are curative in the murine models might be a result of the greater sensitivity of human myeloid progenitors. Using in vitro clonogenic assays, Erickson-Miller et al. *(36)* determined that hematopoietic progenitors of the myeloid lineage from humans, mice, and dogs exhibit differential sensitivity to these compounds. The toxicity of camptothecin analogs to human and animal myeloid progenitors was quantified from the inhibition of marrow CFU-GM colony formation as a result of continuous drug exposure. Camptothecin lactone, topotecan, and 9AC inhibited colony formation in a concentration-dependent manner. The results suggest that because of the greater sensitivity of their myelopoietic tissue, humans cannot tolerate exposures to camptothecins that are curative in murine models. Murine myeloid progenitors were relatively resistant compared to their human counterparts for all the compounds examined. The differences between mice and humans were large, with topotecan and 9-AC, Table 4. The susceptibility of human CFU-GM to drug toxicity is more closely approximated by canine than by murine CFU-GM. This finding explains why even subcurative doses of camptothecins may be severely myelotoxic in patients.

Table 4
The Concentrations of Drug (in mM) Inhibiting CFU-GM Colony Formation from Human,
Canine and Murine Femoral Marrow by 50% (IC_{50}) and 90% (IC_{90})

Compound	$IC_{50}(nM)$			IC_{90} (nM)		
	Human	Murine	Canine	Human	Murine	Canine
CAM lactone	1.7	18	0.5	16	42	7.6
NA+-CAM	n/a	17	n/a	29	67	6.9
TPT	2.8	128	1.7	39	381	7.6
s9-AC	0.6	20	0.3	6.2	66	7.6
ss9-AC	0.3	16	0.6	7.3	43	7.4
(R,S)-9-AC	0.7	75	0.6	16	331	6.9

The average percent inhibition of CFU-GM from 12, six, and three human, canine, and murine marrows, respectively.

(From ref. *36,* with permission.)

7.2. Gastrointestinal Toxicity

For most schedules of administration evaluated clinically, use of irinotecan has been associated with an unexpected and significant incidence of diarrhea, which is now recognized as a dose-limiting toxicity of this compound *(37)*. However, this was not anticipated from studies in rodents, in which diarrhea was not observed. Diarrhea may be caused by abnormalities of intestinal absorption or secretion, because of a change in intestinal flora, increased peristalsis, or drug-induced epithelial damage. The considerable interpatient variability in the severity of diarrhea has made it difficult to explain the mechanism of irinotecan-associated diarrhea. However, this toxicity, is not unique to irinotecan. Diarrhea was the dose-limiting toxicity of topotecan, when administered orally to patients for 21 d. The etiology of this side effect of camptothecins is not yet clear, although several animal models have been established that attempt to simulate irinotecan-induced diarrhea.

7.3. Mouse Models

Ikuno et al *(38)* observed characteristic changes in the intestinal mucosa of irinotecan-treated mice including marked shortening of the villi (villous atrophy), and epithelial vacuolation of the ileum, associated with increased apoptosis, and goblet-cell hyperplasia in the cecum. These structural and functional effects were postulated as the main causes of irinotecan-induced diarrhea, leading to malabsorption and hypersecretion of mucin. The malabsorption in irinotecan-treated mice was believed to be caused by villous atrophy following crypt damage and apotosis of absorptive cells in the small intestine. The goblet-cell hyperplasia associated with excessive production of mucin in the cecum could be another contributing factor to the cause of diarrhea with irinotecan. A mouse model of intestinal toxicity has also been used to identify potential modulators of irinotecan-induced diarrhea. Daily administration of 100 mg/kg irinotecan to mice resulted in loss of villi, epithelial vacuolation, decreased numbers of S-phase cells in the crypts, increased apoptotic cells, and reduced numbers of lymphocytes in the lamina propria. Oral administration of a synthetic bacterial lipopeptide, JBT 3002, encapsulated in phospholipid liposomes prevented irinotecan-induced damage to the intestinal epithelium and lamina propria *(39)*.

7.4. Rat Models

Relatively high concentrations of irinotecan caused eicosanoid-mediated chloride secretion in isolated rat colon *(40)*. Frequently, diarrhea is caused by the active secretion of electrolytes, especially chloride ions, suggesting that this toxicity is independent of the action of irinotecan or the active metabolite, SN-38, on topoisomerase-I. Irinotecan-induced diarrhea was characterized histologically and enzymologically in rats by assessing the relationship between intestinal toxicity and the activity of enzymes involved in the major metabolic pathways of this drug *(41)*. In rodents, irinotecan is converted to its active metabolite SN-38 by carboxylesterase, and one possible mechanism for the diarrhea may include the structural and functional injuries to the intestinal tract resulting from the direct cytotoxic activity of the SN-38. Detoxification of SN-38 occurs by liver glucoronidation, and conjugated SN-38 is secreted into the bile and in the feces. However, it may be further converted/processed to an active SN-38 by β-glucuronidase of the microflora, which resides in the large intestine. In this rat model, histological damage was most severe in the cecum, with markedly decreased size and number of the crypts and superficial mucosal erosion. The segmental differences in the degree of damage showed good correlation with the β-glucuronidase activity in the contents of the lumen, suggesting that this enzyme plays a key role in intestinal toxicity induced by irinotecan. Intestinal-tissue carboxylesterase activity, which also converts irinotecan to its active form, showed poor correlation to the degree of tissue damage. Gut sterilization by administration of antibiotics exerted a protective effect against diarrhea by completely inhibiting the β-glucuronidase activity in intestinal flora, and thus the formation of active SN-38. Rustum and colleagues *(42)* have also developed a rat model of irinotecan-induced gastrointestinal toxicity. In their study, very high dose levels of irinotecan (150–200 mg/kg daily × 3 iv.) resulted in 86–100% lethality in treated animals, and 93–100% incidence of severe diarrhea, associated with serious damage to duodenal villi and colonic crypts. Interleukin-15 (IL-15100–400 µg/kg (3, 8, and 11 ip doses) completely protected against irinotecan-induced delayed diarrhea and lethality. The validity of these rodent models however, must wait for confirmatory clinical trials.

7.5. Hamster Models

The hamster has also been proposed as a model for irinotecan-induced intestinal toxicity *(43)*. Female Syrian hamsters were dosed intraperitoneally with irinotecan (50 mg/kg/d) for 10 d and observed through d 20. By d 5, all treated animals had developed diarrhea and deaths occurred starting on d 7. Histological examination revealed a time-dependent loss of structural integrity of the jejunal and ileal mucosa. The typical columnar morphology of the epithelial cells was lost, and the villi appeared corrugated. The epithelium was thinned and vacuolated in the colon within the first 5 d of treatment. Detection of proliferating-cell nuclear antigen (PCNA), showed an increase in the number of labeled epithelial cells and labeling intensity in treated animals. The labeled cells were located further toward the tips of villi compared to control animals. Increased levels of PCNA and loss of differentiation in cell morphology suggested that irinotecan induces a cell-cycle block in S-G2, with subsequent loss of physiologic

Table 5
Comparison of Irinotecan and SN-38 Systemic Exposure (AUC) between Mice and Humans

Ref.	Lactone irinotecan (ng/mL × h)	Lactone SN-38 (ng/mL × h)	Total irinotecan (ng/mL × h)	Total SN-38 (ng/mL × h)
Mice				
Irinotecan 52.5 mg/kg iv (Bissery et al. [16])	n/a	n/a	62.5	34.5
Irinotecan 10 mg/kg iv [(dX5)2]3 (Stewart et al. [47])	13.0	5.3	n/a	n/a
Humans				
Irinotecan 350 mg/m² iv once every 3 wk (Abigerges et al. [48])	n/a	n/a	34.0	0.45
Irinotecan 100 mg/m²/wk iv for 3 consecutive d every 3 wk (Catimetl et al. [49])	n/a	n/a	27.9	0.96
Irinotecan 150 mg/m²/wk iv for 4 of 6 wk (Rothenberg et al. [50])	5.6	0.24	16.8	0.82
Irinotecan 20 mg/m² iv [(dX5)2]3 (Furman, Stewart, unpublished)	4.0	1.4	n/a	n/a

Total and lactone AUC have been calculated for the cumulative exposure for a 21-d cycle of therapy.

function in hamster intestinal epithelium. Kobayashi et al. *(44)* have also studied the effect of pH on uptake of irinotecan and SN-38 lactone and carboxylate in isolated intestinal cells from Syrian hamsters. From these studies, it is proposed that uptake of lactone is by passive diffusion, yet there may be an energy-dependent accumulation (transport) for carboxylate. Accumulation of irinotecan carboxylate showed saturation kinetics with apparent Km ~ 50 μM in jejunal and ileal cells.

8. INTERSPECIES DIFFERENCES THAT COMPLICATE TRANSLATION OF PRECLINICAL RESULTS

8.1. Interspecies Differences in Drug Metabolism and Disposition

Camptothecins have demonstrated greater activity against model tumors in rodents than against tumors in patients. This seems partly a result of the greater tolerance of mice to the toxic effects of these agents compared to that of humans. Analysis of data from the mouse, rat, and dog showed that predicting the clinical MTD dose for 8 topoisomerase-I inhibitors from rodent data would result in starting clinical trials very close to, or at dose levels exceeding, the human MTD*(45)*. In contrast, initial starting doses based on canine data would have been safe. The plasma systemic exposure, expressed as an area under the concentration-time curve or AUC, for irinotecan and its active metabolite SN-38 in mice *(16,46)* and patients *(47–49)* are presented in Table 5. To facilitate comparison between schedules, systemic exposure has been expressed for each course of therapy, usually in a 21-d time frame at the highest nontoxic dose (HNTD) for mice and the MTD for humans. Not all investigators report both the lactone and total drug. Thus, it is difficult to directly compare the systemic exposure of irinotecan and SN-38 between studies; however, when given once weekly in humans, the systemic exposure to irinotecan and, particularly SN-38, is significantly greater in mice than in humans.

This raises the concern that studies with syngeneic tumors or human xenograft models in mice may over-predict the potential clinical utility of this, as well as other classes of anticancer drugs. For camptothecins the reasons for the interspecies differences are not well understood. However, rather than use the mouse model to predict systemic drug exposures associated with toxicity, we have chosen to use it to determine the systemic exposure associated with antitumor effect against the human-tumor xenograft. For a series of neuroblastoma xenografts, the daily systemic exposure to topotecan that caused objective regressions was determined when the drug was administered 5 d per wk for 2 consecutive wk (30). Partial responses were achieved in each of six independently derived neuroblastoma lines at a daily topotecan lactone systemic exposure of 100 ng/mL*h, whereas complete responses were achieved in four tumor lines. Thus, the results of these studies define the effective antitumor systemic exposure to the camptothecin analog. Current data from our studies in children indicate that exposure of 100 ng/mL*h (achieved after a dose of 0.61 mg/kg in mice) results from a dose of 3 mg/m^2 in children. For irinotecan, dose levels of ~1.25 mg/kg in mice yield SN-38 plasma systemic exposures achieved at doses of 20–30 mg/m^2 administered to children (32). This difference is a consequence of very efficient activation of irinotecan by plasma carboxylesterase in mice. Recently, a strain of mouse, designated Es1^e, deficient in plasma esterases has been identified. Kinetic studies indicated that the activation of irinotecan to SN-38 by Es1^e mouse plasma in vitro is 600-fold less efficient, although extracts from organs indicated no difference in drug metabolism as compared to controls (50). It is proposed that the Es1^e mouse may represent a more representative model of irinotecan drug activation.

8.2. Protein Binding

Systemic exposure to camptothecin analogs represents total drug concentration that consists of both drug bound to plasma protein and unbound drug. For drugs extensively bound to plasma proteins, like SN-38, unbound drug concentrations correlate best with indices of pharmacologic effect. If significant interspecies variability exists in the plasma protein binding, the comparison between unbound drug concentrations and toxicity in humans and animals may be more appropriate than total drug concentration. The relevance of interspecies differences in drug-protein binding is seen with camptothecin analogs. Campothecin exists as a pentacyclic structure with a lactone moiety in the terminal (E) ring. At least against purified topoisomerase-I, the presence of a lactone ring is a structural requirement for activity. Thus, factors influencing the lactone-carboxylate equilibrium may be important determinants of drug activity. In addition to pH, the presence of protein, particularly albumin, has been shown to be important to the stability of the lactone (51,52). Human serum albumin (HSA) had a marked preference for the carboxylate form of camptothecin, greater than serum albumin from five other species. Thus, binding of the carboxylate to albumin drives the equilibrium away from the active lactone form of the drug. However, structural modifications to the camptothecin ring seen with irinotecan, SN-38, and topotecan diminished the interspecies differences in stabilization of the lactone. This contrasts with 9-AC, in which the marked interspecies difference in stabilization of the carboxylate form was similar to that observed with camptothecin. Four hours after intragastric administration to mice of camptothecin or 9-NC, lactone forms comprise 57–81% and 47–95% of the total drug, respectively. In contrast, the lactone comprised only a minor component of total drug levels in plasma from humans treated orally with either drug (53). This interspecies variability in protein stabilization of the carboxylate form is important for translation of data derived in rodents to clinical trials. These results also illustrate the importance of determining the systemic exposure to lactone forms of camptothecin analogs that induce objective regressions in xenograft models. This information may be valuable in understanding and designing phase II clinical trials. Attempts to encapsulate and stabilize lactone forms of camptothecins may also increase the therapeutic utility of drugs such as camptothecin or topotecan (54,55).

9. FUTURE DIRECTIONS

Animal models, and human-tumor xenografts in particular, have predicted dramatic clinical therapeutic activity of camptothecin drugs. Agents such as topotecan and irinotecan, are clearly active in several adult and childhood cancers, as well as myelodysplastic syndromes. However, the response rates anticipated based on xenograft-derived data have not been achieved. For analogs such as 9-aminocamptothecin, clinical results have been quite disappointing. Retrospective analysis of preclinical data for topoisomerase-I inhibitors shows that such differences in results are caused by interspecies differences in drug disposition and host tolerance. For camptothecins, mice tolerate far greater systemic exposure than can be achieved in patients at tolerated levels of toxicity. Furthermore, the remarkable schedule-dependency for antitumor activity seen in many preclinical models has not been adequately addressed in the design of clinical trials. When response rates for xenograft tumors are calculated for doses that yield clinically achievable systemic exposures, these models rather accurately predict the clinical results. For example, based on a plasma systemic exposure of 100 ng/mLh topotecan lactone the predicted response rate is ~60% for neuroblastoma xenografts (30). Similarly, we would anticipate approximately 25% of colon-carcinoma xenografts demonstrating objective responses (≥50% volume regression) using doses of irinotecan that in mice yield clinically achievable systemic exposures for SN-38. However, such information is not available when selecting between analogs at a relatively early stage in development. One way in which equi-efficacious analogs could be distinguished would be to introduce assays of differential species marrow toxicity at an early stage in development. This may allow identification analogs with good antitumor activity, but with little difference in species toxicity.

The topoisomerase-I targeted agents currently in clinical investigation are mainly based on a camptothecin structure. There are many more analogs in preclinical development. One focus has been on stabilization of the E-ring lactone. This has been achieved by increasing the lipophilicity of camptothecins by substitution on the 7-position with bulky alky, alkylamino, and alkylsilyl groups. A more novel approach has been the synthesis of homo-camptothecins, in which a seven-member lactone E-ring has far greater stability. Interestingly, this analog appears to change the sequence specificity of the drug-induced DNA cleavage by topoisomerase-I (56). However, differences in lipophilicity are more likely to result in alterations in the pharmaceutical properties of this class of agent, rendering longer plasma clearance times, and potentially allowing greater systemic exposure to active forms of these drugs. As there is little clinical data to support the value of delivering camptothecins by prolonged continuous infusion, it is uncertain whether analogs with greater lactone stability will be more efficacious. Definitive activity in preclinical models with intrinsic or acquired resistance to current camptothecins would be important in advancing such analogues to clinical testing.

New structures such as protoberberines *(57)*, indolocarbazoles (rebeccamycin analogs), *(58)*, and lipophilic epipodophyllotoxins have emerged as potential dual inhibitors of topoisomerases. Of particular interest is F11782, an ethylidene glucoside ester of epipodophyllotoxin that inhibits the catalytic cycle of both type I and II enzymes, preventing their binding to DNA *(59)*. This agent has demonstrated significantly better activity against both syngeneic and xenograft tumor models than etoposide *(60)*. However, direct comparison with irinotecan and topotecan has not been reported. Demonstration of activity of these newer inhibitors against camptothecin-resistant tumors would be an exciting development. Development and characterization of additional human tumor models resistant to camptothecins would be valuable.

The full curative/therapeutic potential of these drugs will not be realized without the development of approaches to compensate for the dose-limiting neutropenia, and intestinal toxicity. Thus, approaches to reducing myelosuppression, through use of hematopoetic growth factors, reconstitution with peripheral-blood-cell (PBC) progenitors, or protecting marrow through transduction of camptothecin-resistance genes, appear rational. Attempts to modulate intestinal toxicity through administration of interleukin-15, or JBT 3002, or alkalinization of the intestinal lumen *(61)* may allow increased dose intensity, or (rationally) more protracted courses of treatment with these agents. Validation of the current animal models of intestinal toxicity is important. Design of clinical protocols that more accurately recapitulate optimal schedules and drug exposures determined in xenograft models also seems appropriate with these agents, which are highly schedule-dependent in their antitumor activity. Clearly, an understanding of the biochemical/molecular events that determine such dramatic schedule-dependency will help in more effective clinical utilization of these agents, alone or in combination with other cytotoxic agents.

ACKNOWLEDGMENTS

Work from these laboratories was supported by UPHS grants CA23099, CA 32613, CA21765 (Cancer Center Support CORE Grant), and by American Lebanese Syrian Associated Charities (ALSAC).

REFERENCES

1. Trask DK, Muller MT. Stabilization of type I topoisomerase-DNA covalent complexes by actinomycin D. *Proc Natl Acad Sci* 1988; 85:1417–1421.
2. Cancer Medicine, 4th ed. (Morton DL, Holland JF, Frei III E, Bast Jr RC, Kufe DU), Williams and Wilkins, Baltimore, Maryland, Weichselbaum, RR 1997.
3. Giovanella BC, Stehlin JS, Wall ME, Wani MC, Nicholas AW, Liu LF, et al. DNA topoisomerase 1-targeted chemotherapy of human colon cancer xenografts. *Science* 1989; 246:1046–1048.
4. DeWys WD, Humphreys SR, Goldin A. Studies on the therapeutic effectiveness of drugs with tumor weight and survival time indices of Walker 256 carcinosarcoma. *Cancer Chemo Rept* 1968; 52(2):229–242.

5. Gallo RC, Whang-Peng J, Adamson RH. Studies on the antitumor activity, mechanism of action, and cell cycle effects of camptothecin. *J Natl Cancer Inst* 1971; 46:789–795.

6. Gottlieb JA, Guarino AM, Call JB, Oliverio VT, Block JB. Preliminary pharmacologic and clinical evaluation of camptothecin sodium (NSC 100880). *Cancer Chemother Rep* 1970; 54:461–470.

7. Moertel CG, Schutt AJ, Reitemeier RJ, Hahn RG. Phase II study of camptothecin (NSC-100880) in the treatment of advanced gastrointestinal cancer. *Cancer Chemother Rep* 1972; 56:95–101.

8. Kingsbury WD, Boehm JC, Jakas DR, Holden KG, Hecht SM, Gallagher G, et al. Synthesis of water soluble (aminoalkyl) camptothecin analogues: inhibition of topoisomerase I and antitumor activity. *J Med Chem* 1990; 4:98–107.

9. Hsiang YH, Hertzberg R, Hecht S, Liu LF. Camptothecin induces protein-linked DNA breaks via mammalian DNA topoisomerase I. *J Biol Chem* 1985; 260:14873–14878.

10. Chen AY, Liu LF. DNA topoisomerases: essential enzymes and lethal targets *Annu Rev Pharmacol Toxicol* 1994; 34:191–218.

11. Nitiss J, Wang JC. DNA topoisomerase-targeted drugs can be studied in yeast. *Proc Natl Acad Sci USA* 1988; 85:7501–7505.

12. Liu LF. Topoisomerase-I targeted drugs. Mechanism of inhibition and cytotoxicity. In: Taguchi T, Wang JC, eds. 5th World Conference on Clinical Pharmacology and Therapeutics. Highlights of a satellite symposium: Approaches to Cancer Treatment by Topoisomerase-I inhibitors. BIOMEDIS, Tokyo, 1992, pp. 6–9.

13. McCabe FL, Johnson RK. Comparative activity of oral and parenteral topotecan in murine tumor models: efficacy of oral topotecan. *Cancer Investig* 1994; 12:308–313.

14. Kunimoto T, Nitta K, Tanaka T, Uehara N, Baba H, Takeuchi M, et al. Antitumor activity of 7-ethyl-10-[4-(1-piperidino)-1-piperidino]-1-carbonyloxy-camptothecin, a novel water soluble derivative of camptothecin, against murine tumors. *Cancer Res* 1987; 47:5944–5947.

15. Matsuzaki T, Yokokura T, Mutai M, Tsuruo T. Inhibition of spontaneous and experimental metastasis by a new derivative of camptothecin, irinotecan, in mice. *Cancer Chemother Pharmacol* 1988; 21:308–312.

16. Bissery MC, Vrignaud P, Lavelle F, Chabot GG. Experimental antitumor activity and pharmacokinetics of the camptothecin analog irinotecan (CPT-11) *Anti-Cancer Drugs* 1996; 7:437–460.

17. Kawato Y, Furuta T, Aonuma M, Yasuoka M, Yokokura T, Matsumoto K. Antitumor activity of a camptothecin derivative against human tumor xenografts in nude mice. *Cancer Chemother Pharmacol* 1991; 28:192–198.

18. Pantazis P, Hinz HR, Mendoza JT, Kozielski AS, Williams LJ, Stehlin JS Jr., et al. Complete inhibition of growth followed by death of human malignant melanoma cells in vitro and regression of human melanoma xenografts in immunodeficient mice induced by camptothecins. *Cancer Res* 1992; 52:3980–3987.

19. Houghton PJ, Cheshire PJ, Myers L, Stewart CF, Synold TW, Houghton JA. Evaluation of 9-dimethylaminomethyl-10-hydroxycamptothecin against xenografts derived from adult and childhood solid tumors. *Cancer Chemother Pharmacol* 1992; 31:229–239.

20. Pentazis P, Kozielski AJ, Verdeman DM, Petry ER, Giovanella BC. Efficacy of camptothecin congeners in the treatment of human breast carcinoma xenografts. *Oncol Res* 1993; 5:273–281.

21. Houghton PJ, Cheshire PJ, Hallman JC, Bissery MC, Mathieu-Boue A, Houghton JA. Therapeutic efficacy of the topoisomerase I inhibitor 7-ethyl-10-(4-[1-piperidino]-1-piperidino)-carbonyloxy-camptothecin against human tumor xenografts: lack of cross resistance in vivo in tumors with acquired resistance to the topoisomerase inhibitor 9-dimethylaminomethyl-10-hydoxycamptothecin. *Cancer Res* 1993; 53:2823–2829.

22. Komuro H, Li P, Tsuchida Y, Yokomori K, Nakajima K, Aoyama T, et al. Effects of CPT11 (a unique DNA topoisomerase 1 inhibitor) on a highly malignant xeno-transplanted neuroblastoma. *Med Pediatr Oncol* 1994; 23:487–492.

23. Houghton PJ, Cheshire PJ, Hallman JD, Lutz L, Friedman HS, Danks MK, et al. Efficacy of topoisomerase I inhibitors, topotecan and irinotecan, administered at low dose levels in protracted schedules to mice bearing xenografts of human tumors. *Cancer Chemother Pharmacol* 1995; 36:393–403.

24. Emerson DL, Besterman JM, Brown HR, Evans MG, Leitner PP, Luzzio MJ, et al. In vivo antitumor activity of two seven-substituted water soluble camptothecin analogues. *Cancer Res* 1995; 55:603–609.

25. Vassal G, Terrier-Lacombe MJ, Bissery MC, Venuat AM, Gyergyay F, Benard J, et al. Therapeutic activity of CPT-11, a DNA-topoisomerase I inhibitor, against peripheral primitive neuroectodermal tumour and neuroblastoma xenografts. *Br J Cancer* 1996; 74:537–545.

26. Thompson J, Zamboni WC, Cheshire PJ, Lutz L, Luo X, Li Y, et al. Efficacy of systemic administration of irinotecan against neuroblastoma xenografts. *Clin Cancer Res* 1997; 3:423–431.

27. Thompson J, Zamboni WC, Cheshire PJ, Richmond L, Luo X, Houghton JA, et al. Efficacy of oral administration of irinotecan against neuroblastoma xenografts. *Anti-Cancer Drugs* 1997; 8:313–322.

28. Hare CB, Elion GB, Houghton PJ, Houghton JA, Keir S, Marcelli SL, et al. Therapeutic efficacy of the topoisomerase I inhibitor 7-ethyl-10-(4-[1-piperidino]-1-piperidino)-carbonyloxy-camptothecin against pediatric and adult central nervous system tumor xenografts. *Cancer Chemother Pharmacol* 1997; 393:187–191.

29. deSouza PL, Cooper MR, Imondi AR, Myers CE. 9-aminocamptothecin: a topoisomerase I inhibitor with preclinical activity in prostate cancer. *Clin Cancer Res* 1997; 3:287–294. by 9-amino-20(S)-camptothecin. *Cancer Res* 1997; 57:1929–1933.

30. Zamboni WC, Stewart CF, Thompson J, Santana V, Cheshire PJ, Richmond LB, et al. The relationship between topotecan systemic exposure and tumor response in human neuroblastoma xenografts. *J Natl Cancer Inst* 1998; 90:505–511.

31. Thompson J, Stewart CF, Houghton PJ. Animal models for studying the action of topoisomerase I targeted drug. *Biochimica Biophysica Acta* 1998; 1400:301–319.

32. Furman WL, Stewart CF, Poquette CA, Pratt CB, Santana VM, Zamboni WC, et al. Direct translation of a protracted irinotecan schedule from xnograft model to phase I trial in chidren. *J. Clin Oncol* 1999; 17:1815–1824.

33. Fujimori A, Harker WG, Kohlhagen G, Hoki Y, Pommier Y. Mutation at the catalytic site of topoisomerase I in CEM/C2, a human leukemia cell line resistant to camptothecin. *Cancer Res.* 1995; 55:1339–1346.

34. Knab AM, Fertala J, Bjornsti MA. A camptothecin-resistant DNA topoisomerase I mutant exhibits altered sensitivities to other DNA topoisomerase poisons. *J Biol Chem* 1995; 270:6141–6148.

35. Houghton PJ, Stewart CF, Zamboni WC, Thompson J, Luo X, Danks MK, et al. Schedule-dependent efficacy of camptothecins in models of human cancer. *Ann NY Acad Sci USA* 1996; 803:188–201.

36. Erickson-Miller CL, May RD, Tomaszewski J, Osborn B, Murphy MJ, Page JC, et al. Differential toxicity of camptothecin, topotecan and 9-aminocamptothecin to human, canine, and murine myeloid progenitors (CFU-GM) in vitro. *Cancer Chemother Pharmacol* 1997; 39:467–472.

37. Wiseman LR, Markham A. Irinotecan. *Drugs* 1996; 52:606–623.

38. Ikuno N, Soda H, Watanabe M, Oka M. Irinotecan (CPT-11) and characteristic mucosal changes in the mouse ileum and cecum. *J Natl Cancer Inst* 1995; 87:1876–1883.

39. Shinohara H, Killion JJ, Kuniyasu H, Kumar R, Fidler IJ. Prevention of intestinal toxic effects and intensification of irinotecan's thrapeutic efficacy against murine colon cancer liver metastases by oral administration of the lipopeptide JBT 3002. *Clin Cancer Res* 1998; 4:2053–2063.

40. Sakai H, Diener M, Gartmann V, Takeguchi N. Eicosanoid-mediated Cl⁻ secretion induced by the antitumor drug, irinotecan (CPT-11), in the rat. *Naunyn-Schmiedeberg's Arch Pharmacol* 1995; 351:309–314.

41. Takasuna K, Hagiwara T, Hirohashi M, Kato M, Nomura M, Nagai E, et al. Involvement of beta-glucoronidase in intestinal microflora in the intestinal toxicity of the antitumor camptothecin derivative irinotecan hydrochloride (CPT-11). *Cancer Res* 1996; 56:3752–3757.

42. Cao S, Black JD, Troutt AB, Rustum YM. Interleukin 15 offers selective protection from irinotecan-induced intestinal toxicity in a preclinical animal model. *Cancer Res* 1998; 58:3270–3274.

43. Bacon JA, Petrella DK, Cramer CT, Maruyama Y, Ford C, Stapert D, et al. Intestinal toxicity and changes in proliferating cell nuclear antigen (PCNA) levels in hamsters induced by a camptothecin analogue. *The Toxicologist* 1996; (abstract).

44. Kobayashi K, Bouscarel B, Matsuzaki Y, Ceryak S, Kudoh S, Fromm H. pH-dependent uptake of irinotecan and its active metabolite, SN-38, by intestinal cells. *Int J Cancer* 1999; 83:491–496.

45. Roy SK, Clark DL, Zheng H, McGuinn WD, Smith DD, Andrews PA. Predictive value of rodent and non-rodent toxicology studies in support of phase I trials of topoisomerase inhibitors. 737A *Proc American Assoc Cancer Res* 1999; 40:737A.

46. Stewart CF, Zamboni WC, Crom WR, Houghton PJ. Disposition of irinotecan and SN-38 following oral and intravenous irinotecan dosing in mice. *Cancer Chemother Pharmacol* 1997; 40:259–265.

47. Abigerges D, Chabot GG, Armand J, Herait P, Gouyette A, Gandia D. Phase I and pharmacologic studies of the camptothecin analog irinotecan administered every three weeks in cancer patients. *J Clin Oncol* 1995; 13:210–221.

48. Catimel G, Chabot GG, Guastalla JP, Dumortier A, Cote C, Engel C, et al. Phase I and pharmacokinetic study of irinotecan (CPT-11) administered daily for three consecutive days every three weeks in patients with advanced solid tumors. *Annals Oncology* 1995; 6(2):133–140.

49. Rothenberg ML, Kuhn JG, Burris HA, Nelson J, Eckardt JR, Tristan-Morales M, et al. Phase I and pharmacokinetic trial of weekly CPT-11. *J Clin Oncol* 1993; 11:2194–2204.

50. Morton CL, Wierdl M, Oliver L, Ma M, Danks MK, Stewart CF, et al. Activation of CPT-11 in mice: identification and analysis of a highly effective plasma esterase, *Cancer Res* 2000; 60:4206–4210.

51. Burke TG, Mi Z. The structural basis of camptothecin interactions with human serum albumin: impact on drug stability. *J Med Chem* 1994; 37:40–46.

52. Burke TG, Munshi CB, Mi Z, Jiang Y. The important role of albumin in determining the relative human blood stabilities of the camptothecin anticancer drugs [letter] [published erratum appears] *J Pharm Sci* 1995; 84:518–519.

53. Liehr JG, Ahmed AE, Giovanella BC. Pharmacokinetics of camptothecins administered orally. *Ann NY Acad Sci* 1996; 803:157–163.

54. Daud SS, Fetouh MI, Giovanella BC. Antitumor effect of liposome-incorporated camptothecin in human malignant xenografts. *Anti-Cancer Drugs* 1995; 6:83–93.

55. Burke TG, Gao X. Stabilization of topotecan in low pH liposomes composed of distearoylphosphatidylcholine. *J Pharm Sci* 1994; 83:967–969.

56. Bailly C, Lansiaux A, Dassonneville L, Demarquay D, Coulomb H, Huchet M, et al. Homocamptothecin, an E-ring-modified camptothecin analogue, generates new topoisomerase I-mediated DNA breaks. *Biochemistry* 1999; 38:15,556–15,563.

57. Sanders MM, Liu AA, Li TK, Wu HY, Desai SD, Mao Y, et al. Selective cytotoxicity of topoisomerase-directed protoberberines against glioblastoma cells. *Biochem Pharmacol* 1998; 56:1157–1166.

58. Bailly C, Qu X, Chaires JB, Colson P, Houssier C, Ohkubo M, et al. Substitution at the F-ring N-imide of the indolocarbazole antitumor drug NB-506 increases the cytotoxicity, DNA binding, and topoisomerase I inhibition activities. *J Med Chem* 1999; 42:2927–2935.

59. Hill BT, Barrett JM, Perrin D, Gras S, Limouzy A, Chazottes E, et al. Mechanism of action of F 11782, a novel catalytic dual inhibitor of topoisomerase I and II. *Proc Am Assoc Cancer Res* 1999; 40:755A.

60. Kruczynski A, Astruc J, Chazottes E, Ricome C, Berrichon G, Imbert T, et al. Preclinical antitumor activity of F 11782, a novel catalytic dual inhibitor of topoisomerase I and II. *Proc Am Assoc Cancer Res* 1999; 40:757A.

61. Kobayashi K, Takeda Y, Akiyama Y, Soma T, Hand T, Kudo K, et al. Reduced irinotecan-induced side-effects by the oral alkalinization. *Proc Am Assoc Clin Oncol* 1999; 18:1900a.

30 Spontaneous Pet Animal Cancers

Mark W. Dewhirst, DVM, PhD,
Donald Thrall, DVM, PhD,
and E. Gregory MacEwen, DVM

Contents

1. INTRODUCTION

A significant amount of the in vivo work assessing cancer biology or experimental therapeutics is conducted in small laboratory animals. Indeed, the vast majority of this book is based on in vivo laboratory animal systems that have enabled significant advances to be made in the understanding of cancer. Clearly, there are many advantages associated with these models. Alternatively, however, studies of spontaneous cancer can provide information that cannot be obtained elsewhere, except for the study of cancer in humans. Spontaneous tumors in large animals (dogs and cats) can provide a bridge between novel discoveries in the laboratory and implementation of new therapies in humans in a number of novel ways. This chapter reviews some of the basic aspects of spontaneous large animal tumors and provides specific examples of results that have important implications for human cancer therapy.

2. BIOLOGY OF PET ANIMAL CANCERS

2.1. Canine and Feline Cancer Facts

There are many similarities between the biology of canine and feline malignancies and their human tumor counterparts. This section briefly reviews some of these aspects.

2.1.1. Epidemiology

Epidemiologic information about cancer in dogs and cats is limited in comparison to what is known in humans. Incidence data are few, but in a study performed in California in the late 1960s the estimated annual incidence rates for cancer of all sites were approx

From: *Tumor Models in Cancer Research*
Edited by: B. A. Teicher © Humana Press Inc., Totowa, NJ

380 per 100,000 dogs and 150 per 100,000 cats *(1)*. These incidence rates are on the same order of magnitude as estimates of overall cancer incidence in humans. Interestingly, the leading sites of cancer vary between humans and animals. In humans, the leading sites are prostate, breast, lung, and colon *(2)*. In comparison, cancers of the pharynx, breast, testis, and skin are the most common sites in dogs and cats *(1)*. Thus, when spontaneous canine or feline tumors are studied in experimental therapy trials, the models may not be an exact counterpart of a human tumor. However, the response of a spontaneous tumor and its surrounding tumor-perturbed normal tissue bed can be evaluated.

2.1.2. ETIOLOGY

The causes of cancer in dogs and cats are also unclear. Viruses have only been definitively associated with carcinogenesis in two instances. Feline leukemia virus (FeLV) and feline immunodeficiency virus (FIV) have been defined as a cause of hematopoietic neoplasms in cats *(3,4)*, and feline sarcoma virus (FeSV) has been associated with some soft-tissue sarcomas in cats *(5)*. Soft-tissue sarcomas in cats have also been associated with vaccination reactions, with tumors developing secondary to rabies or FeLV vaccines *(6)*. Environmentally, only a few agents have been associated with cancer in dogs: asbestosis and mesothelioma *(7)*, industrial activity and bladder cancer *(8)*, and air pollution and tonsillar carcinoma *(9)*.

Most reports indicate that in the United States the privately owned pet population includes about 55 million dogs and 60 million cats *(10)*. Thus, considering the cancer incidence rates noted here, large numbers of dogs and cats develop new tumors each year. Seemingly, this provides an excellent opportunity for the study of tumor immunology, physiology, and experimental therapies in a spontaneous tumor system. Indeed, some exciting and valuable information has been obtained from the study of tumors in pet animals. However, certain limitations have also come into play that have prevented more widespread investigation of this resource. To understand why it would be informative to study these large animal tumors at all, and why their use has not been more widespread, it is helpful to enumerate the biologic characteristics and the advantages and disadvantages of studying spontaneous tumors, in large animals.

2.2. Comparative View of Rodent Large Animal and Human Tumors

2.2.1. TUMOR: BODY MASS

A localized tumor can have an effect on the overall physiology of the host—e.g., cancer cachexia syndrome *(11)*. These physiologic perturbations, which can relate to the relative size of the tumor, may influence the effects of the experimental therapy or the biology of the tumor. In canine and feline cancer, the relative size of the tumor to the mass of the subject is more similar to that in humans than are rodent tumors. The tumor:body mass index is also important in the assessment of clinical treatments such as radiation therapy, in which geometric relationships are influential in effectively irradiating the tumor and in sparing adjacent normal tissue. The tumor:body mass index has been named as one of two reasons why rodent tumors cannot be taken as literal models of human tumors *(12)*.

2.2.2. GROWTH KINETICS

In rodent tumors, the growth fraction (fraction of cells active in the cell cycle) frequently ranges from 30–50%, while the cell-loss factor (fraction of cells produced by cell division lost from the tumor) varies from 0% to more than 90%. Cell-loss factors tend to be small in small tumors and increase with tumor size. Growth fraction is more variable in human tumors than in rodent tumors and correlates better with clinical volume-doubling time. Further, the cell-loss factor for human tumors has been estimated to have an average value in excess of 50% *(13,14)*. Kinetic data are available for canine lymphomas and osteosarcomas, where it has been shown that potential doubling time (Tpot) has correlated with treatment outcome *(15–17)*. Survey data have also been reported for a variety of canine and feline tumors *(18)*. These data and their clinical characteristics of tumor-growth rates are more consistent with growth kinetics of human tumors than rodent tumors. Thus, perturbations in physiology or response to therapy as a function of kinetic parameters are more similar between canine vs human tumors in comparison to rodent vs human tumors.

2.2.3. IMMUNOGENICITY

Some rodent tumors are highly immunogenic. This immunogenicity may either alter the response of the tumor to the experimental therapy, or necessitate physiologic alteration of the host—i.e., immunosuppression—which could also alter the tumor or therapeutic response. Immunologic factors are of particular importance when studying human tumor xenografts, which necessarily require immunosuppressed hosts such as nude or SCID mice. These factors are not issues when studying canine or feline spontaneous tumors, which are typically not immunogenic. Canine tumors have been studied extensively with a variety of immunotherapeutic approaches, because the challenges to stimulate tumor-specific immune responses are so similar to humans *(19–22)*.

2.2.4. GROWTH RATE AND TIME COURSE OF DISEASE

Rodent tumors grow rapidly, and tumor control assays, for example, can generally be completed within 60–180 d of completing treatment. In human-cancer trials, permanent local control is typically not defined until at least 5 yr after treatment. Considering that most trials are ongoing for 3–5 y, final analysis could conceivably be delayed for as long as 10 yr after beginning the trial. In dogs and cats, where the average life span of 8–12 yr is considerably shorter than in humans, local control can typically be assessed at 2 yr after therapy, and the effects of treatment on overall survival are much shorter than comparable studies in humans. Thus, the window of observation is compressed, and therapy-outcome trials can be completed more expediently.

2.2.5. HETEROGENEITY

Transplanted rodent tumors are more homogeneous between subjects than canine or human tumors. With regard to therapy trials, the homogeneity of rodent tumors could give a false impression of the effectiveness of the therapy being studied. For example, if a population of rodent neoplasms is characterized by low intratumoral pO_2, then it may be justified to move a strategy that successfully improves tumor oxygenation and response to therapy rapidly into human trials. However, in the human population, where intertumoral pO2 heterogeneity will be greater, the overall population effect of the intervention would likely be lower, because tumors with high pO_2 values will not be effected by the intervention. Additionally, in many human trials, characteristics of the tumor or patient that predict for outcome are identified retrospectively. These parameters can then be evaluated in future prospective studies to validate their use as methods to identify either favorably-responding or refractory patients prior to therapy *(23,24)*. The hetero-

geneity of canine/feline tumors provides an opportunity for advances in the field of predictive assays, and also provides a population of tumors in which the response to therapy,
or the biologic-characteristics studies, will have the same effect as that encountered in
human studies. Examples of studies in which this type of analysis has been helpful in the
design of subsequent human trials include the multivariate analyses conducted on phase
III pet animal trials testing radiation ± hyperthermia *(25–27)*.

2.3. Advantages vs Disadvantages of Studying Canine and Feline Tumors

2.3.1. ADVANTAGES

2.3.1.1. Best Conventional Therapy. There are fewer standard (best conventional)
therapies in canine/feline oncology than are defined for treatment of human cancer.
Thus, there is more flexibility in entering patients into trials of new modalities.
Although "standard therapy" is less well defined, it is important that pet animals with
cancer are never denied access to conventional therapy in favor of entering the patient
into a clinical trial. All options for therapy must always be discussed in detail with the
pet owner to enable the owner to make the decision that is best for them. Informed
owner consent is as important in pet animal trials as patient consent is in human trials.
These discussions are time-consuming, and mandate that well-informed clinicians who
are invested in the goals of the project—as well as being familiar with expected outcome from standard therapies—are responsible for pet-owner consultation. The careful
study of new cancer-treatment methods in large animals can provide a way for these
modalities to be applied more efficiently to humans. Therapeutic studies of cancer in
animals can result in continued enthusiasm for a modality that may be discarded
because of incomplete preliminary information gained from human trials. For example,
the therapeutic use of hyperthermia was carefully evaluated in canine trials long before
it was tested in human trials, and the beneficial effects of those canine trials provided
impetus for continued and careful evaluation in humans *(25,28–30)*. It has subsequently been shown in several human trials that hyperthermia improves outcome when
combined with radiation therapy *(31–35)*.

2.3.1.2. Normal Tissue Effects. Often, it is normal tissue toxicity that limits the
effectiveness of cancer therapy. In rodent therapy trials, most emphasis is placed on
tumor response, and few studies provide detailed information about the response of the
tumor as well as acute and late-normal tissue responses. Thus, toxicity may be underestimated. In canine trials, follow-up is typically conducted for months or years after
treatment. This provides an opportunity to assess acute and late-normal tissue
responses and metastasis in addition to local tumor response. Assessment of tumor and
late-normal tissue effects are required before it can be concluded that therapeutic gain
is associated with the new modality. This is part of standard procedure in most pet animal trials *(22,26,28,36–42)*.

2.3.1.3. Serial Biopsy. Serial interventions are usually possible in canine/feline trials. Pet owners are often amenable to having minor procedures, such as multiple or
sequential tumor biopsies, performed. This provides a powerful resource for monitoring intratumoral variation in a parameter, or change in a parameter over time. For
example, multiple biopsies have been used to assess the minimum number of tumor
biopsies needed to estimate the intratumoral distribution of tumor oxygenation *(43)*
and changes in the tumor oxygenation as a function of time after initiation of radiation
therapy *(44)*.

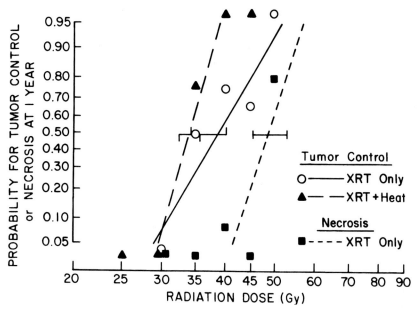

Fig. 1. Radiation dose-effect plots for local control of canine oral squamous-cell carcinomas (SCCs) treated with radiation therapy alone vs combined with local hyperthermia. Also plotted is the dose-effect curve for bone necrosis, the dose-limiting normal tissue for these tumors. Hyperthermia treatment made the slope of the dose-effect curve steeper, with a dose-modifying factor at the 50% probability of control at 1 yr of 1.15. There was no effect of hyperthermia on the dose-effect curve for bone necrosis. Data reproduced with permission of the author and publisher (28).

2.3.1.4. Dose-Response Assays. A dose-response assay is a valuable method of evaluating the effectiveness of a new therapy, because it provides a measure of response quantified as tumor control. Such studies provide a measure of the homogeneity of the response to treatment quantified in terms of the slope of the dose-response curve. As an example, we show radiation-dose response data for local control of canine oral squamous-cell carcinomas (SCCS) with and without the addition of local hyperthermia treatment (28) (Fig. 1). Hyperthermia increased the steepness of the dose effect curve and shifted it to the left. The shift to the left is indicative of the dose-modifying effect of hyperthermia to increase the effectiveness of radiation killing. The steeper slope indicated that underlying sources of heterogeneity in radiation-dose effect, such as hypoxia or distribution of cells in the cell cycle, were being selectively eliminated by the hyperthermia treatment. Dose-response assays are useful for computing the enhancement ratio for radiation combined with other modalities. In the example shown, the dose-modifying effect was a factor of 1.15 at the dose to control 50% of the tumors. At higher control probabilities, the factor would be larger because of the differences in slopes of the dose-response curves. Determination of dose-response assays for tumor and normal tissue in the same subject also allows for quantification of the therapeutic gain factor. In the example shown, there was no detectable change in the normal tissue dose-response curve with the addition of hyperthermia. Thus, the therapeutic gain factor would be greater than 1.0, indicating that the addition of hyperthermia to radiation therapy yielded a greater effect in enhancing antitumor effects than normal tissue damage. By necessity, dose-response assays require the administration of variable doses of a modality, usually radiation. It is also necessary to assign doses randomly. Randomization of humans to receive variable doses of radiation in a dose-response assay is ethically impossible. It is not necessarily the case with canine tumors, and the study of canine tumors in dose-response assays has provided valuable information on the effect of various modifiers of radiation (27,28,36).

2.3.1.5. Host Can Be Studied. By following pets treated in experimental therapy trials for long periods of time after treatment, there is an opportunity to observe the host and the effect of the tumor and treatment on the host. Assessing for systemic metastasis, alterations in metastasis, and scoring normal tissue toxicity are examples of this principle. For example, the combination of local and whole-body hyperthermia was proposed as a way to increase the low end of the temperature distribution in solid tumors during hyperthermia treatments. There is a vast amount of information supporting the theory that the low end of the temperature distribution is predictive for tumor response. However, in a trial that combined local and whole-body hyperthermia as a means to elevate the low end of the temperature distribution in canine sarcomas, the new treatment was found to be associated with an increased risk for metastasis in comparison with local hyperthermia. The hazard ratio for metastasis in dogs receiving local and whole-body hyperthermia was 2.5 (96% confidence interval (CI), 1.2–5.4). Thus, detection of this of unexpected alteration of biologic behavior avoided introduction of a potentially harmful therapy into the human clinic (45).

2.3.1.6. Long-term Follow-Up and Availability for Autopsy. Long-term follow-up after treatment is often difficult in human trials. Patients often return to their referring physician after treatment, and do not return to the trial center. Follow-up by referring physicians who are not familiar with protocol details leads to significant loss of data and/or errors in data recording. Alternatively, patients may not return to trial centers because of lack of interest or concomitant illnesses that prevent them from traveling. In some human trials, loss attributable to follow-up can significantly hamper statistical analysis of data. In our experience conducting prospective clinical trials in dogs over a period of 20 yr, the compliance of owners with the follow-up process is extremely good. This is a result of the fact that the patients and owners are screened via the referral process. Many times the owners themselves or relatives of the owners have been touched by cancer in some way, and their choice to enter their pet into a clinical trial is combined with a strong desire to contribute to new knowledge. In humans, the autopsy rate has been steadily decreasing, and is typically less than 20% (46). Decreasing autopsy rates hamper the ability to fully understand the effect of therapy on the disease, or the effect of the disease on the host. In carefully conducted trials in pet animals, it is typical for the autopsy rate to be >90%—a result of careful consultation with the pet owner. Having such a high autopsy rate provides an opportunity for thorough gross and histologic assessment of the tumor, tumor bed, and other anatomic areas that may have been affected by the tumor or therapy.

2.3.2. DISADVANTAGES OF STUDYING CANINE AND FELINE TUMORS

2.3.2.1. Cost and Support. Studying pet animal tumors requires the direct involvement of a variety of veterinary health care professionals and facilities to manage the treatment and any complications that may arise. Assembling a team of specialized personnel who have a common goal of expanding the knowledge base through the study of naturally occurring disease in pets is difficult. This also requires facilities that are capable of handling the specialized treatments given as part of the protocol, and dealing with complications as they arise. Having specialists available in other disciplines is also an important part of the concept. Additionally, owner costs for treatments administered under the auspices of the investigation are commonly subsidized. This subsidization pertains not only to the initial treatment, but to all follow-up examinations. It is not unusual for the cost of treating an individual animal in a prospective trial to be $3,000–$5,000 over what the owner contributes for the initial diagnosis and staging. Clearly, this is much higher than the cost of treating an individual rodent, but the advantages outlined here justify this expense in some circumstances. Also, this cost is considerably less than the cost of treating a human in a clinical trial. Human medical costs are at least partially defrayed by third-party payers, and this source of support is not widely available in veterinary medicine. Typically, prospective trials involving pet animals are heavily supported through competitive funding sources.

2.3.2.2. Accrual Despite the huge popularity of pet ownership and the relatively high incidence of cancer in dogs and cats, gathering sufficient numbers of patients to meet the objectives of the study is always challenging. Rarely will one veterinary institution access enough patients to complete a randomized phase III trial in a reasonable length of time. Yet the resources of two or more institutions can be pooled, with subjects being entered onto the protocol at more than one treatment site. There is no question that this process increases the complexity of the trial, and heightens the need for flawless quality control, but collaborative pet animal trials have be accomplished, and provide valuable information *(22,27,36,45)*.

3. STAGING OF CANINE AND FELINE TUMORS

3.1. Clinical-Pathologic Characterization

3.1.1. TNM CLASSIFICATION

Companion animals with cancer undergo diagnostic testing and clinical staging similar to the procedures used for human-cancer patients. In addition to a tumor biopsy for histopathological evaluation, these animals are routinely evaluated with a complete physical examination, hematological and biochemical testing, radiographs of primary tumor (when indicated) and thorax, and ultrasound of the abdomen. It is not rare for affected animals to undergo advanced imaging techniques, such as Computed tomography (CT) and (MRI). In 1980, the World Health Organization (WHO) adopted a clinical staging system based on the classic TNM system *(47)*. This system characterizes the primary tumor (designated T) which includes location, size, and invasiveness; the involvement of region lymph-node metastasis (designated N), and distant metastatic disease (designated M). Following the determination of the TNM, animals are assigned a clinical stage (i.e., I, II, III, or IV) based on the extent of tumor. This clinical staging has been critical for design and analysis of clinical trials using animals.

3.1.2. HISTOLOGIC AND BIOLOGIC CHARACTERISTICS

The spontaneous tumors that develop in companion animals are, in many cases, histopathologically identical to the same histogenetic tumor that develops in humans.

Many of these cancers are identical pathologically, and have similar metastatic patterns *(48–50)*. Malignant tumors, such as mammary cancer *(51)*, osteosarcoma, prostate cancer, melanoma *(52)*, and lung cancer will metastasize to regional lymph nodes, lung, liver, kidney, bone, and brain *(21,53–62)*. Tumor-grading systems (i.e., degree of cellular differentiation, mitotic index, extent of local invasion, and lymphatic invasion) have been developed to further characterize malignant potential and prognosis *(51,63–66)*. Non-Hodgkin's lymphomas (NHL), multiple myeloma, and leukemias are quite common in both dogs and cats *(67–74)*. Most NHL are high-grade tumors, and tend to present in advanced clinical stages *(16)*. The leukemias commonly diagnosed include lymphoblastic leukemia and chronic lymphocytic and myelogenous leukemia *(72,73,75)*.

3.1.3. MOLECULAR AND GENOMIC CHARACTERIZATION

All cancer develops as a result of genetic alterations. The two broad classes of genes associated with cancer development and progression have been characterized: as tumor-suppressor genes and tumor oncogenes *(76,77)*. The *p53* tumor-suppressor gene is the most frequently mutated in human cancer *(78,79)*. The prevalence of the *p53* mutation is extremely variable among tumor types, ranging from 0–60% in major human cancers. The spontaneous deamination of 5-methyl cytosine at 5-meCpG dinucleotides, resulting in cytosine to thymidine transitions, is a common source of *p53* mutations, and this has been detected in canine mammary cancer *(80,81)*. In human breast cancer, the frequency of the *p53* mutation ranges from 15–43%, depending on the mutation detection technique used and the proportion of the gene examined *(82–84)*. In one recent study of 40 primary canine mammary carcinomas, 15% were found to have *p53* mutations *(81)*. In addition to canine mammary cancer, *p53* mutations have been detected in oral papilloma, thyroid tumors, osteosarcoma *(85)*, and lymphoma *(86–88)*. Using immunohistochemical assays, overexpression of *p53* has been detected in canine osteosarcoma and feline vaccine-associated sarcomas *(85,87,89)*.

Oncogenes are overexpressed proto-oncogenes, and their cell product results in a gain of function, which contributes to the malignant transformation and the malignant phenotype. Oncogenes that are overexpressed include *c-sis,* which encodes platelet-derived growth factor (PDGF)*(90–93)*. This oncogene has been seen in feline sarcomas associated with FeSV and feline vaccine-associated sarcoma *(6)*. Dysregulated *c-myc* has been detected in several canine and feline cancers *(94–98)*. Mutations in the *Erb-B* gene (epidermal growth-factor receptor) has been identified in a number of human cancers, including mammary, ovarian, and prostate cancer *(99–102)*. These have also been identified in canine mammary tumors *(95,103)*. Other growth-factor receptors detected are the insulin-like growth factor-1 receptor (IGF-1R) and *c-met* (hepatocyte growth-factor receptor) in canine osteosarcoma *(104,105)*. The *ras* signal-transduction pathway is similarly susceptible to mutation-induced constitutive activation *(106)*. *K-ras* mutations are frequently associated with lung adenocarcinomas in humans *(107)*. Similar mutations in *ras* have also been demonstrated in canine lung cancers *(108,109)*. The genetic and molecular events associated with canine and feline cancer are just beginning to be defined. As new genetic and defined mechanism-of-action therapeutic agents become available, it will be essential to reach a better understanding of the molecular characterization associated with companion animal tumors.

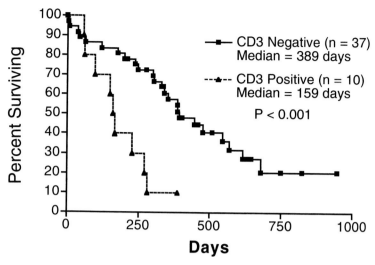

Fig. 2. Kaplan-Meier overall survival for Non-Hodgkin's lympho (NHL) in dogs treated with a modified CHOP protocol, characterized by the immunophenotype CD3-positive (T-cell) and CD3-negative (B-cell) classification. Data abstracted from work of Kurzmann et al., *(38)*.

4. EXPERIMENTAL THERAPEUTICS

4.1. Chemotherapy

A number of spontaneous tumors in dogs can serve as models for chemotherapy testing. These include NHL multiple myeloma, leukemia, mammary carcinoma, advanced bladder cancer, soft-tissue sarcoma, and osteosarcoma. In current clinical oncology practice for humans, chemotherapy is used primarily as the major curative modality for Hodgkin's disease, lymphoma, acute leukemia in children, and testicular cancer. Chemotherapy is used as palliative treatment for many other advanced cancers.

4.1.1. Drug Resistance in Lymphomas

One of the major challenges facing potential curative chemotherapy is the development of acquired drug resistance. Canine NHL is an excellent model to study acquired drug resistance. Dogs with spontaneous NHL are commonly treated with a CHOP protocol, a combination of cyclophosphamide (C), doxorubicin (H, hydroxydaunarubicin), vincristine (O, Oncovin®), and (P) prednisone). Using this CHOP protocol combined with L-asparaginase, dogs with advanced clinical stage and high-grade NHL show high complete remission rates of 80–90% with median survivals of 11–12 mo. Most dogs with NHL have B-cell tumors, which have a better prognosis than the T-cell immunophenotype *(16,67)*(Fig. 2). However, relapse is common, and most animals will eventually die of advanced disease because of multidrug resistance. Both MDR1 gene and P-glycoprotein (Pgp) have been detected in canine lymphoma *(110,111)*. Studies have indicated elevated levels of Pgp in relapsed canine NHL *(111,112)*. Pgp 170 has been detected in 16 of 91 (17.5%) canine lymphomas that were positive for Pgp, using immunohistochemistry *(111)*. Furthermore, in dogs with relapsed lymphoma, Pgp expression was greater and pretreatment Pgp levels were an independent prognostic factor for overall survival for low and high levels of Pgp expression (median

225 d vs 367 days $p = 0.02$)(*111*). These studies provide evidence that canine lymphoma can serve as a good model for chemotherapy drug resistance.

4.1.2. Limb-Sparing in Osteosarcoma

Canine osteosarcoma (OS) is a common malignancy, and is the best model for human osteosarcoma (48–50). Canine OS has been used to test a number of conventional and novel chemotherapeutic agents. Most dogs present with a primary tumor involving a long bone in a limb. At the time of diagnosis, 90+% will have microscopic metastatic disease. This has been determined using amputation alone, which results in a median survival time of 4 mo, with 90% of dogs dying of lung metastasis by 1 yr. A number of surgical adjuvant studies have been performed using cisplatin, carboplatin, doxorubicin, and combined cisplatin and doxorubicin (*38,113–118*). For single-agent chemotherapy, median survivals of 10–12 mo can be expected. Combination chemotherapy has extended survival to 18 mo. However, 75–80% of these treated dogs still ultimately die of drug-resistant metastatic disease.

A novel delivery system has been developed to provide for slow release of relatively low concentrations of cisplatin (*119*). The system is a biodegradable polymer called open-cell polylactic acid (OPLA-Pt). When OPLA-Pt is implanted in dogs, serum pharmacological data reveals an increase approx 30-fold in area under the concentration-time curve (AUC) for systemic platinum exposure, compared to a similar dose of cisplatin administered intravenously. In a clinical trial, 39 dogs with OS treated by amputation and one dose of OPLA-Pt showed median survival of 8 mo and 41% 1-yr survival (*120*).

4.1.3. Liposomal Formulations

Spontaneous tumors in dogs and cats have been used to study other chemotherapeutic delivery systems, such as liposome-encapsulated doxorubicin and cisplatin formulations. Recent studies evaluating sterically stabilized liposome-encapsulated doxorubicin (Stealth® DOXIL) have demonstrated therapeutic efficacy and cutaneous toxicity similar to that seen in human trials (*121,122*). A randomized study to evaluate pyridoxine (vitamin B_6) to prevent the cutaneous toxicity associated with DOXIL was recently published (*37*). This study showed that vitamin B_6 reduced the development of the hand-foot syndrome.

4.1.4. Inhalational Chemotherapy

The dog model has also been used to evaluate inhalational delivery of doxorubicin and Taxol as a therapy for macroscopic and micrometastatic lung cancer (*123*). Recent results of current clinical trials demonstrate antitumor activity in proof-of-principle studies. Furthermore, inhalational doxorubicin has been shown to extend survival in dogs with primary lung carcinoma when compared to surgery alone (Vail, personal communication). In addition, a recent study showed that in dogs with metastatic splenic hemangiosarcoma, treatment with combined inhalational doxorubicin combined with systemic chemotherapy resulted in prolonged survival compared to dogs treated with the same combination chemotherapy without the inhalational doxorubicin (Vail, personal communication).

4.2. Immunotherapy

A number of clinical trials have been conducted using spontaneous tumors in dogs and cats for the evaluation of various immunotherapeutic agents (*22,38,124–130*). The

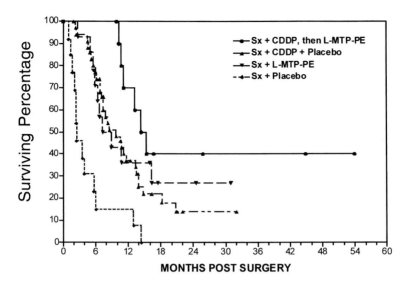

Fig. 3. Kaplan-Meier overall survival for dogs with OS treated as follows: amputation (Sx) followed by cisplatin (CDDP) and L-MTP-PE; CDDP and placebo (liquid equivalent); Sx and L-MTP-PE and Sx and placebo (liquid equivalent). Data abstracted from work of Greenlee et al., *(69)*.

best tumor models for immunotherapy in dogs have been oral melanoma, OS, splenic hemangiosarcoma, and in cats, mammary carcinoma. All these tumors occur with a high frequency, and are excellent models for human cancer because they all develop spontaneous metastasis. A number of randomized clinical trials have been conducted to evaluate a nonspecific immunotherapeutic agent, liposome-encapsulated muramyl-tripeptide phosphatidyl thanilamine (L-MTP-PE) *(22,128,129,131)*. L-MTP-PE is a potent macrophage activator, and has been shown to exhibit antitumor activity in a number of murine tumor models *(132–134)*. L-MTP-PE has been shown to delay the development of metastatic disease and significantly extend survival time in dogs with OS following amputation alone, and in another study, following amputation and chemotherapy *(38,131)* (Fig. 3). In another randomized trial, L-MTP-PE was shown to extend disease-free survival and overall survival in dogs with highly metastatic splenic hemangiosarcoma *(129)*. This surgical adjuvant study showed that L-MTP-PE used with combination chemotherapy was significantly more effective than chemotherapy alone. Oral melanoma is a common tumor seen in dogs, with a similar biologic and metastatic pattern to human oral melanoma. Dogs treated with surgery alone have a median survival of 8–10 mo (clinical-stage-dependent) and death is usually caused by lung metastasis. In a recent randomized trial, L-MTP-PE resulted in 75% long-term survival (>2 yr) in dogs with stage 1 (tumor diameter <2 cm) compared to 20% long-term survival in dogs treated with surgery and placebo (lipid alone) *(22)*. Studies are now underway to determine whether genetically modified autologous tumor vaccines can extend survival in dogs with oral melanoma following surgery *(126,135)*.

4.3. Total Body Hyperthermia Combined with Chemotherapy

Concomitant with the interest in using hyperthermia in combination with radiation for localized solid tumors, there have been a number of studies evaluating chemotherapy in combination with systemic hyperthermia for treatment of disseminated cancer. Canine trials provided considerable information on this subject. The effect of systemic hyperthermia on the toxicity of melphalan *(39)*, doxorubicin *(136)*, cisplatin *(40)*, carboplatin *(42)*, and mitoxantrone *(137)* was evaluated in phase I trials in dogs with spontaneous tumors. In all instances except mitoxantrone and doxorubicin, the maximum tolerated dose (MTD) of the chemotherapeutic agent was reduced through a combination with hyperthermia. Although the MTD for most drugs was reduced, there was still potential for therapeutic gain because of alterations in drug distribution that became apparent in phase I trials. For most drugs studied, the area under concentration vs. time curve (AUC) was reduced with systemic hyperthermia. The lowered AUC resulted from an increase in the volume of distribution and serum clearance. These observations may significantly influence drug delivery to tumor and normal tissue. Thus, phase III trials of chemotherapy ± systemic hyperthermia were conducted in dogs with lymphoma *(41)* and osteosarcoma (Page R., personal communication). Unfortunately, neither trial resulted in evidence for enhanced therapeutic effect. In an important study of lung-tumor metastases from osteogenic sarcoma, it was demonstrated that the altered volume of distribution achieved with whole-body hyperthermia did not result in improved drug delivery to tumor *(138)*. This result may explain the lack of therapeutic benefit for these combinations. Although these trials were negative, they provided important information on a therapeutic strategy that was being considered for use in humans, and defined drug-hyperthermia protocols that were unlikely to provide a benefit.

4.4. Radiation Therapy

4.4.1. Adjuvant Hyperthermia

A number of clinical trials have been conducted to evaluate the effects of radiation therapy alone or in combination with other therapies on local tumor control and normal tissue tolerance. One of the best-studied adjuvants has been hyperthermia. Phase III canine clinical trials *(25,28,29,139)* implicated the potential therapeutic advantage of this combination therapy many years before the first positive phase III human clinical trial was published *(140)*. One primary gain made with the canine trials was in the identification of therapeutically significant prognostic factors and in the assessment of normal tissue damage that could result from therapy *(25,28,29,141)*. Some of the earliest principles of thermal dosimetry were identified in these pet animal trials, and were later confirmed in human trials *(142–146)*. These dosimetric principles are still under investigation today, and prospective trials are testing the therapeutic efficacy of low vs high thermal doses in combination with radiation therapy *(147)*. As an example, we show the relationship between minimum tumor temperature and duration of local control of pet animal tumors following the combination of fractionated radiation and hyperthermia treatment (Fig. 4).

Two trials have examined the combination of total-body hyperthermia in combination with fractionated radiotherapy *(45,148)*. The first trial examined the potential use of total-body hyperthermia in combination with local heating as a means to improve minimum tumor temperatures, since these temperatures had been shown in numerous trials to be important for tumor response and duration of local control. The results of this trial did not lead to human trials for two important reasons. First, there was no evidence that this method of therapy was any better than local hyperthermia alone for

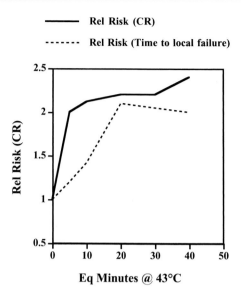

Fig. 4. Relative risk factors for complete response and duration of local control following radiotherapy combined with hyperthermia as a function of minimum thermal isoeffect dose (thermal data converted to equivalent number of minutes at 43°C). The importance of temperature minima in increasing the likelihood for achieving an initial response or durable local control is clear. In multivariate analysis, minimum thermal dose was the most important prognostic factor for both endpoints. Data derived from *(25)*.

achieving local tumor control. Second and more importantly, it was very clear that this combination therapy led to a higher incidence of distant metastases than local heating *(45)*. A second trial combined total-body hyperthermia with radiation therapy to treat brain tumors in dogs. This trial also failed to demonstrate any evidence for improvement in tumor control *(148)*. Although these trials were not positive, they served a very important purpose, because they prevented the instigation of similar human trials, which probably would have led to similar results.

4.4.2. ROLE IN LIMB-SPARING FOR CANINE OSTEOSARCOMA

Canine trials have provided useful information on the role of radiation therapy in combination with intra-arterial or systemic chemotherapy in limb-sparing procedures for osteogenic sarcoma. Radiation is not typically used in humans for limb-sparing procedures, but for tumors located in regions where complete local excision may be difficult, radiation could play an important role in diminishing the likelihood for local recurrence. It has been shown that use of radiation therapy alone had detrimental effects on allograft incorporation, and was also associated with an unacceptable incidence of failure of the internal fixation devices *(149)*. When combined with chemotherapy, lower doses of radiation were found to result in a high percentage of tumor necrosis, and to maintain host bone viability and allograft incorporation.

4.5. Extrapolation of Experimental Therapeutics Trials to Human Studies

Although therapeutic trials in pet animals have yielded important data with respect to the potential therapeutic value of new modalities, there are limits to what this type of trial data can provide. There is no clinical trial using spontaneous pet animal tumors that could replace a human trial, in the event that the modality moves into human studies. Determination of the MTD of a drug in dogs cannot be extrapolated to humans to circumvent the need for phase I studies in humans, for example. Similarly, a positive phase III trial in pets with cancer cannot replace the need for randomized clinical trials in humans. The best that such trials can provide is a rationale for initiating human trials. The positive phase III trials in pet animal tumors combining hyperthermia with radiation therapy provided a strong stimulus to continue development and testing of hyperthermia in humans. The examples of the two total-body hyperthermia trials discussed here represent clear cases in which the initiation of human studies was halted because of negative results.

If positive pet animal trials cannot replace human trials, what is the rationale for doing them as models for human cancer? The real strength of these models lies in what can be learned about the tumor biology as the animals are being treated in a trial. The ability to perform multiple biopsies, imaging procedures, and other diagnostic tests in a well-controlled environment is what sets such trials apart. The high compliance rate and low loss to follow-up confirm the value of such studies. Several examples of how pet animal tumors have been used to study tumor biology are discussed in the following section.

4.5.1. MEASUREMENT OF TUMOR HYPOXIA USING NITROIMADAZOLE-BASED HYPOXIA-MARKER DRUGS

Tumor hypoxia has consistently been shown to be a negative prognostic factor for local tumor control and disease-free survival following radiation therapy. The human clinical trials for which this has been shown include head and neck cancer and cervical carcinoma (150–156). There may also be a tie between the presence of tumor hypoxia and the likelihood of development of distant metastases, as has been indicated in soft-tissue sarcomas and cervical cancer *(153,157)*. The propensity of studies of this type in peripherally accessible tumors has been by necessity. The primary method used to measure hypoxia in tumors is the polarographic electrode, which requires accessibility through the skin for routine use. Clearly, there is a need to be able to measure hypoxia in other more common tumors, such as colorectal cancer and lung cancer. In order to achieve this goal, alternate methods to measure this parameter must be used. One of the more promising methods involves the use of drugs that are selectively bound in viable hypoxic cells. These drugs, now being developed by a number of laboratories, can be used to quantify the percentage of hypoxic cells from biopsy specimens using immuno-histochemistry or flow cytometry *(158,159)*. Radiolabeled analogs can also be detected using nuclear medicine or MR techniques *(160,161)* but these methods are less well-developed. The heterogeneity of tumor hypoxia is a potential limitation for the immunohistochemical and flow-cytometric methods. The primary question is: how much tissue must be analyzed to obtain a strong estimate of the true hypoxic fraction? This question was addressed directly by performing extensive sampling of canine tumors that were labeled with the hypoxia-marker drug CCI 103F. Using a detailed statistical analysis method, a sampling paradigm was established that provides an accurate estimate of the hypoxic fraction throughout the tumor *(43,162)*. Subsequent studies of similar drugs in human tumors have clearly shown very similar patterns of distribution of the drug, thus validating the sampling method. Additional studies from this group have evaluated the interrelationship between hypoxia-marker uptake and cell proliferation *(163,164)* and the lifetime of hypoxic cells *(165)*. All of these data have proven to be valid predictors of what has subsequently been measured in humans. These studies were useful because they provided strong preclinical data to support FDA application for use of these drugs in humans.

4.5.2. TUMOR METABOLISM

It is well-established that the metabolism of tumors is frequently grossly abnormal, characterized most clearly by the propensity toward anaerobic metabolism, lactic acidosis, and hypoxia *(166)*. The relationship between physiologic attributes of poor perfusion, hypoxia, and acidosis with poorer treatment outcome and prognosis highlight the need to evaluate these parameters clinically. In two unique studies, physiologic parameters obtained from both humans and dogs with soft-tissue sarcomas, as assessed by 31-P magnetic resonance spectroscopy, were compared with treatment outcome following thermoradiotherapy *(167,168)*. Magnetic resonance spectroscopy provides data relating to the overall level of metabolic activity, as reflected by levels of ATP, inorganic phosphorus (Pi) and phosphocreatine (PCR), for example. Intracellular pH can also be derived from these data. In humans, thermoradiotherapy was administered preoperatively, and pretreatment intracellular pH was positively correlated with the likelihood of achieving tumor, sterilization, as assessed by histopathologic analysis at the time of resection. In canine subjects, the tumors were treated with definitive thermoradiotherapy, and followed for duration of local control. pH was positively correlated with duration of local control. In a second study, changes in physiologic parameters after the first hyperthermia treatment were assessed. In both the human and canine series, changes in ATP/Pi signal-to-noise ratio correlated with temperatures achieved during heating. In addition, in the canine subjects, reduction in ATP/Pi ratio after the first heat were correlated with temperatures achieved, suggesting that such data could be used to predict the efficiency of heating, if such measurements were taken prior to therapy. In a subsequent study from a different series of animals with soft-tissue sarcomas, it was demonstrated that changes in perfusion and oxygenation of tumors, at 24 h after treatment, were correlated with temperatures achieved during hyperthermia *(169)* (Fig. 5). These results provided a strong rationale for placing an upper limit on allowable temperatures in order to avoid thermally induced hypoxia, which could compromise subsequent fractions of radiation therapy.

4.5.3. REGULATION OF TUMOR pH

The propensity of tumors to use anaerobic metabolism leads to acidification of the extracellular environment. In both rodent and human tumors, extracellular pH (pHe) is reduced, relative to normal tissues *(166)*. Typical values are in the range of 6.8–7.2, compared with values of 7.3–7.4 in normal tissues. This degree of acidification has therapeutic implications. For example, pHe has been correlated with the likelihood of achieving a complete response in human tumors treated with thermoradiotherapy *(170)*. Furthermore, lactate levels, which reflect the degree of anaerobic metabolism in tumors, have been correlated with a higher likelihood of developing distant metastases in humans with head and neck *(171)* or cervical cancer *(172)*. The acidification of the extracellular space is accomplished by active hydrogen ion transporters, which move excess hydrogen from the interior of the cell to the outside. Thus, cells try to maintain a fairly well-controlled intracellular pH. The result of this transport activity is a pH gra-

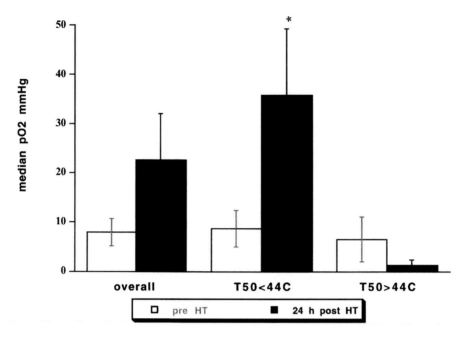

Fig. 5. Relationship between median temperature achieved during first hyperthermia treatment and changes in oxygenation 24 h post-treatment. These data confirmed earlier observations in humans demonstrating that hyperthermia causes reoxygenation of tumors. However, there must be an upper threshold of temperature for this effect to occur. If median temperatures exceed 44°C for 1 h, the improvement in pO2 is lost. This may occur because of vascular damage induced by hyperthermia. Data modified from *(169)*.

dient that develops across the cell membrane. Among its other roles, the pH gradient affects transport of drugs that are either weak acids or weak bases *(173)*. Although considerable work has been done to study the effects of pH gradients on drug accumulation and cytotoxicity in vitro and in rodent model systems, validation that such gradients existed in spontaneous tumors has not been accomplished. Recently, a relatively large series was published in which both parameters were measured in the same canine subjects with soft-tissue sarcomas *(174)*. In general, the existence of the gradients was confirmed for most of the tumors in this series, although the magnitude of the gradient varied considerable from one tumor to the next (Fig. 6). The therapeutic implications of these results were discussed.

4.5.4. MANIPULATION OF TUMOR BLOOD FLOW

Theoretically, if it is possible to improve tumor perfusion, there are practical consequences relating to the potential for improved drug and nutrient delivery. However, nearly all types of vasoactive drugs paradoxically reduce tumor blood flow rather than increasing it. This paradoxical effect is most likely caused by a relative lack of arteriolar input to tumors, combined with the fact that tumor arterioles tend to be maximally dilated under control conditions. Thus, when a vasoactive drug is administered, the vasculature of surrounding normal tissue dilates, and blood is shunted from the tumor (vascular steal). One of the first studies to investigate the effect of hydralazine-induced vascular steal on temperatures during hyperthermia was by Voorhees and Babbs in

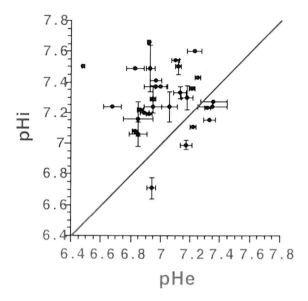

Fig. 6. Relationship between intracellular and extracellular pH in canine soft-tissue sarcomas. Evidence for an overall pH gradient is seen, but the direction and magnitude vary considerably. Data modified from *(174)*.

1982, using a naturally occurring tumor allograft in the dog, called the transmissable venereal tumor *(175,176)*. The results were remarkable enough that a number of subsequent studies were performed in rodent and human tumors to further investigate the feasibility of this approach. A significant clinical limitation was the reluctance of the clinicians to subject normotensive human patients to transient hypotension because of the risks of exacerbation of stroke or myocardial infarct. In a subsequent study, both human and canine patients were treated with hydralazine at doses that caused minimal (human) to moderate (canine) reductions in blood pressure *(177)*. The canine results clearly demonstrated that hypotension was required to see improvement in temperatures during hyperthermia. In a subsequent study, the short-acting vasoactive drug nitroprusside was tested as a means to improve tumor temperatures *(178)*. The logic of using this drug was that blood pressure is more easily controlled than with hydralazine. More recently, the nitric oxide synthase inhibitor, L-NAME, was tested. The potential advantage of this agent is that it reduces tumor blood flow by causing peripheral vasoconstriction and reduced tumor blood flow, without appreciably affecting cardiac output. This agent causes slight hypertension, as opposed to hypotension, and thus would be safer to use clinically. Surprisingly, the drug led to life-threatening acute pancreatitis in the first two clinical subjects in which it was tested, and the trial was terminated early *(179)*. Studies of this agent in normal dogs prior to the initiation of the therapy trial and in the setting of iatrogenically induced septic shock did not lead to this side-effect *(180)*. Careful examination of the history surrounding these two animals identified risk factors for pancreatitis, suggesting that careful screening of patients is necessary if studies with this agent are to be initiated in human trials. The results of this clinical study highlight the importance of studying therapies in older animals, in which where concurrent diseases can affect the spectrum of normal tissue toxicities that may be encountered with cancer therapy.

REFERENCES

1. Dorn C, Taylor D, Schneider R, Hibbard H, Klauber M. Survey of animal neoplasms in Alameda and Contra Costa Counties, California. II. Cancer morbidity in dogs and cats from Alameda county. *J Natl Cancer Inst* 1968; 40:307–318.
2. Greenle R, Murray T, Bolden S, Wingo P. Cancer Statistics, 2000. *CA Cancer J Clin* 2000; 50:7–33.
3. Hardy Jr. W, Hess P, MacEwen E, McClelland A, Zuckerman E, Essex M, et al. Biology of feline leukemia virus in the natural environment. *Cancer Res* 1976; 36:582–588.
4. Shelton G, Grant C, Cotter S, Gardner M, Hardy Jr. W, DiGiacomo R. Feline immunodeficiency virus and feline leukemia virus infections and their relationships to lymphoid malignancies in cats: a retrospective study (1968–1988). *J Acquir Immune Defic Syndr* 1990; 3:623–630.
5. Essex M, Klein G, Snyder S, Harrold J. Correlation between humoral antibody and regression of tumours induced by feline sarcoma virus. *Nature* 1971; 233:195–196.
6. Hendrick M, Goldschmidt M, Shofer F, Wang Y, Somlyo A. Postvaccinal sarcomas in the cat: epidemiology and electron probe microanalytical identification of aluminum. *Cancer Res* 1992; 52:5391–5394.
7. Glickman L, Domanski L, Maguire T, Dubielzig R, Churg A. Mesothelioma in pet dogs associated with exposure of their owners to asbestos. *Environ Res* 1983; 32:305–313.
8. Hayes Jr. H, Hoover R, Tarone R. Bladder cancer in pet dogs: a sentinel for environmental cancer? *J Epidemiol* 1981; 114:229–233.
9. Reif J, Cohen D. The environmental distribution of canine respiratory tract neoplasms. *Arch Environ Health* 1971; 22:136–140.
10. Patronek G, Rowan A. Editorial—Determining dog and cat numbers and population dynamics. *Anthrozoos* 1995; 8:199–205.
11. Puccio M, Nathanson L. The cancer cachexia syndrome. *Semin Oncol* 1997; 24:277–287.
12. Trott K-R. Differences between mouse and human tumors that affect their responses to radiotherapy. In: Kallman R, ed. *Rodent Tumor Models in Experimental Cancer Therapy.* Pergamon Press, New York, NY, 1987. pp. 6–11.
13. Hall E. Cell, Tissue, and Tumor Kinetics. In: Hall E, ed. *Radiobiology for the Radiologist.* 4th ed. J.B. Lippincott Philadelphia, PA, 1994. pp. 191–210.
14. Steel G. *Growth Kinetics of Tumours.* Oxford University Press, Oxford, 1977.
15. Larue SM, Fox MH, Ogilvie GK, Page RL, Getzy DM, Thrall DE, et al. Tumour cell kinetics as predictors of response in canine lymphoma treated with chemotherapy alone or combined with whole body hyperthermia. *Int J Hyperthermia* 1999; 15(6):475–486.
16. Vail DM, Kisseberth WC, Obradovich JE, Moore FM, London CA, MacEwen EG, et al. Assessment of potential doubling time (Tpot), argyrophilic nucleolar organizer regions (AgNOR), and proliferating cell nuclear antigen (PCNA) as predictors of therapy response in canine non-Hodgkin's lymphoma [see comments]. *Exp Hematol* 1996; 24(7):807–815.
17. LaRue SM, Fox MH, Withrow SJ, Powers BE, Straw RC, Cote IM, et al. Impact of heterogeneity in the predictive value of kinetic parameters in canine osteosarcoma. *Cancer Res* 1994; 54(14):3916–3921.
18. Schwyn U, Crompton NE, Blattmann H, Hauser B, Klink B, Parvis A, et al. Potential tumour doubling time: determination of Tpot for various canine and feline tumours. *Vet Res Commun* 1998; 22(4):233–247.
19. MacEwen EG. An immunologic approach to the treatment of cancer. *Vet Clin North Am* 1977; 7(1):65–75.
20. MacEwen EG. Approaches to cancer therapy using biological response modifiers. *Vet Clin North Am Small Anim Pract* 1985; 15(3):667–688.
21. MacEwen EG, Kurzman ID. Canine osteosarcoma: amputation and chemoimmunotherapy. *Vet Clin N Am Small Anim Pract* 1996; 26(1):123–133.
22. MacEwen EG, Kurzman ID, Vail DM, Dubielzig RR, Everlith K, Madewell BR, et al. Adjuvant therapy for melanoma in dogs: results of randomized clinical trials using surgery, liposome-encapsulated muramyl tripeptide, and granulocyte macrophage colony-stimulating factor. *Clin Cancer Res* 1999; 5(12):4249–4258.
23. Crompton N, Ozsahin M, Schweizer P, Larsson B, Luetolf U. Theory and practice of predictive assays in radiation therapy. *Strahlenther Onkol* 1997; 173:58–67.
24. Hall P, Going J. Predicting the future: a critical appraisal of cancer prognosis studies. *Histopathology* 1999; 6:489–494.

25. Dewhirst MW, Sim DA. The utility of thermal dose as a predictor of tumor and normal tissue responses to combined radiation and hyperthermia. *Cancer Res* 1984; 44(10 Suppl):4772s–4780s.

26. Dewhirst MW, Sim DA. Estimation of therapeutic gain in clinical trials involving hyperthermia and radiotherapy. *Int J Hyperthermia* 1986; 2:165–178.

27. McChesney-Gillette S, Dewhirst MW, Gillette EL, Thrall DE, Page RL, Powers BE, et al. Response of canine soft tissue sarcomas to radiation or radiation plus hyperthermia: a randomized phase II study. *Int J Hyperthermia* 1992; 8:309–320.

28. Gillette EL, McChesney SL, Dewhirst MW, Scott RJ. Response of canine oral carcinomas to heat and radiation. *Int J Radiat Oncol Biol Phys* 1987; 13(12):1861–1867.

29. Denman DL, Legorreta RA, Kier AB, Elson HR, White ML, Buncher CR, et al. Therapeutic responses of spontaneous canine malignancies to combinations of radiotherapy and hyperthermia. *Int J Radiat Oncol Biol Phys* 1991; 21(2):415–422.

30. Dewhirst MW, Sim DA, Wilson S, DeYoung D, Parsells JL. The correlation between initial and long-term responses in pet animal tumors to heat and radiation or radiation alone. *Cancer Res* 1983; 43:5735–5741.

31. van der Zee J, González González D, van Rhoon G, van Dijk J, van Putten W, Hart A. Comparison of radiotherapy alone with radiotherapy plus hyperthermia in locally advanced pelvic tumours: a prospective, randomised, multicentre trial. *Lancet* 2000; 355:1119–1125.

32. Vernon C, Hand J, Field S, Machin D, Whaley J, van der Zee J, et al. Radiotherapy with or without hyperthermia in the treatment of superficial localized brest cancer: results from five randomized controlled trials. *Int J Radiat Oncol Biol Phys* 1996; 35:731–744.

33. Valdagni R, Amichetti M. Report of long-term follow-up in a randomized trial comparing radiation therapy and radiation therapy plus hyperthermia to metastatic lymph nodes in stage IV head and neck patients. *Int J Radiat Oncol Biol Phys* 1994; 28(1):163–169.

34. Overgaard J, Gonzalez Gonzalez D, Hulshof MC, Arcangeli G, Dahl O, Mella O, et al. Hyperthermia as an adjuvant to radiation therapy of recurrent or metastatic malignant melanoma. A multicentre randomized trial by the European Society for Hyperthermic Oncology. *Int J Hyperthermia* 1996; 12(1):3–20.

35. Sneed PK, Stauffer PR, McDermott MW, Diederich CJ, Lamborn KR, Prados MD, et al. Survival benefit of hyperthermia in a prospective randomized trial of brachytherapy boost +/– hyperthermia for glioblastoma multiforme. *Int J Radiat Oncol Biol Phys* 1998; 40(2):287–295.

36. McChesney S, Gillette E, Dewhirst M, Withrow S. Influence of WR 2721 on radiation response of canine soft tissue sarcomas. *Int J Radiat Oncol Biol Phys* 1986; 12:1957–1963.

37. Vail DM, Chun R, Thamm DH, Garrett LD, Cooley AJ, Obradovich JE. Efficacy of pyridoxine to ameliorate the cutaneous toxicity associated with doxorubicin containing pegylated (Stealth) liposomes: a randomized, double-blind clinical trial using a canine model. *Clin Cancer Res* 1998; 4(6):1567–1571.

38. Kurzman ID, MacEwen EG, Rosenthal RC, Fox LE, Keller ET, Helfand SC, et al. Adjuvant therapy for osteosarcoma in dogs: results of randomized clinical trials using combined liposome-encapsulated muramyl tripeptide and cisplatin. *Clin Cancer Res* 1995; 1(12):1595–601.

39. Page R, Thrall D, Dewhirst M, Macy D, George S, McEntee M, et al. Phase I study of melphalan alone and melphalan plus whole body hypertherma in dogs withmalignant melanoma. *Int J Hyperthermia* 1991; 7:559–566.

40. Page R, Thrall D, George S, Price G, Heidner G, McEntee M, et al. Quantitative estimation of the thermal dose-modifying factor for cis-diamminedichloroplatinum (CDDP) in tumour-bearing dogs. *Int J Hyperthermia* 1992; 8:761–769.

41. Page R, Macy D, Ogilvie G, Rosner G, Dewhirst M, Thrall D, et al. Phase III evaluation of doxorubicin and whole body hyperthermia in dogs with lymphoma. *Int J Hyperthermia* 1992; 8:187–197.

42. Page R, McEntee M, Williams P, George S, Price G, Novotney C, et al. Effect of whole body hyperthermia on carboplatin disposition and toxicity in dogs. *Int J Hyperthermia* 1994; 10:807–816.

43. Cline JM, Rosner GL, Raleigh JA, Thrall DE. Quantification of CCI-103F labeling heterogeneity in canine solid tumors. *Int J Radiat Oncol Biol Phys* 1997; 37(3):655–662.

44. Thrall DE, McEntee MC, Cline JM, Raleigh JA. ELISA quantification of CCI-103F in canine tumors prior to and during irradiation. *Int J Radiat Oncol Biol Phys* 1994; 28:649–659.

45. Thrall DE, Prescott DM, Samulski TV, Rosner GL, Denman DL, Legorreta RL, et al. Radiation plus local hyperthermia versus radiation plus the combination of local and whole-body hyperthermia in canine sarcomas. *Int J Radiat Oncol Biol Phys* 1996; 34(5):1087–1096.

46. Champ C, Tyler X, Andrews P, Coghill S. Improve your hospital autopsy rate to 40–50 per cent, a tale of two towns. *J Pathol* 1992; 166:405–407.

47. Organization WH. TNM Classification of tumors in domestic animals. Geneva: World Health Organization; 1980.

48. MacEwen EG. Spontaneous tumors in dogs and cats: models for the study of cancer biology and treatment. *Cancer Metastasis Rev* 1990; 9(2):125–136.

49. Withrow SJ, Powers BE, Straw RC, Wilkins RM. Comparative aspects of osteosarcoma. Dog versus man. *Clin Orthop* 1991(270):159–168.

50. Vail DM, MacEwen E. Spontaneous occurring tumors of companion animals as models for human cancer. *Cancer Invest* 2000; 18:767–778.

51. Gilbertson SR, Kurzman ID, Zachrau RE, Hurvitz AI, Black MM. Canine mammary epithelial neoplasms: biologic implications of morphologic characteristics assessed in 232 dogs. *Vet Pathol* 1983; 20(2):127–142.

52. Conroy JD. Melanocytic tumors of domestic animals with special reference to dogs. *Arch Dermatol* 1967; 96(4):372–380.

53. Cooley DM, Waters DJ. Skeletal metastasis as the initial clinical manifestation of metastatic carcinoma in 19 dogs. *J Vet Intern Med* 1998; 12(4):288–293.

54. Brodey RS. The use of naturally occurring cancer in domestic animals for research into human cancer: general considerations and a review of canine skeletal osteosarcoma. *Yale J Biol Med* 1979; 52(4):345–361.

55. Brodey RS, Riser WH. Canine osteosarcoma. A clinicopathologic study of 194 cases. *Clin Orthop* 1969; 62:54–64.

56. Bostock DE. Prognosis after surgical excision of canine melanomas. *Vet Pathol* 1979; 16(1):32–40.

57. Brown NO, Patnaik AK, MacEwen EG. Canine hemangiosarcoma: retrospective analysis of 104 cases. *J Am Vet Med Assoc* 1985; 186(1):56–58.

58. MacEwen EG, Hayes AA, Harvey HJ, Patnaik AK, Mooney S, Passe S. Prognostic factors for feline mammary tumors. *J Am Vet Med Assoc* 1984; 185(2):201–204.

59. Misdorp W, Romijn A, Hart AA. Feline mammary tumors: a case-control study of hormonal factors. *Anticancer Res* 1991; 11(5):1793–1797.

60. Scavelli TD, Patnaik AK, Mehlhaff CJ, Hayes AA. Hemangiosarcoma in the cat: retrospective evaluation of 31 surgical cases. *J Am Vet Med Assoc* 1985; 187(8):817–819.

61. Weijer K, Hart AA. Prognostic factors in feline mammary carcinoma. *J Natl Cancer Inst* 1983; 70(4):709–716.

62. Benjamin SA, Lee AC, Saunders WJ. Classification and behavior of canine mammary epithelial neoplasms based on life-span observations in beagles. *Vet Pathol* 1999; 36(5):423–436.

63. Kurzman ID, Gilbertson SR. Prognostic factors in canine mammary tumors. *Semin Vet Med Surg* (Small Anim) 1986; 1:25–32.

64. Kuntz CA, Dernell WS, Powers BE, Devitt C, Straw RC, Withrow SJ. Prognostic factors for surgical treatment of soft-tissue sarcomas in dogs: 75 cases (1986–1996). *J Am Vet Med Assoc* 1997; 211(9):1147–1151.

65. Bostock DE. The prognosis following the surgical excision of canine mammary neoplasms. *Eur J Cancer* 1975; 11(6):389–396.

66. Vail DM, Powers BE, Getzy DM, Morrison WB, McEntee MC, O'Keefe DA, et al. Evaluation of prognostic factors for dogs with synovial sarcoma: 36 cases (1986–1991). *J Am Vet Med Assoc* 1994; 205(9):1300–1307.

67. Keller ET, MacEwen EG, Rosenthal RC, Helfand SC, Fox LE. Evaluation of prognostic factors and sequential combination chemotherapy with doxorubicin for canine lymphoma. *J Vet Intern Med* 1993; 7(5):289–9.

68. Teska E, van Heerde P, Rutterman G. Prognostic factors for treatment of malignant lymphoma in dogs. *J Am Vet Med Assoc* 1994; 205:1722–1728.

69. Greenlee PG, Filippa DA, Quimby FW, Patnaik AK, Calvano SE, Matus RE, et al. Lymphomas in dogs. A morphologic, immunologic, and clinical study. *Cancer* 1990; 66(3):480–490.

70. Vail DM, Moore AS, Ogilvie GK, Volk LM. Feline lymphoma (145 cases): proliferation indices, cluster of differentiation 3 immunoreactivity, and their association with prognosis in 90 cats. *J Vet Intern Med* 1998; 12(5):349–354.

71. Cuoto C. Clinicopathologic aspects of acute leukemias in the dog. *J Am Vet Med Assoc* 1985; 186:681–685.

72. Leifer C, Matus RE, Saal S, MacEwen E. Chronic myelogenous leukemia in the dog. *J Am Vet Med Assoc* 1983; 183:686–689.

73. Matus RE, Leifer C, MacEwen E. Acute lymphoblastic leukemia in the dog: a review of 30 cases. *J Am Vet Med Assoc* 1983; 183:859–862.

74. Matus RE, Leifer C, MacEwen E, Hurvitz AI. Prognostic factors for multiple myeloma in the dog. *J Am Vet Med Assoc* 1986; 188:1288–1292.

75. Leifer C, Matus RE. Chronic lymphocytic leukemia in the dog: 22 cases. *J Am Vet Med Assoc* 1986; 189:214–217.

76. Benchimol S, Minden M. Viruses, oncogenes and tumor suppressor genes. In: Tannock I, Hill RP, eds. *The Basic Science of Oncology,* 3rd ed. McGraw Hill Co., New York, 1998, pp. 79–105.

77. Krontiris TG. Oncogenes. *N Engl J Med* 1995; 333(5):303–306.

78. Smith ML, Fornace AJ, Jr. The two faces of tumor suppressor p53. *Am J Pathol* 1996; 148(4):1019–1022.

79. Lowe SW, Bodis S, McClatchey A, Remington L, Ruley HE, Fisher DE, et al. p53 status and the efficacy of cancer therapy in vivo. *Science* 1994; 266(5186):807–810.

80. van Leeuwen I, Hellman E, Cornelisse C, van den Burgh B, Rutterman G. p53 mutations in mammary tumor cell lines and corresponding tumor tissue in the dog. *Anticancer Res* 1996; 16:3737–3744.

81. Chu L, Rutterman G, Kong J, Ghahremani M, Schmeing M, Misdorp W, et al. Genomic organization of the canine p53 gene and its mutation status in canine mammary neoplasia. *Breast Cancer Res Treat* 1998; 50:11–25.

82. Hollstein M, Sidransky D, Vogelstein B, Harris CC. p53 mutations in human cancers. *Science* 1991; 253(5015):49–53.

83. Greenblatt MS, Bennett WP, Hollstein M, Harris CC. Mutations in the p53 tumor suppressor gene: clues to cancer etiology and molecular pathogenesis. *Cancer Res* 1994; 54(18):4855–4878.

84. Casey G, Lopez ME, Ramos JC, Plummer SJ, Arboleda MJ, Shaughnessy M, et al. DNA sequence analysis of exons 2 through 11 and immunohistochemical staining are required to detect all known p53 alterations in human malignancies. *Oncogene* 1996; 13(9):1971–1981.

85. van Leeuwen I, Cornelisse C, Misdorp W, Goedegebuure S, Kirpenstein J, Rutterman G. p53 gene mutations in osteosarcomas in the dog. *Cancer Let* 1997; 111:173–178.

86. Veldhoen N, Stewart J, Brown R, Milner J. Mutations of the p53 gene in canine lymphoma and evidence for germ line p53 mutations in the dog. *Oncogene* 1998; 16(2):249–255.

87. Gamblin RM, Sagartz JE, Couto CG. Overexpression of p53 tumor suppressor protein in spontaneously arising neoplasms of dogs. *Am J Vet Res* 1997; 58(8):857–863.

88. Mendoza S, Konishi T, Dernell WS, Withrow SJ, Miller CW. Status of the p53, Rb and MDM2 genes in canine osteosarcoma. *Anticancer Res* 1998; 18(6A):4449–4453.

89. Mayr B, Schaffner G, Kurzbauer R. Mutations in tumor suppressor gene p53 in two feline fibrosarcomas. *Br Vet J* 1995; 151:707–713.

90. Hannink M, Donoghue DJ. Structure and function of platelet-derived growth factor (PDGF) and related proteins. *Biochim Biophys Acta* 1989; 989(1):1–10.

91. Leveen P, Claesson-Welsh L, Heldin CH, Westermark B, Betsholtz C. Expression of messenger RNAs for platelet-derived growth factor and its receptors in human sarcoma cell lines. *Int J Cancer* 1990; 46(6):1066–1070.

92. Liang Y, Robinson DF, Dennig J, Suske G, Fahl WE. Transcriptional regulation of the SIS/PDGF-B gene in human osteosarcoma cells by the Sp family of transcription factors. *J Biol Chem* 1996; 271(20):11,792–11,797.

93. Yang D, Kohler SK, Maher VM, McCormick JJ. v-sis oncogene-induced transformation of human fibroblasts into cells capable of forming benign tumors. *Carcinogenesis* 1994; 15(10):2167–2175.

94. Ahern T, Bird C, Bird A, Wolfe L. Overexpression of c-erbB-2 and c-myc but not c-ras, in canine melanoma cell lines is associated with metastatic potential in nude mice. *Anticancer Res* 1996; 13:1365–1371.

95. Ahern T, Bird A, Bird R, Wolfe L. Expression of the oncogene c-erbB-2 in canine mammary cancers and tumor-derived lines. *Am J Vet Res* 1996; 57:693–696.

96. Inoue M, Wada N. Immunohistochemical detection of p53 and p21 proteins in canine testicular tumours. *Vet Rec* 2000; 146(13):370–372.

97. Inoue M, Shiramizu K. Immunohistochemical detection of p53 and c-myc proteins in canine mammary tumours. *J Comp Pathol* 1999; 120(2):169–175.

98. Forrest D, Onioris D, Lees G, Neil JC. Altered structure and expression of c-myc in feline T-cell tumours. *Virology* 1987; 158(1):194–205.

99. Mellon K, Wright C, Kelly P, Horne CH, Neal DE. Long-term outcome related to epidermal growth factor receptor status in bladder cancer. *J Urol* 1995; 153(3 Pt 2):919–925.

100. Neal DE, Marsh C, Bennett MK, Abel PD, Hall RR, Sainsbury JR, et al. Epidermal-growth-factor receptors in human bladder cancer: comparison of invasive and superficial tumours. *Lancet* 1985; 1(8425):366–368.

101. Porter-Jordan K, Lippman ME. Overview of the biologic markers of breast cancer. *Hematol Oncol Clin N Am* 1994; 8(1):73–100.

102. Lamerz R. Role of tumour markers, cytogenetics. *Ann Oncol* 1999; 10 (Suppl. 4):145–149.

103. Rutterman GR, Foekens JA, Portengen H, Vos JH, Blankenstein MA, Teske E, et al. Expression of epidermal growth factor receptor (EGFR) in non-affected and tumorous mammary tissue of female dogs. *Breast Cancer Res Treat* 1994; 30(2):139–146.

104. MacEwen E, Pastor J, Kutze J, Tsan R, Kurzman ID, Wilson M, et al. Insulin-like growth factor-1 (IGF-1) and IGF-1 receptor expression contributes to the malignant phenotype in osteosarcoma. *Cancer Res* 2000;Submitted.

105. MacEwen E, Kutze J, Carew J, Pastor J, Tsan R, Radinsky R. c-met tyrosine kinase receptor expression and function in human and canine osteosarcoma cells. *Cancer Res* 2000;submitted.

106. Rowinsky EK, Windle JJ, Von Hoff DD. Ras protein farnesyltransferase: a strategic target for anticancer therapeutic development. *J Clin Oncol* 1999; 17(11):3631–3652.

107. Minamoto T, Mai M, Ronai Z. K-ras mutation: early detection in molecular diagnosis and risk assessment of colorectal, pancreas, and lung cancers—a review. *Cancer Detect Prev* 2000; 24(1):1–12.

108. Castagnaro M. Ras gene analysis in mammary tumors of dogs by means of PCR-SSCP and direct genomic analysis. *Anneli dell Instituto Superiore di Sanita* 1995; 31:337–341.

109. Kraegel S, Gumerlock P, Dungworth D, Oreffo V, Madewell BR. K-ras activation in non-small cell lung cancer in the dog. *Cancer Res* 1992; 52:4724–4727.

110. Steingold S, Sharp N, McGahan M, Hughes C, Dunn S, Page RL. Characterization of canine MDR1 mRNA: its abundance in drug resistant cell lines and in vivo. *Anticancer Res* 1998; 18:393–400.

111. Lee J, Hughes C, Fine R, Page RL. P-glycoprotein expression in canine lymphoma: a relevant, intermediate model of multidrug resistance. *Cancer* 1996; 77:1892–1898.

112. Moore AS, Leveille C, Reimann K, Shu H, Arias I. The expression of P-glycoprotein in canine lymphoma and its association with multidrug resistance. *Cancer Invest* 1995; 13:475–479.

113. Straw RC. Tumors of the skeletal system. In: Withrow SJ, ed. *Small Animal Clinical Oncology,* 2nd ed. WB Saunders, Philadelphia, PA, 1996, pp. 1509–1566.

114. Bergman PJ, MacEwen EG, Kurzman ID, Henry CJ, Hammer AS, Knapp DW, et al. Amputation and carboplatin for treatment of dogs with osteosarcoma: 48 cases (1991 to 1993). *J Vet Intern Med* 1996; 10(2):76–81.

115. Mauldin GN, Matus RE, Withrow SJ, Patnaik AK. Canine osteosarcoma. Treatment by amputation versus amputation and adjuvant chemotherapy using doxorubicin and cisplatin. *J Vet Intern Med* 1988; 2(4):177–180.

116. Berg J, Weinstein MJ, Springfield DS, Rand WM. Results of surgery and doxorubicin chemotherapy in dogs with osteosarcoma. *J Am Vet Med Assoc* 1995; 206(10):1555–1560.

117. Chun R, Kurzman ID, Cuoto G, Klausne J, Henry C, MacEwen E. Cisplatin and doxorubicin combination chemotherapy for the treatment of canine osteosarcoma. *J Vet Int Med* 2000; 14:495–498.

118. Berg J, Gebhardt MC, Rand WM. Effect of timing of postoperative chemotherapy on survival of dogs with osteosarcoma. *Cancer* 1997; 79(7):1343–1350.

119. Dernell WS, Withrow SJ, Straw RC, Powers BE, Drekke JH, Lafferty M. Intracavitary treatment of soft tissue sarcomas in dogs using cisplatin in a biodegradable polymer. *Anticancer Res* 1997; 17(6D):4499–4505.

120. Withrow SJ, Straw RC, Brekke J. Slow release adjuvant cisplatin for the treatment of metastatic canine osteosarcoma. *Eur J Musculoskeletal Res* 1995; 4:105–110.

121. Vail DM, Kravis LD, Cooley AJ, Chun R, MacEwen EG. Preclinical trial of doxorubicin entrapped in sterically stabilized liposomes in dogs with spontaneously arising malignant tumors. *Cancer Chemother Pharmacol* 1997; 39(5):410–416.

122. Thamm DH, Vail DM. Preclinical evaluation of a sterically stabilized liposome-encapsulated cisplatin in clinically normal cats. *Am J Vet Res* 1998; 59(3):286–289.

123. Hershey AE, Kurzman ID, Forrest LJ, Bohling CA, Stonerook M, Placke ME, et al. Inhalation chemotherapy for macroscopic primary or metastatic lung tumors: proof of principle using dogs with spontaneously occurring tumors as a model. *Clin Cancer Res* 1999; 5(9):2653–2659.

124. Bostock DE, Gorman NT. Intravenous BCG therapy of mammary carcinoma in bitches after surgical excision of the primary tumour. *Eur J Cancer* 1978; 14(8):879–883.

125. Fox LE, MacEwen E, Kurzman ID. Liposome-encapsulated muramyl tripeptide phosphatidylethanolamine for the treatment of feline mammary adenocarcinoma—a multicenter randomized double blind study. *Cancer Biotherapy* 1995; 10:125–130.

126. Hogge GS, Burkholder JK, Culp J, Albertini MR, Dubielzig RR, Keller ET, et al. Development of human granulocyte-macrophage colony-stimulating factor-transfected tumor cell vaccines for the treatment of spontaneous canine cancer. *Hum Gene Ther* 1998; 9(13):1851–1861.

127. MacEwen EG, Harvey HJ, Patnaik AK, Mooney S, Hayes A, Kurzman I, et al. Evaluation of effects of levamisole and surgery on canine mammary cancer. *J Biol Response Mod* 1985; 4(4):418–426.

128. Teske E, Rutteman GR, v.d. Ingh TS, van Noort R, Misdorp W. Liposome-encapsulated muramyl tripeptide phosphatidylethanolamine (L-MTP-PE): a randomized clinical trial in dogs with mammary carcinoma. *Anticancer Res* 1998; 18(2A):1015–1019.

129. Vail DM, MacEwen E, Kurzman I, Dubielzig RR, Helfand SC, Kisseberth WC, et al. Liposome-encapsulated muramyl tripeptide phosphatidylethanolamine adjuvant immunotherapy for splenic hemangiosarcoma in the dog: a randomized multi-institutional clinical trial. *Clin Cancer Res* 1995; 1:1165–1170.

130. MacEwen EG, Hayes AA, Mooney S, Patnaik AK, Harvey HJ, Passe S, et al. Evaluation of effect of levamisole on feline mammary cancer. *J Biol Response Mod* 1984; 3(5):541–546.

131. MacEwen EG, Kurzman ID, Rosenthal RC, Smith BW, Manley PA, Roush JK, et al. Therapy for osteosarcoma in dogs with intravenous injection of liposome-encapsulated muramyl tripeptide. *J Natl Cancer Inst* 1989; 81(12):935–938.

132. Fidler IJ, Sone S, Fogler WE, Barnes ZL. Eradication of spontaneous metastases and activation of alveolar macrophages by intravenous injection of liposomes containing muramyl dipeptide. *Proc Natl Acad Sci USA* 1981; 78(3):1680–1684.

133. Fidler IJ. Therapy of cancer metastasis by systemic activation of macrophages. *Adv Pharmacol* 1994; 30:271–326.

134. Kleinerman ES, Gano JB, Johnston DA, Benjamin RS, Jaffe N. Efficacy of liposomal muramyl tripeptide (CGP 19835A) in the treatment of relapsed osteosarcoma. *Am J Clin Oncol* 1995; 18(2):93–99.

135. Hogge GS, Burkholder JK, Culp J, Albertini MR, Dubielzig RR, Yang NS, et al. Preclinical development of human granulocyte-macrophage colony-stimulating factor-transfected melanoma cell vaccine using established canine cell lines and normal dogs. *Cancer Gene Ther* 1999; 6(1):26–36.

136. Novotney C, Page R, Macy D, Dewhirst M, Ogilvie G, Withrow S, et al. Phase I evaluation of doxorubicin and whole-body hyperthermia in dogs with lymphoma. *J Vet Int Med* 1992; 6:245–249.

137. Hauck M, Price G, Ogilvie G, Johnson J, Gillette E, Thrall D, et al. Phase I evaluation of mitoxantrone alone and combined with whole body hyhperthermia in dogs with lymphoma. *Int J Hyperthermia* 1995; 12:309–320.

138. Page RL, Lee J, Riviere JE, Dodge RK, Thrall DE, Dewhirst MW. Absence of whole body hyperthermia effect on cisplatin distribution in spontaneous canine tumors. *Int J Radiat Oncol Biol Phys* 1995; 32(4):1097–102.

139. McChesney SL, Withrow SJ, Gillette EL, Powers BE, Dewhirst MW. Radiotherapy of soft tissue sarcomas in dogs. *J Am Vet Med Assoc* 1989; 194(1):60–63.

140. Overgaard J, Gonzalez Gonzalez D, Hulshof MC, Arcangeli G, Dahl O, Mella O, et al. Randomised trial of hyperthermia as adjuvant to radiotherapy for recurrent or metastatic malignant melanoma. European Society for Hyperthermic Oncology [see comments]. *Lancet* 1995; 345(8949):540–543.

141. Dewhirst MW, Winget JM, Edelstein-Keshet L, Sylvester J, Engler M, Thrall DE, et al. Clinical application of thermal isoeffect dose. *Int J Hyperthermia* 1987; 3(4):307–318.

142. Valdagni R, Liu FF, Kapp DS. Important prognostic factors influencing outcome of combined radiation and hyperthermia. *Int J Radiat Oncol Biol Phys* 1988; 15(4):959–972.

143. Kapp DS, Cox RS. Thermal treatment parameters are most predictive of outcome in patients with single tumor nodules per treatment field in recurrent adenocarcinoma of the breast [see comments]. *Int J Radiat Oncol Biol Phys* 1995; 33(4):887–899.

144. Oleson J, Samulski T, Leopold K, Clegg S, Dewhirst M, Dodge R, et al. Sensitivity of hyperthermia trial outcomes to temperature and time: implications for thermal goals of treatment. *Int J Radiat Oncol Biol Phys* 1993; 25:289–297.

145. Seegenschmiedt MH, Martus P, Fietkau R, Iro H, Brady LW, Sauer R. Multivariate analysis of prognostic parameters using interstitial thermoradiotherapy (IHT-IRT): tumor and treatment variables predict outcome. *Int J Radiat Oncol Biol Phys* 1994; 29(5):1049–1063.

146. Dewhirst M. Thermal Dosimetry. In: Seegenschmiedt M, Fessenden P, Vernon C, eds. Thermo-radiotherapy and thermochemotherapy. Springer-Verlag, Berlin, 1995, pp. 123–136.

147. Thrall D, Rosner G, Azuma C, LaRue S, Case B, Samulski T, et al. Using units of CEM 43·C T90, local hyperthermia thermal dose can be delivered as prescribed. *Int J Hyperthermia* 2000; 16:415–428.

148. Thrall D, LaRue S, Powers B, Page R, Johnson J, George S, et al. Use of whole body hyperthermia as a method to heat inaccessible tumours uniformly: a phase III trial in canine brain masses. *Int J Hyperthermia* 1999; 15:383–398.

149. Thrall D, Withrow S, Powers B, Straw R, Page R, Heidner G, et al. Radiotherapy prior to cortical allograft limb sparing in dogs with osteosarcoma: a dose response assay. *Int J Radiat Oncol Biol Phys* 1990; 18:1351–1357.

150. Brizel DM, Sibley GS, Prosnitz LR, Scher RL, Dewhirst MW. Tumor hypoxia adversely affects the prognosis of carcinoma of the head and neck. *Int J Radiat Oncol Biol Phys* 1997; 38(2):285–289.

151. Brizel DM, Dodge RK, Clough RW, Dewhirst MW. Oxygenation of head and neck cancer: changes during radiotherapy and impact on treatment outcome. *Radiother Oncol* 1999; 53(2):113–117.

152. Nordsmark M, Overgaard M, Overgaard J. Pretreatment oxygenation predicts radiation response in advanced squamous cell carcinoma of the head and neck. *Radiother Oncol* 1996; 41:31–39.

153. Hockel M, Schlenger K, Aral B, Mitze M, Schaffer U, Vaupel P. Association between tumor hypoxia and malignant progression in advanced cancer of the uterine cervix. *Cancer Res* 1996; 56(19):4509–4515.

154. Hockel M, Schlenger K, Hockel S, Aral B, Schaffer U, Vaupel P. Tumor hypoxia in pelvic recurrences of cervical cancer. *Int J Cancer* 1998; 79(4):365–369.

155. Fyles AW, Milosevic M, Wong R, Kavanagh MC, Pintilie M, Sun A, et al. Oxygenation predicts radiation response and survival in patients with cervix cancer [published erratum appears in *Radiother Oncol* 1999 Mar;50(3):371]. *Radiother Oncol* 1998; 48(2):149–156.

156. Rofstad EK, Sundfor K, Lyng H, Trope CG. Hypoxia-induced treatment failure in advanced squamous cell carcinoma of the uterine cervix is primarily due to hypoxia-induced radiation resistance rather than hypoxia-induced metastasis. *Br J Cancer* 2000; 83(3):354–359.

157. Brizel DM, Scully SP, Harrelson JM, Layfield LJ, Bean JM, Prosnitz LR, et al. Tumor oxygenation predicts for the likelihood of distant metastases in human soft tissue sarcoma. *Cancer Res* 1996; 56(5):941–943.

158. Varia MA, Calkins-Adams DP, Rinker LH, Kennedy AS, Novotny DB, Fowler WC, Jr., et al. Pimonidazole: a novel hypoxia marker for complementary study of tumor hypoxia and cell proliferation in cervical carcinoma. *Gynecol Oncol* 1998; 71(2):270–277.

159. Evans SM, Jenkins WT, Joiner B, Lord EM, Koch CJ. 2-Nitroimidazole (EF5) binding predicts radiation resistance in individual 9L s.c. tumors. *Cancer Res* 1996; 56(2):405–411.

160. Evans SM, Kachur AV, Shiue CY, Hustinx R, Jenkins WT, Shive GG, et al. Noninvasive detection of tumor hypoxia using the 2-nitroimidazole [18F]EF1. *J Nucl Med* 2000; 41(2):327–336.

161. Chapman JD, Engelhardt EL, Stobbe CC, Schneider RF, Hanks GE. Measuring hypoxia and predicting tumor radioresistance with nuclear medicine assays. *Radiother Oncol* 1998; 46(3):229–237.

162. Thrall DE, Rosner GL, Azuma C, McEntee MC, Raleigh JA. Hypoxia marker labeling in tumor biopsies: quantification of labeling variation and criteria for biopsy sectioning. *Radiother Oncol* 1997; 44(2):171–176.

163. Raleigh JA, Zeman EM, Calkins DP, McEntee MC, Thrall DE. Distribution of hypoxia and proliferation associated markers in spontaneous canine tumors. *Acta Oncol* 1995; 34(3):345–349.

164. Zeman EM, Calkins DP, Cline JM, Thrall DE, Raleigh JA. The relationship between proliferative and oxygenation status in spontaneous canine tumors. *Int J Radiat Oncol Biol Phys* 1993; 27(4):891–898.

165. Azuma C, Raleigh JA, Thrall DE. Longevity of pimonidazole adducts in spontaneous canine tumors as an estimate of hypoxic cell lifetime. *Radiat Res* 1997; 148(1):35–42.

166. Vaupel P, Jain R. Tumor Blood Supply and Metabolic Microenvironment. Gustav Fischer Verlag Stuttgart, 1991,

167. Prescott DM, Charles HC, Sostman HD, Dodge RK, Thrall DE, Page RL, et al. Therapy monitoring in human and canine soft tissue sarcomas using magnetic resonance imaging and spectroscopy. *Int J Radiat Oncol Biol Phys* 1994; 28(2):415–423.

168. Sostman HD, Prescott DM, Dewhirst MW, Dodge RK, Thrall DE, Page RL, et al. MR imaging and spectroscopy for prognostic evaluation in soft-tissue sarcomas. *Radiology* 1994; 190(1):269–275.

169. Vujaskovic Z, Poulson J, Gaskin A, Thrall D, Page R, Charles H, et al. Temperature dependent changes in physiologic parameters of spontaneous canine soft tissue sarcomas after combined radio-therapy and hyperthermia. *Int J Radiat Oncol Biol Phys* 2000; 46:179–185.

170. Engin K, Leeper D, Thistlethwaite A, Tupchong L, McFarlane J. Tumor extracellular pH as a prognostic factor in thermoradiotherapy. *Int J Radiat Oncol Biol Phys* 1994; 29:125–132.

171. Walenta S, Salameh A, Lyng H, Evensen JF, Mitze M, Rofstad EK, et al. Correlation of high lactate levels in head and neck tumors with incidence of metastasis. *Am J Pathol* 1997; 150(2):409–415.

172. Schwickert G, Walenta S, Sundfor K, Rofstad E, Mueller-Klieser W. Correlation of high lactate levels in human cervical cancer with incidence of metastasis. *Cancer Res* 1995; 55:4757–4759.

173. Gerweck LE, Seetharaman K. Cellular pH gradient in tumor versus normal tissue: potential exploitation for the treatment of cancer. *Cancer Res* 1996; 56(6):1194–1198.

174. Prescott DM, Charles HC, Poulson JM, Page RL, Thrall DE, Vujaskovic Z, et al. The relationship between intracellular and extracellular pH in spontaneous canine tumors [In Process Citation]. *Clin Cancer Res* 2000; 6(6):2501–2505.

175. Voorhees WDd, Babbs CF. Hydralazine-enhanced selective heating of transmissible venereal tumor implants in dogs. *Eur J Cancer Clin Oncol* 1982; 18(10):1027–1033.

176. Babbs CF, DeWitt DP, Voorhees WD, McCaw JS, Chan RC. Theoretical feasibility of vasodilator-enhanced local tumor heating. *Eur J Cancer Clin Oncol* 1982; 18(11):1137–1146.

177. Dewhirst MW, Prescott DM, Clegg S, Samulski TV, Page RL, Thrall DE, et al. The use of hydralazine to manipulate tumour temperatures during hyperthermia. *Int J Hyperthermia* 1990; 6(6):971–983.

178. Prescott DM, Samulski TV, Dewhirst MW, Page RL, Thrall DE, Dodge RK, et al. Use of nitroprus-side to increase tissue temperature during local hyperthermia in normal and tumor-bearing dogs. *Int J Radiat Oncol Biol Phys* 1992; 23(2):377–385.

179. Poulson J, Dewhirst M, Gaskin A, Samulski T, Prescott D, Meyer R, et al. Unexpected toxicity associated with nitric oxide synthase inhibition in tumor-bearing dogs. In Vivo 2000; 14:709–714.

180. Kilbourn R, Szabo, C, Traber, DL. Beneficial versus detrimental effects of nitric oxide synthase inhibitors in circulatory shock: Lessons learned from experimental and clinical studies. *Shock* 1997; 7:235–246.

IX EXPERIMENTAL METHODS AND END POINTS

31 In Vivo Tumor Response End Points

Beverly A. Teicher, PhD

Contents

1. INTRODUCTION

The field of cancer research is very fortunate, because only recently has it come the forefront of human scientific endeavor, allowing cancer to take advantage of the experience of others. Before the organized investigation of malignant disease, researchers had worked out scientific methodology and recognized the importance of laboratory models for infectious diseases, allowing rapid progress in antibacterial drug development. Cancer research has also benefited from the early research of the 1950s and 1960s, which took a very orderly and rigorously scientific approach to the development of in vivo models and to the development of the most informative end points available from their experiments.

While the rapidly growing, intraperitoneally implanted murine leukemias are now rarely used as primary tumor models, their value as a foundation of sound scientific in vivo methodology is undiminished. Therefore, this chapter on end points begins with a discussion of murine leukemic ascites tumors.

2. ASCITES TUMORS

The science of preclinical modeling of anticancer therapies began in the 1950s, yet the establishment of guidelines for experimental quality and end point rigor can be attributed in large part to the group headed by Howard Skipper at the Kettering-Meyer Laboratory affiliated with Sloan-Kettering Institute, Southern Research Institute in Birmingham, Alabama. In the mid-1960s, this group published a series of reports on the criteria of "curability" and on the kinetic behavior of leukemic cells in animals and the effects of anticancer chemotherapy. The principles put forth in these reports were derived directly from the behavior of bacterial-cell populations exposed to antibacterial

From: *Tumor Models in Cancer Research*
Edited by: B. A. Teicher © Humana Press Inc., Totowa, NJ

agents, and were based upon experimental findings in mice bearing intraperitoneally implanted L1210 or P388 leukemia *(1–15)*.

The initial assumptions were: 1) One living leukemic cell can be lethal to the host. Therefore, to cure experimental leukemia, it is necessary to kill every leukemic cell in the animal, regardless of the number, anatomic distribution, or metabolic heterogeneity, with treatment that spares the host. 2) The percentage, not the absolute number, of in vivo leukemic-cell populations of various sizes killed by a given dose of a given antileukemic drug is reasonably constant. This phenomenon of a constant fractional (or percentage) drug-kill of a cell population, regardless of the population size, has been repeatedly observed, and may be a general phenomenon. 3) The percentage of experimental leukemic-cell populations of any size killed by single-dose treatment of drug to the host is directly proportional to the dose level of the drug (the higher the dose, the higher the percentage of cell-kill). Thus, it is obviously necessary to kill leukemic cells faster than they are replaced by proliferation of the cells surviving the therapy if a "cure" is to be attempted *(10–12)*.

The exponential killing of cells by drugs with time (mathematically equivalent to "a constant percentage kill of leukemic cells regardless of number") was observed in bacterial-cell populations around 1900 *(16)*, and has been investigated with many antibacterial agents *(17–20)*. Through studies with bacterial cells exposed to anticancer agents, it was confirmed that the first-order kinetics of cell-kill by anticancer agents was similar to that of antibacterial agents *(12)*. The hypothesis that "the percentage, not the absolute number, of cells in populations of widely varying sizes killed by a given dose of a given anticancer drug is reasonably constant" was studied intensively and found, for the most part, to be valid *(12)*.

Skipper and the group at the Kettering-Meyer Laboratory went on to develop the murine L1210 leukemia *(21)*, as well as the murine P388 leukemia *(22)*, into highly sensitive and reasonably quantitative in vivo bioassay systems to study anatomic distribution and the rate of proliferation of leukemic cells, and the effects of chemotherapy in tumor-bearing mice *(14)*. These studies were based on the notion that the principal mechanism by which drug-induced increase in host life span is achieved is through leukemic cell-kill, not "inhibition of growth" of the leukemic-cell population *(23–26)*. Furthermore, leukemic cells that gain access to the brain and other areas of the central nervous system (CNS) are not markedly affected by certain peripherally administered antileukemic drugs. Therefore, if there are leukemic cells in the CNS when treatment is initiated, it is necessary to employ a drug that passes the blood-brain barrier if a "cure" is to be achieved *(27,28)*.

The observation that there was a close relationship between the number of L1210 leukemic cells inoculated into BDF1 mice and the life span of these animals was critical *(23)* (Fig. 1). Thus, it was possible to estimate the average in vivo doubling (or generation) time of L1210 leukemic cells and the approximate lethal number when L1210 leukemia cells were inoculated into the animals by various routes. When the intraperitoneal (ip) route was employed, the average doubling time for the tumor cells was about 0.55 d, and the number of leukemic cells required to be lethal to the host was calculated to be approx 1.5 billion *(23)*. When the L1210 tumor cells were implanted intravenously or intracerebrally, the average doubling time and/or lethal number of cells appeared to be somewhat less. This knowledge was used to develop an in vivo bioassay by ip implantation of unknown numbers of viable L1210 cells from various

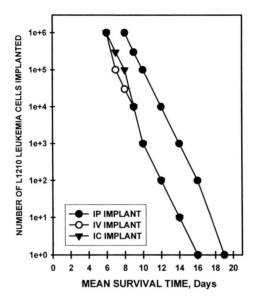

Fig. 1. Mean survival time of mice inoculated with various numbers of murine L1210 leukemia cells injected intraperitoneally, intravenously, or intracranially. These data form the basis for the in vivo bioassay method for determining the number of L1201 cells surviving after treatment of L1210 tumor-bearing mice with therapy. From these survival curves, it was determined that from: 1) ip inoculation the L1210 cell-generation time = 0.55 d; the lethal number of L1210 cells = 1.5×10^9; 2) iv inoculation the L1210 cell-generation time = 0.43 d; and 3) ic inoculation the L1210 cell-generation time = 0.46 d (adapted from ref. *14*).

tissues of chemotherapy-treated L1210 bearing animals into fresh hosts and using the survival time of those animals to estimate the tumor-cell-killing by the chemotherapy. The estimated experimental error in this bioassay procedure was ± 1 log of tumor cells. Thus, the method gave a reasonable order-of-magnitude estimate of the number of leukemic cells in various tissues, and was sensitive to small, absolute numbers of viable L1210 leukemia cells *(14)*.

Antitumor activity in these early murine ascitic leukemia models was assessed on the basis of percent mean or median increase in life span (% ILS), net $\log_{10}$ cell-kill, and long-term survivors *(29,30)*. The percent mean or median increase in life span (% ILS) is derived from the ratio of the survival time of the treated animals (days) compared with the survival time of the untreated control animals (days). Calculations of net $\log_{10}$ cell-kill are made from the tumor doubling time determined from an internal tumor titration consisting of implants from serial 10-fold dilutions *(31)* (Fig. 1). Long-term survivors are excluded from calculations of % ILS and net $\log_{10}$ tumor-cell-kill. To assess net $\log_{10}$ tumor-cell-kill at the end of treatment, the survival time (days) difference between treated and control groups is adjusted to account for regrowth of tumor-cell populations that may occur between individual treatments *(32)*. The net $\log_{10}$ cell-kill is calculated as follows:

Net $\log_{10}$ cell-kill = [(T–C) – (duration of treatment in days)]/3.32 × T_d, where (T–C) is the difference in the median day of death between the treated (T) and the control (C) groups, 3.32 is the number of doublings required for a population to increase 1

$\log_{10}$ unit, and T_d is the mean tumor doubling time (days) calculated from a log-linear least-squares fit of the implant sizes and the median days of death of the titration groups—and is the factor that accounts for any repopulation of the tumor during or after treatment (Fig. 1).

3. SOLID TUMOR

As solid-tumor models were developed, the appropriate end points devised were tumor-growth delay or tumor control of a primary implanted tumor. These assays require that drugs be administered at doses producing tolerable normal tissue toxicity, so that the response of the tumor to the treatment can be observed for a relatively long period of time. Treatment with test compounds can be initiated either prior to tumor development or after a tumor nodule has appeared. If treatment begins the day after or on the day of tumor-cell implant, the experiment is designated a tumor-growth-inhibition study. If treatment begins when an established tumor nodule (50–200 mm^3) is present, the experiment is designated a tumor-growth-delay study. Activity in a tumor-growth-delay study is a much stronger data than activity in a tumor-growth-inhibition study, because it is a better model of clinical disease.

Historically, in primary screening experiments in murine solid-tumor models, the tumor volumes in the treated and control groups were measured with calipers only once, usually when the control tumors reached approx 1 cm^3 in volume (1 g by weight), at which time all of the mice were sacrificed. Alternately, the mice in all of the groups were sacrificed when the tumors of the untreated or vehicle-treated control group reached approx 1 cm^3 in volume, and the tumors were excised and weighed. This traditional protocol design provided no kinetic data regarding tumor growth and response *(33)*. A more informative experimental design includes tumor-volume measurements and body-wt measurements of individual mice twice per wk for the duration of the experiment—one which allows elucidation of the growth pattern of the unmanipulated tumor in the control animals as well as the effect of the drug on the tumor-growth pattern *(33–35)*.

Tumor volumes are usually estimated from measurements of two diameters of the individual tumors:

$$\text{Tumor volume (mm}^3) = (\text{longer diameter} \times \text{shorter diameter}^2) \times 0.5$$

where the diameters are the tumor length and width in mm, usually measured with calipers, respectively. The data from experiments in which tumor-volume measurements are made over a relatively long period of time until the tumors reach a volume of 1.5–2 cm^3 available allow the calculation of the tumor-growth delay and percent T/C at multiple time-points and the exponential tumor-volume doubling time (Fig. 2).

Tumor-growth delay is the difference in days for treated vs control tumors to reach a specified volume, usually 500 mm^3 or 1 cm^3. Therefore, tumor-growth delay is simply T–C in days. T is the mean or median time (in days) required for the treatment group tumors to reach a predetermined size, and C is the mean or median time (in days) for the control group tumors to reach the same size. Animals that are tumor-free at the time of the determination of tumor-growth delay are excluded from these calculations. This value may the single most important criterion of antitumor effectiveness, because it mimics most closely clinical end points and requires observation of the animals through the time of disease progression.

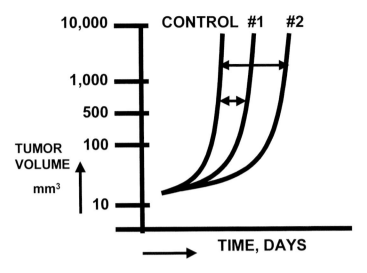

Fig. 2. Schematic representation of the calculation of tumor-growth delay in days. Tumor-growth delay is usually calculated when control tumors reach a volume of 500 mm³ or 1000 mm³.

In some cases, when the tumor is grown in a log-linear manner through the treatment and response phase of the experiment, this information can be converted to the log-cell-kill. The group at the Kettering-Meyer Laboratories applied similar techniques used in the murine leukemia models for obtaining order-of-magnitude estimates of the absolute number or percent of viable cancer cells remaining, and established log_{10} cell-kill methodology for selected experimental solid tumors after a single dose of a drug *(13)*. This work was based upon the assumptions that: 1) The mass of a tumor is in direct proportion to the number of malignant cells in the mass. 2) The cells killed by the cytotoxic agent immediately become nonviable. 3) The cells which remain viable despite treatment begin to grow again, after a relatively short lag, and proliferate at the same average rate as tumor cells in untreated control animals. These assumptions appeared to be valid for two of the three tumors studied in the initial report, which included the hamster Plasmacytoma 1 tumor, the murine Sarcoma 180, and the murine adenocarcinoma 755 tumor. This technique was similar to that developed for L1210 leukemia, an ascites tumor that continues in logarithmic growth until very near the death of the host. Because the untreated control tumor for both Plasmacytomal and Sarcoma 180 grow logarithmically during most of the treatment period, a similar method of estimating cell-killing could be applied to these tumors. Since many solid tumors are not in log phase during most of the host life span, this reasoning cannot be applied to those tumors without modification. Furthermore, many cytotoxic therapies such as radiation therapy do not kill cells destined to die promptly, but kill cells over several generations of proliferation. Thus, this methodology cannot be accurately applied to these agents.

Tumors were implanted subcutaneously by trocar into the right axillary region of hamsters or mice. Slopes were derived from tumor-growth curves for untreated tumor-bearing animals and from % T/C curves for tumors after treatment (Fig. 3). These values were applied to the first-order rate-constant equation to allow determination of the fraction of tumor cells killed or the fraction of viable cells remaining after the treatment.

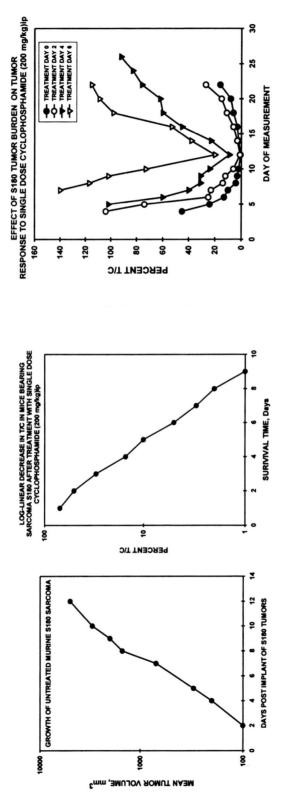

Fig. 3. *Left panel:* Exponential growth of the murine Sarcoma 180 after implantation of a 2 mm³ cube of tumor tissue by subcutaneous (sc) trocar injection. *Center panel:* Effect of day of treatment on the percent T/C response of mice bearing Sarcoma 180 after treatment with a single dose of cyclophosphamide (200 mg/kg) administered by ip injection. *Right panel:* Time course of response of the murine Sarcoma 180 after treatment with a single dose of cyclophosphamide (200 mg/kg) by ip injection on various days post-tumor implantation. (adapted from ref. *13*).

Table 1
Conversion of Log 10 Tumor Kill to An Activity Rating

Antitumor Activity	Duration of Treatment		
	<5 days	5–20 days	>20 days
	Log10-Cell Killing		
	Net	Net/Gross	Net/Gross
Highly Active			
++++	>2.6	>2.0/>2.8	>0.8/>3.4
+++	1.6–2.6	0.8–2.0/2.0–2.8	2.0–2.8/2.5–3.4
++	0.9–1.5	1.3–1.9	1.7–2.4
+	0.5–0.8	0.7–1.2	1.0–1.6
Inactive			
–	<0.5	<0.7	<1.0

An activity rating of +++ to ++++ is needed to effect partial regression (PR) or complete (CR) regression of 100–300 mg transplanted solid tumors of mice. Thus, an activity rating of + or ++ would not be scored as active by usual criteria (adapted from ref. *33*).

For subcutaneously growing tumors, the log_{10} cell-kill is calculated from the following formula:

The log_{10} cell-kill total (gross) = [T–C value in days/(3.32)(T$_d$)]

where T–C is the tumor-growth delay and T$_d$ is the tumor-volume doubling time (in days) of the untreated control tumors in exponential growth over a volume range from approx 100 mm^3 to 1 cm^3. The conversion of the T–C values to log_{10} cell-kill is possible if the tumor maintains a log-linear growth pattern and if the T$_d$ of the tumors regrowing posttreatment approximates the T$_d$ values of the tumors in untreated control mice. The calculations for net log_{10} cell-kill are provided by subtraction of the duration of the treatment period from the T–C value and then dividing by 3.32 × Td *(36,37)*. Corbett et al. *(33)* have used a relative activity rating scale to describe log_{10} cell-kill accounts for the treatment duration (Table 1). The activity of several standard anticancer agents in five rapidly growing murine tumors is provided on Table 2.

For most, solid-tumor-volume behavior is a notoriously unquantitative end point with respect to tumor-cell-kill *(4,38–41)*. A drug-induced regression in tumor mass of no more than 50% may represent a 99.99% reduction in clonogenic cells in a measurable solid-tumor mass (Fig. 2). Many of the human tumor xenograft models now used widely do not conform to the requirement of log-linear growth, and many recently developed anticancer therapies do not kill promptly, with little lag prior to the resumption of log-linear growth in the treated groups (Figs. 4, 5).

Response to therapies in solid-tumor models can also be assessed using excision assays (see Chapter 32). Tumor excision assays or tumor-cell survival assays can be performed if the tumor cells can grow in animals and also in cell culture with a good plating efficiency (1–20% or more). One important difference between excision assays and the *in situ* assays of ILS tumor regression/growth delay, or local tumor control is that excision assays require removal of the tumor from the environment in which it was treated. This difference and the nature of the assay procedure lead to a number of

Table 2
In Vivo Activity of Standard Agents Against Early Mouse Solid Tumors

Antitumor Agent	Colon 38	Mam16/C	Colon 51	Panc 02	Panc 03
Doxorubicin	++	++++	±	–	+++
Paclitaxel	++++	++++	+++	–	++++
Irinotecan	±	+++	+	–	++++
Etoposide	++	+++	+	–	–
Vincristine	–	++	–	–	–
5-Fluorouracil	+++	+++	–	–	–
Cytosine arabinoside	++	++	–	–	–
Cyclophosphamide	±	+++	++	–	++
Cisplatin	±	±	++	–	++
Doubling time (days)	2.3–3.0	1.0–1.2	2.2–2.9	1.2–1.5	2.3–2.8
Metastatic potential	mod/low	very high	high	very high	moderate
Syngeneic host	C57BL/6	C3H	Balb/c	C57BL/6	C57BL/6

(Adapted from ref. *33*).

advantages and disadvantages in using excision assays rather than *in situ* assays. The ability to measure cell survival (cell killing) from the in vivo treatment directly is important because it gives basic information about the ultimate definitive cellular effect. Tumor-excision assays also allow greater accuracy and finer resolution between various therapeutic regimens than *in situ* assays. Perhaps the greatest disadvantage of excision assays is that extended treatment regimens cannot be used because of tumor-cell loss and tumor-cell proliferation over the treatment period (*35,42–49*). Thus, an excision assay provides a static picture of tumor response a short time after treatment.

The murine EMT-6 mammary carcinoma syngeneic to the Balb/c mouse was selected for this study. As an initial therapeutic high-dose study, the EMT-6 tumor was implanted subcutaneously in a hind-leg of the mice, and the animals were treated with standard regimens or single high doses of anticancer drugs. Treatment was begun on d 7 post-tumor-cell implantation, when the tumors were approx 150 mm^3 in volume. All drugs were administered by ip injection (Table 3). The standard treatment cyclophosphamide regimen of 150 mg/kg on alternate days for three doses produced a tumor-growth delay of 6.2 d, but no significant period of tumor regression. The single high-dose cyclophosphamide regimen of 450 mg/kg, however, resulted in a tumor-growth delay of 31.5 d, and regression duration of 9.5 d. The standard murine dose and regimen for melphalan of a single dose of 10 mg/kg produced a tumor-growth delay of about 2.6 d. With administration of peripheral blood cells (PBC) (*42*) on d 8 and rhG-CSF on d 8–20, Balb/c mice bearing the EMT-6 tumor could be treated with a single dose of melphalan of up to 40 mg/kg. This high dose of melphalan produced a tumor-growth delay of approx 9.3 d, and a period of tumor regression of approx 3 d. A standard treatment regimen for thiotepa of 5 mg/kg once daily for 5 d produced a tumor-growth delay of 3.7 d, while a single dose of 40 mg/kg of thiotepa resulted in 6.1 d of tumor-growth delay and a period of approx 2 d when tumors were at or below the original treatment volume. Carboplatin administered at the standard dose of 50 mg/kg produced a tumor-growth delay of 4.5 d, and increasing that dose fivefold to 250 mg/kg

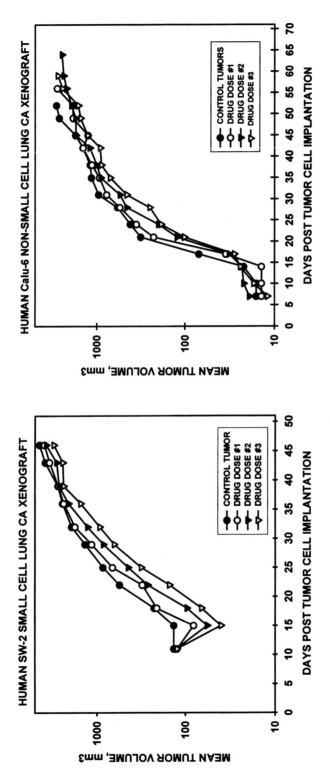

Fig. 4. Growth curves for the human SW-2 SCLC and for the human Calu-6 NSCLC grown as sc xenograft tumors in nude mice. Although small regions of the tumor-growth curves may approach log-linear growth, marked deviations from log-linearity are clear.

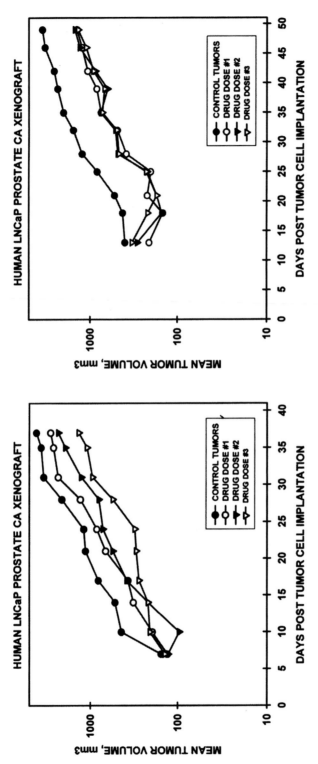

Fig. 5. Growth curves from two different studies for the human LNCaP prostate carcinoma grown as a sc xenograft tumor in nude mice. The control tumors approximate log-linear growth. The drug in the left-hand panel alters tumor growth variously, depending upon dose. After the drug treatment in the right-hand panel, the tumors regain log-linear growth parallel to the control tumors after recovery from the regression phase.

Table 3
Growth Delay of the EMT-6 Tumor After Treatment of Tumor-Bearing Animals
with Each Antitumor Agent at Standard or High Dose

Treatment Group	Tumor Growth Delay (d)[1]	Regression Duration (d)[2]	Total Drug Dose (mg/kg)
Cyclophosphamide (150 mg/kg, d 7,9,11)	6.2 ± 0.5	<1	450
Cyclophosphamide (450 mg/kg, d 7) stem cells[3]	31.5 ± 2.8	9.5	450
Melphalan (10 mg/kg, d 7)	2.6 ± 0.3	<1	10
Melphalan (40 mg/kg, d 7) stem cells	9.3 ± 0.7	3	40
Thiotepa (5 mg/kg, days 7–11)	3.7 ± 0.6	<1	25
Thiotepa (40 mg/kg, d 7) stem cells	6.1 ± 0.6	2	40
Carboplatin (50 mg/kg, d 7)	4.5 ± 0.5	<1	50
Carboplatin (250 mg/kg, d 7) stem cells	9.0 ± 1.0	2	250
5-FU (30 mg/kg, d 7–11)	3.1 ± 0.3	<1	150
5-Fu (275 mg/kg, d 7) stem cells	1.8 ± 0.4	<1	275

[1] Tumor growth delay is the difference in days for treated vs control tumors to reach 500 mm³. Control tumors reach 500 mm³ in 12.2 ± 0.7 days postsubcutaneous implantation.

[2] Tumor regression duration is the number of days that the tumor volume is less than the original treatment volume.

[3] "Stem cells" indicates that animals received 10^7 peripheral blood cells (PBC) intravenously on d 8 and rhG-CSF (2 µg/kg) intraperitoneally twice daily on d8 through 20. (adapted from ref. 42).

with hematopoietic support resulted in a tumor-growth delay of 9.0 d and a period of regression of about 2 d. The antimetabolite 5-fluorouracil (5-Fu) administered in a standard regimen of 30 mg/kg daily for 5 d produced a tumor-growth delay of 3.1 d in the EMT-6 tumor. Administering 5-Fu as a single dose of 275 mg/kg with hematopoietic support resulted in only 1.8 d of tumor-growth delay.

These tumor-growth delay data obtained at high doses allow a comparison to be made between tumor-cell survival (tumor-cell killing) and tumor-growth delay for the same doses of a drug. In Table 4, this analysis is shown for melphalan, thiotepa, and cyclophosphamide. Through 6 logs of cell killing, the relationship holds that a 6.5 mg/kg increase in the dose of melphalan, a direct-acting nitrogen mustard, corresponds to a 1-log increase in tumor-cell killing and 1.7 d of tumor-growth delay of the EMT-6 tumor. For thiotepa, a 10 mg/kg increase in dose corresponds to a 1-log increase in tumor-cell killing and 1.7 d of tumor-growth delay in the EMT-6 tumor. Cyclophosphamide, a prodrug that undergoes metabolic activation primarily in the liver as well as metabolic inactivation primarily in circulation, requires approx 115 mg/kg to produce approx 1 log of tumor-cell killing over the 3-log range of tumor-cell killing examined. However, based on the known tumor-growth delay data (4.2 d) for a single dose of 150 mg/kg of cyclophosphamide, the tumor-growth delay for a dose of 450 mg/kg of cyclophosphamide is underestimated and based on the known tumor-growth-delay data (31.5 d) for 450 mg/kg cyclophosphamide, the tumor-growth delays for the lower doses of cyclophosphamide are overestimated (number in parentheses) (42). Thus, if the tumor remains *in situ,* the response to cyclophosphamide increases nonlinearly with increasing dose, perhaps because the conversion of the prodrug to the active

Table 4
Comparison between Tumor-Cell Survival and Tumor-Growth
Delay for EMT-6 Tumors Treated In Vivo[1]

Dose (mg/kg)	EMT-6 Tumor Surviving Fraction	Emt-6 Tumor Growth Delay (Days)
Melphalan		
n		
9	0.1	1.7
10	**0.05**	**2.6**
15.5	0.01	3.5
22	0.001	5.2
28.5	0.0001	6.9
35	0.00001	8.6
40	**2E-06**	**9.3**
41.5	1E-06	10.3
Thiotepa		
13	0.1	1.7
23	0.01	3.4
25	**0.007**	**3.7**
33	0.001	5.1
40	**0.0002**	**6.1**
43	0.0001	6.8
Cyclophosphamide		
115	0.1	2.9 (10)
150	**0.05**	**4.2 (15)**
270	0.01	5.7 (20)
425	0.001	8.6 (30)
450	**0.0008**	**31.5**
580	0.0001	11.5 (40)

[1] Tumor-cell survival data were reported *(42–49)*. Numbers shown in bold were experimentally determined (adapted from ref. *42*).

metabolite(s) increases in a nonlinear manner with increasing dose of the prodrug. The tumor cells *in situ* go into a long lag phase, thus yielding an incorrect estimate of the number of tumor cells killed by the treatment.

Analysis of tumor-growth delay and tumor-cell-survival data in this murine model system indicates that for two antitumor alkylating agents, melphalan and thiotepa, linearly increasing dose results in linearly increasing tumor-growth delay and log-linearly increasing tumor-cell killing. Analysis of this type of data for carboplatin indicates approx 3.4 days of tumor-growth delay per log tumor-cell killing, and shows that 300 mg/kg increases in drug dose are required to produce log increases in tumor-cell killing. As would be expected for an antimetabolite, administration of 5-Fp as a single high dose was less effective as an antitumor treatment than treatment with the standard 5-Fu regimen of once daily for 5 d. Other chemotherapeutic agents that frequently produce long lag phases in vivo before tumor regrowth become log-linear, and thus produce longer tumor-growth delays for the number of tumor cells killed by the treatments, include cisplatin and BCNU.

4. COMBINATION TREATMENTS: ISOBOLOGRAM ANALYSIS

In the study of multimodality therapy or combined chemotherapy, it is important to determine whether the combined effects of two agents are additive or whether their combination is substantially different than the sum of their parts *(50,51)*. Conceptual foundations for this form of analysis were popularized by Steel and Peckman *(52)*, based on the construction of an envelope of additivity in an isoeffect plot (isobologram). This approach provides a rigorous basis for defining regions of additivity, supra-additivity, sub-additivity, and protection. This method of analysis is based on a clear conceptual formulation of the way that drugs or agents can be expected to show additivity. The first form of additivity is conceptually more simple, and is defined as Mode 1 by Steel and Peckham *(52)*. For a selected level of effect (survival in this case) on a log scale, the dose of Agent A to produce this effect for the survival curve is determined. A lower dose of Agent A is then selected, the difference in effect from the isoeffect level is determined, and the dose of Agent B needed to make up this difference is determined from the survival curve for Agent B. For example, 3 mg of Agent A may be needed to produce 0.1% survival (3 logs of kill), the selected isoeffect. A dose of 2.5 mg of Agent A produces 1.0% survival (2 logs of kill). The Mode I isoeffect point for Agent B would thus be the level of Agent B needed to produce 1 log of kill, to result in the same overall effect of 3 logs of kill. In this instance, we may find that 4 mg of Agent B are needed to produce 1 log of kill.

Mode II additivity is conceptually more complex, but corresponds to the concepts of additivity discussed by Berenbaum *(53)*. For any given level of effect, the dose of Agent A needed to produce this effect is determined from the survival relationship. The isoeffect dose of Agent B is calculated as the amount of Agent B needed to produce this effect, determined from the survival relationship. The isoeffect dose of Agent B is calculated as the amount of Agent B needed to produce the given effect, starting at the level of effect produced by Agent A. For example, 3 mg of Agent A may be needed to produce 0.1% survival (3 logs of kill). A dose of 2.5 mg of Agent A produces 1.0% (2 logs of kill). A dose of 6 mg of Agent B is needed to produce 3 logs of kill, and 2 logs of kill are obtained with Agent B at 5 mg. Thus, the Mode II isoeffect point with Agent A at 2.5 mg is equal to the amount of Agent B needed to take Agent B from 2 logs of kill to 3 logs of kill (6 mg – 5 mg = 1 mg). This can be conceptualized by noting that Agent A should produce 2 logs of kill, and in this case is equal to 5 mg of Agent B. If Agent A + Agent B are identical in their mode of action, then 1 mg more of Agent B should be equivalent in effect to 6 mg of Agent B. Graphically, on a linear dose scale, Mode II additivity is defined as the straight line connecting the effective dose of Agent A alone and the effective dose of Agent B alone. This relationship is also described by the equation:

$$\frac{\text{Dose of A}}{A_e} + \frac{\text{Dose of B}}{B_e} = 1$$

where A_e and B_e are the doses of Agent A and Agent B, respectively, needed to produce the selected effect.

Overall, combinations that produce the desired effect that are within the boundaries of Mode I and Mode II are considered additive. Those displaced to the left are supra-additive, and those displaced to the right are subadditive. Combinations that produce effects, outside the rectangle defined by the intersections of A_e and B_e are protective.

This type of classical isobologram methodology is difficult to use experimentally, because each combination must be carefully titrated to produce a constant level of effect. Dewey et al. *(54)* described an analogous form of analysis for the special case in which the dose of one agent was held constant. Using full survival curves of each agent alone, this method produces envelopes of additive effect for various levels of the variable agent. It is conceptually identical to generating a series of isoeffect curves and then plotting the survivals from a series of these at constant dose of Agent A on a log effect by dose of Agent B coordinate system *(55)*. This approach can often be applied to the experimental situation in a more direct and efficient manner, and isobolograms can be derived describing the expected effect (Mode I and Mode II) for any level of the variable-agent and constant-agent combinations.

It has been recognized that the schedule and sequence of drugs in combination can affect therapeutic outcome. Over the last 15 years, the definition of additivity and therapeutic synergism has evolved with increasing stringency. In the work of Schabel et al. *(56–61)*, Corbett et al. *(62,63)*, and Griswold et al. *(64,65)*, therapeutic synergism between two drugs was defined to mean that "the effect of the two drugs in combination was significantly greater than that which could be obtained when either drug was used alone under identical conditions of treatment." Using this definition, the combination of cyclophosphamide and melphalan administered simultaneously by ip injection every 2 wk was reported to be therapeutically synergistic in the Ridgeway OS growth-delay assay *(56–60)*. Similarly, the combination of cyclophosphamide and melphalan has been reported to be therapeutically synergistic in L1210 and P388 leukemias *(61)*. Cyclophosphamide plus a nitrosourea (BCNU, CCNU, or MeCCNU) have also been reported to be therapeutically synergistic in ILS and growth-delay assays using this definition *(61)*.

In the EMT6 murine mammary carcinoma in vivo, the maximum tolerated combination therapy of thiotepa (5 mg/kg × 6) and cyclophosphamide (100 mg/kg × 3) produced approx 25 d of tumor-growth delay, which was not significantly different than expected for additivity of the individual drugs (Fig. 6) *(46,47,49)*. The survival of EMT6 tumor cells after treatment of the animals with various single doses of thiotepa and cyclophosphamide was assayed. Tumor-cell killing by thiotepa produced a very steep and linear survival curve through 5 logs. The tumor-cell survival curve for cyclophosphamide of 500 mg/kg gave linear tumor-cell kill through almost 4 logs. In all cases, the combination treatment tumor-cell survivals fell well within the envelope of additivity (Fig. 7). Both of these drugs are somewhat less toxic toward bone-marrow cells by the granulocyte-macrophage colony-forming unit (GM-CFU) in vitro assay method than to tumor cells. The combination treatments were sub-additive or additive in bone-marrow GM-CFU killing. When bone marrow is the dose-limiting tissue, there is a therapeutic advantage to the use of this drug combination *(46–50)*.

The Lewis Lung Carcinoma (LLC) arose spontaneously as a carcinoma of the lung of a C57BL mouse in 1951 in the laboratory of Dr. Margaret R. Lewis at the Wistar Institute. The LLC was among the earliest transplantable tumors used to identify new anticancer agents. Sugiura and Stock found that the LLC produced tumors 100% of the time, yielding a very malignant carcinoma. These investigators at the Sloan-Kettering Institute for Cancer Research used the LLC in combination with several other transplantable tumors to determine the antitumor activity of a series of phosphoramides from which the antitumor alkylating agent thiotepa emerged *(66–68)*. Twenty years

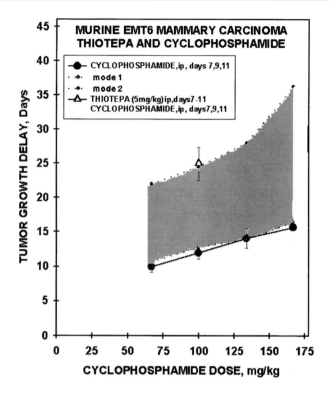

Fig. 6. Isobologram for the growth delay of the EMT6 murine mammary carcinoma treated with combinations of thiotepa and cyclophosphamide. Tumor treatments with cyclophosphamide alone are shown as solid circles. The dotted area represents the envelope of additivity for treatments with thiotepa and cyclophosphamide. Combination treatment of 5 mg/kg thiotepa × 6 + 100 mg/kg cyclophosphamide × 3 is shown as open triangle. Points represent three independent experiments (7 animals/group; 21 animals/point); bars represent the standard error of the mean (SEM) (adapted from ref. *46*).

later, DeWys, working at the Strong Memorial Hospital of the University of Rochester School of Medicine, standardized techniques for following primary tumor growth by tumor-volume measurements for assessing the response of lung metastases to a therapeutic intervention *(69)*. DeWys observed the Gompertsian pattern of primary tumor growth, effects of tumor burden on therapeutic efficacy, and the effects of the presence of the primary tumor on the growth rate of the lung metastases *(70)*. G. Gordon Steel and co-investigators continued working with the LLC and in the mid- and late 1970s developed culture colony-formation techniques, lung-colony formation techniques, and limiting-dilution techniques to assess tumor response to new anticancer drugs and radiation therapy *(71,72)*.

This syngeneic tumor system mimics the human disease because from the primary tumor it metastasizes to lungs, bone and liver. It is nonimmunogenic, and is grown in a host with a fully functional immune system. The rate of tumor growth is relatively rapid, with a tumor-volume doubling time of 2.5 d—and it is lethal in 21–25 d. Although this growth rate is rapid, it is in line with the life span of the host, which is about 2 yr.

Gemcitabine (LY18801; 2′,2′-difluorodeoxycytidine) is an analog of the natural pyrimidine. The mechanism of action and metabolism of gemcitabine have been well-

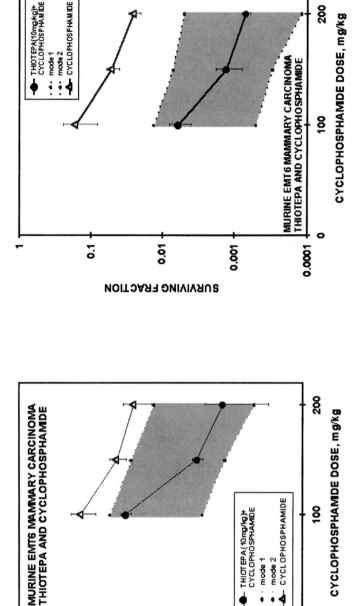

Fig. 7. Isobolograms for the combination treatment of the EMT6 tumor in vivo with 10 or 15 mg/kg thiotepa and various doses of cyclophosphamide. The survival curve for EMT6 tumors exposed to cyclophosphamide only is shown with open triangles. The dotted area represents the envelope of additivity for the combination treatment. Tumor-cell survivals for the combination treatments are shown in solid circles (adapted from ref. *46*).

characterized *(73,74)*. Deoxycytidine kinase (dCK) activates gemcitabine to gemcitabine monophosphate, gemcitabine diphosphate, and gemcitabine triphosphate. The triphosphate competes with deoxycytidine triphosphate for incorporation into DNA, and results in chain termination 1 basepair beyond the point of insertion *(74,75)*. The addition of a basepair after gemcitabine triphosphate protects this lesion from excision by exonucleases. Gemcitabine cytotoxicity is proportional to the intracellular concentration of gemcitabine triphosphate and its incorporation into DNA. The diphosphate of gemcitabine exerts a time- and concentration-dependent inhibition of the enzyme ribonucleotide reductase, thereby diminishing intracellular deoxycytidine triphosphate and enhancing the incorporation of gemcitabine triphosphate into DNA *(73)*. In cell culture, gemcitabine produces accumulation of cells in the S phase of the cell cycle *(73,76,77)*. Gemcitabine is active against a number of solid tumors in vitro, and has demonstrated activity against many solid-tumor models, including the CX-1 human colon-cancer xenograft and the LX-1 human lung carcinoma xenograft in nude mice *(75–78)*. In Phase I human trials, gemcitabine has been evaluated in a variety of schedules. The greatest efficacy with the least toxicity has been demonstrated with a weekly schedule *(73)*. In Phase II human trials, gemcitabine has demonstrated activity against small-cell lung, non-small-cell lung, breast, ovarian, pancreatic, myeloma, prostatic, renal, and bladder cancer *(79,80)*. Gemcitabine has demonstrated a 22% objective tumor response rate in a database of 331 patients diagnosed with non-small-cell lung cancer (NSCLC), who received the drug on a weekly schedule in a dose range of 800 mg/m^2 to 1250 mg/m^2.

Vinorelbine (navelbine) is a new, semisynthetic vinca alkaloid, and its antitumor activity is related to its ability to depolymerize microtubules that dissolve the mitotic spindles *(81–86)*. Its activity in cell culture was equal to or greater than other vinca alkaloids *(86)*. Vinorelbine was as effective as vinblastine against the A2780 human ovarian-carcinoma cell line, and was more cytotoxic than other vinca alkaloids against a human bronchial epidermoid carcinoma *(83)*. In a variety of human tumor-cell lines (leukemia, NSCLC, small-cell lung cancer (SCLC), colon, breast, melanoma, and brain), vinorelbine was cytostatic at nanomolar concentrations that are significantly below achievable plasma levels *(82,86)*. In a number of in vivo studies exploring activity in rodent-tumor models and human tumor xenografts in athymic mice, vinorelbine demonstrated efficacy against P388, L1210, B16, and M5076 in vivo in murine models and in animals with human tumor xenografts. Phase I human trials have shown that in a weekly intravenous (iv) administration, the maximum tolerated dose (MTD) of vinorelbine was 30 mg/m^2. This dose was the recommended amount to be used in subsequent Phase II human trials employing a weekly schedule *(85,87,88)*. Phase II human trials employing weekly schedules of vinorelbine have demonstrated activity against SCLC, NSCLC, and ovarian and breast cancer *(86)*. Vinorelbine as a single agent was studied in nonrandomized Phase II human trials as first-line therapy in NSCLC using a weekly schedule, and showed good activity with 23 responders out of 70 evaluable patients producing a response rate of 32.8%. The median duration of response was 34 wk *(86–89)*.

Gemcitabine was an active anticancer agent in animals bearing the LLC. Gemcitabine was well-tolerated by the animals over the dosage range from 40 mg/kg × 3 to 80 mg/kg × 3 (Fig. 8). Navelbine was administered in three different well-tolerated regimens with total doses of 10, 15, and 22.5 mg/kg. Both gemcitabine and navelbine pro-

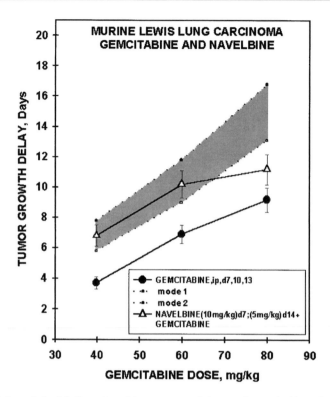

Fig. 8. Growth delay of the LLC produced by a range of doses of gemcitabine alone or along with navelbine (15 mg/kg total dose). The dotted area is the envelope of additivity determined by isobologram analysis. The bars are SEM.

duced increasing tumor-growth delay with increasing dose of the drug. To assess the efficacy of the drug combination, the intermediate dosage regimen of navelbine was combined with each dosage level of gemcitabine. These combination regimens were tolerated, and the tumor-growth delay increased with increasing dosages of gemcitabine. Isobologram methodology *(50)* was used to determine whether the combinations of gemcitabine and navelbine achieved additive antitumor activity (Fig. 8). At gemcitabine doses of 40 mg/kg and 60 mg/kg, the combination regimens achieved additivity, with the experimental tumor-growth delay falling within the calculated envelope of additivity. At the highest dose of gemcitabine, the combination regimen produced less than additive tumor-growth delay *(51)*.

The untreated control animals in this study had a mean number of 35 lung metastases on d 20. Gemcitabine was highly effective against disease metastatic to the lungs, so that the mean number of lung metastases on d 20 was decreased to 1.0–1.5 or 3–4% of the number found in the untreated controls. Each of the navelbine regimens decreased the number of lung metastases on d 20 to 10 or 11, or to about 30% of the number found in the untreated control animals. The combination regimens were highly effective against LLC metastatic to the lungs, with a mean number of <1–0 metastases found on d 20. These results support the notion that gemcitabine and navelbine may be an effective anticancer drug combination against NSCLC *(51)*.

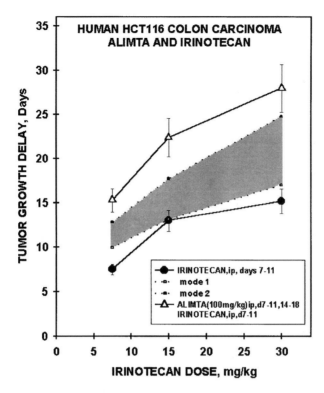

Fig. 9. Growth delay of human HCT116 colon carcinoma growth as a xenograft in nude mice after treatment with irinotecan (7.5, 15, or 30 mg/kg) intraperitoneally on days 7–11 after tumor-cell implantation alone or along with ALIMTA (100 mg/kg) intraperitoneally on d 7–11 and d 14–18. The points are the mean values of two experiments with five animals per group per experiment; bars indicate the SEM. The dotted area represents the envelope of additivity by isobologram analysis (adapted from ref. *95*).

The human HCT116 colon carcinoma was selected for the initial study of ALIMTA (N-[4-[2-(2-amino-3,4-dihydro-4-oxo-7H-pyrrolo[2,3-d]pyrimidin-5-yl)ethyl]-benzoyl]-L-glutamic acid; LY231514) in combination treatment because the HCT116 tumor is responsive to ALIMTA, and because antitumor activity of ALIMTA has been observed in patients with colon cancer *(90–94)*. Treatment of nude mice bearing subcutaneously implanted HCT116 colon tumors with ALIMTA (100 mg/kg) twice daily for 5 ds produced a tumor-growth delay of 2.7 ± 0.3 ds. Irinotecan administered daily for 5 ds produced increasing tumor-growth delay with increasing dose of the drug (Fig. 9) *(95)*. Treatment of HCT116 tumor-bearing animals with ALIMTA and irinotecan resulted in greater than additive tumor growth for the two drugs, reaching 27 ds when the irinotecan dose was 30 mg/kg. No toxicity was observed when a full standard dose of ALIMTA was administered with a full standard dose of irinotecan.

Irinotecan (CPT-11) is a synthetic analog of the plant alkaloid camptothecin, which exerts its antitumor activity through inhibition on the DNA-unwinding enzyme topoisomerase I, resulting in a strand break in the DNA *(96,97)*. Cell-culture studies have shown that combinations of raltitrexed and SN-38, the active metabolite of irinotecan, can produce synergistic tumor-cell killing *(98)*. The combination of ALIMTA and irinotecan can result in synergistic antitumor effect against the human HCT116 colon carcinoma across all the doses of irinotecan examined. In general terms, this may reflect the fixing of the sublethal damage of one of the drugs by the other, or may reflect enhancement of one of the drug targets by the other drug *(99)*. Exposure to irinotecan may increase the proportion of tumor cells in S phase, as has been shown on exposure of HL-60 cells to camptothecin in cell culture *(99)*, thus increasing the portion of tumor cells that are susceptible to the cytotoxic action of ALIMTA.

CONCLUSION

The tumor response end points described in this chapter are well-established, and reflect clinical outcomes in the human disease. Although the value of the particular tumor lines and the value of the mouse as a host remain topics for discussion; response end points, survival end points, and tumor-cell-killing end points are well-coordinated with clinical investigations.

REFERENCES

1. Skipper HE. Historic milestones in cancer biology: a few that are important in cancer treatment (revisited). *Semin Oncol* 1979; 6:506–514.
2. Skipper HE. Thoughts on cancer chemotherapy and combination modality therapy *JAMA* 1974; 230:1033–1035.
3. Skipper HE. Successes and failures at the preclinical level; where now? *Seventh National Cancer Conference Proc.* JB Lippincott Company, Philadelphia, PA, pp. 1973, 109–121.
4. Skipper HE. Kinetics of mammary tumor cell growth and implications for therapy. *Cancer* 1971; 28:1479–1499.
5. Skipper HE. Cancer chemotherapy is many things: G.H.A. Clowes memorial lecture. *Cancer Res* 1971; 31:1173–1180.
6. Skipper HE. Improvement of the model systems. *Cancer Res* 1969; 29:2329–2333.
7. Skipper HE. Biochemical, biological, pharmacologic, toxicologic, kinetics and clinical (subhuman and human) relationships. *Cancer* 1968; 21:600–610.
8. Skipper HE. Criteria associated with destruction of leukemia and solid tumor cells in animals. *Cancer Res* 1967; 27:2636–2645.
9. Himmelfarb P, Thayer PS, Martin H. Growth of colonies of murine leukemia L1210 in vitro. *Cancer Chemother Rep* 1967; 51:451–453.
10. Wilcox WS, Schabel FM, Skipper HE. Experimental evaluation of potential anticancer agents XV. On the relative rates of growth and host kill of "single" leukemia cells that survive in vivo cytoxan therapy. *Cancer Res* 1966; 26:1009–1014.
11. Moore GE, Sandberg AA, Ulrich K. Suspension cell culture and in vivo and in vitro chromosome constitution of mouse leukemia 1210. *J Natl Cancer Inst* 1966; 36:405–421.
12. Pittilo RF, Schabel FM, Wilcox WS, Skipper HE. Experimental evaluation of potential anticancer agents. XVI. Basic study of effects of certain anticancer agents on kinetic behavior of model bacterial cell populations. *Cancer Chemother Rep* 1965; no. 47:1–26.
13. Wilcox WS, Griswold DP, Laster WR, Schabel FM, Skipper HE. Experimental evaluation of potential anticancer agents. XVII. kinetics of growth and regression after treatment of certain solid tumors. *Cancer Chemother Rep* 1965; no. 47:27–39.
14. Skipper HE, Schabel FM, Wilcox WS, Laster WR, Trader MW, Thompson SA. Experimental evaluation of potential anticancer agents. XVIII. Effects of therapy on viability and rate of proliferation of leukemia cells in various anatomic sites. *Cancer Chemother Rep* 1965; 47:41–64.
15. Skipper HE. The effects of chemotherapy on the kinetics of leukemic cell behavior. *Cancer Res* 1965; 25:1544–1550.
16. Chick H. An investigation of the laws of disinfection. *J Hyg* (London) 1908; 8:92–158.
17. McCulloch EC. *Disinfection and Sterilization,* 2nd ed. Lea and Febiger, Philadelphia, PA, 1945.
18. Davis BD. *Bacterial and Mycotic Infections in Man,* 3rd ed. Dubos RJ, ed. J B Lippincott Company, Philadelphia, PA, 1958,

19. Porter JR. *Bacterial Chemistry and Physiology.* John Wiley and Sons Inc., New York, NY, 1947.
20. Wyss O. Chemical factors affecting growth and death. In: Werkman CH, Wilson PW, eds. *Bacterial Physiology* Academic Press, Inc., New York, NY, 1951,
21. Law LW, Dunn TB, Boyle PJ, Miller JH. Observations on the effects of a folic-acid antagonists on transplantable lymphoid leukemias in mice. *J Natl Cancer Inst* 1949; 10:179–195.
22. Evans VJ, LaRock JF, Yosida TH, Potter M. A new tissue culture isolation and explanation of the P388 lymphocytic neoplasm in a chemically characterized medium. *Exp Cell Res* 1963; 32:212–217.
23. Skipper HE, Schabel FM, Wilocox WS. Experimental evaluation of potential anticancer agents. XIII. On the criteria and kinetics associated with "curability" of experimental leukemia. *Cancer Chemother Rep* 1964; 35:1–111.
24. Skipper HE. Perspectives in cancer chemotherapy: therapeutic design. *Cancer Res* 1964; 24:1295–1302.
25. Frei E III. Potential for eliminating leukemic cells in childhood acute leukemia (Abstr) *Proc Amer Assoc Cancer Res* 1964; 5:20.
26. Hananian J, Holland JF, Sheehe P. Intensive chemotherapy of acute lymphocytic leukemia in children (Abstr) *Proc Am Assoc Cancer Res* 1965; 6:26.
27. Rall DP. Experimental studies of the blood-brain barrier. *Cancer Res* 1965; 25(9):1572–1577.
28. Thomas LB. Pathology of leukemia in the brain and meninges: postmortem studies of patients with acute leukemia and of mice inoculated with L1210 leukemia. *Cancer Res* 1965; 25(9):1555–1571.
29. Bibby MC. Making the most of rodent tumor systems in cancer. *Br J Cancer* 1999; 79:1633–1640.
30. Waud WR. Murine L1210 and P388 leukemias. In: Teicher B, ed. *Anticancer Drug Development Guide: Preclinical Screening, Clinical Trials and Approval.* Humana Press Inc., Totowa, NJ, 1998, pp. 59–74.
31. Schabel FM Jr, Griswold DP Jr, Laster WR Jr, Corbett TH, Lloyd HH. Quantitative evaluation of anti-cancer agent activity in experimental animals. *Pharmacol Ther* (A) 1977; 1:411–435.
32. Lloyd HH. Application of tumor models toward the design of treatment schedules for cancer chemotherapy. In: Drewinko B, Humphrey RM, eds. *Growth Kinetics and Biochemical Regulation of Normal and Malignant Cells.* Williams & Wilkins, Baltimore, MD, 1977, 455–469.
33. Corbett T, Valeriote F, LoRusso P, Polin L, Panchapor C, Pugh S, et al. In vivo methods for screening and preclinical testing. In: Teicher B, ed. *Anticancer Drug Development Guide: Preclinical Screening, Clinical Trials and Approval.* Humana Press Inc., Totowa, NJ, 1998, pp. 75–99.
34. Plowman J, Dykes DJ, Hollingshead M, Simpson-Herren L, Alley MC. Human tumor xenograft models in NCI drug development. In: Teicher B, ed. *Anticancer Drug Development Guide: Preclinical Screening, Clinical Trials and Approval.* Humana Press Inc., Totowa, NJ, 1998, pp. 101–125.
35. Teicher BA. Preclinical models for high-dose therapy. In: Teicher B, ed. *Anticancer Drug Development Guide: Preclinical Screening, Clinical Trials and Approval.* Humana Press Inc., Totowa, NJ, 1998, pp. 145–182.
36. Corbett TH, Valeriote FA. Rodent models in experimental chemotherapy. In: Kallman RF, ed. *The Use of Rodent Tumors in Experimental Cancer Therapy: Conclusions and Recommendations.* Pergamon, Press, New York, New York. 1987, 233–247.
37. Corbett TYH, Valeriote FA, Polin L, et al. Discovery of solid tumor active agents using a soft agar colony formation disk-diffusion assay. In: Valeriote FA, Corbett TH, Baker LH, eds. *Cytotoxic Anti-cancer Drugs: Models and Concepts for Drug Discovery and Development.* Kluwer Academic Publishers, Boston, MA, 1992, pp. 33–87.
38. Griswold DP, Jr., Schabel FM, Jr., Wilcox WS, Simpson-Herren L, Skipper HE. Success and failure in the treatment of solid tumors. I. Effects of cyclophosphamide (NSC-26271) on primary and metastatic plasmacytoma in the hamster. *Cancer Chemother* 1968, Rep 52:345–387.
39. Hermens AF, Barendsen GW. Changes of cell proliferation characteristics in a rat rhabdomyosarcoma before and after x-irradiation. *Eur J Cancer* 1969; 5:173–189.
40. Laster WR, Jr., et al. Success and failure in the treatment of solid tumors. II. Kinetic parameters and "cell cure" of moderately advanced carcinoma 755. *Cancer Chemother Rep* 1969; 53:169–188.
41. van Putten LM, Lelieveld P. Factors determining cell killing by chemotherapeutic agents in vivo. I. Cyclophosphamide. *Eur J Cancer* 1970; 6:313–321.
42. Teicher BA, Northey D, Yuan J, Frei E, III. High-dose therapy/stem cell support: Comparison of mice and humans. *Int J Cancer* 1996; 65:695–699.
43. Rockwell SC. Characteristics of a serially transplanted mouse mammary tumor and its tissue-culture-adapted derivative. *J Natl Cancer Inst* 1972; 49(3):735–749.

44. Teicher BA. Preclinical models for high dose therapy. In: Armitage JO, Antman KH, eds. *High-dose Cancer Therapy: Pharmacology, Hematopoietins, Stem Cells.* Williams and Wilkins, Baltimore, MD, 1992, pp. 14–42.

45. Teicher BA, Herman TS, Holden SA, Wang Y, Pfeffer MR, Crawford JM, et al. Tumor resistance to alkylating agents conferred by mechanisms operative only in vivo. *Science* 1990; 247:1457–1461.

46. Teicher BA, Holden SA, Cucchi CA, Cathcart KNS, Korbut TT, Flatow JL, et al. III. Combination of N,N′,N″-triethylenethiophosphoramide and cyclophosphamide in vitro and in vivo. *Cancer Res* 1988; 48:94–100.

47. Teicher BA, Holden SA, Eder JP, Brann TW, Jones SM, Frei E III. Preclinical studies relating to the use of thiotepa in the high-dose setting alone and in combination. *Semin Oncol* 1990; 17:18–32.

48. Teicher BA, Holden SA, Jones SM, Eder JP, Herman TS. Influence of scheduling on two-drug combinations of alkylating agents in vivo. *Cancer Chemother Pharmacol* 1989; 25:161–166.

49. Teicher BA, Waxman DJ, Holden SA, Wang Y, Clarke L, Alvarez Sotomayor E, et al. Evidence for enzymatic activation and oxygen involvement in cytotoxicity and antitumor activity of N,N′,N″-triethylenethiophosphoramide. *Cancer Res* 1989; 49:4996–5001.

50. Teicher BA, Herman TS, Holden SA, Eder JP. Chemotherapeutic potentiation through interaction at the level of DNA. In: Chou T-C, Rideout DC, eds. *Synergism and Antagonism in Chemotherapy.* Academic Press, Orlando, FL, 1991, pp. 541–583.

51. Teicher BA, Frei E III. Laboratory models to evaluate new agents for the systemic treatment of lung cancer. In: Skarin AT, ed. *Multimodality Treatment of Lung Cancer.* New York, Marcel Dekker, Inc., NY, 2000, pp. 301–336.

52. Steel GG, Peckham MJ. Exploitable mechanisms in combined radiotherapy-chemotherapy: the concept of additivity. *Int J Radiat Oncol Biol Phys* 1979; 5:85–91.

53. Berenbaum MC. Synergy, additivism and antagonism in immunosuppression. *Clin Exp Immunol* 1977; 28:1–18.

54. Dewey WC, Stone LE, Miller HH, Giblak RE. Radiosensitization with 5-bromodeoxyuridine of Chinese hamster cells x-irradiated during different phases of the cell cycle. *Radiat Res* 1977; 47:672–688.

55. Deen DF, Williams MW. Isobologram analysis of x-ray-BCNU interactions in vitro. *Radiat Res* 1979; 79:483–491.

56. Schabel FM, Trader MW, Laster WR, Wheeler GP, Witt MH. Patterns of resistance and therapeutic synergism among alkylating agents. *Antibiot Chemother* (Basel) 1978; 23:200–215.

57. Schabel FM, Griswold DP, Corbett TH, Laster Wr, Mayo JG, Lloyd HH. Testing therapeutic hypotheses in mice treated with anticancer drugs that have demonstrated or potential clinical utility for treatment of advanced solid tumors of man. *Methods Cancer Res* 1979; 17:3–51.

58. Schabel FM Jr. Concepts for systemic treatment of micrometastases. *Cancer* 1975; 35:15–24.

59. Schabel FM, Jr., Griswold DP, Jr., Corbett TH, Laster WR, Jr. Increasing the therapeutic response rates to anticancer drugs by applying the basic principles of pharmacology. *Cancer* 1984; 54:1160–1167.

60. Schabel FM Jr., Simpson-Herren L. Some variables in experimental tumor systems which complicate interpretation of data from in vivo kinetic and pharmacologic studies with anticancer drugs. *Antibiot Chemother* 1978; 23:113–127.

61. Schabel FM Jr., Griswold DP Jr., Corbett TH, Laster WR. Increasing therapeutic response rates to anticancer drugs by applying the basic principles of pharmacology. *Pharmacol Ther* 1983; 20:283–305.

62. Corbett TH, Griswold DP Jr., Roberts BJ, Peckham JC, Schabel FM, Jr. Evaluation of single agents and combinations of chemotherapeutic agents in mouse colon carcinomas. *Cancer* 1977; 40:2660–2680.

63. Corbett TH, Griswold DP, Jr., Wolpert MK, Venditti JM, Schabel, FM, Jr. Design and evaluation of combination chemotherapy trials in experimental animal tumor systems. *Cancer Treat Rep* 1979; 63:799–801.

64. Griswold DP Jr., Corbett TH, Schabel FM, Jr. Cell kinetics and the chemotherapy of murine solid tumors. *Antibiot Chemother* 1980; 28:28–34.

65. Griswold DP, Corbett TH, Schabel FM, Jr. Clonogenicity and growth of experimental tumors in relation to developing resistance and therapeutic failure. *Cancer Treat Rep* 1981; 65 (Suppl. 2):51–54.

66. Sugiura K, Stock C. Studies in a tumor spectrum. III. The effect of phosphoramides on the growth of a variety of mouse and rat tumors. *Cancer Res* 1955; 15:38–51.

67. Sugiura K, Stock C. Studies in a tumor spectrum. I. Comparison of the action of methylbis(2-chloroethyl)amine and 3-bis(2-chloroethyl) aqminomethyl-4-methoxymethyl-5-hydroxy-6-methyl-pyridine on the growth of a variety of mouse and rat tumors. *Cancer* 1952; 5:282–315.

68. Sugiura K, Stock C. Studies in a tumor spectrum. II. The effect of 2,4,6-triethyleneimino-s-triazine on the growth of a variety of mouse and rat tumors. *Cancer* 1952; 5:979–991.

69. DeWys W. A quantitative model for the study of the growth and treatment of a tumor and its metastases with correlation between proliferative state and sensitivity to cyclophosphamide. *Cancer Res* 1972; 32:367–373.

70. DeWys W. Studies correlating the growth rate of a tumor and its metastases and providing evidence for tumor-related systemic growth-retarding factors. *Cancer Res* 1972; 32:374–379.

71. Steel GG, Adams K. Stem-cell survival and tumor control in the Lewis lung carcinoma. *Cancer Res* 1975; 35:1530–1535.

72. Steel GG, Nill RP, Peckhyam MJ. Combined radiotherapy-chemotherapy of Lewis lung carcinoma. *Int J Radiat Oncol Biol Phys* 1978; 4:49–52.

73. Gemcitabine HCl (LY188011 HCl) clinical investigational brochure. Eli Lilly and Company, Indianapolis, IN, October 1993.

74. Huang P, Chubb S, Hertel L, Plunkett W. Mechanism of action of 2′,2′-difluorodeoxycytidine triphosphate on DNA synthesis (Abstr 2530). *Proc Am Assoc Cancer Res* 1990; 31:426.

75. Hertel L, Boder G, Kroin J. Evaluation of the antitumor activity of gemcitabine 2′,2′-difluoro-2′-deoxycytidine. *Cancer Res* 1990; 50:4417–4422.

76. Bouffard D, Fomparlwer L, Momparler R. Comparison of the antineoplastic activity of 2′,2′-difluorodeoxycytidine and cytosine arabinoside against human myeloid and lymphoid leukemia cells. *Anticancer Drugs* 1991; 2:49–55.

77. Heinemann V, Hertel L, Grindey G, Plunkett W. Comparison of the cellular pharmacokinetics and toxicity of 2′,2′-difluorodeoxycytidine and 1-beta-D-arabinofuranosyl cytosine. *Cancer Res* 1988; 48:4024–4031.

78. Eckhardt I, VonHoff D. New drugs in clinical development in the United States. *Hematol Oncol Clin N Amer* 1994; 8:300–332.

79. Anderson H, Lund B, Bach F. Single-agent activity of weekly gemcitabine in advanced non-small cell lung cancer: a Phase 2 study. *J Clin Oncol* 1994; 1821–1826.

80. Gatzemeier U, Shapard F, LeChevalier T, et al. Activity of gemcitabine in patients with non-small cell lung cancer: a multicentre, extended Phase II study. *Eur J Cancer* 1996; 32A:243–248.

81. Bertelli P, Mantica C, Farina G, Cobelli S, LaVerde N, Gramegna G, et al. Treatment of non-small cell lung cancer with vinorelbine. *Proc Am Soc Clin Oncol* 1994; 13:362.

82. Bore P, Rahmani R, VanCamfort J. Pharmacokinetics of a new anticancer drug, navelbine, in patients. *Cancer Chemother Pharmacol* 1989; 23:247–251.

83. Cros S, Wright M, Morimoto M. Experimental antitumor activity of navelbine. *Semin Oncol* 1989; 16(Suppl.):15–20.

84. Cvitkovic E. The current and future place of vinorelbine in cancer therapy. *Drugs* 1992; 44(Suppl. 4):36–45.

85. Marquet P, Lachatre G, Debord J. Pharmacokinetics of vinorelbine in man. *Eur J Clin Pharmacol* 1992; 42:545–547.

86. Navelbine (vinorelbine tartrate) clinical investigational brochure. Burroughs Wellcome Co., October 1995.

87. Fumoleau P, Delgado F, Delozier T, et al. Phase II trial of weekly intravenous vinorelbine in first line advanced breast cancer chemotherapy. *J Clin Oncol* 1993; 11:1245–1252.

88. Jehl F, Quoix E, Leveque D. Pharmacokinetics and preliminary metabolite fate of vinorelbine in human as determined by high performance liquid chromatography. *Cancer Res* 1991; 51:2073–2076.

89. Lepierre A, Lemarie E, Dabouis G, Garnier G. A Phase 2 study of navelbine in the treatment of non-small cell lung cancer. *Am J Clin Oncol* 1991; 14:115–119.

90. Shih C, Thornton DE. Preclinical pharmacology studies and the clinical development of a novel multi-targeted antifolate, MTA (LY231514). In: Jackman AL, ed. *Anticancer Drug Development Guide: Antifolate Drugs in Cancer Therapy*. Humana Press, Totowa, NJ, 1998, pp. 183–201.

91. Rinaldi DA, Burris HA, Dorr FA, et al. Initial Phase I evaluation of the novel thymidylate synthase inhibitor, LY231514, using the modified continual reassessment method for dose escalation. *J Clin Oncol* 1995; 13:2842–2850.

92. McDonald AC, Vasey PA, Adams L, et al. A phase I and pharmacokinetic study of LY231514, the multitargeted antifolate. *Clin Cancer Res* 1998; 4:605–610.

93. Takimoto CH. Antifolates in clinical development. *Semin Oncol* 1997; 24 (Suppl. 18):40–51.

94. Brandt DS, Chu E. Future challenges in the clinical development of thymidylate synthase inhibitor compounds. *Oncol Res* 1997; 9:403–410.

95. Teicher BA, Alvarez E, Liu P, Lu K, Menon K, Dempsey J, et al. MTA (LY231514) in combination treatment regimens using human tumor xenografts and the EMT6 murine mammary carcinoma. *Semin Oncol* 1999; 26 (Suppl.6):55–62.

96. Giovanella BC. Topoisomerase I inhibitors. In: Teicher BA, ed. *Cancer Therapeutics: Experimental and Clinical Agents.* Humana Press, Totowa, NJ, 1997, pp. 137–152.

97. Chabot GC. Clinical pharmacokinetics of irinotecan. *Clin Pharmacokinet* 1997; 33:245–259.

98. Aschele C, Baldo C, Sobrero AF, et al. Schedule-dependent synergism between ZD1694 (ralititrexed) and CPT-11 (irinotecan) in human colon cancer in vitro. *Clin Cancer Res* 1998; 4:1323–1330.

99. O'Reilly S, Rowinsky EC. The clinical status of irinotecan (CPT-11), a novel water soluble camptothecin analogue: *Crit Rev Oncol Hematol* 1996; 24:47–70.

32 Tumor-Cell Survival

Sara Rockwell, PhD

CONTENTS

INTRODUCTION
SELECTION OF TUMOR-HOST SYSTEMS
CELL-SURVIVAL ASSAYS
ANALYSIS OF CELL-SURVIVAL DATA
CONCLUSIONS
REFERENCES

1. INTRODUCTION

The development of assays for measuring the survival of individual tumor cells revolutionized the study of experimental cancer therapy by enabling researchers to move from assessing the gross responses of tumors to measuring the survival of cells in the critical, clonogenic tumor-cell populations *(1)*. The development and use of these assays formed the basis for many of our modern concepts of tumor biology, from the concept of logarithmic cell kill to considerations of cell-proliferation kinetics. The first major step in this revolution in cancer biology was made by Puck and Marcus, who developed a cell-culture assay for cloning individual HeLa cells, derived from a human carcinoma of the cervix, and then used this assay to determine the changes in cell survival in cultures given graded doses of radiation *(2,3)*. Assays for measuring the viability of cells suspended from tumors in vivo followed rapidly. The first cell-survival curve for tumors treated in vivo was obtained in 1959 Hewitt and Wilson, using a quantitative tumor transplantation assay (the TD50 assay) to measure the survival of cells harvested from leukemia infiltrates in the livers of mice after treatment with graded doses of radiation *(4)*. Over the next few years, Hewitt's TD50 assay was extended and used to study the quantitative transplantation and radiation responses of a wide variety of hematologic malignancies and solid tumors *(5,6)*. The techniques were also refined and extended to produce true clonogenic assays for tumor-cell survival, in which the clonogenicity of individual tumor cells was tested by preparing tumor-cell suspensions, counting the tumor cells, and determining the ability of individual tumor cells to proliferate to form macroscopic clones *(6)*. For some tumors, this can be done by injecting known numbers of tumor cells intravenously into recipient mice, allowing the cells to lodge in the spleen *(7)* or the lung *(8)*, waiting for the individual cells to grow into macroscopic tumors, and counting the number of tumors. In a few tumor systems, the

From: *Tumor Models in Cancer Research*
Edited by: B. A. Teicher © Humana Press Inc., Totowa, NJ

suspended cells can be plated at low densities in cell culture, so that individual tumor cells will grow into macroscopic colonies, allowing the measurement of cell survival by colony-formation assays analogous developed by Puck and Marcus *(9,10)*. The final step in this revolution in cancer biology came in 1961, when Till and McCulloch *(11)* described their spleen-colony assay for measuring the survival of bone-marrow stem cells. Clonogenic assays for other normal cell populations followed *(12)*, allowing the toxicities of antineoplastic agents to be evaluated in terms of the responses of the critical clonogenic stem-cell populations within the dose-limiting normal tissues.

The conceptual basis of all these cell-survival assays is simple: the cell population of interest is harvested, and the individual cells are isolated and tested for their ability to proliferate indefinitely. In practice, however, the process of making this measurement is fraught with problems and potential artifacts. The techniques used in these measurements, and their problems and limitations, are the subject of this chapter.

2. SELECTION OF TUMOR-HOST SYSTEMS

As in all studies with experimental rodent tumors, the tumor-host system used with cell-survival assays must be chosen with care, to ensure that it provides an appropriate model for the proposed studies *(1,5,6,10,13,14)*. Because the assays require quantitative comparisons of cells suspended from treated and control tumors, they require the use of matched tumors grown in carefully matched recipients. For most rodent systems, the ideal host is the inbred strain and subline in which the tumor originated *(5,14)*, so that immunologic incompatibilities between tumor and host are minimized. It can sometimes be difficult, or even impossible, to find truly syngeneic hosts for a particular tumor line. Some commonly used tumor lines arose in non-inbred lines or in mouse substrains which have been lost *(5,6,15,16)*. Some of the common, commercially available mouse strains (e.g., Balb/c, C57/BL, and C3H) have been maintained in various places as genetically separate breeding stock for several decades, and the resultant sublines have diverged over dozens or hundreds of generations to have markedly different phenotypes *(15,16)*. This is an even more serious problem for the investigator who wishes to use tumors originating in genetically altered mice or who wishes to study tumors transplanted into genetically manipulated hosts, as many transgenic and knockout mouse lines are only partially inbred. Although these lines are well-defined at the loci of interest, they may have other genetic differences that influence the behavior of implanted tumors. For investigators studying human tumors xenografted into immune-deficient rodents *(17–19)*, the choice of host can also be difficult. It must first be remembered that xenografts of established human tumor-cell lines in mice are inevitably imperfect models for the primary human cancers from which the cells were isolated. The tumor cells have been heavily selected for their ability to grow rapidly in vitro or in mice, and their patterns of differentiation and proliferation are very different from those in the original tumor. The different drug pharmacokinetics in mice and humans will also produce differences in tumor responses. Moreover, the stromal cells and vasculature within the tumors originate from the mice, and those tumor responses that reflect the interactions of tumor cells with the host may therefore reflect the characteristics of the murine host, rather than those of the human tumor cells. This may raise special problems when human tumors are treated in SCID mice, because the DNA-repair-deficient phenotype of the SCIDs leads to unusual radiation and drug sensitivity in the host and tumor bed *(19)*. The athymic *nu/nu* (nude) mutation exists in a number of genetic backgrounds, and the available nude strains can be quite different. The presence of genetic heterogeneity in the hosts within or between experiments can result in experimental variability that can compromise the validity and precision of the experiments. This problem is even more serious for assays such as the lung-colony and spleen-colony assays, which use recipient mice as hosts for the analysis of tumor-cell survival.

Other sources of host variability should also be considered *(13,20)*. Sex and age may be important. The use of immature animals (less than 2.5 mo) can be problematic. The rapid growth and changing physiology of these young animals can result in large experimental variations from small differences in age. Rapidly growing tumors also produce stress and disease in small, fast-growing animals more quickly than in adult animals. Because many vendors ship very young mice, the investigator must balance the costs and problems of holding mice to maturity before use with the benefits of the more stable model system that results from this practice. Stress resulting from shipping, recaging, environmental problems, or experimental manipulations can also introduce experimental variability, and should be avoided or considered in the experimental design *(13,20)*.

The health and microbiological status of the animals are also major considerations. Active and prior infections with many bacteria, viruses, and parasites have been shown to alter tumor transplantation, tumor growth, and tumor responses to therapy *(13,20)*. Moreover, many common murine viruses and some bacteria have been found to infect tumor tissue and tumor cells, and can be passaged with the tumor cells in vitro or in vivo. Even subclinical or "nonpathogenic" infections can have effects of considerable experimental significance. Some murine viruses, such as Minute Virus of Mice or Killam's Rat Virus, replicate in and selectively kill proliferating cells in vivo and in culture, thereby altering the proliferative patterns of tumor cells, changing their response to cycle-active therapy, and compromising cell-survival assays. Tumor-cell lines infected with human or murine pathogens have been implicated as a source of active infection in mice inoculated with the tumors, and in some cases have been a source of infections that have spread through animal colonies—and have resulted in illness among people in proximity to the colonies *(13,21)*. Murine or human viruses carried by human tumor-cell lines can also compromise the use of the tumors in experimental cancer-therapy studies, and offer even greater risks of illness in the immune-deficient hosts and for investigators.

Another factor that influences the choice of model system for tumor-cell survival studies is the question of whether a human tumor xenograft or a syngeneic animal tumor offers a better model system *(6,19)*. For example, human tumor cells are sometimes critical in studies of species-specific cytokines, antibodies, or gene-therapy approaches. In other studies, it may be more important that the tumor and host are syngeneic, so that immunological incompatibilities or cross-species differences in signaling pathways are avoided. In this case, a murine system will be the better model.

3. CELL-SURVIVAL ASSAYS

3.1. Implications of Clonogenic Cell Survival

Clonogenic assays measure the ability of individual cells to proliferate indefinitely, forming colonies of hundreds or thousands of cells. In tumors, this is the critical measure of cell viability: only a clonogenic cell has the ability to cause a recurrence or to create a metastasis. A cell that is intact and metabolically active but incapable of proliferation is unimportant in cancer therapy, because it will not contribute to the growth, recurrence, or metastasis of the malignancy. Conversely, there are resting, clonogenic cells within tumors, which are not proliferating at the time of assay, but which can be called back into indefinite proliferation to cause growth, recurrence, or metastases *(14,22–24)*. These resting, clonogenic cells must be forced into proliferation during the clonogenic assay. Clonogenic assays differ fundamentally from assays that follow tumor growth, that examine cellular integrity (e.g., by Trypan blue exclusion), or that measure cell proliferation directly (by changes in cell number or by BUdR or 3HTdR incorporation) or indirectly (by measures of protein content or metabolism). The latter assays consider all of the cells in the tumor (clonogenic and nonclonogenic, alive, dying, and sometimes dead), and therefore offer only indirect, and sometimes misleading, measures of the responses of the critical clonogenic cell populations in treated tumors *(14,25)*.

3.2. Measuring Clonogenicity

In a clonogenic assay, individual tumor cells are isolated and tested for their ability to proliferate indefinitely. This can be done in several ways. Some tumor cells that have been selected for or adapted to growth in cell culture will form colonies when plated at low densities in vitro *(6,9,10)*. Cell-culture assays can be used to assay the clonogenicity of cells suspended from these tumors. When cells from some hematologic malignancies are injected intravenously, the cells lodge in the spleen and the clonogenic cells grow to form small tumors *(7)*. Similarly, cells of many solid tumors lodge in the lung when injected intravenously, and the clonogenic cells form "lung colonies" *(8)*. In vitro colonies, spleen colonies, and lung colonies are the most common assays for clonogenic cell survival. In the end point dilution technique originally developed by Hewitt and Wilson *(4)*, graded doses of tumor cells are injected into animals, and the pattern of tumor development is used to calculate the TD50, or the number of cells needed to produce tumors in 50% of the sites injected. Although the TD50 technique is in some ways the most physiologic test of the clonogenicity of cells from solid tumors, it also suffers from the limitation of requiring that very large numbers of recipient animals be followed for several months for tumor development *(4,5,14)*.

3.2.1. IDENTIFYING CLONOGENIC CELLS

A primary requirement of a clonogenic assay is that it must distinguish clonogenic cells (cells with a capacity for prolonged or unlimited proliferation) from cells that can undergo only one or a few divisions. This is critical when the assay is used to study the effects of radiation or drugs that damage DNA and produce mitotic death. Cells killed by these agents will continue to proliferate after treatment, with cell-proliferation patterns that are at first indistinguishable from those of the cells that will survive; eventually all of the cells in these "abortive clones" will cease proliferation, die, and lyse. However, up to five cell divisions may occur before this happens *(26,27)*. The lower threshold for colony size must therefore be set high enough that abortive clones are not counted among the surviving cells, even when the dying cells undergo abortive mitoses and become multinucleate "giant cells." This is not a problem with the in vivo assays, which count tumors containing millions of cells, but can be a problem in some cell-culture systems. A threshold size of 50 cells is often used for colonies in cell-culture

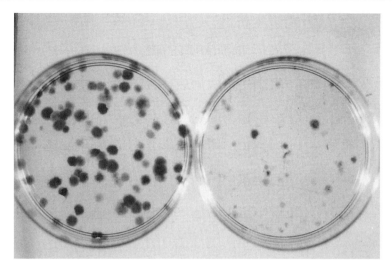

Fig. 1. Petri dishes from an experiment determining a dose-response curve for EMT6 cells treated with radiation. Left: control plate, 150 cells plated. Right: heavily irradiated cells (10 Gy); 10,000 cells plated.

assays, because it has been found to distinguish between cells surviving and dying from low doses of X-rays *(28)*. The assay must consider the fact that treatments with many cytotoxic or cytostatic agents will injure the surviving cells and cause them to proliferate more slowly than usual *(26–30)*. Colonies developing from heavily treated tumors therefore grow more slowly than control colonies *(30)*, and the incubation time and colony size threshold must be chosen to allow detection of all of the slowly growing clonogens in the treated cultures (*see* Fig. 1).

The requirements described here create some stringent requirements for cell-culture systems that are used to measure clonogenic cell survival. Additional requirements are imposed by the fact that it is important to detect all of the clonogens, so that quiescent clonogens or slowly growing clonogens are not overlooked. Considerable work may be needed to optimize the cell-culture system so that the viability of cells suspended from control and treated tumors can be assayed reproducibly and reliably.

3.2.2. Motion Artifacts

For colonies developing on the surface of Petri dishes, covered by liquid medium, it is critical that the system be optimized so that the cultures can sit undisturbed for the full duration of the colony-formation assay. As cells in these cultures enter mitosis, they become round and nearly detach from the Petri dish (Fig. 2); the daughter cells do not reattach firmly to the surface of the dish until they are well into G1 *(29)*. If the dishes are moved or the medium is changed during the incubation, mitotic cells will become dislodged from the growth surface and settle elsewhere on the dish, producing smaller "satellite" colonies. The presence of these extraneous colonies can completely invalidate the clonogenic assay.

3.2.3. Cell-Density Problems

The requirements of the cloning assay system become increasingly severe as the intensity of the treatments being tested increases. In many rapidly growing transplanted

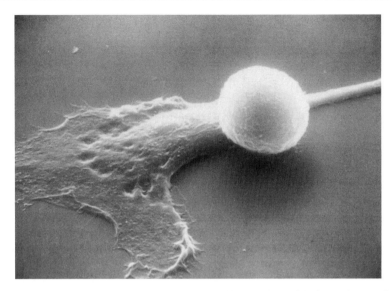

Fig. 2. Scanning electron microscope photo of an EMT6 cell culture. The interphase cells in the culture are spread out on and firmly attached to the growth surface. A mitotic cell is also shown; note that this mitosis is rounded and only loosely attached. Moving the cultures during incubation for clonogenic assays results in the release of mitotic cells from the surface of the culture dish; these cells will settle on other areas of the surface, initiating "satellite colonies" that compromise the validity of the clonogenic assay.

mouse tumor lines, a high proportion of cells are clonogenic *(4,5,8–10,23,24,31,32)*. In the EMT6 system, for example, the plating efficiency of cells explanted from solid tumors is generally about 35%: 35 colonies will form for every 100 cells plated *(10)*. When untreated EMT6 cells are plated into a 60-mm Petri dish for colony formation, only 250 cells are needed to produce approx 100 colonies in the dish. However, if one wishes to assay the survival of cells from tumors treated with a large dose of radiation that reduces the survival of the cells by four logs (producing a surviving fraction of 10^{-4}), it would be necessary to plate 2.5 million cells in the dish to obtain 100 colonies. Some tumors contain only small numbers of clonogenic stem cells (as low as one in 1,000 or even one in 100,000 cells) *(24)*. It may be difficult, or even impossible, to develop reliable clonogenic assays for some of these tumors.

It has been consistently found that the ability of cells to survive, proliferate, and form colonies in vitro varies with the number of cells in the culture. At very high cell densities, the cells will rapidly deplete the medium; as a result, cell proliferation in the cultures will cease. All colony-formation assays must be done below this density. For this reason, it is critical that all measurements of cell survival be based on actual colony formation. Estimates of cell survival which are calculated from the fact that, for example, no colonies were formed when 10^7 cells were plated may only mean that the cell density was high enough to preclude cell growth in the cultures. Other technical problems, such as contamination of the suspension with bacteria or other microorganisms, can also prevent colony formation. At very low densities, especially in suboptimal media, some cell types are unable to proliferate to form colonies. Conditioned media or the use of radiation-sterilized feeder layers can be used to improve the plating efficiency in such cases *(2,10,28,31)*. However, when this occurs, great care must be taken to ensure that similar numbers of cells (feeder layer cells plus experimental cells) are plated in *all* groups, to ensure the linearity of the assay.

3.2.4. COLONY-DENSITY PROBLEMS

The linearity of the assay system also varies with the number of colonies forming in the dish—too many live cells may result in a confluent monolayer of cells, in which individual colonies cannot be distinguished. At slightly lower cell numbers, colonies may be visible, but these colonies will overlap and will be difficult to distinguish. They may also be small, because medium exhaustion near the end of the incubation has inhibited their growth. These problems will result in an underestimate of clonogenic cells. Each clonogenic assay system must be tested to establish the range of colony numbers over which colony number increases linearly with the number of cells plated. Colony numbers in this range should always be used to analyze cell survival. In practical terms, this means that in many experiments, several different dilutions of a cell suspension may need to be plated, so that a group with colony numbers lying within the linear range of the assay can be used in the analysis.

3.2.5. COUNTING THE COLONIES

At the end of the incubation period, the colonies are counted. This process is simplified if the colonies can be fixed and stained to allow the colonies to be visualized more readily. Magnifying the culture so that the individual cells in the colonies are visible can also be valuable, especially in heavily treated cultures. This allows the counter to assess whether a small colony contains 50 or more cells, and to distinguish true colonies from abortive clones containing a small number of giant cells, and from clumps of debris. Size alone may not be sufficient to distinguish true colonies from debris and abortive clones; in such cases, automated image analysis systems may prove problematic. It is also important to remember that the progeny of untreated cells may grow more rapidly than the progeny of heavily treated cells *(28,30)*. As a result, colonies in heavily treated cultures may be smaller and more poorly defined than colonies in untreated control cultures (Fig. 1). Because some subjectivity is inherent in the enumeration of colonies, it is important that all the colonies within an experiment be counted by a single, objective observer, preferably one blinded to the treatments received by the cells in the different Petri dishes.

3.3. Tumor-Cell Suspensions

3.3.1. PREPARING THE SUSPENSION

Preparation of single-cell suspensions is a critical step in the process of performing a clonogenic assay. This process may be as simple as harvesting the fluid containing the tumor cells, in the case of blood-borne leukemias or ascites tumors growing as single cells in the peritoneal cavity. However, preparing a high-quality single-cell suspension may prove very challenging for tumors in which the malignant cells are growing in solid tumors supported by a rich stromal bed. In this case, it is usually necessary to use a combination of mechanical disruption and enzymatic treatment to release the cells from the surrounding matrix *(5,6,10,33–37)*.

In the process used for EMT6 tumors *(10)*, the tumor is removed from the host, using careful sterile techniques to ensure the sterility of the tissue being removed, and

placed in a watch glass with a few drops of a calcium- and magnesium-free Hanks'
Balanced Salt Solution (HBSS), containing 0.2% trypsin. The tissue is then minced
into a fine brei. In our laboratory, this is done by mincing the tissue with a small pair of
curved surgical scissors; it can also be done by chopping the tumor with a single-edged
razor blade. We then place the brie in a fluted trypsinizing flask with 100 mL of the
trypsin solution, at 37°C, and incubate the mixture for 15 min, using a magnetic stir-
ring apparatus to provide continuous gentle agitation. We then filter the mixture, to
remove any intact chunks of tumor tissue, and collect the cells by centrifugation, which
is performed at 4°C to halt the action of the trypsin. There are many possible variations
to this procedure (7–10,31–37), and considerable experimentation may be necessary to
optimize the procedure to the specific tumor used. Various concentrations of trypsin,
other proleolytic enzymes (such as protease or collagenase), or enzyme cocktails have
proven optimal in different systems. Some investigators add ethelenediamine
tetraacetic acid (EDTA) to the enzyme cocktail. The duration of the enzymatic treatment may need to be shorter or longer. Some fragile cell lines require that the action of
the proteolytic enzyme be stopped completely by the addition of inhibitors or serum at
the end of a brief incubation.

The intensity of the suspension procedure reflects an important balance (34,36,37).
It is important to prepare a suspension containing a large population of tumor cells,
which is representative of the total tumor-cell population. An inadequately intensive
procedure will result in low cell yield. On the other hand, both the mincing and enzymatic treatment will kill tumor cells, and too intensive a treatment will decrease the
number and viability of cells in the suspension. Because cells in and near necrotic areas
may be more readily released, an inadequate suspension protocol may result in suspensions enriched in cells from these populations. Conversely, an overly aggressive protocol may kill the cells suspended early in the process, resulting in a suspension which
contains large numbers of dead cells, and which may be enriched in cells from the most
fibrous regions of the tumor.

3.3.2. COUNTING THE CELLS

The quality of the tumor-cell suspension is evaluated during the counting process. In
my laboratory, an aliquot of the suspension is counted, using a hemacytometer, under
phase-contrast microscopy. Trypan blue is used to identify those cells that have lost
their ability to exclude this vital dye and are in the process of dying. Phase-contrast is
used because the edge effects of this imaging approach aid in identifying stained cells,
and also aid in distinguishing tumor cells from blood cells, macrophages, and stromal
cells, which inevitably contaminate tumor-cell suspensions. In some tumors,
macrophages comprise the majority of the cells in the tumor-cell suspension (37). As
these other cells are irrelevant to the clonogenic assay of tumor-cell survival, it is critical that the cell count be based only on counts of the tumor cells. Trypan blue-stained
and Trypan blue-excluding tumor cells should be counted separately, so that the quality
of the suspension can be assessed. In our hands, Trypan blue-stained cells generally
comprise fewer than 10% of the suspended tumor cells: a number higher than this is
considered to indicate a potential problem with the preparation of the cell suspension.
Although we routinely use a Coulter Counter to count cells in our cell culture and
hematology experiments, we do not use this instrument to count primary tumor-cell
suspensions, because it does not adequately distinguish our tumor cells from

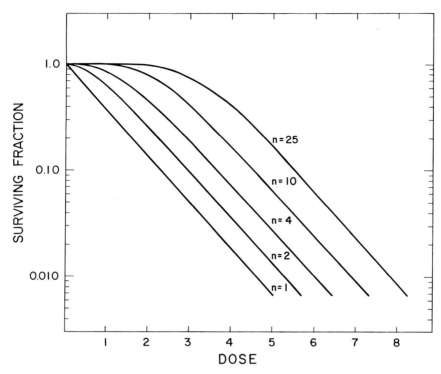

Fig. 3. Effect of multiplicity on survival curves. The linear survival curve is a model survival curve for a hypothetical cell population, assayed as single cells. The survival curves marked $n=2$, $n=4$, $n=10$, and $n=25$ show the theoretical survival curves that would be measured if these cells were assayed in clusters containing 2, 4, 10, or 25 cells, respectively. Reprinted from ref. *39.*

macrophages and other stromal cells, and does not provide the quality control inherent in the analysis of Trypan blue staining.

3.3.3. THE IMPORTANCE OF SINGLE-CELL SUSPENSIONS

The tumor-cell suspension must also be examined visually and microscopically for the presence of multi-cell clumps. The rigorous use of a clonogenic assay depends on the fact that the suspension plated for analysis contains only single cells *(39,40)*. Small bits of tissue or clumps of cells containing two or more viable tumor cells will, of course, form colonies. However, their response to treatment will be different than that of single cells, because it will be necessary to kill every cell in the clump to prevent this clump from growing into a colony *(28,39,40)*. Clumps will therefore be dramatically more resistant to treatment with drugs and radiation than single cells would be. If the "single-cell suspensions" prepared from tumors are contaminated with multicellular aggregates, the dose-response curves measured using the suspensions will erroneously suggest marked resistance, especially after intensive treatments (Figs. 3,4).

3.4. Scheduling Problems in Clonogenic Assays

One of the major problems in designing experiments using clonogenic assays is the question of when the assay should be performed *(37,41)*. The radiobiologists who developed the clonogenic assays had a great advantage in this respect, because the time

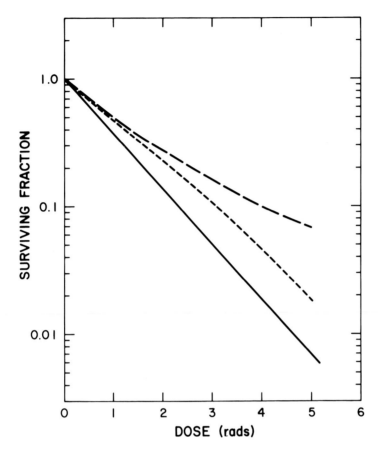

Fig. 4. Effect of small numbers of clusters and clumps on a survival curve. The solid line represents the single-cell survival curve replotted from Fig. 3. Long dashes: theoretical survival curves for a suspension composed of 75% single cells, 5% each of clusters containing 2, 4, 10, or 25 cells, and 5% clumps which are large enough to be counted as colonies. Short dashes: curve obtained if all large clumps are excluded from the colony count with complete accuracy. Although the majority of the colonies in the untreated cultures arise from single cells, the survival curve at high doses is dominated by the colonies arising from multicell clumps and clusters. Reprinted from ref. *39*.

at which a treatment with X-rays is completed can be defined with certainty as the time the X-ray machine turned off, allowing the assay to be performed, unambiguously, "immediately after treatment." When clonogenic assays are used to measure the effect of drugs administered to animals, the "end" of the treatment is more poorly defined. The end of the injection of the drug is clearly not the end of treatment. Rather, the duration of the treatment will be determined by the kinetics of the distribution of the drug and the pharmacokinetics of the drug and its active metabolites. For some drugs, the lifetime of the active species is short, and treatment will effectively end minutes after administration of the drug. In other cases, however, cytotoxic species may be present for hours or days, and cells would continue to be killed throughout this period. The decision of when to perform the clonogenic assay is therefore a significant one.

Complicating this decision is the fact that many different processes occurring in the treated tumors may impact the measurement of tumor-cell survival. Cells may repair potentially lethal damage after treatment with radiation or drugs, and cell survival will increase as a result of the repair if the time of assay is delayed for some hours after treatment *(42)*. Cells will also proliferate after treatment. If the proliferation patterns of the surviving and dying cells are different, the surviving fractions measured by clonogenic assays may be inaccurate if treatment is delayed long enough to allow significant proliferation (24 h or more). Cell death may also complicate measurements of cell survival. For radiation and radiomimetic drugs, the major mechanism of cell death is generally mitotic death, which may occur days after treatment *(26,27)*. However, in some tumors, apoptosis may be a major cause of death even for these treatments, and the death and cell lysis occurring with this mode of death take place soon after treatment and may complicate cell-survival assays *(43)*. Similarly, it may be difficult to measure the cytotoxicity produced by agents such as hyperthermia or certain drugs that kill cells by rapid pathways involving membrane injury and lysis. With such agents, the dying tumor cells may lyse and disappear from the tumor during or soon after treatment, and the cell suspensions prepared from the tumors would appear to have high surviving fractions unless careful analyses of the yields had been performed to detect the fact that cells had died and disappeared before the suspension was counted *(44)*.

Analyses of the yields of cells from treated and control tumors can help to identify and correct for changes in the number of tumor cells after treatment. However, these analyses also raise experimental problems *(44)*. First, they depend absolutely on the assumption that the treated and control tumors are the same size, and contain the same number of cells, at the time of treatment. Therefore, they require the use of very carefully matched tumors throughout the experiments. Second, the cell yield can vary dramatically with small variations in the suspension procedure, and cell-yield measurements are quite variable relative to surviving fraction measurements. Moreover, these analyses will not completely identify and account for the various processes occurring in the treated tumors, and therefore cannot completely correct surviving fractions made several hours or days after treatment.

These problems indicate significant limitations in the use of clonogenic assays for the measurement of cell survival after treatments with agents that produce rapid cell death, or after prolonged or fractionated treatment regimens that continue over several days. In such cases, tumor growth or tumor-cure assays may be preferable.

4. ANALYSIS OF CELL-SURVIVAL DATA

Many articles and books have been written on the analysis of data from clonogenic assays and on the analysis and interpretation of the resulting dose-response curves *(28,45,46)*. Much of this discussion is beyond the scope of this chapter, but a few important points of experimental design and analyses should be mentioned. The first is the importance of including appropriate untreated controls in each experiment. In most tumors, many of the cells are inherently not clonogenic. As a result, the "plating efficiency" or "cloning efficiency" (colonies/100 cells plated) is generally well below 100%. The plating efficiency may also vary from experiment to experiment, because of differences in techniques, sera, reagents, etc. The cloning efficiencies of cells from treated tumors therefore should always be analyzed by using the plating efficiencies of cells from control tumors assayed on the same day to calculate the surviving fractions. In cases in which the treatment protocol, as well as the treatment agent, may be stress-

Table 1
Artifact Resulting from the Use of Arithmetic Means to Analyze Ratios*

Experiment	1	2	3	4	5	6	Mean
Colonies/100 cells, control	100	100	100	50	50	50	75
Colonies/100 cells, treated	50	50	50	100	100	100	75
Surviving Fraction	0.5	0.5	0.5	2.0	2.0	2.0	1.0[a]
							1.0[b]
							1.25[c]

* The mean cloning efficiencies for the control cells and treated cells are identical. Calculating the mean of the surviving fractions using arithmetic formulations leads to the erroneous conclusion that the viability of the treated cultures in these experiments was greater than that of control cultures. This error is seen with remarkable frequency in the literature.

[a] calculated from the means of the cloning efficiencies

[b] geometric mean

[c] arithmetic mean

ful or toxic or may have physiologic effects that could alter the viability of the tumor cells, it is also wise to include sham-treated or vehicle-treated controls in the experimental matrix.

Another common problem is the inclusion of "surviving fractions" estimated from plates in which no colonies have developed. As described above, there are numerous experimental problems and artifacts that can prevent colony formation, even when clonogenic cells have been plated. All analyses therefore should be based on actual colony counts, from dishes that have colonies.

Some common errors occur in the analysis of cell-survival data. One lies in the calculation of error limits. All too frequently, investigators assume that standard errors can be calculated by using the counts in the 3–4 replicate Petri dishes plated from one cell suspension. In fact, these dishes do not represent independent observations: the only source of variability in the dishes is the ability of the investigator to plate equal quantities of cells into each dish. Variabilities resulting from heterogeneity in tumors, heterogeneity in treatments, or differences in the preparation of the cell suspension or in the counting process are not considered. Error limits should therefore be based on independent observations of the surviving fractions, preferably made in independent experiments.

Another common problem is the question of whether arithmetic means or geometric means are the appropriate metric to use with cell-survival data. Surviving fractions are ratios, and geometric means are the appropriate means for use with ratios (47). The use of arithmetic means with ratios leads to an analytic artifact frequently seen in the analysis of survival data after relatively nontoxic or ineffective treatments: the calculated mean surviving fractions will artifactually be greater than 1.0 (i.e., greater than the control value). An example of this is provided in Table 1. Moreover, in many experimental therapeutic studies, the surviving fraction varies exponentially with the intensity of treatment. In such cases, the individual surviving fractions determined in replicate experiments are generally log-normally distributed, and the geometric means are again the appropriate metric in such cases.

As described here, clonogenic assays are often used to determine dose-response curves that span surviving fractions extending over two or more orders of magnitude. In such cases, the data should be graphed using logarithmic axes to display the surviving fractions, so that the full range of the dose-response relationship can be visualized. Linear plots and linear analyses do not allow adequate display and consideration of surviving fractions lower than 10–20%.

CONCLUSIONS

The use of clonogenic assays that measure the ability of individual cells to undergo indefinite proliferation produced a revolution in experimental cancer therapy, beginning in the 1950s *(1)*. This revolution began with the demonstration that a single viable cancer cell was sufficient to cause a tumor, a metastasis, or a recurrence *(4)*, a concept that underlies current cancer therapy. The similarity of the dose-response curves for cells in culture, tumor cells in vivo, and clonogenic cells from normal tissues in vivo demonstrated the utility of in vitro studies in the evaluation of anticancer modalities. Since that time, cell-survival assays have been used widely and effectively to study the effects of antineoplastic therapies on tumors and normal tissues, and to examine their efficacies, toxicities, and therapeutic ratios in animal model systems. Cell-survival assays have proved to be invaluable in the development of improved anticancer therapies. The process of performing rigorous, reproducible studies of the survival of cells from solid tumors in vivo is more complicated than it might at first appear. Careful consideration must be given to a variety of technical factors and to many areas of the experimental design when cell-survival assays are used to study the effects of radiation, drugs, or other antineoplastic agents.

REFERENCES

1. Rockwell S. Experimental radiotherapy: a brief history. *Radiat Res* 1998; 150:S157–S169.
2. Puck TT, Marcus PI. A rapid method for viable cell titration and clone production with HeLa cells in tissue culture: the use of x-irradiated cells to supply conditioning factors. *Proc Natl Acad Sci USA* 1955; 41:432–437.
3. Puck TT, Marcus PI. Action of X rays on mammalian cells. *J Exp Med* 1956; 103:653–666.
4. Hewitt HB, Wilson CW. A survival curve for mammalian cells irradiated *in vivo*. *Nature* 1959; 183:1060–1061.
5. Hewitt HB. The choice of animal tumors for experimental studies of cancer therapy. *Adv Cancer Res* 1978; 27:149–200.
6. Kallman RF, ed. *Rodent Tumor Models in Experimental Cancer Therapy*. Pergamon Press, New York, NY, 1987.
7. Bruce WR, Meeker BE, Valeriote FA. Comparison of the sensitivity of normal hematopoietic and transplanted lymphoma colony-forming cells to chemotherapeutic agents administered *in vivo*. *J Natl Cancer Inst* 1966; 37:233–245.
8. Hill RP, Bush RS. A lung colony assay to determine the radiosensitivity of cells of a solid tumour. *Int J Radiat Biol* 1969; 15:435–444.
9. Barendsen GW, Broerse JJ. Experimental radiotherapy of a rat rhabdomyosarcoma with 15 MeV neutrons and 300 kV x-rays. Effects of single exposures. *Eur J Cancer* 1969; 5:373–391.
10. Rockwell S. *In vivo-in vitro* tumor systems: new models for studying the response of tumors to therapy. *Lab Anim Sci* 1977; 27:831–851.
11. Till JE, McCulloch EA. A direct measurement of the radiation sensitivity of normal mouse bone marrow cells. *Radiat Res* 1961; 14:213–222.
12. Hendry JH, Potten CS, Moore JV, Hune WJ, eds. *Assays of normal tissue injury, and their cellular interpretations. Br J Cancer* 1986; 53:Suppl. VII.

13. Rockwell S. Maintenance of tumor systems and appropriate treatment techniques for experimental tumors. In: Kallman RF, ed. *Rodent Tumors in Experimental Cancer Therapy* Pergamon Press, New York, NY, 1987; pp. 29–36.

14. Kallman RF, Rockwell S. Effects of radiation on animal tumor models. In: Becker FF, ed. *Cancer: A Comprehensive Treatise,* Vol. 6. Plenum Publishing, New York, NY, 1977, pp. 225–279.

15. Keeler CE. *The Laboratory Mouse. Its Origin, Heredity, and Culture.* Harvard University Press, Cambridge, MA, 1931.

16. Foster HL, Small JD, Fox JG, eds. *The Mouse in Biomedical Research. IV. Experimental Biology and Oncology.* Academic Press, New York, NY, 1982.

17. Steel GG, Courtenay VD, Peckham MJ. The response to chemotherapy of a variety of human tumor xenografts. *Br J Cancer* 1983; 47:1–13.

18. Rofstad EK. Human tumor xenografts in radiotherapeutic research. *Radiother Oncol* 1985; 3:35–46.

19. Taghian AG, Suit HD. Animal systems for translational research in radiation oncology. *Acta Oncologica* 1999; 38:829–838.

20. Pakes SP, Lu YS, Meunier PC. Factors that complicate animal research. In: Fox JG, Cohen BJ, Loew FM, eds. *Laboratory Animal Medicine* Academic Press, Orlando, FL, 1984, pp. 649–666.

21. Hotchin J, Sikora E, Kinch W, Hinman A, Woodall. Lymphocytic choriomeningitis in a hamster colony causes infection of hospital personnel. *Science* 1974; 185:1173–1174.

22. Mendelsohn ML. The growth fraction: a new concept applied to tumors. *Science* 1960; 132:1496.

23. Barendsen GW, Roelse H, Hermens AF, Madhuizen HT, Van Peperzeel HA, Rutgers DH. Clonogenic capacity of proliferating and non-proliferating cells of a transplantable rat rhabdomyosarcoma in relation to its radiosensitivity. *J Natl Cancer Inst* 1973; 51:1521–1526.

24. Steel GG. *Growth Kinetics of Tumours.* Clarendon Press, Oxford. 1977.

25. Moulder JE, Rockwell S. Comparison of tumor assay methods. In: Kallman RF. ed. *Rodent Tumor Models in Experimental Cancer Therapy.* Plenum Press, New York, NY, 1987, pp. 272–278.

26. Elkind MM, Han A, Volz KW. Radiation response of mammalian cells grown in culture. IV. Dose dependence of division delay and post-irradiation growth of surviving and non-surviving Chinese hamster cells. *J Natl Cancer Inst* 1963; 30:705–721.

27. Hurwitz C, Tolmach LJ. Time-lapse cinemicrographic studies of HeLa S3 cells. *Biophys J* 1969; 9:607–633.

28. Elkind MM, Whitmore GF. *The Radiobiology of Cultured Mammalian Cells.* Gordon and Breach, New York, NY, 1967.

29. Terasima T, Tolmach LJ. Variations in several responses of HeLa cells to x-irradiation during the division cycle. *Biophys J* 1963; 3:11–33.

30. Kallman RF. The growth kinetics of clonogenic tumor cells that survive radiation therapy. In: *Effects of Therapy on Biology and Kinetics of the Residual Tumor. Part B: Clinical Aspects,* Wiley Liss Inc, New York, NY, 1990, pp. 55–65.

31. Martin DF, Rockwell S, Fischer JJ. Development of an *in vitro* assay for the survival of cells suspended from BA1112 rat sarcomas. *Eur J Cancer Clin Oncol* 1983; 19:791–797.

32. Rosenblum ML, Knebel KD, Wheeler KT, Barker M, Wilson CB. Development of an *in vitro* assay for the evaluation of *in vivo* chemotherapy of a rat brain tumor. *In Vitro* 1975; 11:264–273.

33. Waymouth C. Obtaining cell suspensions from animal tissues. In: Pretlow TG, Pretlow TP, eds. *Cell Separation: Methods and Selected Applications,* Vol. I Academic Press, New York, NY, 1982, pp. 1–29.

34. Rasey JS, Nelson NJ. Effect of tumor disaggregation on results of *in vitro* cell survival assay after *in vivo* treatment of the EMT6 tumors: X-rays, cyclophosphamide, and bleomycin. *In Vitro* 1990; 16:547–553.

35. Raaphorst GP, Sapareto SA, Freman ML, Dewey WC. Changes in cellular heat and/or radiation sensitivity observed at various times after trypsinization and plating. *Int J Radiat Biol* 1979; 35:193–197.

36. Pallavicini MG. Characterization of cell suspensions from solid tumors. In: Kallman RF, ed. *Rodent Tumor Models in Experimental Cancer Therapy* Pergamon Press, New York, NY, 1987, pp. 76–81.

37. Wheeler KT, Wallen CA. Timing: an important variable in colony-formation assays. In: Kallman RF, ed. *Rodent Tumor Models in Experimental Cancer Therapy.* Pergamon Press, New York, NY, 1987, pp. 84–89.

38. Stewart CC, Beetham KL. Cytocidal activity and proliferative ability of macrophages infiltrating the EMT6 tumor. *Int J Cancer* 1978; 22:152–159.

39. Rockwell S. Effects of clumps and clusters on survival measurements with clonogenic assays. *Cancer Res* 1985; 45:1601–1607.

40. Selby P, Buick RN, Tannock I. A critical appraisal of the "human tumor stem-cell assay." *N Engl J Med* 1983; 308:129–134.

41. Twentyman PR. Timing of assays: an important consideration in the determination of clonogenic cell survival both *in vitro* and *in vivo*. *Int J Radiat Oncol Biol Phys* 1979; 5:1213–1220.

42. Hahn GM, Rockwell S, Kallman RF, Gordon LF, Frindel E. Repair of potentially lethal damage *in vivo* in solid tumor cells after x-irradiation. *Cancer Res* 1974; 34:351–354.

43. Olive PL, Durand RE. Apoptosis: an indicator of radiosensitivity *in vitro? Int J Radiat Biol* 1997; 71:695–707.

44. Stephens TC. Measurement of tumor cell surviving fraction and absolute numbers of clonogens per tumor in excision assays. In: Kallman RF, ed. *Rodent Tumor Models in Experimental Cancer Therapy.* Pergamon Press, New York, NY 1987, pp. 90–94.

45. Alper T. *Cellular Radiobiology.* Cambridge University Press, Cambridge UK. 1979.

46. Alper T, ed. Cell survival after low doses of radiation: Theoretical and clinical implications. (Proceedings of the 6th LH Gray Conference), Institute of Physics/John Wiley & Sons, New York, NY, 1975.

47. Zar JH. Biostatistical Analysis. Prentice-Hall, Upper Saddle River, NJ, 1984.

33 Apoptosis in Vivo

L. Clifton Stephens, DVM, PhD
and Raymond E. Meyn, PhD

CONTENTS

1. INTRODUCTION AND HISTORICAL PERSPECTIVE

Although apoptosis is a complex and highly regulated process with numerous and varied biological consequences, it is typically described as a sequence of morphological events that can be easily recognized histologically. In fact, the initial identification and subsequent characterization of apoptosis were based on microscopic observations of its occurrence in vivo. Rudolph Virchow (1821–1902) is recognized as the father of modern pathology. He fostered the idea of the cellular basis of disease, and recognized that cell death was a fundamental process for development and that cell death played a role in maintaining homeostasis. As pathologists, Virchow and other nineteenth-century microscopists appreciated the roles and morphologies of cell death in disease, and it was recognized that such features as the appearance and distribution of dead cells were variable. In Virchow's era and throughout most of the twentieth century, necrosis was the exclusive term for cell death, although morphological variations from "typical" necrosis sometimes acquired distinctive names, such as tingible bodies in lymphoid germinal centers, Councilman bodies in the liver, shrinkage necrosis, piecemeal necrosis, karyolytic bodies, zeiosis, and necrobiosis. The biological significance of distinctive morphologies of cell death was first brought to the attention of the scientific community in the early 1970s by an experimental pathologist who not only recognized that not all dead cells look the same, but also took this observation further by deducing that this could mean that mechanisms for cell death could also differ *(1)* This Australian pathologist, Professor John Kerr, made these seminal observations, and with his colleagues also devised the name *apoptosis* to distinguish the process from necrosis *(2)* Kerr's sound morphological observations and interpretations based on those observa-

From: *Tumor Models in Cancer Research*
Edited by: B. A. Teicher © Humana Press Inc., Totowa, NJ

tions are the foundations for the explosion of apoptosis research. His remarks published in 1980 in a symposium proceedings were prophetic, not only for radiation biologists but for all research in fundamental cellular processes: "…it is possible that an understanding of the general controls of initiation and inhibition of apoptosis at the molecular level may help define the critical targets and ultimate effector mechanisms in radiation-induced cell death" *(3)* As detailed in this chapter, some aspects of that prophecy have come true in the intervening years.

2. RECOGNITION AND QUANTIFICATION OF APOPTOSIS

2.1. Morphological Assessment In Vivo

Morphology of in vivo apoptosis, as initially described by Kerr in conventionally prepared tissue sections, is reliable for recognition and quantification of this mode of cell death. Identification of apoptosis in tissue sections has been facilitated by an immunohistochemical method described by Gavrieli et al. *(4),* in which DNA breaks in apoptotic nuclei are marked by dUTP-biotin transferred to the free 3′ end of cleaved DNA. Because terminal deoxynucleotidyl transferase is employed to transfer dUPT-biotin by nick-end labeling, the convenient acronym, "TUNEL" is used to depict this procedure, which has become the standard technique for the study of apoptosis in tissue sections.

The in vivo morphology of apoptosis is identical regardless of species, cell, or tissue type, and whether it occurs in normal tissue or tumors. The appearance is not influenced by cause, which encompasses apoptosis associated with physiological processes, pathological conditions, and responses to therapeutic modalities including drugs, ionizing radiation, hyperthermia, and gene therapy. Spontaneous and radiation-induced apoptotic bodies appear histologically the same in all of the normal tissues we have studied, including serious glands, thymus, intestine, and mammary gland. As far as tumors are concerned, the morphology of background and induced apoptosis are the same in carcinomas, lymphomas, and sarcomas of man and animals. With the recognition of the regulation of apoptosis by the expression of oncogenes and tumor-suppressor genes, studies of these parameters in conjunction with determination of the proliferation and apoptotic indices are providing insights into the interplay of cell proliferation and cell death on in vivo tumorigenesis in such tissues as the human colorectum *(5–7)* and rodent models of breast cancer *(8–10)* and lymphoma *(11,12).*

Having emphasized the constancy of the morphology of apoptosis in vivo, an additional critical factor relating to the detection of this mode of cell death is timing. Apoptosis is ephemeral—it occurs rapidly and is removed quickly. An understanding of the kinetics is critical for successful in vivo investigation of apoptosis. We have utilized radiation in studies of the propensity of normal cells and tumor cells to undergo apoptosis in vivo in large part because of the precision of time zero.

Implicit in the light-microscopic study of in vivo apoptosis is an appreciation of the distribution, size, shape, and staining characteristics of dead cells. Apoptosis can be seen and distinguished from necrosis in sections of tissue fixed in buffered formalin, processed by conventional methods, embedded in paraffin, and stained by hematoxylin and eosin (H&E). Cell death by apoptosis typically involves scattered individual cells as opposed to necrosis, which can involve confluent groups of cells. Cells undergoing apoptosis shrink and lose contact with neighboring cells, so that they are often surrounded by a narrow empty halo. Necrotic cells have a tendency to swell. Apoptotic bodies are smaller than normal cells and necrotic cells. Nuclei in both apoptotic and necrotic cells can be characterized as pyknotic and karyorrhexic. Wylie et al. *(13,14)* propose that the commonality of pyknosis and karyorrhexis may have obscured the recognition of apoptosis as a distinctive process. In apoptosis, the condensed and densely stained pyknotic chromatin becomes packed into smooth, round, or curved profiles situated in close apposition to the nuclear membrane. These cells shrink into a dense, rounded mass, becoming a single apoptotic body—or the nucleus may break up, which is known as karyorrhexis—and the cell emits processes or buds that contain nuclear fragments surrounded by a narrow rim of cytoplasm. These processes tend to break off and become apoptotic bodies, which may remain free, or become phagocytized by macrophages or neighboring cells.

A routine H&E is superior to a poor TUNEL for the detection of apoptosis in tissue sections. However, a properly prepared TUNEL section that is suitably counterstained allows one to employ the features used with H&E—namely, distribution, structure (nuclear fragment surrounded by narrow rim of cytoplasm), shape, and size—and have the added parameter of the positive peroxidase reaction to draw attention to apoptotic cells. A good counterstain is important, so that morphology can be appreciated and with scrutiny of the morphology in TUNEL sections, one can differentiate apoptosis from necrotic cells, autolytic cells, and debris that can all show positive reactions *(15)*. It is helpful to utilize positive controls—e.g. sections of lymph node with follicular hyperplasia, to develop familiarity with the appearance of positive TUNEL staining.

2.2. Quantification of Apoptosis In Vitro

Quantification of apoptosis in vitro on the basis of morphological assessment can be done by a variety of techniques including those described above for histological sections. However, many different staining options are available, including a number of fluorescent indicators of either chromatin configuration, Hoechst 33342, or propidium iodide, or fluorescent-based TUNEL detection of fragmented DNA. Cells growing or placed on microscope slides can then be examined under a fluorescent microscope and detached cells, perhaps more conveniently, by flow cytometry *(16,17)*. In addition to detecting apoptosis on the basis of changes at the DNA level, cell-surface changes indicative of apoptosis can also be used. The early stages of apoptosis are characterized by cell-surface membrane blebbing and translocation of phosphatidyl serine (PS) from the inner to the outer surface of the plasma membrane *(18)*. The externalized PS can be labeled using a fluorescent tagged binding protein, Annexin V, which can be quantified using fluorescent indicators by either microscopy or flow cytometry *(19)*. Several manufacturers offer kits based on TUNEL or Annexin V for apoptosis quantification.

Prior to the advent of these methods, apoptosis in vitro was routinely assessed on the basis of a highly characteristic pattern of DNA fragmentation. The DNA of a cell is enzymatically cleaved by a specific endonuclease during apoptosis into oligonucleotides with sizes that are multiples of the internucleosomal distance, 180 basepairs *(20)*. These produce a "ladder pattern" when separated by agarose gel electrophoresis. Such a pattern is highly diagnostic of apoptosis in vitro. The shortcomings of this method are that it is not very quantitative, and some cell systems are inefficient in producing this type of low molecular weight DNA fragmentation. It is now understood that the endonuclease responsible for this characteristic DNA fragmentation is activated through a cascade of proteolytic steps mediated by a family of cysteine proteases referred to as caspases *(21)*. Thus, caspase activity itself is now used as a marker for apoptosis in vitro, and kits are available for the detection of this activity as well.

3. APOPTOSIS IN TUMOR BIOLOGY

3.1. The Role of Apoptosis in Tumor Development

The failure of cells to undergo apoptosis is now associated with the pathogenesis of several human diseases, including cancer, autoimmune disorders, and certain viral infections *(22)*. In the case of cancer, tumors are usually clonal in origin—they arise from normal cells that have acquired a series of mutations in critical genes that control proliferation, survival, adhesion, and mobility *(23)*. Thus, several sequential mutations are required to convert a normal cell into a tumor cell. A popular idea is that one of the earliest mutations may involve the disregulation of proliferation, which may in turn allow a clonal expansion of cells that are available as targets for further oncogenic lesions. However, abnormal cell proliferation is probably recognized by the host activating a response to eliminate the nascent tumor cell by triggering its apoptosis. In this case, apoptosis may represent a mechanism for protecting the host from inappropriate cell expansion, thereby maintaining homeostasis *(22)*. Eventually, the emerging tumor cell counteracts this attack through additional mutations that suppress or inhibit the apoptotic pathway. Therefore, tumor cells are typically characterized with regard to their genetic lesions by one or more mutations in genes involved in the regulation of apoptosis, i.e., many tumor-suppressor genes and oncogenes have critical roles in apoptosis.

3.2. Genetic Regulation of Apoptosis

Bcl-2 was one of the first genes that was shown to have a major regulatory activity in apoptosis. Originally identified as a result of its location at the site of the t(14:18) chromosome translocation present in human B-cell follicular lymphoma, overexpression of bcl-2 in transgenic animal models was shown to mimic the pattern of human lymphoma development *(24)*. Other studies demonstrated that bcl-2 acts to promote cell survival rather than cell proliferation, by suppressing cell death *(25)*. More recently it has been revealed that bcl-2 is the prototypic member of a large and growing family of genes. The protein products of these genes share homology in four conserved domains: BH1, BH2, BH3, and BH4. Interestingly, some members of this family of proteins, such as bax, bak, and bcl-X_S, are pro-apoptotic, and other members of the family, such as bcl-2, Mcl-1, and bcl-X_L, are anti-apoptotic *(26)*. Although these proteins function as individual proteins, some of their activities are mediated through dimerization at the site of their BH3 domains. These proteins form hetero- and homodimers in the cell, and their pro- vs anti-apoptotic activity appears to be dependent on the ratio of bax-like to bcl-2-like composition of the dimers *(27)*.

In spite of the fact that the role of bcl-2 in apoptosis was discovered more than 10 years ago, its mechanism has remained elusive. Clues related to its activity have come through analysis of the DNA sequence of the gene encoding bcl-2. Many bcl-2 family members have a hydrophobic stretch of amino acids at the C-terminal region, suggesting membrane localization. Indeed, bcl-2 protein appears to be localized in cellular membranes, including the endoplasmic reticulum, nuclear envelope, and mitochondrial membrane *(26)*. Recently, the focus of research has been on the possible function of bcl-2 in the mitochondrial membrane. The importance of mitochondria in apoptosis was not initially appreciated, but it is now generally recognized that mitochondria fulfill an essential role in the execution of apoptosis *(28)*. It appears that mitochondria respond to apoptosis-inducing signals from other parts of the cell by releasing factors that activate caspases, the cysteine proteases that carry out the degradative part of apoptosis. Cytochrome c is one such factor released from the mitochondria in cells undergoing apoptosis *(29)*. Cytochrome c participates in the activation of caspase 3, one of the caspases central to the apoptotic process. Release of cytochrome c and activation of caspase 3 do not take place in bcl-2 expressing cells *(30)*. This ability to effectively block apoptosis has a profound influence on tumor-cell development, and also influences cancer therapy. Since many therapeutic agents kill cells through apoptosis, bcl-2-expressing tumor cells are highly resistant to these modalities *(31)*.

Another very important gene, discovered at about the same time as bcl-2 and also now known to play a very centralized role in controlling apoptosis propensity, to be highlighted in this discussion, is *p53*. P53 is a transcription factor that particularly responds to DNA damage *(32)*. Normally, *p53* protein is expressed at very low levels because of targeted degradation, but the levels of protein rise following irradiation or other DNA-damaging insults, forcing the cell into either growth arrest or apoptosis *(33)*. Cells from transgenic animals, in which both alleles have been knocked out, are unable to carry out G1-arrest or apoptosis after irradiation *(34,35)*. As a direct effect of the loss of these functions, cells with nonfunctional *p53* have increased risk for malignant transformation when exposed to genotoxic/carcinogenic agents. *P53* is the most frequently mutated gene in human cancer and its role in cancer progression when mutated is apparently related to the inability of cells sustaining DNA damage to be eliminated by apoptosis, leading to the idea of *p53* as "guardian of the genome" *(36)*. *P53*'s role in apoptosis was discovered when cells engineered to overexpress *p53* underwent spontaneous apoptosis *(37)*, immediately suggesting a gene-therapy strategy for cancer that has been exploited to some success *(38)*. The ability of *p53* to exert a growth arrest in G1 phase is most likely a result of the transcription of genes that regulate the cell cycle. One such gene is the cyclin-dependent kinase inhibitor *p21 (39)*. A role for *p53*-mediated transcriptional regulation of apoptosis is less clear, but the expression of at least one gene that promotes apoptosis—bax—is known to be controlled by *p53 (40)*. Furthermore, *p53* may repress the transcription of anti-apoptotic genes, and there is some evidence to suggest that nontranscriptional mechanisms may also be involved *(41)*.

Although the focus of this section on genes that control apoptosis in tumors has been on two of the most universal—*p53* and bcl-2—numerous other tumor-suppressor genes and oncogenes can also be involved in specific types of tumor cells. A long list of such genes would include c-*myc, ras, raf,* E2F, Rb, and Mdm2. Discussion of these other genes is outside of the scope of this chapter, but it should be apparent that disregulation of the apoptotic mode of cell death is a critical event in tumor progression, perhaps as important as disregulation of controls on cell proliferation. Loss of apoptotic propensity confers a subsequent tumor resistance to cancer-treatment modalities that kill cells by apoptosis.

4. APOPTOSIS IN CANCER THERAPY

4.1. Response of Normal Tissue to Cytotoxic Therapy

Investigation of apoptotic cell death in vivo in normal organs has been the subject of specific research and as a by-product of cytotoxic therapy of tumors. For all modalities of cancer treatment, and in particular, localized and systemic cytotoxic therapies in particular, there is significant concern for concurrent injury of normal tissue. It is now well-established that death of tumor cells and normal cells by apoptosis is a major response to virtually all cancer-therapy modalities, including radiotherapy, chemotherapy, immunotherapy, hyperthermia, hormone ablation, photodynamic therapy, and, most recently, gene therapy. However, the contribution of apoptosis in determining the curability of tumors and the sensitivity of normal tissues to exposure to the cytotoxic insults are largely unknown. A better understanding of apoptosis in tumors and normal tissues should lead to improvement of treatment regimens. Chemotherapy or radiation can accentuate the apoptotic elimination of cells from normal tissues comprised either of rapidly proliferating cells or long-lived cell populations. Apoptotic bodies are normally observed in lymphoid germinal centers and in the involuting thymic cortex. Lymphocyte apoptosis is greatly increased by glucocorticoids, chemotherapy, and radiation. Nonlymphoid tissues with a structure regulated by apoptosis include glandular epithelium in which hormones or growth factors control hyperplasia and involution (e.g., the mammary gland, uterus, and prostate), complex differentiated epithelium with long-lived stem cells (e.g., skin and intestine), and rapidly proliferating cell populations (e.g., bone marrow and gonads). These tissues, like lymphoid tissues, display increased apoptosis when exposed to cytotoxic injury.

Our initial interest in apoptosis was based on the investigation of a common problem encountered by our clinical colleagues in patients receiving radiotherapy for cancer of the head and neck regions. The acute clinical responses of salivary glands and lacrimal glands are similar. When radiation treatment fields encompass the major salivary glands or lacrimal glands, many patients experience dryness of oral or conjunctival mucous membranes during the first or second wk of therapy. The associated complications are distressing, and sometimes serious for afflicted patients. The need to understand the pathogenesis of these sequelae in these patients has prompted our investigations with a primate model. We found that differentiated serous acinar cells of salivary glands and lacrimal glands die by apoptosis after radiation exposure, and loss of these cells by apoptosis is responsible for many of the oral and ocular complications experienced by patients receiving radiotherapy for cancer of the head and neck *(42–46)*. As we have shown in the major serous glands, it has become well-established that enhanced apoptosis—in sites such as the lymphoid tissues, crypt cells of the gut, hair follicles, bone marrow, and testicles—is responsible for many of the adverse side-effects cancer patients experience because it is certain that extensive apoptosis is damaging to the normal function of these tissues *(47–50)*.

The mammary gland is comprised of ducts and acini such as the salivary glands and lacrimal glands, but mammary acinar cells do not display the remarkable extent of apoptosis that serous cells exhibit following irradiation. However, the propensity for apoptosis, or lack of proclivity to undergo apoptosis, is being studied in the mammary gland in the context of tumorigenesis. As mentioned in the previous section, the tumor-suppressor gene *p53* maintains the integrity of the genome by stimulating apoptosis in cells that have sustained DNA damage. The *p53* gene is frequently altered in human cancers, including breast cancer. We used radiation as a DNA-damaging agent to test the role of *p53* in controlling apoptosis in preneoplastic mouse mammary glands *(8,9)*. The results of in vivo experiments were consistent with the hypothesis that normal *p53* function is important if mammary cells with DNA damage are to be deleted by apoptosis. Additional in vivo experiments reinforcing the central roles of *p53* and other proteins such as *p21* in fundamental radiation responses, including cell-growth arrest and apoptosis, used knockout mice that were null for the *p53* or *p21* alleles to study the response of skin to radiation *(49)*. They demonstrated that the radiation-induced apoptosis in hair follicles was fully dependent on *p53*, and growth arrest in the epidermis was only partially dependent on *p53*, but fully dependent on *p21*.

If genetic polymorphisms in humans that determine levels of cytotoxic therapy-induced damage to normal tissue were identified, predictive assays might be developed to ascertain which patients are likely to suffer unacceptable injury from standard treatment doses. Identification and quantification of in vivo apoptosis has been the basis of research directed at understanding the effects of genetic polymorphisms on radiosensitivity of the intestine *(51)* and thymus *(52,53)*. Radiation exposure of the intestine results in rapid apoptotic death of cells lining the crypts *(47)*. This accounts for acute malabsorption syndromes that are regularly encountered following abdominal irradiation in clinical radiation oncology practice. But, as is the case for most normal tissue reactions to radiation, interindividual differences in response and sensitivity are frequently observed. Differences in susceptibility to crypt-cell apoptosis between strains of inbred mice indicate that heritability plays a role in the variability of apoptosis in these animals, and supports the notion that genetic predisposition influences the response of patients *(51)* Although no adverse clinical syndromes are associated with irradiation of the thymus, study of in vivo apoptosis in the thymus confirms further the heritability of the propensity for apoptosis in another cell type and indicates the suitability of the murine model for identifying genes controlling apoptotic cell death *(52,53)*.

4.2. Apoptosis in Tumors Responding to Cytotoxic Therapy

The occurrence of apoptosis in solid tumors responding to cytotoxic treatments in vivo was initially demonstrated many years ago. Searle et al. reported in 1975 that certain chemotherapy agents induced apoptosis in model tumors growing in mice *(54)*. The work in this area prior to 1980 was reviewed by Kerr and Searle, and in that article they illustrate examples of apoptosis following irradiation of a model tumor in vivo *(3)*. These seminal observations by Kerr and his colleagues stimulated our interest in systematically assessing apoptosis in solid tumors treated in vivo with various cancer therapeutic agents. To that end, we have quantified apoptosis in a variety of transplantable murine tumors treated in vivo with several different chemotherapy agents and ionizing radiation. In all of these investigations, the percentage of cells with the features of apoptosis was determined from H&E stained histological sections of the treated tumors using the morphological criteria described in Subheading 2.1.

Since very little had been done up until that time, the intent of our first study was to simply establish whether apoptosis was a feature of irradiated tumors *(55)*. Thus, two transplantable murine tumors were chosen based on prior data showing that the hepatocarcinoma, HCa-1, was very resistant to radiation, with a TCD_{50} (the single dose of radiation required to cure 50% of tumors) of >80 gy, and that an ovarian adenocarcinoma, OCa-1, was moderately sensitive, with a TCD_{50} of about 53 gy. Tumors growing in the hind legs of mice were treated with a series of high doses of radiation and followed for relatively long periods after irradiation, because we had no preconception about the dose response and kinetics for radiation-induced apoptosis in vivo. The results showed that apoptosis occurred in the OCa-1 tumor, but not in the HCa-1 tumor. In the OCa-1 tumor, the maximum percentage of apoptosis occurred at 6 h, and fell with longer times. The dose response was already on a plateau with the lowest dose used—25 gy. The findings prompted a more detailed examination of apoptosis in the OCa-1 model (56). There we found that the dose response for radiation-induced apoptosis plateaus at about 30–35% apoptotic cells following doses of 7.5 gy or more. In addition, the apoptosis peaks very soon after irradiation, about 4 h, and then drops dramatically.

These first two series of experiments enabled the following conclusions to be drawn: 1) some tumors are susceptible to apoptosis but others are not. 2) apoptotic index peaks quickly after irradiation and then falls as the apoptotic bodies are phagocytosed. 3) low doses of radiation preferentially induce apoptosis. 4) there is a relatively large proportion of cells that are apparently resistant to apoptosis, even within tumors that display apoptosis after irradiation. These conclusions were borne out in an expanded study of 15 different murine tumors intended to provide a clearer picture about the heterogeneity in response (57). In this study, we confirmed that some types of tumors, namely adenocarcinomas of the mammary gland and ovaries and lymphomas, display an apoptotic response to radiation in vivo, whereas other types of tumors—squamous-cell carcinomas (SCCs), hepatocarcinomas, and fibrosarcomas—do not. Fortunately, other laboratory data related to the radiation response of these tumors were available, allowing us to determine correlations of in vivo apoptotic response to tumor response. This analysis indicated that when radiation-induced apoptosis for all of the tumors was plotted against the respective tumor's TCD_{50} value and specific growth delay, those tumors that responded by apoptosis tended to have lower TCD_{50} values ($0.1<p<0.2$) and longer specific growth delays ($p<0.05$). Interestingly, the most significant correlation was produced when the spontaneous levels of apoptosis present in untreated tumors was plotted against the levels of radiation-induced apoptosis for each given tumor ($p<0.001$). This suggests that pretreatment apoptosis levels may predict treatment response, and we subsequently tested this hypothesis in other studies of specimens from patients who had received radiotherapy for bladder cancer (58), carcinoma of the cervix (59), or lymphoma (60).

Although these correlations may seem to indicate that apoptosis was important in tumor response to radiation, they do not prove such a relationship. Moreover, as discussed in detail elsewhere, the fact that under the best of conditions solid tumors in this series only achieved 30–35% apoptotic indices indicates that radiation-induced apoptosis cannot account for the sensitivity of the tumors, and other modes of cell death must also be involved. This does not rule out a role for apoptosis in tumor response, but suggests that apoptosis is perhaps only one of several mechanisms responsible for tumor response to therapy.

In light of the interesting results described here for apoptosis assessed in irradiated murine tumors, we have focused some attention on apoptosis induced in tumors treated in vivo by chemotherapy agents. In the first of these studies, we examined two murine tumors previously shown to be sensitive to radiation-induced apoptosis, MCa-4 and OCa-1, for apoptotic response to cyclophosphamide using the same methodological approach *(61)*. The kinetics of apoptosis development were determined as a function of time after treatment with single injections of the mice with 200 mg/kg. The apoptotic index peaked between 10–18 h in both tumor models, and then slowly declined to background levels by 5 d. The dose-response relationships illustrated that apoptosis could be observed at much lower doses of cyclophosphamide. A very similar analysis to this was repeated using the same tumor models with another chemotherapy agent, cisplatin *(62)*. As with cyclophosphamide, the kinetics of cisplatin-induced apoptosis was very broad, peaking between 10 and 20 h, then declining to background levels by 5 d. For both cyclophosphamide and cisplatin, the dose-response curves for apoptosis induction did not correlate well with the tumor growth-delay measurements made on tumors treated with the same doses—substantial apoptosis was observed under conditions where this dose of drug only produced a slight delay in growth. Higher doses of drug did not greatly enhance apoptosis, but did enhance growth delay and cause tumor regression. Thus, we concluded that, as with radiation, apoptosis may be important in tumor response to these chemotherapeutic agents, but it may not be the only parameter that governs response. Indeed, we speculated that since the kinetics of apoptosis is spread out over such a long period, factors such as tumor-cell proliferation may also come into play.

To extend the investigation of apoptosis in vivo as a response to cancer chemotherapy agents, we completed a series of experiments in which we compared the apoptotic response of the MCa-4 and OCa-1 tumors to eight different agents *(63)*. In addition, we compared 7 different murine tumors for their apoptotic response to cyclophosphamide, cisplatin, and radiation. The chemotherapy drugs used for the first part of this analysis were cyclophosphamide, cisplatin, adriamycin, 5-FU, ara-C, etoposide, camptothecin, melphalan, and fludarabine. All of these agents produced substantial apoptosis in both MCa-4 and OCa-1 tumors at the doses used and times measured—8 and 24 h. Two of the agents, camptothecin and etoposide, appeared to be especially potent. The other part of the analysis, in which the apoptotic responses of seven different tumors were compared, produced a striking pattern. Tumors previously shown to be responsive to radiation, MCa-4, OCa-1, and the TH lymphoma also had an apoptotic response to cyclophosphamide and cisplatin, and tumors previously shown to be resistant to radiation-induced apoptosis, SSC-7, FSA, NFSA, and SA-NH were cross-resistant to CY and CP. This observation is certainly consistent with the theory presented in Subheading 3.2, which suggests that intrinsic factors such as expression patterns of tumor-suppressor genes and oncogenes control apoptosis propensity and may at least partially influence tumor response to therapy. The caveat to this theory was also illustrated in this same study, because several of the tumors that displayed no apoptotic response to either cisplatin or cyclophosphamide did display a growth delay following the same treatments. Thus, factors other than apoptosis must be important in determining tumor response to therapy.

As emphasized in this chapter, tumor-suppressor genes and oncogenes regulate apoptosis pathways and, although these pathways have been elucidated in in vitro cell systems, it seems safe to conclude that they regulate apoptosis in vivo as well. Based on the patterns of tumor apoptosis induced by cancer-therapeutic agents in vivo observed in various murine tumors, we attempted to test the influence of one of the most important of these genes in a system we derived from one of these tumors. Of the various tumors used in our studies, one in particular, the TH-lymphoma, displayed high levels of apoptosis in response to all agents examined. We placed cells derived from this tumor into cell culture, and have used them in a variety of other investigations. Although these cells initially retained a substantial apoptotic response in vitro, they eventually became resistant *(64)*. We subsequently derived apoptosis-sensitive, LY-as, and apoptosis-resistant LY-ar sublines from the original cell population, and have determined that the resistant line has a 30-fold overexpression of bcl-2 *(65)*. Thus, there is a correlation between apoptosis propensity and bcl-2 expression in this set of two lines. In other in vitro investigations, we have demonstrated that the resistant line does not undergo apoptosis in response to radiation, CP, adriamycin, or VP-16 whereas the sensitive line does *(66)*. Since these lines were derived from a syngeneic strain of mice, we investigated whether transplantable tumors derived from these lines would respond similarly. LY-ar and LY-as tumors were grown in syngeneic mice and the mice were then given adriamycin, VP-16, CP, CY, camptothecin, or ara-C *(67)*. Some tumors were sectioned for analysis of apoptosis, and others were left to grow to assess growth delay. Interestingly, the analysis of apoptosis in the treated tumors indicated that the propensity for apoptosis in vivo was identical to that expressed by these same lines when treated in vitro, i.e. the LY-ar tumors had less apoptosis in every case compared to the LY-as tumors. However, the tumor growth-delay effects of these chemotherapy agents were not predicted by the apoptotic indices from tumors receiving the same treatment. Indeed, for some drugs, the LY-ar tumors were more sensitive than the LY-as tumors. Thus, despite considerable interest in using apoptotic indices as predictors of treatment outcome, these findings suggest that such relationships in vivo are complicated by other factors such as tumor-cell heterogeneity, host effects and drug pharmacokinetics.

SUMMARY AND CONCLUSIONS

This chapter presents a broad overview of apoptosis as it relates to in vivo systems, with special emphasis on tumor models used in cancer research. The biochemical and molecular aspects of the apoptosis pathway are necessarily investigated using cultured cell systems growing in vitro. These types of questions are more difficult to address using in vivo models. In general, much less has been done with regard to apoptosis in vivo. Although we have taken the opportunity to highlight some of our own work in this chapter, cancer researchers now generally recognize the need to extrapolate from the in vitro studies to the more clinically relevant in vivo situation. Realizing that apoptosis occurs in response to therapeutic treatments, the critical question at the moment concerns finding out whether this apoptotic response represents a determinant of therapeutic response. Perhaps even more importantly, tumor cells are most likely resistant to apoptosis mediated by cytotoxic agents because they have turned off this pathway for cell deletion as part of their progression to malignancy. Therefore, strategies designed to restore apoptosis to resistant tumors are currently being explored in a number of laboratories. These would include the use of so-called death cytokines such as TRAIL[68], or gene-therapy strategies that restore wild-type p53 function *(38)*. When used in combination with conventional therapeutic agents, radiation, and chemotherapy, these new strategies may enhance apoptosis in a synergistic manner, producing an enhanced therapeutic effect. By necessity, these new strategies must be tested in preclinical model systems. However, once these treatments are applied to patients, assessing apoptosis in vivo and correlating it with other tumor markers—including, ultimate, response—should provide important insight into the role of apoptosis in human cancer.

REFERENCES

1. Kerr JFR. Shrinkage necrosis: a distinct mode of cell death. *J Pathol* 1971; 105:13–20.
2. Kerr JFR, Wyllie AH, Currie AR. Apoptosis: a basic biological phenomenon with wide ranging implications in tissue kinetics. *Br J Cancer* 1972; 26:239–257.
3. Kerr JFR, Searle J. Apoptosis: its nature and kinetic role. In: Meyn RE, Withers HR, eds. *Radiation Biology in Cancer Research.* New York, Raven Press, NY, 1980, pp. 367–384.
4. Gavrieli Y, Sherman Y, Ben-Sasson SA. Identification of programmed cell death in situ via specific labeling of nuclear DNA fragmentation. *J Cell Biol* 1992; 119(3):493–501.
5. Sinicrope FA, Raun SB, Cleary KR, Stephens LC, Levin B. bcl-2 and p53 oncoprotein expression during colorectal tumorigenesis. *Cancer Res* 1995; 55:237–241.
6. Sinicrope FA, Roddey G, McDonnell TJ, Shen Y, Cleary KR, Stephens LC. Increased apoptosis accompanies neoplastic development in human colorectum. *Clin Cancer Res* 1996; 12:1999–2006.
7. Sinicrope FA, Roddey G, Lemoine M, et al. Loss of *p21$^{WAF1/Cip1}$* protein expression accompanies progression of sporadic colorectal neoplasms but not hereditary nonpolyposis colorectal cancers. *Clin Cancer Res* 1998; 4:1251–1261.
8. Meyn RE, Stephens LC, Mason KA, Medina D. Radiation-induced apoptosis in normal and pre-neoplastic mammary glands in vivo: significance of gland differentiation and p53 status. *Int J Cancer* 1996; 65:466–472.
9. Medina D, Stephens LC, Bonilla PJ, et al. Radiation-induced tumorigenesis in preneoplastic mouse mammary glands in vivo: significance of p53 status and apoptosis. *Mol Carcinog* 1998; 22(3):199–207.
10. Sivaraman L, Stephens LC, Markaverich BM, et al. Hormone-induced refractoriness to mammary carcinogenesis in Wistar-Furth rats. *Carcinogenesis* 1998; 19(9):1573–1581.
11. Marin MC, Hsu B, Stephens LC, Brisbay S, McDonnell TJ. The functional basis of c-myc and bcl-2 complementation during multistep lymphomagenesis in vivo. *Exp Cell Res* 1995; 217(2):240–247.
12. Hsu B, Marin MC, el-Naggar AK, Stephens LC, Brisbay S, McDonnell TJ. Evidence that c-myc mediated apoptosis does not require wild-type p53 during lymphomagenesis. *Oncogene* 1995; 11(1):175–179.
13. Wyllie AH, Kerr JFR, Currie AR. Cell death: the significance of apoptosis. *Int Rev Cytol* 1980; 68:251–306.
14. Wyllie AH. Apoptosis and the regulation of cell numbers in normal and neoplastic tissues: an overview. *Cancer Metastasis Rev* 1992; 11:95–103.
15. Grasl-Kraupp B, Ruttkay-Nedecky B, Koudelka H, Bukowska K, Bursch W, Schulte-Hermann R. In situ detection of fragmented DNA (TUNEL assay) fails to discriminate among apoptosis, necrosis, and autolytic cell death: a cautionary note. *Hepatology* 1995; 21(5):1465–1468.
16. Dive C, Gregory CD, Phipps DJ, Evans DL, Milner AE, Wyllie AH. Analysis and discrimination of necrosis and apoptosis (programmed cell death) by multiparameter flow cytometry. *Biochim Biophys Acta* 1992; 1133:275–285.
17. Gorczyca W, Gong J, Darzynkiewicz Z. Detection of DNA strand breaks in individual apoptotic cells by the in situ terminal deoxynucleotidyl transferase and nick translation assays. *Cancer Res* 1993; 53(8):1945–1951.
18. Fadok VA, Voelker DR, Campbell PA, Cohen JJ, Bratton DL, Henson PM. Exposure of phosphatidylserine on the surface of apoptotic lymphocytes triggers specific recognition and removal by macrophages. *J Immunol* 1992; 148(7):2207–2216.
19. Koopman G, Reutelingsperger CP, Kuijten GA, Keehnen RM, Pals ST, van Oers MH. Annexin V for flow cytometric detection of phosphatidylserine expression on B cells undergoing apoptosis. *Blood* 1994; 84(5):1415–1420.
20. Wyllie A. Glucocorticoid-induced thymocyte apoptosis is associated with endogenous endonuclease activation. *Nature* 1980; 284:555–556.
21. Cohen GM. Caspases: the executioners of apoptosis. *Biochem J* 1997; 326:1–16.

22. Thompson CB. Apoptosis in the pathogenesis and treatment of disease. *Science* 1995; 267:1456–1462.

23. Evan G. Cancer-A matter of life and cell death. *Int J Cancer* 1997; 71:709–711.

24. McDonnell T, Korsmeyer S. Progression from lymphoid hyperplasia to high grade lymphoma in mice transgenic for the t(14;18). *Nature* 1991; 349:254–256.

25. Vaux D, Cory S, Adams J. Bcl-2 gene promotes haemopoietic cell survival and cooperates with c-*myc* to immortalize pre-B cells. *Nature* 1988; 335:440–442.

26. Adams JM, Cory S. The Bcl-2 protein family: arbiters of cell survival. *Science* 1998; 281:1322–1326.

27. Korsmeyer S, Shutter J, Veis D, Merry D, Oltvai Z. Bcl-2/Bax: a rheostat that regulates an anti-oxidant pathway and cell death. *Semin Cancer Biol* 1993; 4:327–332.

28. Susin SA, Zamzami N, Kroemer G. Mitochondria as regulators of apoptosis: doubt no more. *Biochim Biophys Acta* 1998; 1366:151–165.

29. Liu X, Kim NC, Yang J, Jemmerson R, Wang X. Induction of apoptotic program in cell-free extracts: requirement for dATP and cytochrome c. *Cell* 1996; 86:147–157.

30. Yang J, Liu X, Bhalla K, et al. Prevention of apoptosis by Bcl-2: release of cytochrome c from mitochondria blocked. *Science* 1997; 275:1129–1131.

31. Voehringer DW, Meyn RE. Reversing drug resistance in Bcl-2-expressing tumor cells by depleting glutathione. *Drug Resist Updates* 1998; 1:345–351.

32. Lu X, Lane DP. Differential induction of transcriptionally active p53 following UV or ionizing radiation: defects in chromosome instability syndromes? *Cell* 1993; 75:765–778.

33. Kastan MB, Onyekwere O, Sidransky D, Vogelstein B, Craig RW. Participation of p53 protein in the cellular response to DNA damage. *Cancer Res* 1991; 51:6304–6311.

34. Lowe SW, Schmitt EM, Smith SW, Osborne BA, Jacks T. p53 is required for radiation-induced apoptosis in mouse thymocytes. *Nature (London)* 1993; 362:847–849.

35. Clarke AR, Purdie CA, Harrison DJ, et al. Thymocyte apoptosis induced by p53-dependent and independent pathways. *Nature (London)* 1993; 362:849–852.

36. Lane DP. p53, guardian of the genome. *Nature (London)* 1992; 358:15–16.

37. Yonish-Rouach E, Resnitzky D, Lotem J, Sachs L, Kimchi A, Oren M. Wild-type p53 induces apoptosis of myeloid leukaemic cells that is inhibited by interleukin-6. *Nature (London)* 1991; 352:345–347.

38. Spitz FR, Nguyen D, Skibber JM, Meyn RE, Cristiano RJ, Roth JA. Adenoviral-mediated wild-type p53 gene expression sensitized colorectal cancer cells to ionizing radiation. *Clin Cancer Res* 1996; 2:1665–1671.

39. El-Deiry WS, Tokino T, Veculescu VE, et al. WAF1, a potential mediator of p53 tumor suppression. *Cell* 1993; 75:817–825.

40. Miyashta T, Reed J. Tumor suppressor p53 is a direct transcriptional activator of the human bax gene. *Cell* 1995; 80:293–299.

41. Gottlieb TM, Oren M. p53 and apoptosis. *Seminars in Cancer Biology* 1998; 8(5):359–368.

42. Stephens L, King G, Peters L, Ang K, Schultheiss T, Jardine J. Acute and late radiation injury in rhesus monkey parotid glands: evidence of interphase cell death. *Am J Pathol* 1986; 124:469–478.

43. Stephens LC, King GK, Peters LJ, Ang KK, Schultheiss TE, Jardine JH. Unique radiosensitivity of serous cells in rhesus monkey submandibular glands. *Am J Pathol* 1986; 124(3):479–487.

44. Stephens LC, Ang KK, Schultheiss TE, King GK, Brock WA, Peters LJ. Target cell and mode of radiation injury in Rhesus salivary glands. *Radiother Oncol* 1986; 7:165–174.

45. Stephens LC, Schultheiss TE, Ang KK, Gray KN. Acute radiation injury of ocular adnexa. *Arch Ophthalmol* 1988; 106:389–391.

46. Stephens LC, Schultheiss TC, Price RE, Ang KK, Peters LJ. Radiation apoptosis of serous acinar cells of salivary and lacrimal glands. *Cancer* 1991; 67:1539–1543.

47. Hendry J, Potten C. Intestinal cell radiosensitivity: a comparison for cell death assayed by apoptosis or loss of clonogenicity. *Int J Radiat Biol* 1982; 42:621–628.

48. Cece R, Cazzaniga S, Morelli D, et al. Apoptosis of hair follicle cells during doxorubicin-induced alopecia in rats. *Lab Invest* 1996; 75(4):601–609.

49. Song S, Lambert PF. Different responses of epidermal and hair follicular cells to radiation correlate with distinct patterns of p53 and p21 induction. *Am J Pathol* 1999; 155(4):1121–1127.

50. Kerr JFR, Winterford CM, Harmon BV. Apoptosis—Its significance in cancer and cancer therapy. *Cancer* 1994; 73:2013–2026.

51. Weil MM, Stephens LC, Amos CI, Ruifrok AC, Mason KA. Strain difference in jejunal crypt cell susceptibility to radiation-induced apoptosis. *Int J Radiat Biol* 1996; 70(5):579–585.

52. Weil MM, Amos CI, Mason KA, Stephens LC. Genetic basis of strain variation in levels of radiation-induced apoptosis of thymocytes. *Radiat Res* 1996; 146(6):646–651.

53. Weil MM, Xia X, Lin Y, Stephens LC, Amos CI. Identification of quantitative trait loci controlling levels of radiation-induced thymocyte apoptosis in mice. *Genomics* 1997; 45(3):626–628.

54. Searle J, Lawson TA, Abbott PJ, Harmon B, Kerr JFR. An electron-microscope study of the mode of cell death induced by cancer chemotherapeutic agents in populations of proliferating normal and neoplastic cells. *J Pathol* 1975; 116:129–138.

55. Stephens LC, Ang KK, Schultheiss TE, Milas L, Meyn RE. Apoptosis in irradiated murine tumors. *Radiat Res* 1991; 127:308–316.

56. Stephens LC, Hunter NR, Ang KK, Milas L, Meyn RE. Development of apoptosis in irradiated murine tumors as a function of time and dose. *Radiat Res* 1993; 135:75–80.

57. Meyn RE, Stephens LC, Ang KK, et al. Heterogeneity in the development of apoptosis in irradiated murine tumours of different histologies. *Int J Radiat Biol* 1993; 64:583–591.

58. Chyle V, Pollack A, Czerniak BA, et al. Apoptosis and downstaging after preoperative radiotherapy for muscle-invasive bladder cancer. *Int J Radiat Oncol Biol Phys* 1996; 35:281–287.

59. Wheeler JA, Stephens LC, Eifel P, et al. ASTRO Research Fellowship: apoptosis as a predictor of tumor response to radiation in stage IB cervical carcinoma. *Int J Radiat Oncol Biol Phys* 1995; 32:1487–1493.

60. Logsdon ME, Meyn RE, Besa PC, et al. Apoptosis and the BCL-2 gene family—patterns of expression and prognostic value in stage I and II follicular center lymphoma. *Int J Radiat Oncol Biol Phys* 1999; 44(1):19–29.

61. Meyn RE, Stephens LC, Hunter NR, Milas L. Induction of apoptosis in murine tumors by cyclophosphamide. *Cancer Chemother Pharmacol* 1994; 33:410–414.

62. Meyn RE, Stephens LC, Hunter NR, Milas L. Kinetics of cisplatin-induced apoptosis in murine mammary and ovarian adenocarcinomas. *Int J Cancer* 1995; 65:466–472.

63. Meyn RE, Stephens LC, Hunter NR, Milas L. Apoptosis in murine tumors treated with chemotherapy agents. *Anticancer Drugs* 1995; 6:443–450.

64. Story MD, Voehringer DW, Malone CG, Hobbs ML, Meyn RE. Radiation-induced apoptosis in sensitive and resistant cells isolated from a mouse lymphoma. *Int J Radiat Biol* 1994; 66:659–668.

65. Mirkovic N, Voehringer DW, Story MD, McConkey DJ, McDonnell TJ, Meyn RE. Resistance to radiation-induced apoptosis in Bcl-2-expressing cells is reversed by depleting cellular thiols. *Oncogene* 1997; 15:1461–1470.

66. Story MD, Meyn RE. Modulation of apoptosis and enhancement of chemosensitivity by decreasing cellular thiols in a mouse B-cell lymphoma cell line that overexpresses bcl-2. *Cancer Chemother Pharmacol* 1999; 44:362–366.

67. Story MD, Mirkovic N, Hunter N, Meyn R. Bcl-2 expression correlates with apoptosis induction but not tumor growth delay in transplantable murine lymphomas treated with different chemotherapy drugs. *Cancer Chemother Pharmacol* 1999; 44:367–371.

68. French LE, Tschopp J. The trail to selective tumor death. *Nat Med* 1999; 5(2):146, 147.

34

Transparent Window Models and Intravital Microscopy

Imaging Gene Expression, Physiological Function, and Drug Delivery in Tumors

Rakesh K. Jain, PhD, Lance L. Munn, PhD, and Dai Fukumura, PhD, MD

CONTENTS

1. INTRODUCTION

The past 30 years have witnessed spectacular advances in our understanding of the molecular origins of cancer and other diseases. These advances have led to the identification of various genes associated with angiogenesis and oncogenesis, and to the development of a vast array of therapeutic agents. The grand challenges now are to relate the expression of these genes to their function in an intact organism, and to deliver these novel therapeutics to their targets in vivo *(70)*. Currently, gene expression, physiological function, and drug delivery are usually measured with techniques that are either destructive or have poor spatial resolution (millimeter to centimeter). The former have limited ability to provide insight into the dynamics, and the latter preclude visualization at the cellular and subcellular levels (1–10 µm).

Intravital microscopy of tumors in various organs grown in transparent windows can overcome these limitations and offer powerful insight into tumor physiology and drug delivery. Furthermore, the recent availability of in vivo reporters such as green fluorescent protein (GFP), as well as transgenic mice and cell lines, is likely to present new opportunities for unexpected discoveries.

From: *Tumor Models in Cancer Research*
Edited by: B. A. Teicher © Humana Press Inc., Totowa, NJ

Depending on the thickness of the preparation, either trans- or epi-illumination can be used to visualize all tissue or only its superficial regions. Based on the method, the tissue preparations can be divided into three broad categories: **chronic-transparent windows** such as the rabbit-ear chamber; dorsal skinfold chamber in mice, rats, hamsters, and rabbits; cranial windows in mice and rats; hamster-cheek-pouch-window (Fig. 1); **acute (exteriorized) tissue preparations** such as the hamster cheek pouch; mouse, rat or rabbit mesentery; mouse or rat liver; mouse or rat pancreas; air sac in mice and rats (Fig. 2); and *in situ* preparations such as the chick chorioallantoic membrane (CAM); corneal pocket or iris implant in the eye; mouse ear; or mouse-tail lymphatics (Fig. 3). Each of these preparations can be used to study normal tissue or an implanted tumor. The tumor source can be a suspension of cancer cells or a fragment of tumor tissue. For some applications, a gel containing defined growth factor(s) or engineered cells can be implanted in these tissue preparations *(73)*. Each preparation has its strengths and weaknesses. Thus, a combination of several methodologies is usually required to examine the effect of tissue microenvironment on gene expression, physiology, and drug delivery.

In this chapter, each section begins with a brief historical perspective followed by brief descriptions of the surgical procedures for making various tissue preparations.[a] We then outline the computer-assisted analyses/techniques used to extract parameters of interest from images acquired by intravital microscopy. Finally, we highlight key insights obtained from such approaches and possibilities for the future.

2. CHRONIC WINDOW PREPARATIONS

In 1924, Sandison developed the first transparent window (chamber) for implantation in the ear of a rabbit *(119)*. This chronic preparation allowed continuous, noninvasive, long-term monitoring of angiogenesis during wound healing *(22,23)*. Ide and colleagues *(64)* were the first to study angiogenesis in this window, using Brown-Pearce carcinoma.

In the 1940s, Algire adapted the Sandison chamber to the dorsal skin in mice, and conducted pioneering studies of angiogenesis during wound healing and tumor growth *(1–4)*. Similar chronic windows have been developed for the dorsal skin of other rodents such as rats and hamsters for the hamster cheek pouch, and for the cranium of the mouse and rat (*see* Table 1 for references).

Each of these chronic windows has its advantages and disadvantages. For example, the rabbit-ear chamber is perhaps the most optically clear. However, rabbits are expensive to purchase and maintain, and the granulation tissue takes 4–6 wk to mature before a tumor can be implanted in the window. Mice, hamsters, and rats are less expensive, and because of their smaller body wt (etc.), require smaller quantities of reagents. From the surgical point of view, rats and hamsters are easier to work with compared to mice, but the latter have many advantages. The easy availability of immunodeficient and genetically engineered mice as well as murine reagents has made mice the most

---

[a] All surgical procedures described in this Chapter should be performed under appropriate anesthesia (please refer to individual references for details) and with full approval by the institutional animal care and use committee. During the surgical procedure or intravital microscopy, animal body-core temperature should be maintained constant at 36–37°C, using a heating device.

Table 1
Examples of Various Intravital Preparations for Tumor Studies

Models	Species	Tumor	Year	References
Chronic window preparations				
Ear chamber	rabbit	Brown-Pearce CA*	1939	(64)
		VX2 CA-intra-arterial injection	1958	(135)
		VX2 CA-multifocal growth	1984	(29,114)
Dorsal skin chamber	mouse	various CAs, SAs*, melanomas	1943	(1,2)
		hepatoma 134	1961	(78)
		mammary CA	1971	(117)
	nude mouse	human amelanotic melanoma	1984	(34)
	SCID mouse	human tumor xenograft	1992	(91)
	hamster	amelanotic melanoma	1981	(5)
	rat	ascites hepatoma	1971	(136)
		rhabdomyosarcoma	1977	(118)
		rat SA	1979	(32,33)
		rat mammary CA	1989	(27)
Cranial window	rat and mouse	various rodent and human tumors	1994	(140)
Acute (exteriorized) preparations				
Cheek pouch	hamster	chemically induced SAs	1950	(97)
		human tumors	1952	(21,129)
		melanomas, CA, human angiopericytoma	1965	(52)
		malignant neurilemmoma	1973	(31)
Mesentery	rabbit	VX2 CA – intra-arterial injection	1961	(142)
	rat	murine colon CA	1990	(113,137)
Cremaster muscle	rat	Walker 256 CA, chondrosarcoma	1986	(59)
Liver	mouse	human adenocarcinoma	1997	(44)
Mammary gland	mouse	human mammary CA	1998	(107)
Pancreas	mouse	human pancreatic CA	1999	(122,133)
Lung	mouse	Lewis Lung CA	2000	(45)
In situ preparations				
Eye anterior chamber	frog	renal CA	1939	(96)
	guinea pig	human tumor	1952	(53)
Anterior chamber/ iris assays	rabbit	mouse mammary tumor	1976	(49)
		mouse mammary papilloma	1977	(13)
		hyperplastic rat mammary grand	1977	(99)
Comeal micropocket assay	rabbit	Brown-Pearce CA, VX2 CA	1974	(7,48)
	mouse	murine mammary CA and SA	1979	(109)
Tail lymphatics	mouse	murine fibrosarcoma	2000	(89)
Specialized models				
Individual microvessel perfusion	mouse	human adenocarcinoma	1996	(94)
Angiogenesis gel assay	mouse	various angiogenesis factors	1996	(25)
GFP used to track cancer cells	mouse	CHO cells, murine mammary CA, human adenocarcinoma	1997	(18,20, 92,110)
GFP used as an intravital gene reporter in transparent windows	transgenic mouse	murine mammary and liver CA	1998	(42)

* CA: carcinoma, SA: sarcoma

commonly used laboratory animals for cancer research. The dorsal chamber in mice is the most widely used chamber preparation because the surgery is less involved than some of the other preparations, and because of its longer history. The cranial window can be kept for up to 1 yr, compared to 30–40 d for the dorsal window, and along with the cheek pouch, is an immuno-privileged site. The main disadvantage of the cranial window is that the visualization of microvessels requires, in most cases, epi-illumination and the injection of a contrast agent such as fluorescent marker.

2.1. Procedures

2.1.1. RABBIT-EAR CHAMBER

Transparent chambers are surgically implanted in the ears of male New Zealand white rabbits (2–3 kg body wt) using the following procedure *(114,141)*.

1. The animal's ear is shaved, and four holes are punched in the ear, avoiding large blood vessels. The four holes consist of three outer perforations, which are used to position the chamber, and a central puncture (5.4-mm diameter) for housing the transparent window with the newly developing tissue.
2. The epidermis on both sides of the ear around the puncture is carefully retracted. A molded plate is placed on the inside of the ear and aligned with the existing holes, and a thin (approx 200 µm) cover of mica glass is positioned on the outside of the cartilage. The molded plate and the mica glass, which sandwich the central puncture to form the chamber, are fastened to each other by three threaded rods and six hex nuts.
3. The retracted skin is then pulled taut over the edges of the mica glass and molded plate to protect the exposed area. A light covering of antiseptic is administered, and two plastic covers are mounted to enclose and protect the chamber.
4. Granulation tissue grows in the chamber (thickness, 40 ± 5 µm; diameter, 5.4 mm) at an average of 8 d, and reaches maturity at approx 40 d postoperation. At this time, the chamber is ready for normal (granulation) tissue study or tumor implantation.
5. For tumor implantations *(114)* the cover glass, which forms the top plate of the transparent chamber, is carefully removed and a tumor, excised from the flank of a tumor-bearing host, is minced and placed in 0.9% NaCl solution and spread uniformly over the cover glass.
6. The cover glass is replaced flush against the intact normal tissue.
7. If this procedure causes tissue damage, the damaged tissue should be excluded from the study. Angiogenic response is observed 3–4 d post implant, and the tumor-bearing chamber is ready for intravital microscopy approx 10 d post implant.
8. For intravital microscopy, the animal is placed in a dorsal recumbent position in a cradle which restricts head movement while still maintaining proper circulation to the chamber. The ear containing the chamber is extended horizontally to the specimen plane of an intravital microscope. The chamber is secured to the microscope stage with an aluminum adapter *(114)*.

2.1.2. DORSAL-SKIN CHAMBER PREPARATION

Dorsal-skin chambers are implanted in mice using the following procedure *(91)*.

1. Prior to chamber implantation, the entire back of the animal is shaved and depilated, and two symmetrical titanium frames (weight 3.2. g)—mirror images of each other—are used to sandwich the extended double layer of skin.
2. One layer of skin is removed in a circular area approx 15 mm in diameter, and the remaining layer, consisting of epidermis, subcutaneous (sc) tissue, and striated muscle, is covered with a glass coverslip incorporated into one of the frames.

3. Following implantation of the transparent access chamber, animals are allowed to recover from microsurgery and anesthesia for 48 h before tumor implantation or in vivo microscopy studies.
4. For implantation of tumor cells/tissue or matrix gel, the animals are positioned in a transparent polycarbonate tube (inner diameter: 25 mm).
5. The coverslip of the chamber is carefully removed, and 2 μL of dense tumor-cell suspension (~2×10^5 cells), a small piece (1 mm in diameter) of tumor tissue or 20 μL of matrix gel is implanted at the center of the dorsal chamber. A new coverslip is then placed in the chamber.
6. The growth of the tumor and angiogenesis are monitored on a regular basis after implantation. The measurements of functional parameters are made when tumors have reached the desired size.
7. To obtain microcirculatory parameters, the mouse is positioned in a polycarbonate tube of approx 25 mm inner diameter, and tumors are observed with an intravital fluorescence microscope equipped with an intensified CCD camera, a regular CCD camera, a photomultiplier tube, and a S-VHS videocassette recorder.

2.1.3. CRANIAL WINDOW PREPARATION

Cranial windows are implanted in mice using the following procedure *(140)*.

1. The head of the animal is fixed by a stereotactic apparatus.
2. A longitudinal incision of the skin is made between the occiput and forehead. Then the skin is cut in a circular manner on top of the skull, and the periosteum underneath is scraped off to the temporal crests.
3. A 6-mm circle is drawn over the frontal and parietal regions of the skull bilaterally. Using a high-speed drill with a burr-tip, 0.5 mm in diameter, a groove is made on the margin of the drawn circle. This groove is made thinner by cautious and continuous drilling of the groove until the bone flap becomes loose.
4. Using a malis dissector, the bone flap is separated from the dura mater underneath. After removal of the bone flap, gelfoam is placed on the cutting edge, and the dura mater is continuously superfused with physiological saline.
5. A nick is made close to the sagittal sinus. Iris microscissors are passed through the nick. The dura and arachnoid membranes are cut completely from the surface of both hemispheres, avoiding any damage to the sagittal sinus.
6. A piece of the tumor tissue, 1 mm in diameter, or 20 μL of matrix gel is placed at the center of the window. The window is sealed with a 7-mm cover-glass, which is glued to the bone with histocompatible cyanoacrylate glue.
7. The growth of the tumor and angiogenesis are monitored on a regular basis after implantation.
8. The measurements of functional properties are made when tumors have reached the desired size. The animals are anesthetized and put on a polycarbonate plate. The surface of the cranial window is adjusted to be flat and perpendicular to the objective lens.

2.1.4. ANGIOGENESIS GEL ASSAY

Instead of using tumor fragments, a polymer matrix (gel/sponge) containing a known amount of angiogenic factor(s) or cells can be glued/attached to a vascular bed *(25,30,35,81,98,112,115,116)*. The structure and function of new vessels penetrating the matrix can be measured in a variety of ways *(35,67,69)*. The matrix implant technique combined with the microcirculatory preparations in the dorsal skin-fold chambers and the cranial windows in immunodeficient mice allow investigation into the

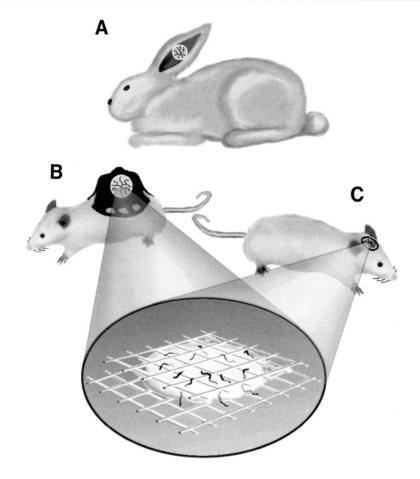

Fig. 1. Chronic window preparations. Rabbit ear chamber (A), mouse dorsal-skin chamber (B), cranial window (C), and gel implantation models (D) are used for high-resolution longitudinal observation of tumor growth, angiogenesis, physiological processes, and gene expression. Adapted from ref. *69.*

effect of different growth factors sequestered in the matrix on angiogenesis into the polymer gels *(25)* (Fig. 1). As a direct application of this method, we demonstrated that the angiogenesis in these gels placed in the cranial windows can be suppressed by a tumor grown elsewhere in the animal *(51,56,123).*

A common problem associated with various assays of vascularization into matrix implants is the nonspecific host response to the matrix implantation. A significant angiogenic response has been observed without any stimulation with exogenous growth factors *(25,112).* Therefore, caution should be exercised when interpreting the data. Only the amount of angiogenesis relative to the controls should be considered as the response to the exogenous angiogenic factors.

The following procedure describes the gel assay *(25)* (Fig. 1):

1. A known amount of growth factor (e.g., 60 ng of human recombinant basic fibroblast growth factor (bFGF) or vascular endothelial growth factor (VEGF) is mixed with 2.4 µL of 0.1% bovine serum albumin, 6.5 mg sucralfate, 17.6 µL vitrogen 100 (a type 1

collagen), neutralized to pH 7.4 by addition of 1 part sodium bicarbonate solution (11.76g/dL), and 1 part 10 × minimal essential medium to 8 parts vitrogen.

2. 20 μL of this mixture (3,000 ng/mL bFGF or VEGF) is sandwiched between two nylon meshes (3×3-mm).

3. 8–10 d following cranial-window implantation, the coverslip is removed, and the collagen gel is transferred onto the pial surface. The cranial window is closed again with a glass coverslip, avoiding pressure on the gel and air bubbles in the preparation.

4. For quantification of angiogenesis in the gel, mice are anesthetized with ketamine/xylazine (90 mg/9 mg per kg body wt) and positioned on a stereotactic apparatus.

5. Under a dissecting microscope, the number of squares in the top nylon mesh containing at least one vessel is counted with a 2× objective. Angiogenic response is determined as the number of squares containing at least one vessel divided by the total number of squares.

3. ACUTE (EXTERIORIZED) PREPARATIONS

For visualization of tumors grown in internal organs, it is necessary to surgically exteriorize these organs to place them on a microscope stage. The mesentery of mice, rats, and cats has been extensively used for intravital microscopy of microcirculation *(60,62,82–84,105)*. Since only two layers of thin membrane cover the microvessels in the mesentery, this model provides the best optical quality for in vivo microcirculation studies. On the other hand, preparation of intact mesenteric microcirculation requires extremely careful technique and much experience, because the mesentery is quite vulnerable to physical stress. Furthermore, repeated or long-term observation is not feasible. In addition to normal vessels, mesentery can be used to study peritoneal dissemination of tumors *(137,142)*.

It is generally accepted that the host microenvironment influences tumor biology, including gene expression, angiogenesis, physiological functions, tumor growth, invasion, metastasis, and responses to antitumor treatments. Therefore, the use of orthotopic tumor models is necessary to obtain rigorous understanding in tumor pathophysiology and design of antitumor treatments *(37)*. Orthotopic tumor models include the liver *(44,108)*, pancreas *(133)*, and the mammary gland *(107)*. These preparations have provided unprecedented insights into the effect of host-tumor interactions on tumor biology and response to therapy.

3.1. Procedures

3.1.1. MESENTERY

The following procedure can be used for mice and rats *(71)*.

1. Animals fast for 24 h prior to the observation.

2. After the anesthesia and hair removal of abdominal skin, the abdomen is opened with a midline incision. The ileocecal portion is exteriorized and the intestinal loop is gently developed onto the thin glass part of a polyacrylate stage using a saline-immersed cotton swab, avoiding direct contact with and and tension to the mesentery.

3. The intestine is gently straightened and fixed by cotton sponges immersed in warmed saline, so that the mesentery does not unfold. The mesentery is kept moist and warm by superfusion with warm saline (37°C).

4. The mesenteric microcirculation is observed with an inverted or upright intravital microscope using a 20–40 × objective lens with transillumination or epifluorescence illumination in combination with appropriate tracers.

3.1.2. LIVER TUMOR PREPARATION

The liver is the most common and critical site for distant metastasis of colorectal carcinomas. The liver-tumor metastasis model is prepared by performing a splenic injection of tumor cells *(44)*.

1. A small incision is made in the left lateral flank, the spleen is exteriorized, and tumor cells ($1–5 \times 10^6$ cells in 100 µL) injected into the spleen just under the capsule.
2. The spleen is replaced into the peritoneal cavity. The two layers of incision (skin and abdominal wall) are closed with metal wound-clips.
3. The metal clips are removed 1 wk later.
4. Three to four weeks after the tumor-cell injection, the abdominal wall is opened with a midline incision for examination. The functional parameters are measured on tumor foci of approx 3–5 mm in diameter.
5. The main liver lobe with metastatic tumors is gently exteriorized and held by a liver support device. This liver support allows adjustment of the three-dimensional position and angle of the top surface.
6. A circular glass coverslip is fixed by cyanoacrylate adhesive onto the bottom surface of the liver lobe, and this cover glass is fixed to the liver support with denture adhesive cream.
7. The top tissue surface is adjusted flat and perpendicular to the objective lens.
8. The circular glass coverslip, attached to the metal ring support, is gently applied onto the top surface of the tumor or normal liver tissue.

3.1.3. PANCREATIC TUMOR PREPARATION

Pancreatic cancer has a poor prognosis, and treatment strategies conducted from pre-clinical research have not succeeded in extending patient survival appreciably. This newly developed abdominal window allows both direct intravital microscopy and chronic observation during pancreatic tumor growth and the response to treatment *(133)*.

1. For tumor implantation, a portion of the skin and the abdominal wall of the left flank are cut in a linear manner, and a small left lateral laparotomy is performed, matching the position of pancreas and avoiding damage to the vasculature.
2. The tail and body of the pancreas are gently exteriorized from the abdominal cavity.
3. A small piece of tumor is fixed to the serosal side of the pancreas with a 5-0 prolene suture.
4. The abdominal wall and the skin are sutured and closed.
5. When tumors become 6–8 mm in diameter (approx 4 wk after tumor implantation), an abdominal-wall window is implanted to observe tumor microcirculation.
6. To implant the abdominal-wall window, the skin and abdominal wall over the pancreas are reopened, and the tail and body of the pancreas with a growing tumor (located near the spleen) are gently exteriorized.
7. A portion of normal pancreas is sutured to the outer side of the abdominal wall with a 5-0 prolene suture to keep the pancreas and the tumor outside the abdominal cavity.
8. A titanium ring with 8 holes around the edge is attached with sutures to the abdominal wall. This holds the pancreas and tumor inside the window.
9. A circular glass coverslip (11 mm in diameter) is placed on top to seal the window.
10. For the subsequent intravital microscopy, mice are anesthetized, and the tail vein is cannulated for intravenous (iv) injection of fluorescent tracers.
11. The mice are placed inside a plastic tube (25-mm inside diameter) with a slit of 14 mm × 37 mm width.

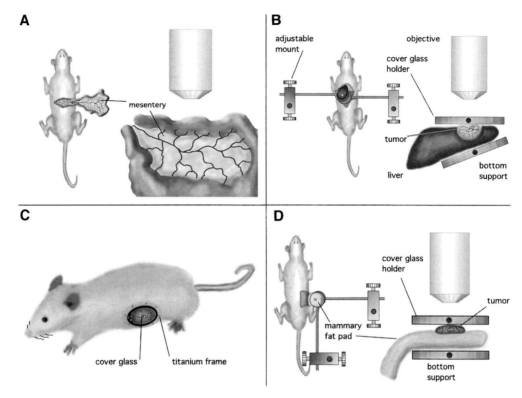

Fig. 2. Acute tissue preparations. Mesentery (A), mouse liver (B), pancreas (C), and mammary fat-pad models (D) are used for acute observations and/or organ-specific tumor microcirculation. Tumor size, angiogenesis and physiological parameters, and gene expression are determined by intravital microscopy.

12. The abdominal window fits in the slit of the plastic tube, and is fixed by an adhesive tape.

3.1.4. MAMMARY FAT-PAD TUMOR PREPARATION

Breast cancer is a leading cause of death in women. The mouse mammary fat pad serves as an orthotopic site for breast cancer (Fig. 2) *(107)*.

1. Breast carcinoma cells are injected into the mammary fat pad just inferior to the nipple of female mice.
2. Four to six weeks later, tumors grow to ~5–8 mm in diameter. A midline incision is made through the skin and fascia, and a flap is gently elevated by blunt dissection with care to avoid disruption of the vasculature and irritation of the tumor vessels.
3. The flap is then placed on a specially designed stage developed for the liver preparation, and a glass coverslip is placed over the tumor to allow intravital microscopy and analysis of microvascular parameters.

4. *IN SITU* PREPARATIONS

The anterior chamber of the eye is a natural site for observing tumor growth, and implantation on the iris and in a corneal pocket are two assays used extensively for this purpose *(7,13,48–50,79,99,109,125)*. Of the two assays, the corneal pocket is more

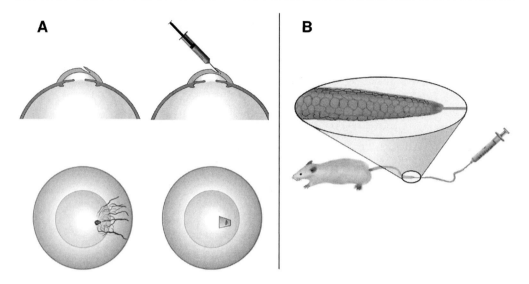

Fig. 3. *In situ* preparations. Cornea pocket assay (A) and mouse tail lymphatic model (B) are *in situ* preparations to study angiogenesis and lymphangiogenesis. (Adapted from ref. *73*).

widely used (for review, see ref. *(79)*. Because of the three-dimensional nature of vessel growth, it is difficult to quantify the vascular response, except in the early stages when the vessel length/number can be assessed. Some investigators have quantified the vascular response by perfusing the cornea with colloidal carbon, and then measuring vascular length using computer-assisted image analysis *(79)*.

Originally developed for rabbits, the corneal micropocket assay (Fig. 3) has been also adapted for rats and mice *(109,121)*. Although it is less expensive to use rats and mice than rabbits, surgery becomes more difficult as the size of the eye gets smaller. Since the rat/mouse cornea is thinner than in rabbits, the three-dimensional growth of vessels is limited in these rodent models.

The CAM is also commonly used with the shell intact, or partially or completely removed *(6,39,87,112)*. This is an inexpensive and widely used angiogenic assay. To eliminate the inflammatory response developed in the 7- to 8-d-old CAM, the vitelline membrane of 4-d-old chick embryo has also been used *(128)*. Because of the difficulty in precisely quantifying newly formed vessels, the CAM assay has been used primarily for screening purposes. However, Nguyen et al. have modified this assay for easy quantification *(112)*. The CAM has also proven useful for analyzing the efficiency of metastatic cell extravasation and colonization *(80)*, and for studying the kinetics of gene expression in metastasizing cells *(124)*.

Finally, lymphatic microvasculature has been studied by adapting lymphangiography to the mouse tail *(9,74,90,127)*. In this technique, a high mol-wt tracer bound to (FITC) is injected into the interstitial compartment of the tail tissue (Fig. 3). The tracer is absorbed by the local lymphatic vessels and carried proximally to the base of the tail. By implanting tumor in the tail, the structure and function of the lymphatics at the tumor periphery can be monitored *(89)*.

4.1. Procedures

4.1.1. Corneal Pocket Assay

The following procedure for the corneal pocket assay in rabbits *(48)* can be used for mice, with modifications *(109)*.

1. After anesthesia and retrobulbar infiltration with 2% Xylocaine, the eye is moved forward and secured in position by a fold clamped in the lower lid.
2. A superficial incision, 1.5 mm long, is made with a surgical blade in the corneal dome to one side of its center. Intra-ocular tension is reduced by draining a small amount of aqueous humor from the anterior chamber through a 27-gauge needle.
3. A malleable iris spatula (1.5 mm width) is inserted, and an oblong pocket is fashioned within the corneal stroma. Peripheral pockets end 1–2 mm from the limbus.
4. A small piece of minced tumor or gel (5–10 µL) is deposited in the bottom of the pocket, which then seals spontaneously.
5. Eyes with corneal implants are observed with a stereomicroscope. Tumor and new-vessel growth are measured *en face* with an ocular micrometer at 10×. A green filter allows clearer definition of fine vascular channels developing within the cornea.

4.1.2. Chick Chorioallantoic Membrane

1. Fertilized White Leghorn chick eggs are incubated at 37°C and 60% relative humidity for 8–12 d *(17,102,112,124)*.
2. To apply tumor cells or a matrix gel implant, large vessels in the CAM are identified, a window (~1 cm^2) is cut with an electric drill in the shell over the CAM, and either a small section or the entire shell is removed, leaving the CAM intact. In studies in which the CAM is removed entirely from the shell, it is carefully placed in a Petri dish.
3. Tumor cells *(17)* or matrix implant *(112)* are placed on top of the CAM or fluorescence-labeled tumor cells are injected into CAM vein ($1–4 \times 10^5$ cells in 0.1 mL) *(102,124)*.
4. Angiogenesis in the gel or tumor growth is determined with a dissecting-microscope *(17,112)*.
5. Surviving tumor cells are visualized by intravital microscopy with epifluorescence illumination *(102,124)*.

4.1.3. Tail Lymphatics

Female *nu/nu* mice are used for normal and tumor lymphangiography as aggressiveness of this gender (fewer tail wounds, which interrupt the lymphatic network). In the *nu/nu* mice, there is also no need for hair removal prior to observation. As a precaution, however, the animals are housed separately prior to observation in order to prevent bite wounds in the tail.

1. For studies of tumor growth in the tail model, a single-cell suspension of tumor cells must be prepared: tumor tissue is harvested, minced and digested by trypsin until a uniform solution is formed.
2. For tumor implantation, a 26-gauge needle is used to inject the single-cell suspension, intradermally puncturing the tail skin approx 1 cm from the distal tip. Great care is taken to avoid lacerating the tail veins. Approximately 0.2 mL of single-cell suspension is injected into the tail.
3. The mouse is monitored for tumor growth in the tail (~ 4 wk depending on growth rate).
4. For microlymphangiography, the mouse is placed on cover sponges and its tail is taped to a metal board using double-stick tape. A strip of tape is place over the hips to secure the mouse to the metal board.

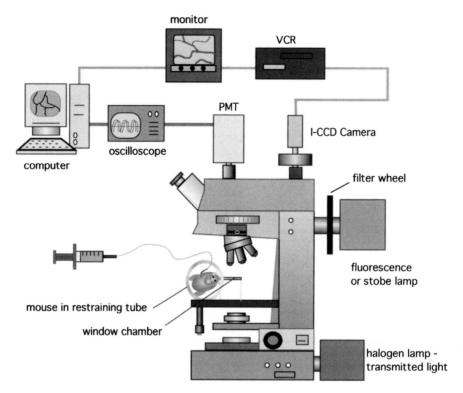

Fig. 4. Intravital microscopy work station. Mouse tumor models are observed using intravital microscopy. With appropriate tracer molecules and/or engineered vectors/cells and computer-assisted image analysis, one can monitor tumor size, vessel density, vessel diameter, RBC velocity, leukocyte endothelial interaction, vascular permeability, tissue pO_2, pH, gene-promoter activity, enzyme activity, and delivery of drugs, including genes.

5. A 30-gauge needle connected to a constant pressure source is used to inject fluorescein-5-isothiocyanate (FITC) dextran (2 million MW) into the interstitial space of the distal tail. The injection is made superficially into the skin above the tumor. Using a syringe, the pressure can be increased to allow filling of peri-tumor lymphatics.
6. The mouse tail is visualized by fluorescence intravital microscopy. The images are captured, digitized, and analyzed.

5. INTRAVITAL MICROSCOPY AND IMAGE ANALYSIS

5.1. Intravital Microscopy Work Station

The microscopy workstation consists of an upright or inverted microscope equipped with transillumination and fluorescence epi-illumination, a flashlamp excitation device, two independent outlet ports, two separate eyepiece units, a motorized X-Y stage with a ±1.0-μm lateral resolution, a set of fluorescence filters, a motor-controlled filter wheel, a CCD camera, an intensified CCD camera, a video monitor, a photomultiplier tube, a dual-trace digital oscilloscope, a video recorder, and a frame-grabber board for image digitization (Fig. 4) *(11,44,58)*.

To obtain tumor size, tumor dimensions are measured at low magnification. To obtain microcirculatory parameters, randomly selected areas (3–6 locations/tumor or

Day 5 **Day 10** **Day 15** **Day 20**

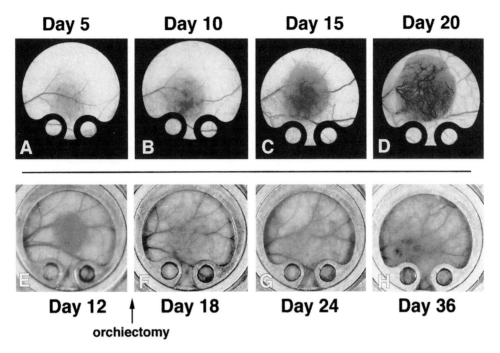

Day 12 ↑ **Day 18** **Day 24** **Day 36**

orchiectomy

Fig. 5. Tumor growth and angiogenesis in a human colon carcinoma (A-D) and regression in a Shionogi mouse mammary carcinoma in the dorsal skin chamber (E-H). Panels A-D: At d 5 after tumor-cell implantation, enlargement of host vessels is observed and by d 10, occasional hemorrhage and sprout formation occurs. At d 15, tumor growth and further angiogenesis become apparent. By d 20, the tumor is fully vascularized. (Adapted from ref. *91*) Panels E-H: (E) 12-d tumor prior to orchiectomy; 3 d (F) and 9 d (G) after orchiectomy, the tumor vessels regress and the tumor shrinks. A second wave of angiogenesis is evident in (H). (Adapted from ref. *72*).

animal) are investigated using a long working-distance objective with appropriate magnification. The parameters that can routinely be measured include: tumor size, angiogenesis, hemodynamics, vascular permeability, leukocyte endothelial interactions, interstitial pH interstitial and microvascular pO_2, interstitial diffusion, convection and binding, and gene-promoter activity.

5.2. Tumor Growth and Regression

To measure two-dimensional tumor size, low-power transillumination or epiillumination images are digitized and analyzed using an image-processing system *(72)*. Tumor volume is calculated from the two-dimensional tumor surface area and depth, if available *(134)* (Fig. 5).

5.3. Vascular Parameters

5.3.1. ANGIOGENESIS AND HEMODYNAMICS

To visualize microvessels, 100 µL of FITC-Dextran (MW 2 million, 10 mg/mL) is injected into the tail vein of mice. During each observation period, FITC-fluorescence images are recorded for 60 s, and the videotapes are analyzed off-line using the following methods.

1. The vessel diameter in μm (D) is measured using an image-shearing device *(75)*.
2. The red-blood cell (RBC) velocity (V_{RBC}) is measured by temporal correlation velocimetry, using a four-slit apparatus connected to a personal computer *(65)*.
3. The mean blood-flow rate of individual vessels (Q) is calculated using D and the mean V_{RBC} (V_{mean}). $Q = \pi/4 \times V_{mean} \times D^2$, where $V_{mean} = V_{RBC}/a$ (a = 1.3, for blood vessels < 10 μm; linear extrapolation 1.3 < a < 1.6 for blood vessels 10 and 15 μm; and a = 1.6 for blood vessels > 15 μm) *(95)*.
4. The functional vessel density, a measure of angiogenesis, defined as the total length of vessels per unit area (cm/cm^2), and the tortuosity, defined as the mean length of non-branching segment (μm), are analyzed using an image-processing system *(43,44,73)*. The vessel volume density, defined as the total volume of vessels per unit area ($\mu m^3/\mu m^2$), is calculated from vessel data and length data *(55)*.
5. Fractal dimensions of vessels can be measured as described elsewhere *(8,46)*.

5.3.2. VASCULAR PERMEABILITY

The effective vascular permeability can be measured using the following procedure *(43,106,139,140)*.

1. After bolus injection of a fluorescent tracer (e.g., Rho or Cy5-labeled bovine serum albumin (BSA) or other molecule, 10 mg/mL; 0.1 mL/25 g body wt), the fluorescence intensity of the tumor tissue is intermittently measured for 20 min.
2. The value of P is calculated as $P = (1-HT) V/S \{1/(I_o - I_b) * dI/dt + 1/K\}$, where I is the average fluorescence intensity of the whole image, I0 is the value of I immediately after the filling of all vessels by the fluorescent tracer, and Ib is the background fluorescence intensity. The average hematocrit (HT) of tumor vessels is estimated independently *(14)*. V and S are the total volume and surface area of vessels within the tissue volume covered by the surface image, respectively. The time constant of clearance of the tracer from plasma (K) is measured independently *(140)*.

5.3.3. LEUKOCYTE ENDOTHELIAL INTERACTIONS

The flux of leukocytes, as well as the number of rolling and adhering leukocytes, is measured as follows *(41)*.

1. Mice are injected with a bolus (20 μL) of 0.1% rhodamine-6G in 0.9% saline through the tail vein and leukocytes are visualized via an intensified CCD camera and recorded on S-VHS tape.
2. The numbers of rolling (Nr) and adhering (Na) leukocytes are counted for 30 s along a 100-μm segment of a vessel. The total flux of cells for 30 s is also measured (Nt).
3. The equations for calculating the ratio of rolling cells to total flux (rolling count), the density of adhering leukocytes (adhesion density), and the shear rate for each vessel are as follows: rolling count (%) = $100 \times Nr/Nt$, adhesion density (cells/mm²) = $10^6 \times Na/\pi \times D \times 100$ μm), Shear rate = $8 \times Vmean/D$.

5.4. Extravascular Parameters

5.4.1. INTERSTITIAL pH MEASUREMENTS

Fluorescence ratio imaging microscopy (FRIM) for pH, its implementation, application to thick tissues, and calibration are performed as previously described (Fig. 6) *(24,58)*.

1. The cell-impermeant form of the pH-sensitive fluorochrome 2′,7′-*bis*-(2-carboxyethyl)-5,6-carboxyfluorescein (BCECF; 0.7 mg/kg intravenously is used.

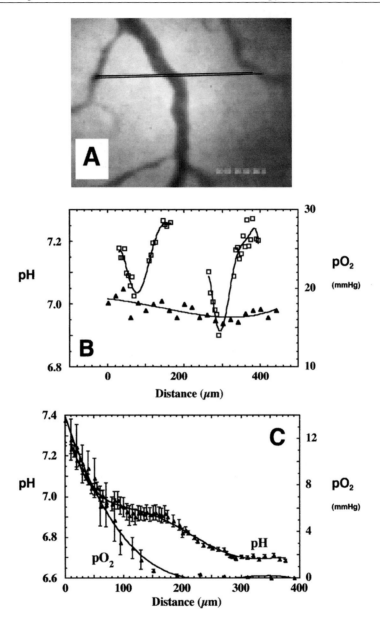

Fig. 6. Noninvasive, intravital pO_2 and pH measurements. **(A)** Trans-illumination image of a LS174T tumor grown in the dorsal-skin chamber; **(B)** Corresponding interstitial pH (open symbols) and pO_2 (closed symbols) profiles; and **(C)** Average profiles of interstitial pO_2 and pH when moving away from the blood vessel wall (SEM shown, n=24 profiles, N=7 tumors). Solid bar in **(A)** represents the scanning line (400 μm). (Adapted from ref. *58*).

2. Emission intensities (570 nm) are imaged through the CCD camera port following sequential excitations at 440 and 495 nm. A sampling depth of ≤25 μm and a lateral spatial resolution of 5 μm are obtained using a 400-μm pinhole in the light excitation pathway and a 40X water-immersion objective.

3. The X-Y stage is cycled through the same locations for dynamic measurements.
4. The ratio of intensities is converted into pH using the calibration curves.

5.4.2. INTERSTITIAL AND MICROVASCULAR pO₂ MEASUREMENTS

The technique is based on the O_2-dependent phosphorescence quenching of albumin-bound palladium meso-tetra (4-carboxyphenyl) porphyrin *(58,130–132)*.

1. The porphyrin probe is injected (60 mg/kg) into the mouse tail vein.
2. The phosphorescence signal resulting from flashlamp excitation (540 nm) of the tissue is detected at ≥630 nm using the photomultiplier tube and averaged on the oscilloscope prior to computer storage.
3. The X-Y stage is cycled through the same tumor locations used for the pH measurements.
4. The illumination field is reduced to a 100-μm spot, and a 10×10 μm² slit is placed in the light emission pathway. This reduces the sampling depth to ≤25 μm and gives a lateral spatial resolution of 10 μm, similar to the pH measurements.
5. A second eyepiece, placed between the slit and the collecting tube, allows refocusing on the region of interest prior to measurements of phosphorescence decay.
6. Phosphorescence measurements are valid within interstitial spaces as well as blood vessels.
7. Data are converted to pO_2 values according to a standard calibration method *(85)*.

Calibration tests have revealed an excellent linearity ($r^2 \geq 0.99$) between pO_2 (0–60 mmHg) and the inverse of lifetime values. Moreover, the pO_2 calibration curves do not show any dependence on the pH of the solution (pH range: 6.60–7.40), which makes this porphyrin an ideal probe for use in tumors. We have also shown that sequential measurements of pH and pO_2 in tissues in vivo are possible (Fig. 6), since the presence of the pH probe (BCECF) does not affect lifetime measurements of the pO_2 probe (porphyrin) *(58)*.

5.4.3. INTERSTITIAL DIFFUSION, CONVECTION, AND BINDINGS

Fluorescence recovery after photobleaching (FRAP) with spatial Fourier analysis, its implementation, application to thick tissues, and calibration performed as described in *(10,11)*.

1. A fluorescently labeled molecule of interest is infused into the tumor interstitium either through extravasation or low-pressure microinfusion.
2. A brief (~milliseconds) flash of focused laser light bleaches out a subpopulation of the fluorescent molecules.
3. Consecutive images of the bleached region are generated via epifluorescence and captured on the CCD camera as unbleached fluorophore diffuse back into the bleached region. During the bleaching flash, the camera is shuttered to avoid damage to the electronics.
4. Spatial Fourier analysis of the fluorescence recovery images is performed as described in *(10,11,19)* to extract diffusion coefficients, convection velocity, and binding parameters.

5.4.4. GENE EXPRESSION: PROMOTER ACTIVITY VIA GFP IMAGING

To monitor gene-promoter activity in stromal and tumor cells, a fluorescent reporter gene driven by the promoter of interest is introduced into mice *(42)* and/or tumor cells *(40)*. Once the gene is activated, the corresponding cells become fluorescent and the fluorescence intensity is measured. Currently, the most commonly used reporter gene is

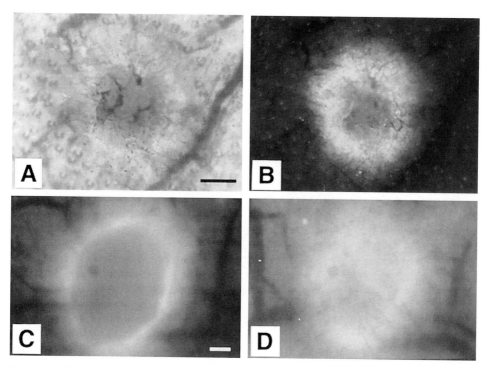

Fig. 7. VEGF promoter activity during wound healing and tumor growth. Transillumination **(A)** and GFP fluorescence image **(B)** of a wound 2 wk after the wound creation in the ear of ^VEGF^EGFP mice; and GFP images of murine hepatoma Hcal grown in the dorsal skin chamber in the ^VEGF^EGFP mice 2 wk **(C)** and 3 wk **(D)** after the implantation. Mice bearing ^VEGF^EGFP transgene show cellular green fluorescence around the healing margins and throughout granulation tissue of superficial ulcerative wounds (A,B). Implantation of solid tumors in the transgenic mice leads to an accumulation of green fluorescence, resulting from tumor induction of VEGF promoter activity in host stromal cells. With time, the fluorescent cells invade the tumor and can be seen throughout the tumor mass (C, D). In both, wound and tumor models, the predominant GFP-positive cells are fibroblasts *(42)*. The finding that the VEGF promoter of nontransformed cells is strongly activated by the tumor microenvironment points to a need to analyze and understand stromal-cell collaboration in tumor angiogenesis. The bars in panels A and C indicate 500 μm for A/B and C/D, respectively (Adapted from ref. *42*).

GFP. However, as other variants of GFP become available, the possibility of monitoring multiple genes at once or gene activation in different cell populations will become practical. GFP fluorescence (emission: 509 nm) is imaged through the intensified CCD camera following excitation at 488 nm (Fig. 7). In order to obtain quantitative data on the promoter activity in vivo, a deconvolution algorithm must be used to account for the kinetics of GFP decay and the relationship between protein levels and the fluorescence emitted by GFP.

6. NOVEL INSIGHTS

Our laboratory has a long-standing tradition of developing techniques to measure physiological parameters from intravital microscopy. Some of these developments are listed in Table 2, and the resulting novel insights are summarized here.

Table 2
Examples of Non-Invasive Techniques Developed in Authors' Laboratory

Technique	References
Vascular parameters	
Microvascular permeability of normal and neoplastic tissues	*(47)*
Microvascular permeability of albumin, tumor vascular surface area, and vascular volume	*(139)*
Pore cut-off size of tumor vessels	*(61,138)*
Perfusion of single-tumor microvessels: Application to vascular permeability measurement	*(93,94)*
Effect of RBCs on leukocyte-endothelial interactions	*(104)*
Extravascular parameters	
Fluorescence ratio imaging of pH gradients: calibration and application in normal and tumor tissues	*(100,101)*
Noninvasive measurement of microvascular and interstitial oxygen profiles in a human tumor xenograft	*(131)*
Simultaneous high-resolution measurements of interstitial pH and pO_2 gradients in solid tumors in vivo	*(58)*
Direct measurement of interstitial diffusion and convection of albumin in normal and neoplastic tissues using fluorescence photobleaching	*(19)*
Fluorescence photobleaching with spatial Fourier analysis for measurement of diffusion and binding in tumors	*(10,11)*
Flow velocity in the superficial lymphatic network of the mouse tail	*(9,90,127)*
Gene expression using intravital reporter	*(42)*
Cell identification using endogenous GFP	*(18)*

The ability to deliver therapeutic agents to all regions of a tumor is governed by the tumor blood supply. Using in vivo microscopy, we and others have unequivocally demonstrated that the structure and function of tumor vessels is heterogeneous *(27,29,32,91)*, and suggested the possibility that the presence of cancer cells of the vessel wall may contribute to this heterogeneity *(18,120)*. Furthermore, our finding that cancer cells co-opt the host cells into making VEGF, a potent angiogenic molecule, reveals the importance of host cells *(42,134)*: host cells are not passive bystanders, but are active participants in tumor angiogenesis, growth, and response to therapy.

These concepts bring together a number of key observations made in our laboratory: 1) Angiogenesis, pO_2, pH, permeability, and pore cut-off size in tumor vessels vary from one tumor to the next, from one region to the next within the same tumor, from one day to the next, and from one anatomical site to the next *(44,58,140)*. 2) The production of angiogenic inhibitors, similar to angiogenic stimulators, is dependent on the site of primary tumor growth *(51)* and changes in response to treatment *(56)*. 3) Surprisingly, in a hormone-dependent tumor, hormone withdrawal causes apoptosis of endothelial cells prior to that of cancer cells by downregulating the production of VEGF by cancer cells. A second wave of angiogenesis is then driven by VEGF, presumably, from host cells *(72)*. 4) One would expect anti-angiogenic therapy to impair drug delivery by inducing vessels regression. However, in the initial phases, these therapies may prune immature vessels and induce a normal vascular network with more mature vessels, thus explaining the potential synergism between anti-angiogenic and cytotoxic therapies *(55,72,86)*.

Lymphangiography of a fibrosarcoma in the mouse tail model has shown that the lymphatics are impaired within the tumor mass, and yet enlarged at the tumor periphery *(89)*. The former contributes to interstitial hypertension in tumors, a barrier to drug delivery *(68)*. The latter, presumably induced by VEGF-C, facilitates lymphatic metastasis *(74)*. The impairment of intratumor lymphatics presumably results from solid stress generated by proliferating cancer cells *(57)*. Releasing this solid stress should thus open lymphatics, lower pressure, and increase delivery of agents across tumor vessels *(54)*.

Once a therapeutic agent has extraveseted from a blood vessel, it must migrate through the interstitial matrix to reach cancer cells *(66)*. Using FRAP, our lab has provided the first—and to our knowledge, the only measurements of interstitial diffusion, convection, and binding in vivo *(11,19)*. Furthermore, we showed that the anomalous assembly of collagen in tumors can prevent the penetration of therapeutic agents *(111)*. This finding identified collagen synthesis as a potential target for improving the delivery of macromolecules.

In an attempt to understand heterogeneous localization of activated lymphocytes to tumor vessels, we discovered that angiogenic agents regulate adhesion molecules on the vasculature. This finding provided the first link between the disparate fields of angiogenesis and adhesion. For example, we showed that VEGF upregulates while bFGF downregulates adhesion molecules on the vasculature *(26,103)*. This is one of the rare occasions in which two molecules act synergistically for one function but antagonistically for another. This finding also provides a new mechanism of immune evasion by bFGF.

7. FUTURE PERSPECTIVES

Intravital microscopy has provided useful insight into angiogenesis and tumor biology *(16,36,38,76)*. However, two key challenges remain: first, the most widely used microscopy techniques are surface-weighted. Given the heterogeneous nature of tumors, we need dynamic information about the internal environment of tumors. Confocal microscopy can provide images up to a few hundred micrometers in depth *(28,126)*. The advent of multi-photon microscopy is likely to change this limit to over 500 micrometers, depending on the tissue and tracer used *(15,77,88)*. Other optical methods such as optical coherence tomography can image deeper regions, but are still in the development phase, and not widely available *(12,63)*. With more research in this area, we may some day be able to obtain dynamic images of the whole tumor with high spatial resolution.

The second limitation of window models is that they are currently restricted to the study of transplanted (as opposed to spontaneous) tumors. In principle, it should be possible to place windows on spontaneous tumors, but this has not been done yet. Alternatively, mice could be engineered with tissue-specific promoters, so that tumors spontaneously arise in regions where the windows described in this chapter can be used.

With these improvements in microscopy and animal models, in vivo microscopy will continue to offer new opportunities for unexpected discoveries in tumor biology as well as cancer detection and treatment.

ACKNOWLEDGMENTS

The work described here was supported by grants from the National Institutes of Health, National Science Foundation, American Cancer Society, United States Army, National Foundation for Cancer Research, and the Whitaker Foundation.

This chapter is based on two previous related reviews:

1. Jain RK, Schlenger K, Hockel M and Yuan F. Quantitative angiogenesis assays: progress and problems. *Nat Med* 1997; 3:1203–1208.
2. Jain RK, Munn LL, Fukumura D, Melder RJ. *In vitro* and *in vivo* quantification of adhesion between leukocytes and vascular endothelium. *In:* Morgan and Yarmush, eds. *Methods in Molecular Medicine—Tissue Engineering Methods and Protocols,* Vol. 18. Humana Press, Totowa, NJ, 1998, pp. 553–575.

We thank the publishers for allowing us to reproduce the relevant material. We also thank Drs. A. Kadambi, E. Brown, Y. Izumi, F. Yuan, and T. Padera for their helpful input in preparing this chapter.

REFERENCES

1. Algire GH. An adaptation of the transparent chamber technique to the mouse. *J Natl Cancer Inst* 1943; 4:1–11.
2. Algire GH. Microscopic studies of the early growth of a transplantable melanoma of the mouse, using the transparent-chamber technique. *J Natl Cancer Inst* 1943; 4:13–20.
3. Algire GH, Chalkley HW. Vascular reactions of normal and malignant tissues in vivo. I. Vascular reactions of mice to wounds and to normal and neoplastic transplants. *J Natl Cancer Inst* 1945; 6:73–85.
4. Algire GH, Legallis Y. Growth and vascularization of transplanted mouse melanomas. NY *Acad Sci Ann* 1948; 4:159–175.
5. Asaishi K, Endrich B, Gotz Y, Messmer K. Quantitative analysis of microvascular structure and function in the amelanotic melanoma A-Mel-3. *Cancer Res* 1981; 41:p. 1898–1904.
6. Auerbach R, Arensman R, Kubai L, Folkman J. Tumor-induced angiogenesis: lack of inhibition by irradiation. *Int J Cancer* 1975; 15:241–245.
7. Ausprunk DH, Folkman J. Migration and proliferation of endothelial cells in preformed and newly formed blood vessels during tumor angiogenesis. *Microvasc Res* 1977; 14:53–65.
8. Baish JW, Jain RK. Fractals and Cancer. *Cancer Res* 2000; 60:3683–3688.
9. Berk DA, Swartz MA, Leu AJ, Jain RK. Transport in lymphatic capillaries. II. Microscopic velocity measurement with fluorescence photobleaching. *Am J Physiol* 1996; 270(1 Pt 2):H330–H337.
10. Berk NDA, Yuan F, Leunig M, Jain RK. Fluorescence photobleaching with spatial Fourier analysis: measurement of diffusion in light-scattering media. *Biophys J* 1993; 65(6):2428–2436.
11. Berk DA, Yuan F, Leunig M, Jain RK. Direct in vivo measurement of targeted binding in a human tumor xenograft. *Proc Nat Acad Sci USA* 1997; 94:1785–1790.
12. Boppart S, Herrmann J, Pitris C, Stamper D, Brezinski M, Fujimoto J. High resolution optical coherence tomography-gulded laser ablation of surgical tissue. *J Surgical Res* 1999; 82:275–284.
13. Brem SS, Gullino PM, Medina D. Angiogenesis: a marker for neoplastic transformation of mammary papillary hyperplasia. *Science* 1977; 195:880–882.
14. Brize, DM, Klitzman B, Cook JM, Edwards J, Rosner G, Dewhirst MW. A comparison of tumor and normal tissue microvascular hematocrits and red cell fluxes in a rat window chamber model. *Int J Radiat Oncol Biol Phys* 1993; 25:269–276.
15. Brown EB, Campbell RB, Tsuzuki Y, Xu L, Carmeliet P, Fukumura D, et al. In vivo measurement of gene expression, angiogenesis, and physiological function in tumors using multiphoton laser scanning microscopy. Nat Med 2001; *in press.*
16. Carmeliet P, Jain RK. Angiogenesis in cancer and other diseases. *Nature* 2000; 407:249–257.
17. Chambers AF, Shafir R, Ling V. A model system for studying metastasis using the embryonic chick. *Cancer Res* 1982; 42:4018–4025.

18. Chang YS, di Tomaso E, McDonald DM, Jones RC, Jain RK, Munn LL. Mosaic blood vessels in tumors: frequency of cancer cells in contact with flowing blood. *Proc Natl Acad Sci USA* 2001; 97:14608–14613.

19. Chary SR, Jain RK. Direct measurement of interstitial convection and diffusion of albumin in normal and neoplastic tissues by fluorescence photobleaching. *Proc Natl Acad Sci USA* 1989; 86(14):5385–5389.

20. Chishima T, Miyagi Y, Wang X, Yamaoka H, Shimada H, Moossa AR, Hoffman RM. Cancer invasion and micrometastasis visualized in live tissue by green fluorescent protein expression. *Cancer Res* 1997; 57:2042–2047.

21. Chute RN, Sommers SC, Warren S. Heterotransplantation of human cancer. II. Hamster cheek pouch. *Cancer Res* 1952; 12:912–914.

22. Clark ER, Clark EL. Observations on living preformed blood vessels as seen in a transparent chamber inserted into the rabbit's ear. *Am J Anat* 1932; 49:441–477.

23. Clark ER, Kirby-Smith HT, Rex RO, Williams RG. Recent modifications in the method of studying living cells and tissues in transparent chambers inserted in the rabbit's ear. *Anat Rec* 1930; 47:187–211.

24. Dellian M, Helmlinger G, Yuan F, Jain RK. Fluorescence ratio imaging and optical sectioning: effect of glucose on spatial and temporal gradients. *Br J Cancer* 1996; 74:1206–1215.

25. Dellian M, Witwer BP, Salehi HA, Yuan F, Jain RK. Quantitation and physiological characterization of angiogenic vessels in mice: effect of basic fibroblast growth factor, vascular endothelial growth factor/vascular permeability factor, and host microenvironment. *Am J Pathol* 1996; 149:59–72.

26. Detmar M, Brown LF, Schön MP, Elicker BM, Richard L, Velasco P, et al. Increased microvascular density and enhanced leukocyte rolling and adhesion in the skin of VEGF transgenic mice. *J Investig Dermatol* 1998; 111:1–6.

27. Dewhirst MW, Tso CY, Oliver R, Gustafson CS, Secomb TW, Gross JF. Morphologic and hemodynamic comparison of tumor and healing normal tissue microvasculature. *Int J Radiat Oncol Biol Phys* 1989; 17:91–99.

28. Dirnagl U, Villringer A, Einhaupl K. In vivo confocal laser scanning microscopy of the cerebral microcirculation. *J Microscopy* 1992; 65:147–157.

29. Dudar TE, Jain RK. Differential response of normal and tumor microcirculation to hyperthermia. *Cancer Research* 1984; 44(2):605–612.

30. Dvorak HF, Harvey VS, Estrella P, Brown LF, McDonagh J, Dvorak AM. Fibrin containing gels induce angiogenesis. Implications for tumor stroma generation and wound healing. *Lab Investig* 1987; 57:673–686.

31. Eddy HA, Casarett GW. Development of the vascular system in the hamster malignant neurilem-moma. *Microvasc Res* 1973; 6:63–82.

32. Endrich B, Intaglietta M, Reinhold HS, Gross JF. Hemodynamic characteristics in microcirculatory blood channels during early tumor growth. *Cancer Res* 1979; 39:17–23.

33. Endrich B, Reinhold HS, Gross JF, Intaglietta M. Tissue perfusion inhomogeneity during early tumor growth in rats. *J Natl Cancer Inst* 1979; 62:387–395.

34. Falkvoll KH, Rofstad EK, Brustad T, Marton P. A transparent chamber for the dorsal skin fold of athymic mice. *Exp Cell Biol* 1984; 52:260–268.

35. Fan T-PD, Polverini PJ. In vivo models of angiogenesis. In: Bicknell R, Lewis CE, Ferrara N, eds. Tumor angiogenesis. Oxford University Press, Oxford 1997, pp. 5–18.

36. Ferrara N, Alitaro K. Clinical application of angiogenic growth factors and their inhibitors. *Nat Med* 1999; 5:1359–1364.

37. Fidler IJ. Modulation of the organ microenvironment for treatment of cancer metastasis. *J Natl Cancer Inst* 1995; 87:1588–1592.

38. Folkman J. Tumor angiogenesis. In: Holand JF, et al., eds. Cancer Medicine, 5th ed. B.C. Decker Inc., Ontario, 2000, pp. 132–152.

39. Friedlander M, Brooks PC, Shaffer PW, Kincaid CM, Varner JA, Cheresh DA. Definition of two angiogenic pathways by distinct alpha v integrins. *Science* 1995; 270(5241):1500–1502.

40. Fukumura D, Gohongi T, Ohtaka K, Stoll B, Chen Y, Seed B, Jain RK. Regulation of VEGF promoter activity in tumors by tissue oxygen and pH levels. *Proc Am Assoc Cancer Res* 1999; 40:722.

41. Fukumura D, Salehi HA, Witwer B, Tuma RF, Melder RJ, Jain RK. Tumor necrosis factor a-induced leukocyte adhesion in normal and tumor vessels: Effect of tumor type, transplantation site, and host strain. *Cancer Res* 1995; 55:4824–4829.

42. Fukumura D, Xavier R, Sugiura T, Chen Y, Park E, Lu N, et al. Tumor induction of VEGF promoter in stromal cells. *Cell* 1998; 94:715–725.

43. Fukumura D, Yuan F, Endo M, Jain RK. Role of nitric oxide in tumor microcirculation: blood flow, vascular permeability, and leukocyte-endothelial interactions. *Am J Pathol* 1997; 150(2):713–725.

44. Fukumura D, Yuan F, Monsky WL, Chen Y, Jain RK. Effect of host microenvironment on the microcirculation of human colon adenocarcinoma. *Am J Pathol* 1997; 151:679–688.

45. Funakoshi N, Onizuka M, Yanagi K, Ohshima N, Tomoyasu M, Sato Y, et al. A new model of lung metastasis for intravital studies. *Microvasc Res* 2000; 59(3):361–367.

46. Gazit Y, Berk DA, Leunig M, Baxter LT, Jain RK. Scale-invariant behavior and vascular network formation in normal and tumor tissue. *Physical Review Letters* 1995; 75(12):2428–2431.

47. Gerlowski LE, Jain RK. Microvascular permeability of normal and neoplastic tissues. *Microvasc Res* 1986; 31(3):288–305.

48. Gimbrone MAJ, Cotran RS, Leapman SB, Folkman J. Tumor growth and neovascularization: an experimental model using the rabbit cornea. *J Natl Cancer Inst* 1974; 52:413–427.

49. Gimbrone MAJ, Gullino PM. Angiogenic capacity of preneoplastic lesions of the murine mammary gland as a marker of neoplastic transformation. *Cancer Res* 1976; 36:2611–2620.

50. Gimbrone MAJ, Leapman SB, Cotran RS, Folkman J. Tumor dormancy in vivo by prevention of neovascularization. *J Exp Med* 1972; 136:261–276.

51. Gohongi T, Fukumura D, Boucher Y, Yun C-O, Soff GA, Compton C, et al. Tumor-host interactions in the gallbladder suppress distal angiogenesis and tumor growth: involvement of transforming growth factor b1. *Natl Med* 1999; 5(10):1203–1208.

52. Goodall CM, Sanders AG, Shubik P. Studies of vascular patterns in living tumors with a transparent chamber inserted in hamster cheek pouch. *J Natl Cancer Inst* 1965; 35:497–521.

53. Greene HSN. The significance of heterologous transplantability of human cancer. *Cancer* 1952; 5:24–44.

54. Griffon-Etienne G, Boucher Y, Brekken C, Suit HD, Jain RK. Taxane-induced apoptosis decompress blood vessels and lowers interstitial fluid pressure in solid tumors: Clinical implications. *Cancer Res* 1999; 54:3776–3782.

55. Hansen-Algenstaedt N, Stoll BR, Padera TP, Hicklin DJ, Fukumura D, Jain RK. Tumor oxygeneation during VEGF-R2 blockage, hormone ablation, and chemotherapy. *Cancer Res* 2000; 60:4556–4560.

56. Hartford AC, Gohongi T, Fukumura D, Jain RK. Irradiation of a primary tumor, unlike surgical removal, enhances angiogenesis suppression at a distal site: potential role of host-tumor interaction. *Cancer Res* 2000; 60:2128–2131.

57. Helmlinger G, Netti PA, Lichtenbeld HC, Melder RJ, Jain RK. Solid stress inhibits the growth of multicellular tumor spheroids. *Nat Biotechnol* 1997; 15(8):778–783.

58. Helmlinger G, Yuan F, Dellian M, Jain RK. Interstitial pH and pO_2 gradients in solid tumors in vivo: high-resolution measurements reveal a lack of correlation. *Nat Med* 1997; 3(2):177–182.

59. Heuser LS, Miller FN. Differential macromolecular leakage from the vasculature of tumors. *Cancer* 1986; 57:461–464.

60. Higuchi H, Kurose I, Fukumura D, Han JY, Saito H, Miura S, et al. Active oxidants mediate IFN-alpha-induced microvascular alterations in rat mesentery. *J Immunol* 1997; 158:4893–4900.

61. Hobbs SK, Monsky WL, Yuan F, Roberts WG, Griffith L, Torchilin VP, et al. Regulation of transport pathways in tumor vessels: role of tumor type and microenvironment. *PNAS* 1998; 95(8):4607–4612.

62. House SD, Lipowsky HH. In vivo determination of the force of leukocyte endothelium adhesion in the mesentaric microvasculature of the cat. *Cir Res* 1988; 63:658–666.

63. Huang D, Swanson EA, Lin CP, Schuman JS, Stinson WG, Chang W, et al. Optical coherence tomography. *Science* 1991; 254:1178–1181.

64. Ide AG, Baker NH, Warren SL. Vascularization of the Brown-Pearce rabbit epithelioma transplant as seen in the transparent ear chamber. *Am J Roentgenol* 1939; 42:891–899.

65. Intaglietta M, Tompkins WR. Microvascular measurements by video image shearing and splitting. *Microvas Res* 1973; 5(3):309–312.

66. Jain RK. Transport of molecules in the tumor interstitium: a review. *Cancer Res* 1987; 47:3038–3050.

67. Jain RK. Determinants of tumor blood flow: a review. *Cancer Res* 1988; 48:2641–2658.

68. Jain RK. Barriers to drug delivery in solid tumors. *Sci Am* 1994; 271(1):58–65.

69. Jain RK. 1996 Landis Award Lecture: delivery of molecular and cellular medicine to solid tumors. *Microcirculation* 1997; 4:1–23.

70. Jain RK. The next frontier of molecular medicine: delivery of therapeutics. *Nat Med* 1998; 4(6):655–657.

71. Jain RK, Munn LL, Fukumura D, Melder RJ. In vitro and in vivo quantification of adhesion between leukocytes and vascular endothelium. In: *Methods in molecular medicine,* Vol. 18: Tissue Engineering methods and protocols. Morgan JR, Yarmush ML, eds. 1998, Humana Press Inc., Totowa NJ, p. 553–575.

72. Jain RK, Safabakhsh N, Sckell A, Chen Y, Jiang P, Benjamin L, et al. Endothelial cell death, angiogenesis, and microvascular function after castration in an androgen-dependent tumor: role of vascular endothelial growth factor. *Proc Natl Acad Sci USA* 1998; 95(18):10820–10825.

73. Jain RK, Schlenger K, Hockel M, Yuan F. Quantitative angiogenesis assays: progress and problems. *Nat Med* 1997; 3(11):1203–1208.

74. Jeltsch M, Kaipainen A, Joukov V, Meng X, Lakso M, Rauvala H, et al. Hyperplasia of lymphatic vessels in VEGF-C transgenic mice. *Science* 1997; 276(5317):1423–1425.

75. Kaufman AG, Intaglietta M. Automated diameter measurement of vasomotion by cross-correlation. *Int J Microcirc Clin Exp* 1985; 4(1):45–53.

76. Kerbel RS. Tumor angiogenesis: past, present and the near future. *Carcinogenesis* 2000; 21:505–515.

77. Kleinfeld D, Mitra PP, Helmchen F, Denk W. Fluctuations and stimulus-induced changes in blood flow observed in individual capillaries in layers 2 through 4 of rat neocortex. *Proc Natl Acad Sci USA* 1998; 95:15,741–15,746.

78. Kligerman MM, Henel DK. Some aspects of the microcirculation of a transplantable experimental tumor. *Radiology* 1961; 76:810–817.

79. Klintworth GK. In: Corneal angiogenesis: A Comprehensive Critical Review. Springer Verlag, New York, NY, 1991.

80. Koop S, MacDonald I, Luzzi K, Schmidt E, Morris V, Grattan M, et al. Fate of melanoma cells entering the microcirculation: over 80% survive and extravasate. *Cancer Res* 1995; 55(12):2520–2523.

81. Kowalski J, Kwan HH, Prionas SD, Allison AC, Fajardo LF. Characterization and applications of the disc angiogenesis system. *Exp Mol Pathol* 1992; 56(1): p. 1–19.

82. Kubes P, Suzuki M, Grangen DN. Nitric oxide: an endogenous modulator of leukocyte adhesion. *Proc Natl Acad Sci USA* 1991; 88:4651–4655.

83. Kurose I, Fukumura D, Miura S, Suematsu M, Sekizuka E, Nagata H, et al. Nitric oxide mediates vasoactive effects of endothelin-3 on rat mesenteric microvascular beds in vivo. *Angiology* 1993; 44:483–490.

84. Kurose I, Miura S, Fukumura D, Tsuchiya M. Mechanisms of endothelin-induced macromolecular leakage in microvascular beds. *Eur J Pharmacol* 1993; 250:85–94.

85. Lahiri S, Rumsey WL, Wilson DF, Iturriaga R. Contribution of in vivo microvascular pO_2 in the cat carotid body chemotransduction. *J Appl Physiol* 1993; 75(3):1035–1043.

86. Lee CG, Heijn M, diTomaso E, Griffon-Etienne G, Ancukiewicz M, Koike C, et al. Anti-VEGF treatment augments tumor radiation response under normoxic or hypoxic conditions. *Cancer Res* 2000; 60:5565–5570.

87. Leighton J. The spread of cancer. pathogenesis, experimental methods, interpretations. Academic Press, New York, NY, 1967.

88. Lendvai B, Stern EA, Chen B, Svoboda K. Experience-dependent plasticity of dendritic spines in the developing rat barrel cortex in vivo. *Nature* 2000; 404:876–881.

89. Leu AJ, Berk DA, Lymboussaki A, Alitaro K, Jain RK. Absent of functional lymphatics within a murine sarcoma: a molecular functional evaluation. *Cancer Res* 2000; 60:4324–4327.

90. Leu AJ, Berk DA, Yuan F, Jain RK. Flow velocity in the superficial lymphatic network of the mouse tail. *Am J Physiol* 1994; 267(4 Pt 2):H1507–H1513.

91. Leunig M, Yuan F, Menger MD, Boucher Y, Goetz AE, Messmer K, et al. Angiogenesis, microvascular architecture, microhemodynamics, and interstitial fluid pressure during early growth of human adenocarcinoma LS174T in SCID mice. *Cancer Res* 1992; 52:6553–6560.

92. Li C-Y, Shan S, Huang Q, Braun RD, Lanzen J, Hu K, et al. Initial stages of tumor cell-induced angiogenesis: evaluation via skin window chambers in rodent models. *J Natl Cancer Inst* 2000; 92:143–147.

93. Lichtenbeld HC, Ferarra N, Jain RK, Munn LL. Effect of local anti-VEGF antibody treatment on tumor microvessel permeability. *Microvasc Res* 1999; 57(3):357–362.

94. Lichtenbeld HC, Yuan F, Michel CC, Jain RK. Perfusion of single tumor microvessels: application to vascular permeability measurement. *Microcirculation* 1996; 3(4):349–357.

95. Lipowsky HH, Zweifach BW. Applications of the "two-slit" photometric technique to the measurement of microvascular volumetric flow rates. *Microvasc Res* 1978; 15:93–101.

96. Luckè B, Schlumberger H. The manner of growth of frog carcinoma, studied by direct microscopic examination of living intraocular transplants. *J Exp Med* 1939; 70:257–268.

97. Lutz BR, Fulton GP, Patt DI, Handler AH. The growth rate of tumor transplants in the cheek pouch of the hamster (Mesocricetus auratus). *Cancer Res* 1950; 10:231–232.

98. Mahadevan V, Hart IR, Lewis GP. Factors influencing blood supply in wound granuloma quantitated by a new in vivo technique. *Cancer Res* 1989; 49:415–419.

99. Maiorana A, Gullino PM. Acquisition of angiogenic capacity and neoplastic transformation in the rat mammary gland. *Cancer Res* 1978; 38:4409–4414.

100. Martin GR, Jain RK. Fluorescence ratio imaging measurement of pH gradients: calibration and application in normal and tumor tissues. *Microvasc Res* 1993; 46(2):216–230.

101. Martin GR, Jain RK. Noninvasive measurement of interstitial pH profiles in normal and neoplastic tissue using fluorescence ratio imaging microscopy. *Cancer Res* 1994; 54(21):5670–5674.

102. McDonald IC, Schmidt EE, Morris VL, Chambers AF, Groom AC. Intravital videomicroscopy of the chorioallantoic microcirculation: a model system for studying metastasis. *Microvasc Res* 1992; 44:185–199.

103. Melder RJ, Koenig GC, Witwer BP, Safabakhsh N, Munn LL, Jain RK. During angiogenesis, vascular endothelial growth factor and basic fibroblast growth factor regulate natural killer cell adhesion to tumor endothelium. *Nat Med* 1996; 2(9):992–997.

104. Melder RJ, Yuan J, Munn LL, Jain RK. Erythrocytes enhance lymphocyte rolling and arrest in vivo. *Microvasc Res* 2000; 59(2):316–322.

105. Milstone DS, Fukumura D, Padget RC, O'Donnell PE, Davis VM, Benavidez OJ, et al. Mice lacking E-selectin show normal numbers of rolling leukocytes but reduced leukocyte stable arrest on cytokine-activated microvascular endothelium. *Microcirculation* 1998; 5:153–171.

106. Monsky WL, Fukumura D, Gohongi T, Ancukiewicz M, Werch HA, Torchilin VP, et al. Augmentation of transvascular transport of macromolecules and nanoparticles in tumors using vascular endothelial growth factor. *Cancer Res* 1999; 59:4129–4135.

107. Monsky WL, Fukumura D, Gohongi T, Chen Y, Yuan F, Kristensen C, Jain RK. Novel orthotopic models demonstrate effect of host microenvironment on human mammary carcinoma microcirculation. *Proc Am Assoc Cancer Res,* 1998; 39:376–377.

108. Morris VL, MacDonald IC, Koop S, Schmidt EE, Chambers AF, Groom AC. Early interactions of cancer cells with the microvasculature in mouse liver and muscle during hematogenous metastasis: videomicroscopic analysis. *Clinical Experimental Metastasis* 1993; 11(5):377–390.

109. Muthukkaruppan VR, Auerbach R. Angiogenesis in the mouse cornea. *Science* 1979; 205:1416–1418.

110. Naumov GN, Wilson SM, MacDonald IC, Schmidt EE, Morris VL, Groom AC, et al. Cellular expression of green fluorescent protein, coupled with high-resolution in vivo videomicroscopy, to monitor steps in tumor metastasis. *J Cell Sci* 1999; 112:1835–1842.

111. Netti PA, Berk DA, Swartz MA, Grodzinsky AJ, Jain RK. Role of extracellular matrix assembly in interstitial transport in solid tumors. *Cancer Res* 2000; 60:2497–2503.

112. Nguyen M, Shing Y, Folkman J. Quantitation of angiogenesis and antiangiogenesis in the chick embryo chorioallantoic membrane. *Microvasc Res* 1994; 47(1):31–40.

113. Norrby K, Jakobsson A, Sörbo J. Quantitative angiogenesis in spreads of intact rat mesenteric windows. *Microvasc Res* 1990; 39:341–348.

114. Nugent LJ, Jain RK. Extravascular diffusion in normal and neoplastic tissues. *Cancer Res* 1984; 44(1):238–244.

115. Passaniti A, Taylor RM, Pili R, Guo Y, Long PV, Haney JA, et al. A simple, quantitative method for assessing angiogenesis and antiangiogenic agents using reconstituted basement membrane, heparin, and fibroblast growth factor. *Lab Invest* 1992; 67(4):519–528.

116. Plunkett ML, Hailey JA. An in vivo quantitative angiogenesis model using tumor cells entrapped in alginate. *Lab Invest* 1990; 62:510–517.

117. Reinhold HS. Improved microcirculation in irradiated tumours. *Eur J Cancer* 1971; 7:273–280.

118. Reinhold HS, Blachiwiecz B, Blok A. Oxygenation and reoxygenation in "Sandwich" tumours. *Bibl Anat* 1977; 15:270–272.

119. Sandison JC. A new method for the microscopic study of living growing tissues by the introduction of a transparent chamber in the rabbit's ear. *Anat Rec* 1924; 28:281–287.

120. Sasaki A, Melder RJ, Whiteside TL, Herberman RB, Jain RK. Preferential localization of human adherent lymphokine-activated killer cells in tumor microcirculation. *J Natl Cancer Inst* 1991; 83(6):433–437.

121. Schlenger K, Höckel M, Schwab R, Frischmann-Berger R, Vaupel P. How to improve the uterotomy healing. I. Effects of fibrin and tumor necrosis factor-a in the rat uterotomy model. *J Surg Res* 1994; 56:235–241.

122. Schmidt J, Ryschich E, Maksan S, Werner J, Gebhard M, Herfarth C, et al. Reduced basal and stimulated leukocyte adherence in tumor endothelium of experimental pancreatic cancer. *Int J Pancreatol* 1999; 26(3):173–179.

123. Sckell A, Safabakhsh N, Dellian M, Jain RK. Primary tumor size-dependent inhibition of angiogenesis at a secondary site: an intravital microscopic study in mice. *Cancer Res* 1998; 58:5866–5869.

124. Shioda T, Munn L, Fenner M, Jain R, Isselbacher K. Early events of metastasis in the microcirculation involve changes in gene expression of cancer cells: tracking mRNA levels of metastasizing cancer cells in the chick embryo chorioallantoic membrane. *Am J Pathol* 1997; 150(6):2099–2112.

125. Sholley MM, Ferguson GP, Seibel HR, Montour JL, Wilson JD. Mechanisms of neovascularization. Vascular sprouting can occur without proliferation of endothelial cells. *Lab Invest* 1984; 51:624–634.

126. Suzuki T, Yanagi K, Ookawa K, Hatakeyama K, Ohshima N. Blood flow and leukocyte adhesiveness are reduced in the mirocirculation of a peritoneal disseminated colon carcinoma. *Ann Biom Eng* 1998; 26:803–811.

127. Swartz MA, Berk DA, Jain RK. Transport in lymphatic capillaries. I. Macroscopic measurements using residence time distribution theory. *Am J Physiol* 1996; 270(1 Pt 2):H324–H329.

128. Taylor CM, Weiss JB. The chick vitelline membrane as a test system for angiogenesis and antiangiogenesis. *Int J Microcirc Clin Exp* 1984; 3:337.

129. Toolan HW. Transplantable human neoplasms maintained in cortisone-treated laboratory animals: H.S. #1; H.Ep.#1; H.Ep. #2; H.Ep. #3; and H.Emb.Rh.#1. *Cancer Res* 1954; 14:660–666.

130. Torres Filho IP, Intaglietta M. Microvessel PO2 measurements by phosphorescence decay method. *Am J Physiol* 1993; 265(4 Pt 2):H1434–H1438.

131. Torres Filho IP, Leunig M, Yuan F, Intaglietta M, Jain RK. Noninvasive measurement of microvascular and interstitial oxygen profiles in a human tumor in SCID mice. *Proc Natl Acad Sci USA* 1994; 91(6):2081–2085.

132. Tsai AG, Friesenecker B, Mazzoni MC, Kerger H, Buerk DG, Johnson PC, et al. Microvascular and tissue oxygen gradients in the rat mesentery. *Proc Natl Acad Sci USA* 1998; 95(12):6590–6595.

133. Tsuzuki Y, Carreira CM, Jain RK, Fukumura D. Pancreas microenvironment promotes VEGF expression and tumor growth: novel window model for pancreas tumor angiogenesis and microcirculation. *Proc Am Assec Canc Res* 2001; 42:109.

134. Tsuzuki Y, Fukumura D, Oosthuyse B, Carmeliet P, Jain RK. VEGF modulation by targeting HIF1α→HRE→VEGF cascade differentially reglates vascular response and growth rate in tumors. *Cancer Res* 2000; 60:6248–6252.

135. Wood S. Pathogenesis of metastasis formation observed in vivo in the rabbit ear chamber. *Arch Pathol* 1958; 66:550–568.

136. Yamaura H, Suzuki M, Sato H. Transparent chamber in the rat skin for studies on microcirculation in cancer tissue. *Gann* 1971; 62:177–185.

137. Yanagi K, Ohsima N. Angiogenic vascular growth in the rat peritoneal disseminated tumor model. *Microvasc Res* 1996; 51:15–28.

138. Yuan F, Dellian M, Fukumura D, Leunig M, Berk DA, Torchilin VP, et al. Vascular permeability in a human tumor xenograft: molecular size dependence and cutoff size. *Cancer Res* 1995; 55(17):3752–3756.

139. Yuan F, Leunig M, Berk DA, Jain RK. Microvascular permeability of albumin, vascular surface area, and vascular volume measured in human adenocarcinoma LS174T using dorsal chamber in SCID mice. *Microvasc Res* 1993; 45:269–289.

140. Yuan F, Salehi HA, Boucher Y, Vasthare US, Tuma RF, Jain RK. Vascular permeability and microcirculation of gliomas and mammary carcinomas transplanted in rat and mouse cranial window. *Cancer Res* 1994; 54:4564–4568.

141. Zawicki DF, Jain RK, Schmid-Schoenbein GW, Chien S. Dynamics of neovascularization in normal tissue. *Microvasc Res* 1981; 21:27–47.

142. Zeidman I. The fate of circulating tumor cells. 1. Passage of cells through capillaries. *Cancer Res* 1961; 21:38–39.

Index